New Frontiers in Urinary Tract Infections

New Frontiers in Urinary Tract Infections

Edited by Jameson Lopez

hayle medical

New York

Hayle Medical,
750 Third Avenue, 9th Floor,
New York, NY 10017, USA

Visit us on the World Wide Web at:
www.haylemedical.com

ISBN: 978-1-63241-778-7

The publisher's policy is to use permanent paper from mills that operate a sustainable forestry policy. Furthermore, the publisher ensures that the text paper and cover boards used have met acceptable environmental accreditation standards.

Printed in China.

Cataloging-in-Publication Data

New frontiers in urinary tract infections / edited by Jameson Lopez.
p. cm.
Includes bibliographical references and index.
ISBN 978-1-63241-778-7
1. Urinary tract infections. 2. Urinary organs--Diseases. 3. Urinary tract infections--Diagnosis.
4. Urinary tract infections--Treatment. I. Lopez, Jameson.
RC900 .N49 2019
616.63--dc23

Table of Contents

Preface

Urinary tract infections (UTI) are the most frequently occurring bacterial infection in women. It affects the lower and the upper urinary tract. Uropathogenic Escherichia coli bacteria from the gut are the causative agent of 80-85% of acquired UTI, while Staphylococcus saprophyticus contributes to 5-10% of the cases. The bacteria enter the bladder through the urethra. Infections may also occur via the lymph and blood. After entry into bladder, E. coli attaches to the bladder wall and forms a biofilm thus evading the body's immune response. Some of the risk factors associated with the incidence of UTI are the female anatomy, diabetes, obesity, sexual intercourse and family history. UTIs can be concerning in pregnant women as it increases the risk of kidney infections. A kidney infection during pregnancy may lead to pre-eclampsia or premature birth. Prescription of antibiotics such as nitrofurantoin, trimethoprim/sulfamethoxazole (TMP/SMX) or fluoroquinolone can be the treatment method for most UTIs. However complicated UTIs require more aggressive evaluation, treatment and follow-up. This book aims to shed light on some of the unexplored aspects of urinary tract infections and the recent researches in such conditions. It presents researches and studies performed by experts across the globe on UTIs. This book, with its detailed analyses and data, will prove immensely beneficial to professionals and students involved in this area at various levels.

This book is the end result of constructive efforts and intensive research done by experts in this field. The aim of this book is to enlighten the readers with recent information in this area of research. The information provided in this profound book would serve as a valuable reference to students and researchers in this field.

At the end, I would like to thank all the authors for devoting their precious time and providing their valuable contribution to this book. I would also like to express my gratitude to my fellow colleagues who encouraged me throughout the process.

Editor

Palmitate Induced IL-6 and MCP-1 Expression in Human Bladder Smooth Muscle Cells Provides a Link between Diabetes and Urinary Tract Infections

Andreas Oberbach[1¶], Nadine Schlichting[1,4¶], Matthias Blüher[1], Peter Kovacs[2], Holger Till[3], Jens-Uwe Stolzenburg[4], Jochen Neuhaus[4*]

1 Department of Medicine, University of Leipzig, Leipzig, Germany, **2** Faculty of Medicine, Interdisciplinary Centre for Clinical Research, University of Leipzig, Leipzig, Germany, **3** Department of Pediatric Surgery, University of Leipzig, Leipzig, Germany, **4** Department of Urology, University of Leipzig, Leipzig, Germany

Abstract

Background: Urinary tract infections (UTI) are more frequent in type-2 diabetes mellitus patients than in subjects with normal glucose metabolism. The mechanisms underlying this higher prevalence of UTI are unknown. However, cytokine levels are altered in diabetic patients and may thus contribute to the development of UTI. Increased levels of free fatty acids (FFA), as observed in obese patients, can induce IL-6 production in various cell types. Therefore we studied the effects of the free fatty acid palmitate and bacterial lipopolysaccharide (LPS) on interleukin-6 (IL-6) and monocyte chemotactic protein-1 (MCP-1) expression and secretion in cultured human bladder smooth muscle cells (hBSMC).

Methodology/Principal Findings: Biopsies were taken from patients undergoing cystectomy due to bladder cancer. Palmitate or LPS stimulated hBSMC were analysed for the production and secretion of the IL-6, gp80, gp80soluble, gp130, MCP-1, pSTAT3, SOCS3, NF-κB and SHP2 by quantitative PCR, ELISA, Western blotting, and confocal immunofluorescence. In signal transduction inhibition experiments we evaluated the involvement of NF-κB and MEK1 in IL-6 and MCP-1 regulation. Palmitate upregulates IL-6 mRNA expression and secretion via NF-κB dependent pathways in a concentration- and time-dependent manner. MCP-1 was moderately upregulated by palmitate but was strongly upregulated by LPS involving NF-κB and MEK1 dependent pathways. Soluble IL-6 receptor (gp80soluble) was downregulated by palmitate and LPS, while membrane-bound gp80 was moderately upregulated. LPS increased SOCS3 and SHP2, whereas palmitate only induced SOCS3. Secondary finding: most of the IL-6 is secreted.

Conclusions/Significance: Bacterial infection (LPS) or metabolic alterations (palmitate) have distinct effects on IL-6 expression in hBSMC, (i) short term LPS induced autocrine JAK/STAT signaling and (ii) long-term endocrine regulation of IL-6 by palmitate. Induction of IL-6 in human bladder smooth muscle cells by fatty acids may represent a pathogenetic factor underlying the higher frequency and persistence of urinary tract infections in patients with metabolic diseases.

Editor: Joanna Mary Bridger, Brunel University, United Kingdom

Funding: This work was supported by grants from Deutsche Forschungsgemeinschaft (DFG) BL 580/3-1 (MB), the Clinical Research group "Atherobesity" KFO 152: project BL 833/1-1 (MB), the Interdisciplinary Centre of Clinical Research (IZKF) Leipzig at the Faculty of Medicine of the University of Leipzig (Project N06 to PK and project B24 to MB). The funders had no role in study design, data collection and analysis, decision to publish, or preparation of the manuscript.

Competing Interests: The authors have declared that no competing interests exist.

* E-mail: jochen.neuhaus@medizin.uni-leipzig.de

¶ These authors contributed equally to this work.

Introduction

Urinary tract infections (UTI) are more frequent in patients with diabetes mellitus than in subjects with normal glucose metabolism and take a more severe course [1,2]. Women with diabetes require longer and more aggressive antimicrobial treatment for UTI, and have more recurrences of their UTI than non-diabetic women. The hospitalization due to complications of the UTI occurs significantly more often in women with diabetes [3]. Urine cytokine levels and an increased adherence of the microorganisms to the uroepithelial cells seem to be the main predictors of increased prevalence of both asymptomatic and symptomatic bacteriuria in diabetic patients [4]. Whereas some authors suggest glucosuria as diabetes-specific variable potentially associated with symptomatic infection [5], no association between bacteriuria and indicators of glycemic control, such as the blood glucose level and the glycosylated hemoglobin value, have been found by others [6]. In addition to chronic hyperglycemia, altered fatty acid metabolism belongs to the metabolic alterations associated with type-2 diabetes [7]. However, it is not known whether alterations in circulating free fatty acids (FFA) may contribute to the increased UTI frequency in patients with diabetes.

Bacterial UTI lead to upregulation of cytokines and growth factors and recruitment of inflammatory cells by LPS [8,9]. IL-6 was shown to be the single most prominent cytokine detected in the urine patients with UTI [10]. Low-grade chronic inflammation is reflected by a 2–3-fold increase in the systemic levels of certain cytokines [11] as well as C-reactive protein (CRP), and an association has been confirmed between low-grade systemic inflammation and type-2 diabetes [12].

There is growing evidence that increased levels of FFA can induce IL-6 production in various cell types, and might therefore be involved in the pathophysiology of UTI [13–15]. Elevated FFAs in obese patients may provide a mechanistic link between increased fat mass and the development of insulin resistance, glucose intolerance, and beta-cell dysfunction that promote the onset of diabetes [7,16]. Palmitate induced accumulation of IL-6 is regulated dependently of c-Jun N-terminal kinase in 3T3-L1 adipocytes [17], but is regulated via NF-κB in myotubes [13], pointing to the existence of potential tissue/cell specific regulatory mechanisms in inflammation. In addition, palmitate could regulate monocyte chemotactic protein-1 (MCP-1) expression in adipose tissue [18], human vascular umbilical vein cells (HUVEC) and rat vascular smooth muscle cells [19].

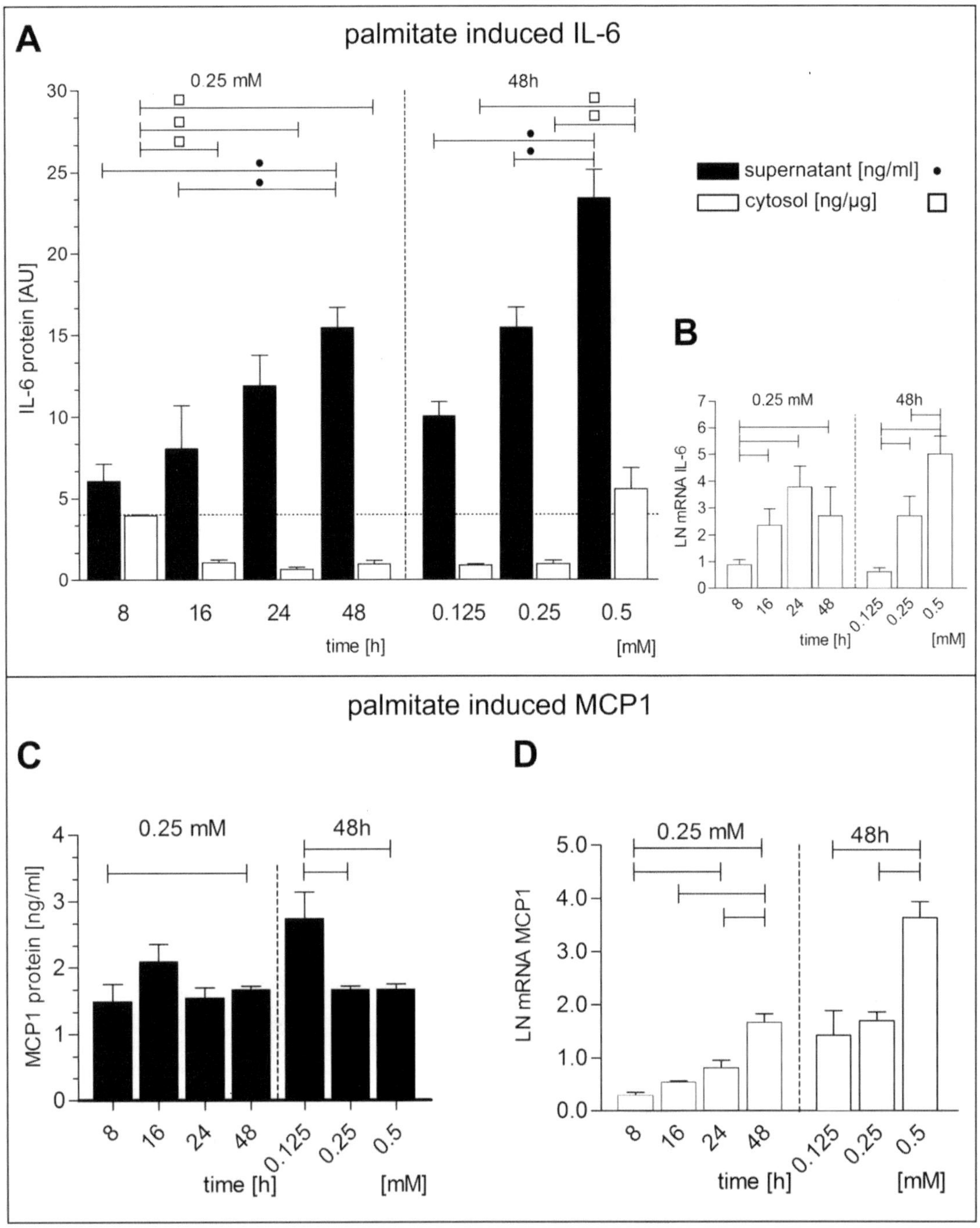

Figure 1. Palmitate effects on IL-6 and MCP-1 mRNA and protein levels. Time- and concentration- dependent regulation of IL-6 and MCP-1 protein (A, C) and mRNA (B, D). IL-6 protein content (A) was measured in cytosol (white bars, ng/µg) and supernatant (black bars, ng/ml), while MCP-1 protein was measured exclusively in supernatant (C, ng/ml). All bars indicate difference to medium control. For each measurement a medium treated control was used. Data are shown as mean and SEM. Significant differences are indicated by lines. mRNA (B, D) was normalized to natural logarithm LN.

The aim of the present study was to investigate IL-6 and MCP-1 regulation in hBSMC by acute bacterial infection (LPS stimulation) and metabolic alterations (palmitate) as potential risk factor for chronic bladder inflammation.

Results

Treatment of hBSMC with FFA palmitate (up to 48 hrs) resulted in significantly increased IL-6 protein concentrations in the supernatant, but not in the cytosol (Fig. 1A) A similar pattern was observed for palmitate stimulated IL-6 mRNA expression (Fig. 1B). Increased IL-6 secretion into the medium was dependent on palmitate concentration and time.

In contrast, stimulation with LPS led to IL-6 protein upregulation in the supernatant while levels decreased with time in the cytosol (Fig. 2A). There was no concentration- dependent regulation of IL-6 mRNA (Fig. 2B). In addition total IL-6 expression was only about 25% of IL-6 protein produced upon palmitate stimulation (Fig. 2A).

While MCP-1 showed similar regulation of the mRNA (Fig. 1D), this concentration- and time-dependent upregulation was not

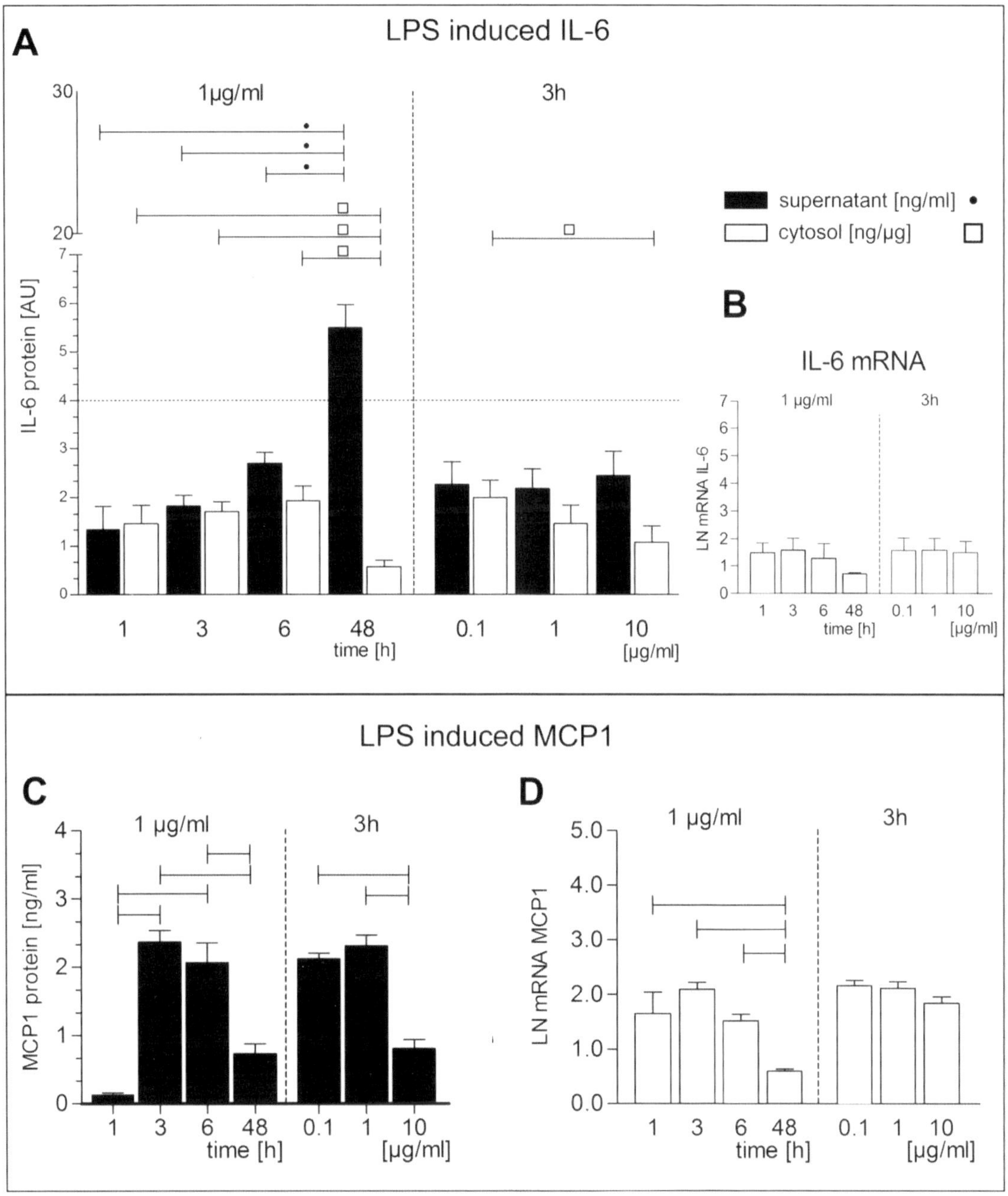

Figure 2. LPS effects on IL-6 and MCP-1 mRNA and protein levels. Time- and concentration- dependent regulation of IL-6 and MCP-1 protein (A, C) and mRNA (B, D). IL-6 protein content (A) was measured in cytosol (white bars, ng/µg) and supernatant (black bars, ng/ml), while MCP-1 protein was measured exclusively in supernatant (C, ng/ml). All bars indicate difference to medium control. For each measurement a medium treated control was used. Data are shown as mean and SEM. Significant differences are indicated by lines. Post-hoc Bonferroni test was used after ANOVA. Significance level was $p<0.05$. mRNA (B, D) was normalized to natural logarithm LN.

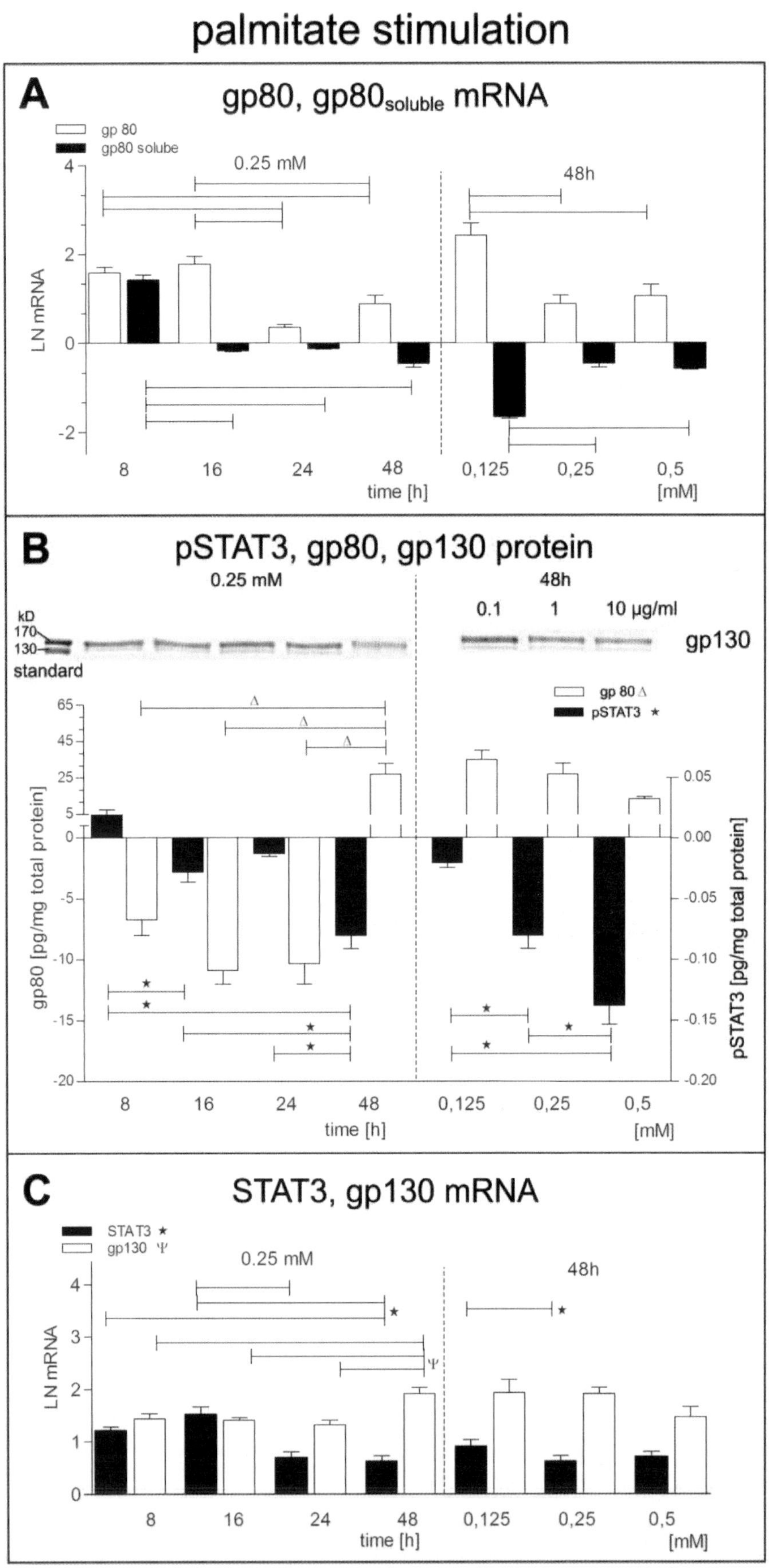
palmitate stimulation
A
gp80, gp80soluble mRNA
gp 80
gp80 solube
0.25 mM
48h
LN mRNA
8
16
24
48
time [h]
0,125
0,25
0,5
[mM]
B
pSTAT3, gp80, gp130 protein
0.25 mM
48h
0.1
1
10 µg/ml
kD
170
130
standard
gp130
gp 80 Δ
pSTAT3 ★
gp80 [pg/mg total protein]
pSTAT3 [pg/mg total protein]
8
16
24
48
time [h]
0,125
0,25
0,5
[mM]
C
STAT3, gp130 mRNA
STAT3 ★
gp130 Ψ
0.25 mM
48h
LN mRNA
8
16
24
48
time [h]
0,125
0,25
0,5
[mM]

Figure 3. Palmitate effects on the expression of IL-6 receptor subunit gp80, $gp80_{soluble}$, gp130 and pSTAT3. (A) Membrane gp80 receptor mRNA (white bars), soluble gp80 mRNA (black bars). (B) Protein expression of gp80 (white bars) and pSTAT3 (black bars) was measured by ELISA, and membrane gp130 receptor was analysed by Western blot. (C) Gp130 mRNA (white bars), STAT3 mRNA (black bars). Data are shown as mean and SEM. mRNA was normalized to natural logarithm LN.

reflected by MCP-1 protein content. Protein expression was constant over 48 hrs and was highest at low palmitate concentration (Fig. 1C). Upon LPS stimulation the MCP-1 protein in the supernatant and in the cytosol decreased time- and concentration-dependent (Fig. 2C). *MCP-1* mRNA showed a comparable downregulation with time but only moderate decrease with increasing concentrations of LPS (Fig. 2D).

We found a transient upregulation of the mRNA of IL-6 receptor protein gp80 and its soluble form $gp80_{soluble}$ (Fig. 3A). After 16 hrs of incubation the gp80 mRNA was still high while the mRNA of $gp80_{soluble}$ was significantly downregulated. This opposite regulatory effect on mRNA levels was most prominent with low palmitate concentration (0.125 mM) but was still present at higher concentrations (Fig. 3A). Gp80 protein was significantly downregulated as early as after 8 hrs incubation lasting up to 24 hrs. However, after 48 hrs incubation with 0.25 mM palmitate the effect was reversed. This high level expression of gp80 was concentration-independent (Fig. 3B).

The effects of LPS stimulation on *gp80* and $gp80_{soluble}$ mRNA are comparable to palmitate induced regulation (Fig. 4A, C), except for a significant initial upregulation of gp80 and $gp80_{soluble}$ after 8 hrs. After 48 hrs there was an opposite regulation of cytosolic gp80 protein, which was increased by palmitate (0.25 mM) but decreased by LPS (1 µg/ml). Prominent downregulation of pSTAT3 protein was evident in LPS stimulated cells on a short time scale up to 6 hrs (Fig. 4B), whereas there was an upregulation of pSTAT3 protein after 8 hrs of palmitate stimulation (Fig. 3B).

The membrane IL-6 receptor protein gp130 showed only moderate mRNA upregulation (Fig. 3C). Both, *STAT3* mRNA and protein were significantly downregulated after 24 hrs incubation with 0.25 mM palmitate, which was the most effective concentration at 48 hrs, too (Fig. 3B, C). Confocal imaging revealed perinuclear enrichment of pSTAT3 after 48 hrs stimulation with 1 µg/ml LPS (Fig. 5A2) and even more prominent with 0.25 mM palmitate (Fig. 5A3).

SOCS3, SHP2

Since SOCS3 and SHP2 are important regulators of IL-6 signaling pathways, we further examined their regulation by palmitate and LPS. *SOCS3* mRNA and SOCS3 protein increased after 48 hrs of palmitate treatment (Fig. 6A, B). *SHP2* mRNA and SHP2 protein levels decreased (Fig. 6C, D). Interestingly, LPS caused upregulation of *SOCS3* mRNA in the first 6 hrs of treatment, but levels returned to baseline level after 48 hrs, while SOCS protein content was highest after 48 hrs (Fig. 6E, F). SHP2 mRNA and protein levels were unaltered after LPS treatment (Fig. 6G, H). These findings were confirmed by confocal immunofluorescence. We found highest immunoreactivity for pSTAT3, SOCS3, and SHP2 after palmitate treatment, while the changes were only moderate in LPS treated cultures (Fig. 5).

NF-κB p65 regulation and activation

NF-κB p65 is the main transcription factor regulating IL-6 gene expression [20]. We found concentration- and time-dependent downregulation of the NF-κB p65 mRNA (Fig. S1A, B) and pNF-κB p65 protein (Fig. 7A, B). This was in striking contrast to the effect of LPS, which led to concentration-dependent upregulation of both, NF-κB p65 mRNA (Fig. S1B) and pNF-κB p65 protein (Fig. 7B).

In double confocal immunofluorecence experiments we found time-dependent translocation of NF-κB p65 into the nuclei as evidence of NF-κB activation after 48 hrs of LPS (1 µg/ml) and palmitate (0.25 mM) stimulation. We found more NF-κB p65 in nuclei of palmitate stimulated cells than after LPS stimulation. To quantify this translocation we performed dot blot analysis using a specific antibody against phosphorylated (Ser536) activated NF-κB p65. Basic ratio was 2.7±0.66 (mean±SD) in medium control and moderate higher in LPS stimulated cells (3.5±0.92), while the ratio was significant higher after 48 h of palmitate stimulation (5.7±1.1).

Pathway analysis by inhibition of NF-κB (MG132) or MEK1 (PD98059) showed that IL-6 was regulated via NF-κB, but not via MEK1, whereas MCP-1 was regulated via NF-κB and MEK1 dependent pathways (Fig. 7D, E).

Discussion

Here we studied the effects of palmitate and LPS on human bladder smooth muscle cells with the aim to elucidate potential novel mechanisms underlying the observation that urinary tract infections are more frequent in patients with diabetes mellitus and take a more severe course [1,2]. Defects in the local urinary cytokine secretions and an increased adherence of pathogenic microorganisms to the uroepithelial cells have been discussed as mechanisms for increased prevalence of UTI in patients with diabetes [4]. In a proteom study Yohannes et al. [21] found significant alterations in rat detrusor muscle after streptozotocin-induced diabetes, suggesting that diabetes depending bladder dysfunction may involve dysregulation of structural cell integrity, cell adhesion, proliferation and inflammation [21].

It is well known that during acute infection LPS triggers intracellular signaling cascades via Toll-like receptor TLR4 that rapidly induce inflammatory cytokines that initiate a variety of overlapping immune responses [22].

However, fatty acids and their metabolites act also directly and indirectly to regulate metabolism and immune function through their interactions with specific enzymes [23]. Exaggerated and prolonged postprandial hyperlipidemia is an important characteristic of diabetic dyslipidemia [7,24].

In the present study we report that palmitate treated human bladder smooth muscle cells (hBSMC) are a source of MCP-1 and IL-6. We used specific inhibitors to interfere with the signaling cascade. We found regulation of IL-6 via NF-κB, which is in line with the regulation of IL-6 by palmitate stimulation in human skeletal muscle cells as reported earlier [13].

Unexpectly, pNF-κB p65 protein content was significantly lower in palmitate stimulated cells as compared to medium control (Fig. 7A). This finding needs further investigation, since on the other hand we found short-term upregulation of pNF-κB p65 by LPS (Fig. 7B). One might suggest that the palmitate stimulus is much stronger than LPS and might therefore lead to increased protein turn-over.

MCP-1 also showed NF-κB dependent regulation as recently reported for IL1β stimulated human aorta smooth muscle cells

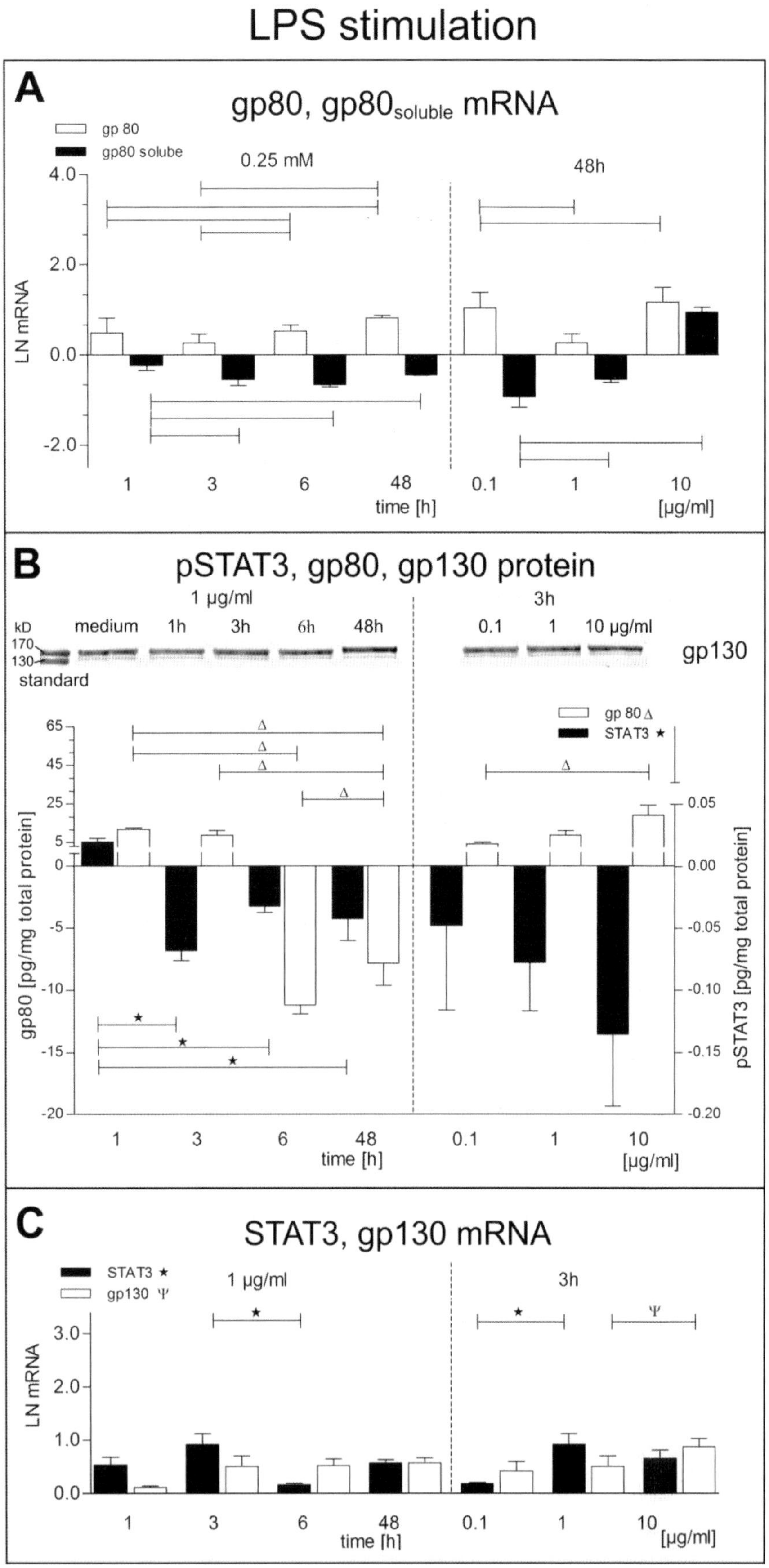
LPS stimulation
A
gp80, gp80soluble mRNA
gp 80
gp80 solube
0.25 mM
48h
LN mRNA
time [h]
[μg/ml]
B
pSTAT3, gp80, gp130 protein
1 μg/ml
3h
kD
medium 1h 3h 6h 48h
0.1 1 10 μg/ml
gp130
standard
gp 80 Δ
STAT3 ★
gp80 [pg/mg total protein]
pSTAT3 [pg/mg total protein]
time [h]
[μg/ml]
C
STAT3, gp130 mRNA
STAT3 ★
gp130 Ψ
1 μg/ml
3h
LN mRNA
time [h]
[μg/ml]

Figure 4. LPS effects on the expression of IL-6 receptor subunit gp80, gp80$_{soluble}$, gp130 and pSTAT3. (A) Membrane gp80 receptor mRNA (white bars), soluble gp80 mRNA (black bars). (B) Protein expression of gp80 (white bars) and pSTAT3 (black bars) was measured by ELISA, and membrane gp130 receptor was analysed by Western blotting. (C) Gp130 mRNA (white bars), STAT3 mRNA (black bars). Data are shown as mean and SEM. mRNA was normalized to natural logarithm LN.

[25]. However, MCP-1 was downregulated by MEK1 inhibitor (PD98059) in hBSMC, indicating regulation via MEK1 pathway in contrast to IL-6. It is well known that MCP-1 promotes migration of monocytes [26] and this mechanism has also been proposed for bladder inflammation [27]. MCP-1 is also related to insulin resistance and the risk of metabolic syndrome [28].

In hBSMC we found higher secretion of MCP-1 after LPS than after palmitate stimulation. In contrast IL-6 secretion was much

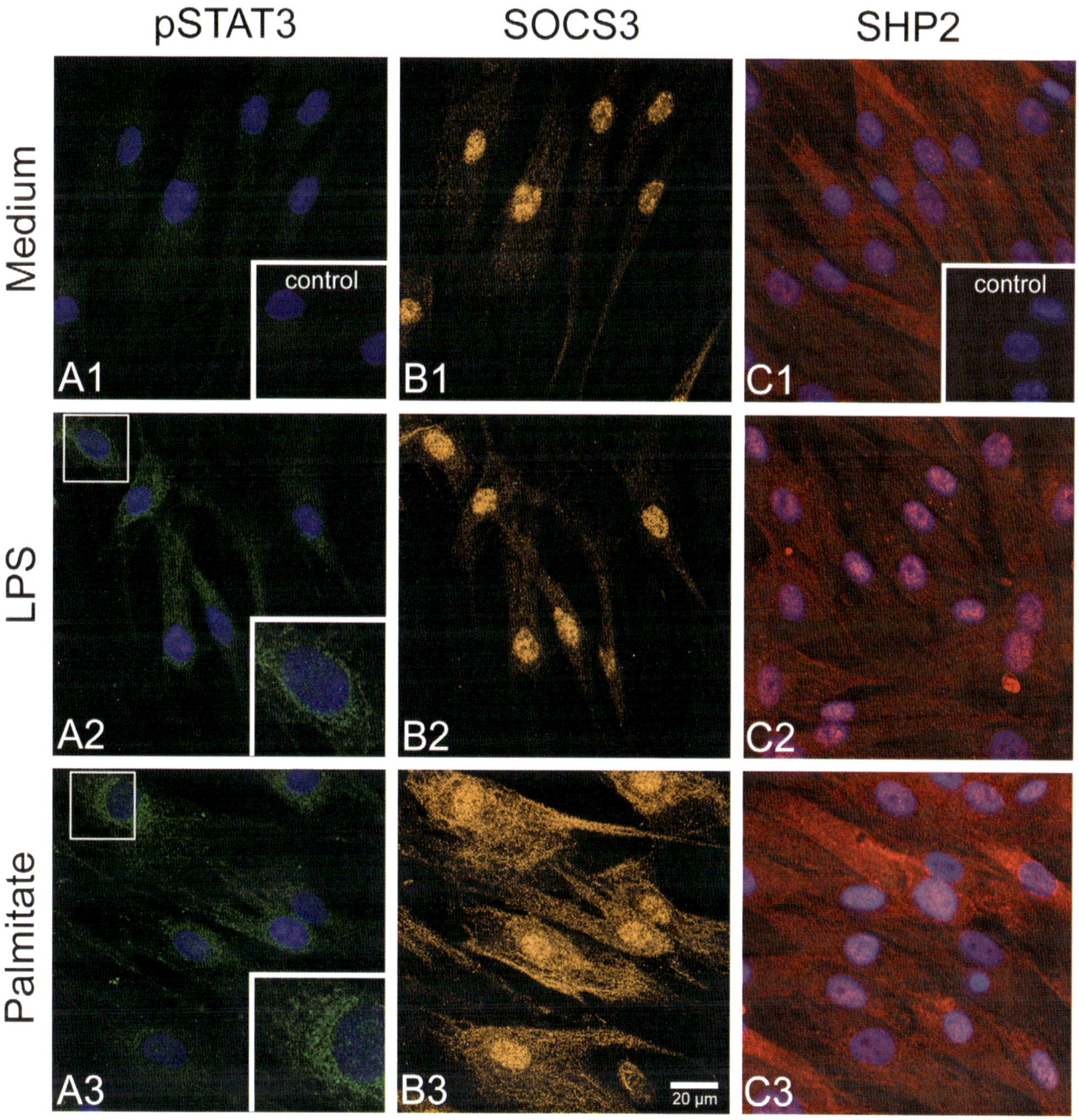

Figure 5. Confocal immunofluorescence of cultures treated for 48 hrs with 1 µg/ml LPS or 0.25 mM palmitate. (A1–C1) Medium control; (A2–C2) LPS treated; (A3–C3) palmitate treated. Cells were double labelled for pSTAT3 (green) and SOCS3 (orange). Monoclonal SHP2 (red) antibody was used in single labelling experiments. Nuclei were stained with DAPI (blue) recorded with standard fluorescence and merged into the confocal images. The scale bar in B3 applies to all images except the insets, which have been enlarged two times.

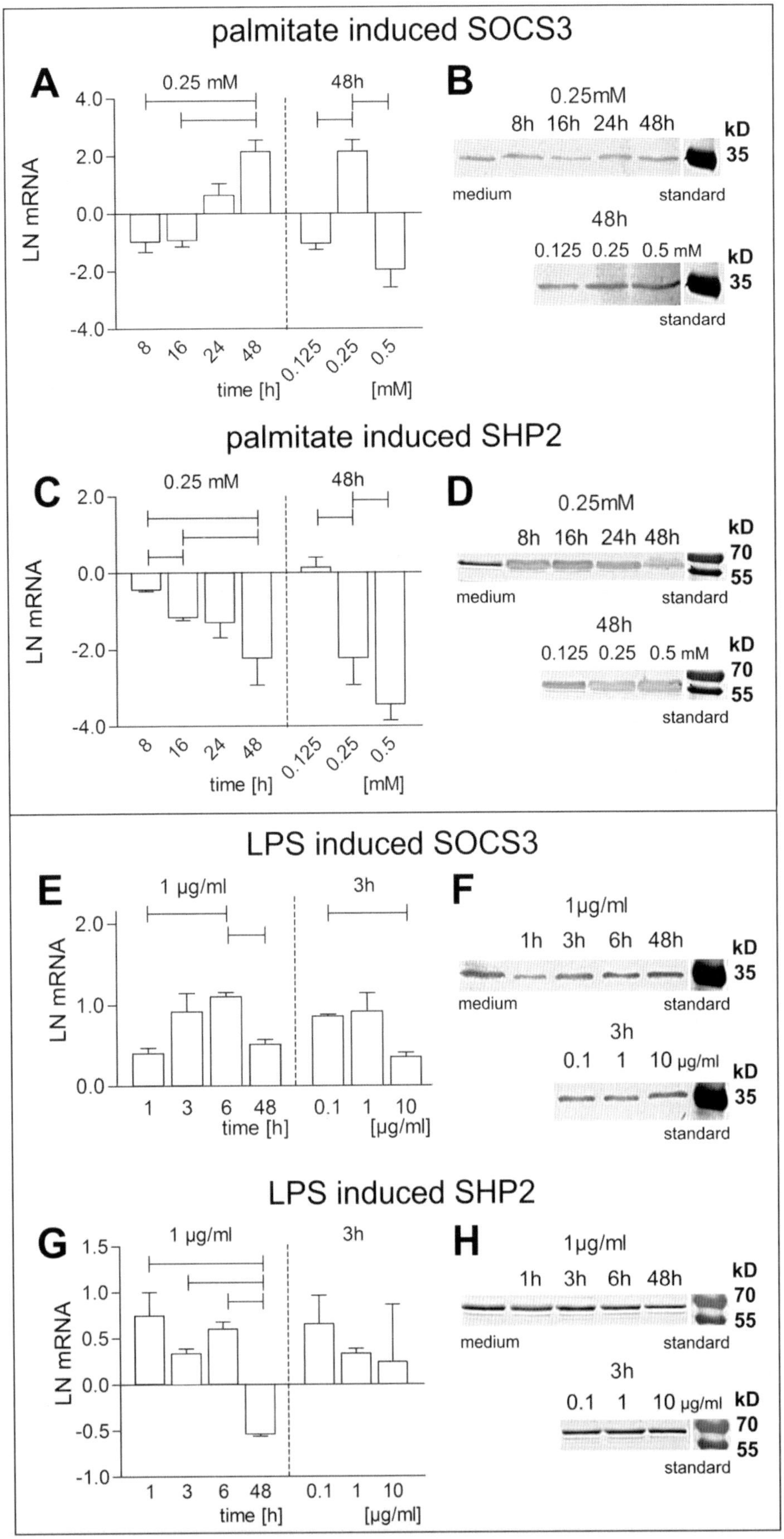
palmitate induced SOCS3
A
0.25 mM
48h
LN mRNA
time [h]
[mM]
B
0.25mM
8h 16h 24h 48h
kD
35
medium
standard
48h
0.125 0.25 0.5 mM
palmitate induced SHP2
C
D
70
55
LPS induced SOCS3
E
1 µg/ml
3h
[µg/ml]
F
1µg/ml
1h 3h 6h 48h
0.1 1 10 µg/ml
LPS induced SHP2
G
H

Figure 6. Palmitate and LPS effects on SOCS3 and SHP2. Time- and concentration- dependent palmitate effects on SOCS3 mRNA (A), SHP2 mRNA (C), SOCS3 protein expression (B), and SHP2 protein expression (D). LPS effects on SOCS3 mRNA (E), SHP2 mRNA (F), SOCS3 protein expression (G), and SHP2 protein expression (H). Protein content was analysed in the cytosol using Western blotting analysis. All bars indicate difference to medium control. For each measurement a medium treated control was used. Data are shown as mean and SEM. Significant differences are indicated by lines. mRNA was normalized to natural logarithm LN.

higher in palmitate stimulated cells than after LPS treatment (Fig. 1, Fig. 2). To the best knowledge of the authors this is the first study to show that the vast amount of palmitate stimulated IL-6 is secreted. Only basic cytosolic amounts are detectable (Fig. 1). This supports the view that the human bladder smooth muscle cells are involved in immunological processes and may have endocrine function. To examine possible regulatory function of IL-6 onto bladder smooth muscle cells we studied the IL-6 receptor pathway in hBSMC.

The IL-6 signaling cascade depends on the common cytokine receptor family gp130 subunit and the IL-6 receptor specific gp80 subunit forming a hexameric receptor-IL-6 complex. Gp80 exists in a membrane-bound and soluble form, produced as alternative splice variant [29]. For long-term autocrine stimulation by IL-6 the whole receptor complex is needed. We could show, that gp80 mRNA and protein were time-dependent down-regulated by both, palmitate and LSP (Fig. 3, 4). This implies preferential exocrine cytokine signaling by BSMC.

We found short term upregulation of pSTAT3 in LPS and palmitate stimulated cells, but long term downregulation of pSTAT3 (Fig. 3, 4) in conjunction with upregulation of SOCS3 (Fig. 5), which implies negative feedback to IL-6 signaling as reported by Croker et al. [30]. Hence it is evident that both, LSP and palmitate also induced short-term autocrine regulation of IL-6 receptor pathway. However, conditional knockout studies have shown that SOCS3 depletion can induce a number of inflammatory and metabolic disorders [30]. Therefore, upregulation of SOCS3 could be a protection mechanism for the hBSMC to cope with chronically elevated IL-6. At present it is not known which genes are regulated by pSTAT3 in hBSMC.

In conclusion, there is a short-term autocrine IL-6 signaling of BSMC, but a long-term exocrine IL-6 signaling providing cytokine stimulation to local or invading cells equipped with the IL-6 receptor complex.

Our study provides evidence for the urinary bladder smooth muscle cells being an immunologically active tissue, which can be triggered by inflammatory conditions, but which is especially sensitive to metabolic alterations as provoked by the saturated FFA palmitate. In the light of our findings, chronically elevated FFA could well be a risk factor for urinary infections and idiopathic bladder inflammation in diabetes.

Materials and Methods

Cell Culture

Human bladder smooth muscle cell (hBSMC) cultures were established from human detrusor muscle after radical cystectomy of tumour patients. Written informed consent was obtained from all patients. The study was approved by the ethics committee of the University of Leipzig (Reg.No. 773). Cells were grown in SMC Growth Medium 2 (PromoCell, Heidelberg, Germany) and subcultured up to the forth passage (P4). At 80% confluence cells were treated with palmitate or with LPS. Palmitate was used in combination with 2% bovine serum albumin (BSA) as carrier of free fatty acids. Medium treated cells were used as control. For pathway analyses, cells were preincubated for 1 h with 20 µM PD98059 (Map Kinase Kinase/Erk Kinase 1 inhibitor) or 40 µM MG123 (proteasome inhibitor; Calbiochem, San Diego, USA). If not indicated otherwise all chemicals were from Sigma-Aldrich, Steinheim, Germany.

RNA Extraction and Real Time PCR

Total RNA was isolated with RNeasy Mini kit (Qiagen, Hilden, Germany). Quantitative PCR was performed with the ABI 7500 Real Time PCR Instrument (Applied Biosystems, Foster, USA) using the Brilliant SYBR Green QPCR Core Reagent kit (Stratagene, La Jolla, USA) and custom primers (MWG-Biotech, Ebersberg, Germany; Table 1). Human 36B4 (acidic ribosomal phosphoprotein P0) served as internal standard.

Western Blotting

Cells were washed with PBS and scrapped off in 1× lyses buffer (Cell Signaling, Danvers, USA) supplemented with 1 mM PMSF and 1/100 volume protease inhibitor cocktail (Sigma-Aldrich). After sonication, the cell extracts were cleared by centrifugation. 75 µg of total protein were separated by sodium dodecyl sulfate polyacrylamide (10%) gel electrophoresis and transferred to polyvinylidene fluoride (PVDF) membrane by tank blotting (Mini-PROTEAN II; BioRad, Munich, Germany). Blots were incubated with primary antibodies for 2 h at room temperature or over night at 4°C. Detection and visulization was done with horseradish peroxidase-conjugated anti-rabbit or anti-mouse IgG (1:1000) for 1 h at room temperature and DAB (FAST 3,3′-diaminobenzidine tablets) as a substrate.

Dot Blot Analysis

Nuclear and cytosolic extracts were prepared according to Yerneni et al. 1999 [31]. 2 µg total protein of nuclear or cytosolic extracts were transferred in duplicates on nitrocellulose membrane by Dot Blotting (Dot Blot 96 System, Biometra, Goettingen, Germany). After blocking with Odyssee blocking buffer (Licor Biosciences, Bad Homburg, Germany) for 1 h the membranes were incubated with anti-Phospho-NF-κB p65 (Ser536) rabbit IgG (1:1000; Cell Signaling, Danvers, USA) over night at 4°C. Detection was done with anti-rabbit IRDye 680 (1:5000; Licor Biosciences) for 2 h. Membranes were scanned with Odyssey Infrared Imager and evaluated by Odyssey Infrared Imaging Software 3.0 (Licor Biosciences). Total protein was visualized by SYPRO Ruby blot stain (BioRad).

Enzyme-linked Immunosorbent Assay (ELISA)

Intracellular and secreted IL-6 was quantified by Quantikine human IL-6 immunoassay (R&D Systems, Minneapolis, MN). Cell extracts were diluted 1:10 with calibrator diluent. IL-6 in cell culture supernatants were measured after being centrifuged in 1:100 diluted samples. IL-6 receptor (gp80) and activated transcription factors (NF-κB, pSTAT3) were determined in undiluted cell extracts by Quantikine human IL-6 sR immunoassay (R&D Systems) and by PathScan Phospho-NF-κB p65 (pNF-κB; Ser536) and PathScan Phospho-STAT3 (pSTAT3; Tyr705) Sandwich ELISA (Cell Signaling). MCP-1 was measured in cell culture supernatants and cell extracts by Quantikine human CCL2/MCP-1 immunoassay (R&D Systems). For quantification

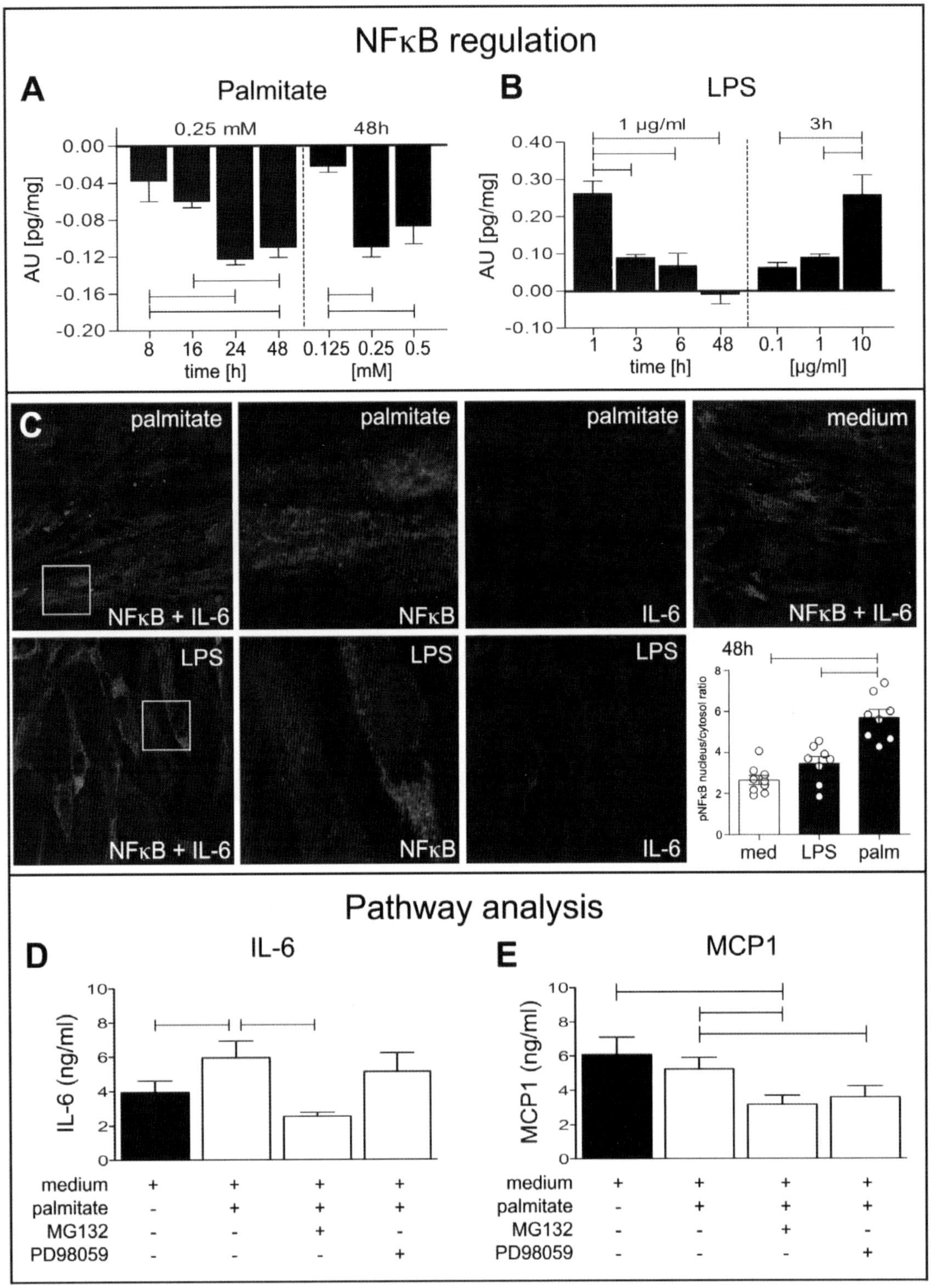

Figure 7. Gene regulation and pathway analysis. Time- and concentration-dependent palmitate and LPS effects on pNF-κB protein expression (A, B). Protein content of pNF-κB was measured in cytosol (A, black bars) and is indicated as difference to medium control (AU in pg/mg) by ELISA. All bars indicate difference to medium control (A, B). For each measurement a medium treated control was used. Confocal double immunofluorescence images demonstrate nuclear translocation of NF-κB (green) and IL-6 (red). Nuclei are depicted by DAPI (blue). Dot blot analysis of phosphorylated NF-κB are shown as ratio of nuclear pNF-κB protein content to cytosolic pNF-κB protein content related to total protein content. Cells were stimulated for 48 h either with 0.25 mM palmitate or with 1 μg/ml LPS (C). Pathway analysis of palmitate induced IL-6 (D) and MCP-1 (E) regulation. Protein content was measured by ELISA in supernatants (ng/ml). Cells were stimulated with palmitate (0.5 mM) and inhibitor of proteasomal degradation of NF-κB (MG132, 40 μM) or MEK1 (PD98059, 20 μM) for 48 hrs. Medium control is indicated as black bar (D, E). Data are shown as mean and SEM. Significant differences are indicated by lines.

Table 1. List of primer pairs used for quantitative PCR.

primer	sequence 5′→3′	product length (bp)	binding site
IL-6 forward	GGT ACA TCC TCG ACG GCA TCT	81	exon 2
IL-6 reverse	GTG CCT CTT TGC TGC TTT CAC		exon 3
gp80 forward	GGG GGA AGC ACC ATA ACT TT	232	exon 10
gp80 reverse	ATC TGG GAC TTC AGG CAC AC		exon 10
soluble gp80 forward	CTC CCA GGT TCA AGA AGA CG	183	exon 8/10
soluble gp80 reverse	TGT GGC TCG AGG TAT TGT CA		exon 10
gp130 forward	TGT AGA TGG CGG TGA TGG TA	246	exon 17
gp130 reverse	CCC TCA GTA CCT GGA CCA AA		exon 17
STAT3 forward	TGT GCG TAT GGG AAC ACC TA	170	exon 24
STAT3 reverse	AGA AGG TCG TCT CCC CCT TA		exon 24
SOCS1 forward	CTG GGA TGC CGT GTT ATT TT	245	exon 2
SOCS1 reverse	TAG GAG GTG CGA GTT CAG GT		exon 2
SOCS3 forward	TGG TCA GCT GGT CTC CTT TT	231	exon 2
SOCS3 reverse	CCC ATC CAG GCT GAG TAT GT		exon 2
SH-P2 forward	TGG CCA GAC AGA AGC ACA G	165	exon 3
SH-P2 reverse	GGC TCT GAT CTC CAC TCG TC		exon 3
NF-κB p50 forward	ACA AAT GGG CTA CAC CGA AG	238	exon 23
NF-κB p50 reverse	ATG GGG CAT TTT GTT GAG AG		exon 24
NF-κB p65 forward	CCT GGA GCA GGC TAT CAG TC	213	exon 5
NF-κB p65 reverse	ATC TTG AGC TCG GCA GTG TT		exon 7
MCP1 forward	CCC CAG TCA CCT GCT GTT AT	171	exon 2
MCP1 reverse	TGG AAT CCT GAA CCC ACT TC		exon 3
h36B4 forward	AAC ATG CTC AAC ATC TCC CC	397	exon 6
h36B4 reverse	CCG ACT CCT CCG ACT CTT C		exon 8

the cell culture supernatants were diluted 2 fold and the cell extracts 5 fold with calibration buffer.

Immunocytochemistry

Cells cultured on cover slips were fixed in 4% buffered paraformaldehyde and incubated overnight at 4°C with primary antibodies (Table 2). Indirect immunofluorescence was performed with secondary antibodies conjugated with Alexa Fluor 488, Alexa Fluor 555 or Alexa Fluor 633 fluorescent dye (1:500; Invitrogen, Karlsruhe, Germany). Cell nuclei were stained with 4′,6-diamidino-2-phenylindoldihydro-chloride (DAPI). The cells were analysed at a confocal laser scanning microscope LSM-5 Pascal (Carl Zeiss, Jena, Germany).

Statistical Analysis

Complete data analysis was performed using Prism 5.0 (GraphPad Software, La Jolla, USA) statistical software. The data are presented as the mean +/− SEM from at least three independent experiments. Statistical differences were analyzed by ANOVA. A p-value <0.05 was considered statistically significant.

Table 2. List of antibodies used for immunocytochemistry.

antigen	host	type	source	dilution
human IL-6	mouse	monoclonal, IgG_{2a}	Acris, Herford, Germany	1:100
human CD126 (IL-6R)	mouse	monoclonal, IgG_1	Acris, Herford, Germany	1:100
human gp130	rabbit	polyclonal, IgG	Santa Cruz Biotechnology, Heidelberg, Germany	1:100
human pSTAT3 (Tyr705)	mouse	monoclonal, IgG_1	Cell Signaling Technology, Danvers, USA	1:100
human SOCS3 (H-103)	rabbit	polyclonal, IgG	Santa Cruz Biotechnology, Heidelberg, Germany	1:100
human SH-PTP2 (C-18)	rabbit	polyclonal, IgG	Santa Cruz Biotechnology, Heidelberg, Germany	1:100
human NF-κB p65 (F-6)	mouse	monoclonal, IgG_1	Santa Cruz Biotechnology, Heidelberg, Germany	1:100

Supporting Information

Figure S1 Gene regulation of NF-κB p65. Time- and concentration-dependent palmitate and LPS effects on NF-κB p65 mRNA expression (A, B). All bars indicate difference to medium control. For each measurement a medium treated control was used. Data are shown as mean and SEM. Significant differences are indicated by lines. mRNA was normalized to natural logarithm LN.

Acknowledgments

The authors want to thank Mrs. A. Weimann for the technical assistance.

Author Contributions

Conceived and designed the experiments: AO NS JN. Performed the experiments: AO NS JN. Analyzed the data: AO NS PK JN. Contributed reagents/materials/analysis tools: AO MB PK HT JUS JN. Wrote the paper: AO NS MB PK JUS JN.

References

1. Benfield T, Jensen JS, Nordestgaard BG (2007) Influence of diabetes and hyperglycaemia on infectious disease hospitalisation and outcome. Diabetologia 50: 549–554.
2. Stapleton A (2002) Urinary tract infections in patients with diabetes. Am J Med 113 Suppl 1A: 80S–84S.
3. Schneeberger C, Stolk RP, Devries JH, Schneeberger PM, Herings RM, et al. (2008) Differences in the pattern of antibiotic prescription profile and recurrence rate for possible urinary tract infections in women with and without diabetes. Diabetes Care 31: 1380–1385.
4. Hoepelman AI, Meiland R, Geerlings SE (2003) Pathogenesis and management of bacterial urinary tract infections in adult patients with diabetes mellitus. Int J Antimicrob Agents 22 Suppl 2: 35–43.
5. Harding GK, Zhanel GG, Nicolle LE, Cheang M (2002) Antimicrobial treatment in diabetic women with asymptomatic bacteriuria. N Engl J Med 347: 1576–1583.
6. Geerlings SE, Stolk RP, Camps MJ, Netten PM, Collet TJ, et al. (2000) Risk factors for symptomatic urinary tract infection in women with diabetes. Diabetes Care 23: 1737–1741.
7. Wilding JP (2007) The importance of free fatty acids in the development of Type 2 diabetes. Diabet Med 24: 934–945.
8. Bouchelouche K, Alvarez S, Horn T, Nordling J, Bouchelouche P (2006) Human detrusor smooth muscle cells release interleukin-6, interleukin-8, and RANTES in response to proinflammatory cytokines interleukin-1beta and tumor necrosis factor-alpha. Urology 67: 214–219.
9. Saban MR, Hellmich H, Nguyen NB, Winston J, Hammond TG, et al. (2001) Time course of LPS-induced gene expression in a mouse model of genitourinary inflammation. Physiol Genomics 5: 147–160.
10. Otto G, Braconier J, Andreasson A, Svanborg C (1999) Interleukin-6 and disease severity in patients with bacteremic and nonbacteremic febrile urinary tract infection. J Infect Dis 179: 172–179.
11. Ross R (1999) Atherosclerosis—an inflammatory disease. N Engl J Med 340: 115–126.
12. Festa A, D'Agostino RJ, Tracy RP, Haffner SM (2002) C-reactive protein is more strongly related to post-glucose load glucose than to fasting glucose in non-diabetic subjects; the Insulin Resistance Atherosclerosis Study. Diabet Med 19: 939–943.
13. Weigert C, Brodbeck K, Staiger H, Kausch C, Machicao F, et al. (2004) Palmitate, but not unsaturated fatty acids, induces the expression of interleukin-6 in human myotubes through proteasome-dependent activation of nuclear factor-kappaB. J Biol Chem 279: 23942–23952.
14. Staiger H, Staiger K, Stefan N, Wahl HG, Machicao F, et al. (2004) Palmitate-induced interleukin-6 expression in human coronary artery endothelial cells. Diabetes 53: 3209–3216.
15. Chavez JA, Summers SA (2003) Characterizing the effects of saturated fatty acids on insulin signaling and ceramide and diacylglycerol accumulation in 3T3-L1 adipocytes and C2C12 myotubes. Arch Biochem Biophys 419: 101–109.
16. Eitel K, Staiger H, Rieger J, Mischak H, Brandhorst H, et al. (2003) Protein kinase C delta activation and translocation to the nucleus are required for fatty acid-induced apoptosis of insulin-secreting cells. Diabetes 52: 991–997.
17. Davis JE, Gabler NK, Walker-Daniels J, Spurlock ME (2009) The c-Jun N-terminal kinase mediates the induction of oxidative stress and insulin resistance by palmitate and toll-like receptor 2 and 4 ligands in 3T3-L1 adipocytes. Horm Metab Res 41: 523–530.
18. Chakrabarti SK, Cole BK, Wen Y, Keller SR, Nadler JL (2009) 12/15-lipoxygenase products induce inflammation and impair insulin signaling in 3T3-L1 adipocytes. Obesity (Silver Spring) 17: 1657–1663.
19. Ishikado A, Nishio Y, Yamane K, Mukose A, Morino K, et al. (2009) Soy phosphatidylcholine inhibited TLR4-mediated MCP-1 expression in vascular cells. Atherosclerosis 205: 404–412.
20. Ajuwon KM, Spurlock ME (2005) Palmitate activates the NF-kappaB transcription factor and induces IL-6 and TNFalpha expression in 3T3-L1 adipocytes. J Nutr 135: 1841–1846.
21. Yohannes E, Chang J, Christ GJ, Davies KP, Chance MR (2008) Proteomics analysis identifies molecular targets related to diabetes mellitus-associated bladder dysfunction. Mol Cell Proteomics 7: 1270–1285.
22. Akira S, Uematsu S, Takeuchi O (2006) Pathogen recognition and innate immunity. Cell 124: 783–801.
23. Zhao S, Yang YN, Song JG (2004) Ceramide induces caspase-dependent and -independent apoptosis in A-431 cells. J Cell Physiol 199: 47–56.
24. Stampfer MJ, Rimm EB (1996) Folate and cardiovascular disease. Why we need a trial now. JAMA 275: 1929–1930.
25. Lim JH, Um HJ, Park JW, Lee IK, Kwon TK (2009) Interleukin-1beta promotes the expression of monocyte chemoattractant protein-1 in human aorta smooth muscle cells via multiple signaling pathways. Exp Mol Med 41: 757–764.
26. Reape TJ, Groot PH (1999) Chemokines and atherosclerosis. Atherosclerosis 147: 213–225.
27. Bouchelouche K, Andresen L, Alvarez S, Nordling J, Nielsen OH, et al. (2006) Interleukin-4 and 13 Induce the Expression and Release of Monocyte Chemoattractant Protein 1, Interleukin-6 and Stem Cell Factor From Human Detrusor Smooth Muscle Cells: Synergy With Interleukin-1beta and Tumor Necrosis Factor-alpha. J Urol 175: 760–765.
28. Kanda H, Tateya S, Tamori Y, Kotani K, Hiasa K, et al. (2006) MCP-1 contributes to macrophage infiltration into adipose tissue, insulin resistance, and hepatic steatosis in obesity. J Clin Invest 116: 1494–1505.
29. Rose-John S, Scheller J, Elson G, Jones SA (2006) Interleukin-6 biology is coordinated by membrane-bound and soluble receptors: role in inflammation and cancer. J Leukoc Biol 80: 227–236.
30. Croker BA, Krebs DL, Zhang JG, Wormald S, Willson TA, et al. (2003) SOCS3 negatively regulates IL-6 signaling in vivo. Nat Immunol 4: 540–545.
31. Yerneni KK, Bai W, Khan BV, Medford RM, Natarajan R (1999) Hyperglycemia-induced activation of nuclear transcription factor kappaB in vascular smooth muscle cells. Diabetes 48: 855–864.

2

Incidence of Hospital-Acquired Pneumonia, Bacteraemia and Urinary Tract Infections in Patients with Haematological Malignancies, 2004–2010

Catherine Huoi[1], Philippe Vanhems[1,2], Marie-Christine Nicolle[1], Mauricette Michallet[3], Thomas Bénet[1,2]*

1 Infection Control and Epidemiology Unit, Edouard Herriot Hospital, Hospices Civils de Lyon, Lyon, France, **2** Epidemiology and Public Health Group, Centre National de la Recherche Scientifique, Unité Mixte de Recherche 5558, University of Lyon 1, Lyon, France, **3** Haematology Department, Edouard Herriot Hospital, Hospices Civils de Lyon, Lyon, France

Abstract

Objective: This study charted incidence trends of hospital-acquired (HA) pneumonia, bacteraemia and urinary tract infections (UTI) in a haematology department.

Methods: Prospective surveillance of hospital-acquired infections (HAI) was undertaken in a 42-bed haematology department of a university hospital. All patients hospitalized ≥48 hours between 1st January 2004 and 31st December 2010 were included. Definitions of HAI were based on a standardized protocol. The incidence was the number of events per 1000 patient-days at risk; only the first HAI was counted. Multivariate Poisson regression was fitted to assess temporal trends.

Results: Among 3 355 patients (58 063 patient-days at risk) included, 1 055 (31%) had HAI. The incidence of HA pneumonia, HA bacteraemia and HA UTI was respectively 3.3, 12.0 and 2.9 per 1000 patient-days at risk. HA bacteraemia incidence increased by 11% (95% confidence interval: +6%, +15%, $P<0.001$) per year, independently of neutropenia, central venous catheterization (CVC) and haematological disease. The incidences of HA pneumonia and HA UTI were stable. The most frequently isolated pathogens were *Aspergillus spp.* (59.2%) for pneumonia, coagulase-negative *Staphylococcus* (44.2%) for bacteraemia and enterobacteria (60%) for UTI.

Conclusion: The incidence of bacteraemia increased, indicating that factors other than CVC exposure, including chemotherapy with its impact on the immune system, could explain this trend. Further analytic studies are needed to explore the factors that could explain this trend.

Editor: Vishnu Chaturvedi, California Department of Public Health, United States of America

Funding: The authors have no support or funding to report.

Competing Interests: The authors have declared that no competing interests exist.

* E-mail: thomas.benet@chu-lyon.fr

Introduction

Patients with haematological malignancies are at high risk of hospital-acquired infections (HAI) because the severity of their underlying illness often requires aggressive treatment: chemotherapy, bone marrow or peripheral blood stem cell transplantation. This could lead to severe and prolonged immunosuppression, increasing the risk of infection and possibly worsening the prognosis [1,2]. Mortality attributable to hospital-acquired (HA) bacteraemia in patients with cancer ranges between 10 and 20% [3–5], whereas mortality from HA pneumonia is much higher, between 40 and 60% [6–8]. Over the past few decades, major progress has been made in the curative treatment of haematological malignancies which has resulted in reduced overall mortality [9–12], but also longer neutropenia and higher risk of infectious complications [13,14].

HAI are important adverse events in the disease history of patients with haematological malignancies, sometimes culminating in death; they are also responsible for longer hospital stay and increased healthcare costs [15,16]. However, few studies have examined the incidence of HAI in this adult patient population as most surveillance have focused only on bone marrow transplant patients or children [13,17–25]. For example, Engelhart et al. noted an incidence of 25.3 HAI per 1000 patient-days at risk [20], and Urrea et al. reported 17.7 HAI per 1000 patient-days among paediatric haematology/oncology patients [21]. To the best of our knowledge, trends in HAI incidence in the general population of adult patients with haematological malignancies have been poorly investigated. The objectives of this prospective surveillance were: 1) to track trends in the incidence of HA pneumonia, bacteraemia and urinary tract infections (UTI) in patients with haematological malignancies; 2) to identify the common etiological pathogens for these infections.

Methods

Setting

Prospective surveillance of HA pneumonia, bacteraemia and UTI was implemented at the 42-bed haematology department of Edouard Herriot University Hospital in Lyon, France, between 1st January 2004 and 31st December 2010. This 1000-bed hospital is composed of 3 haematology adult acute care units. Each of these units can accommodate 14 patients in single rooms. In total, 16 rooms are equipped with laminar airflow (LAF), 14 rooms with positive pressure isolation and high-efficiency particulate air (HEPA) filtration, and 12 have no specific air system. Patients with acute myeloid leukaemia (AML) or acute lymphoid leukaemia (ALL) were selectively admitted in the department, whereas patients with lymphoma were more often admitted to another hospital.

Data Sources

All patients hospitalized ≥48 hours in the haematology department between 1st January 2004 and 31st December 2010 were included in the surveillance. A standardized data sheet was filled for each patient, based on clinical observation and microbiological results. It recorded demographic and medical data: patient age, gender, dates of admission and discharge, diagnosis of the haematological disease, reason for admission. The main risk factors of infection were also recorded: neutropenia (<500 neutrophils/mm^3) and its length, exposure to central venous catheterization (CVC), length of stay, hospitalization in non protected room. Surveillance was based on a local, standardized protocol derived from the French national protocol for HAI surveillance [26].

Table 1. Characteristics of patients hospitalized in the Haematology Department, Edouard Herriot Hospital, Lyon (France), 2004–2010.

Characteristics	**Year**							*P*	**Overall (n = 3355)**
	2004 (n = 617)	**2005 (n = 547)**	**2006 (n = 546)**	**2007 (n = 437)**	**2008 (n = 393)**	**2009 (n = 413)**	**2010 (n = 402)**		
At admission									
Gender, male	366 (59.3)	317 (58)	298 (54.6)	233 (53.3)	212 (53.9)	225 (54.5)	222 (55.2)	0.37	1,873 (55.8)
Age, years[a]	50.8 (15.9)	47.8 (16.1)	48.9 (15.8)	50.0 (15.4)	48.7 (15.6)	47.8 (14.9)	46.5 (15.6)	<0.001	48.8 (15.7)
Haematological disease								<0.001	
Acute myeloid leukaemia	299 (49.6)	252 (46.8)	260 (47.6)	249 (57.2)	230 (58.8)	208 (50.7)	206 (51.4)		1,704 (51.3)
Acute lymphoid leukaemia	118 (19.6)	124 (23.1)	93 (17)	64 (14.7)	97 (24.8)	128 (31.2)	115 (28.7)		739 (22.2)
Chronic lymphocytic leukaemia	13 (2.2)	8 (1.5)	6 (1.1)	11 (2.5)	6 (1.5)	7 (1.7)	2 (0.5)		53 (1.6)
Chronic myeloid leukaemia	28 (4.6)	11 (2)	14 (2.6)	8 (1.8)	5 (1.3)	4 (1)	5 (1.2)		75 (2.3)
Lymphoma	12 (2)	31 (5.8)	15 (2.8)	7 (1.6)	3 (0.8)	6 (1.5)	3 (0.7)		77 (2.3)
Myeloma	71 (11.8)	68 (12.6)	56 (10.3)	35 (8.1)	19 (4.9)	36 (8.8)	30 (7.5)		315 (9.5)
Myelodysplasia	19 (3.1)	15 (2.8)	22 (4)	18 (4.1)	4 (1)	8 (1.9)	4 (1.0)		90 (2.7)
Other	43 (7.1)	29 (5.4)	80 (14.7)	43 (9.9)	27 (6.9)	13 (3.2)	36 (9.0)		271 (8.1)
Reason for admission								<0.001	
Induction chemotherapy	139 (23.2)	102 (18.7)	117 (21.5)	112 (25.6)	81 (20.9)	71 (17.2)	85 (21.3)		707 (21.3)
Consolidation chemotherapy	146 (24.4)	147 (27.0)	119 (21.8)	111 (25.5)	119 (30.8)	148 (35.9)	146 (36.7)		936 (28.2)
Transplantation	86 (14.4)	87 (16.0)	65 (11.9)	70 (16)	63 (16.3)	79 (19.2)	72 (18.1)		522 (15.7)
Palliative	11 (1.8)	15 (2.7)	15 (2.75)	13 (3.0)	8 (2.1)	6 (1.5)	4 (1)		72 (2.2)
Infection suspicion	62 (10.4)	51 (9.4)	41 (7.5)	30 (6.9)	28 (7.2)	15 (3.6)	23 (5.8)		250 (7.5)
Graft rejection suspicion	9 (1.5)	11 (2)	9 (1.7)	10 (2.3)	8 (2.1)	9 (2.2)	7 (1.7)		63 (1.9)
Relapse suspicion	39 (6.5)	57 (10.4)	36 (6.6)	23 (5.3)	11 (2.8)	13 (3.1)	11 (2.8)		190 (5.7)
Other	106 (17.7)	75 (13.8)	143 (26.2)	67 (15.3)	69 (17.8)	71 (17.2)	50 (12.6)		581 (17.5)
During hospitalization									
Neutropenia (neutrophils <0.5G/L)	374 (66.9)	315 (59.4)	302 (58.3)	293 (70.1)	262 (71.8)	255 (72.2)	262 (74.9)	<0.001	2,063 (66.7)
Central venous catheterization	432 (88.9)	401 (80.2)	412 (87.1)	363 (87.9)	336 (96.6)	304 (96.5)	326 (97.6)	<0.001	2,574 (89.7)
Protected room[b]	241 (47.3)	246 (46.2)	313 (61.3)	282 (64.5)	276 (70.2)	273 (66.1)	278 (69.2)	<0.001	1,909 (56.9)
Length of stay, days[a]	23.3 (17.9)	23.2 (16.8)	24.6 (23.6)	29.3 (26.3)	28.8 (19.9)	27.2 (22.6)	28.3 (19.4)	<0.001	26.0 (21.1)
Length of neutropenia, days[a]	20.6 (14.4)	20.0 (12.2)	21.9 (14.3)	20.6 (11.9)	20.8 (11.9)	19.9 (12.9)	22.4 (12.0)	<0.001	20.9 (12.9)
Deceased	20 (3.7)	29 (5.5)	26 (4.9)	31 (7.4)	25 (6.6)	16 (4.1)	12 (3.3)	<0.001	159 (5.0)

Notes: Data are n (%), unless specified otherwise.
[a]Mean (SD).
[b]Protected room: laminar airflow or positive pressure isolation or high-efficiency particulate air filtration.

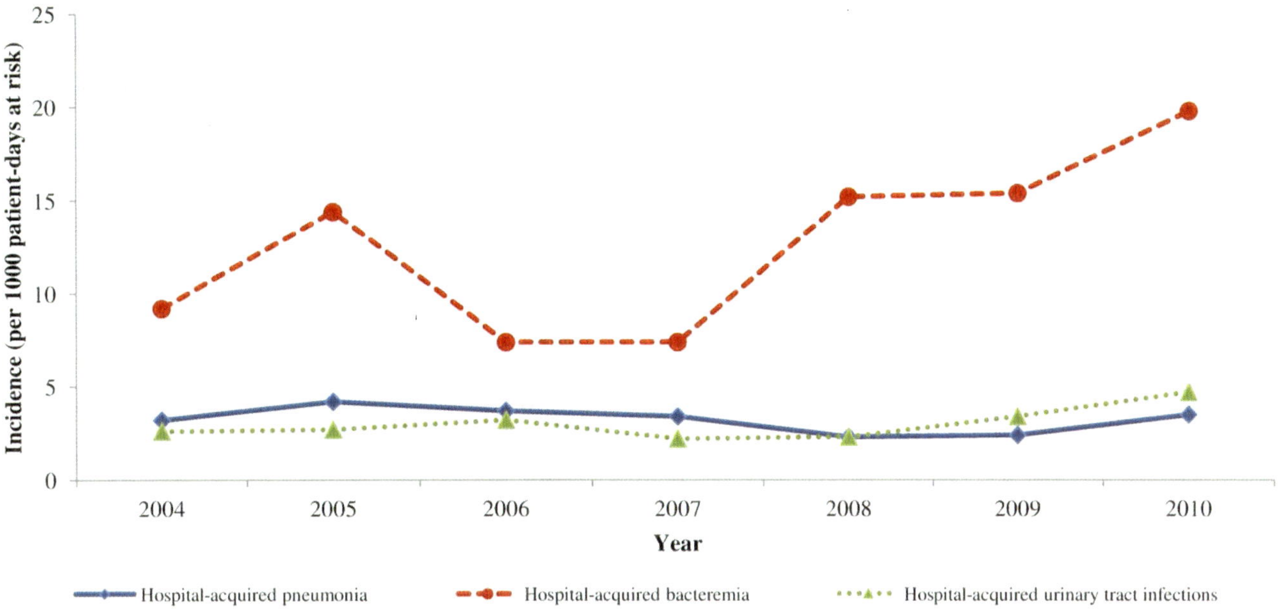

Figure 1. Trends in the incidence of hospital-acquired infections, Haematology Department, Edouard Herriot Hospital, Lyon (France) 2004–2010.

HAI Diagnosis

The case definition of HA pneumonia was: 1) chest X-rays or chest computed tomography-scans exhibiting lung infiltrates; and 2) temperature >38°C or leukocyte count >12 000/mm^3 or <4 000/mm^3; and 3) at least 1 of the following: (a) sputum change, (b) suggestive auscultation, (c) low oxyhaemoglobin saturation, or (d) increased pulmonary oxygen consumption; and 4) confirmation of pneumonia diagnosis by: (a) the practitioner in charge of the patient; and/or (b) microbial identification of the potential causal microorganism. The etiological agents were isolated from sputum, or directed bronchoalveolar lavage, or protected specimen by telescopic brush or protected distal tracheal specimen by catheter, or histological sample [27].

The case definition of HA bacteraemia was: 1) at least 1 positive blood culture justified by clinical signs for most microorganisms; or 2) at least 2 positive blood cultures justified by clinical signs, at 2 different times, separated by less than 48 hours from each other, when the microorganism was 1 of the following: coagulase-negative *Staphylococci*, *Bacillus spp.* (except *Bacillus anthracis*), *Corynebacterium spp.*, *Propionibacterium spp.*, *Micrococcus spp.* [27].

The case definition of HA UTI was: 1) at least 1 of the following clinical signs/symptoms: fever (>38°C), urgency, increased urinary frequency, dysuria, burning on urination or pain in the lower abdomen, with no other recognized cause; and 2) a positive urine culture (≥10^5 microorganisms/mm^3) with 1 or 2 different pathogens isolated in case of urinary catheter exposure in the previous 7 days, or leukocyturia (≥10^4 leukocytes/mm^3) and positive urine culture (≥10^3 microorganisms/mm^3) with 1 or 2 different pathogens isolated if any urinary catheter was in place in the previous 7 days [27].

The causative microorganism for each infection was recorded. Only the first HAI per hospital stay that occurred ≥48 hours after patient admission was considered. Also, patient-days at risk were censored at first HAI, if it occurred.

Statistical Analysis

Discrete variables were described as number and percentage, and continuous variables, as mean and standard deviation (SD). The HAI attack rate was the number of HAI per 100 patients, HAI incidence was the number of HAI per 1000 patients-days of hospitalization at risk. Poisson regression was fitted to assess temporal trends of HA pneumonia, bacteraemia and UTI incidence. The number of HAI was the dependent variable and the number of patient-days at risk was the offset. The independent variable of interest was the year of hospitalization. Potential confounders were: patient age, gender, neutropenia during hospital stay, CVC during hospital stay, diagnosis at admission, and main treatment received during hospitalization. Variables with $P<0.15$ after univariate analysis were entered in the initial multivariate model; then, a backward step-wise process was initiated, the models were compared with the likelihood ratio test. The significance level was $P<0.05$; all tests were 2-tailed. Statistical analysis was performed with Stata 10.0 (Stata Corp.). Data were recorded with EpiInfo, version 6.0. All data were analyzed anonymously.

Results

Patient Characteristics

From 2004 to 2010, 3 355 patients, accounting for 58 063 patient-days at risk, were included. The mean duration of hospital stay was 26 days (SD: 21.1 days). Overall, 1 873 (55.8%) were men and 1 482 (44.2%) were women (men/women gender ratio = 1.26). Mean age was 48.8 years (SD: 15.7 years). Patient characteristics are reported in Table 1. In total, 51.3% (n = 1704) had AML, 22.2% (n = 739) had ALL, and 9.5% (n = 315) had multiple myeloma. During their hospitalization, 66.7% of patients (n = 2 063) had neutropenia for a mean duration of 20.9 days (SD: 12.9 days). Most patients (89.7%, n = 2 574) had CVC and 56.9% (n = 1 909) were hospitalized in a protected room. In-hospital mortality was 5% (n = 159).

Table 2. Annual incidence of hospital-acquired infections, Haematology Department, Edouard Herriot Hospital, Lyon (France) 2004–2010.

Characteristics	2004	2005	2006	2007	2008	2009	2010	Overall
Pneumonia, n (attack rate[a])								
Overall population	33 (5.4)	35 (6.4)	36 (6.6)	32 (7.3)	17 (4.3)	16 (3.9)	22 (5.5)	191 (5.7)
AML patients	28 (9.4)	27 (10.7)	24 (9.2)	24 (9.6)	13 (5.7)	9 (4.3)	14 (6.8)	139 (8.2)
ALL patients	0 (0)	3 (2.4)	8 (8.6)	2 (3.1)	1 (1.0)	2 (1.6)	3 (2.6)	19 (2.6)
Other patients	5 (2.7)	5 (3.1)	4 (2.1)	6 (4.9)	3 (4.7)	5 (6.8)	5 (6.3)	33 (3.7)
Pneumonia incidence rate[b] (95% CI)								
Overall	3.2 (2.2–4.5)	4.2 (3.0–5.8)	3.7 (2.7–5.1)	3.4 (2.4–4.7)	2.3 (1.4–3.6)	2.4 (1.4–3.8)	3.5 (2.3–5.3)	3.3 (2.8–3.8)
AML patients	4.9 (3.3–6.9)	6.0 (4.1–8.7)	4.2 (2.8–6.2)	4.0 (2.6–5.9)	3.0 (1.7–5.0)	2.3 (1.1–4.3)	4.1 (2.3–6.7)	4.2 (3.5–4.9)
ALL patients	0 (–)	2.0 (0.5–5.5)	5.2 (2.4–9.9)	1.8 (0.3–5.8)	0.6 (0.0–2.8)	1.2 (0.2–3.9)	2.0 (0.5–5.4)	1.8 (1.1–2.7)
Other patients	1.6 (0.6–3.6)	2.4 (0.8–4.7)	1.6 (0.5–3.9)	2.5 (1.0–5.3)	2.5 (0.6–6.7)	4.0 (1.5–8.9)	3.8 (1.4–8.5)	2.4 (1.6–3.3)
Bacteremia, n (attack rate[a])								
Overall population	95 (15.4)	119 (21.8)	71 (13.0)	70 (16.0)	112 (28.5)	104 (25.2)	123 (30.6)	694 (20.7)
AML patients	61 (20.4)	70 (27.8)	44 (16.9)	45 (18.1)	75 (32.6)	60 (28.8)	75 (36.4)	430 (25.2)
ALL patients	17 (14.4)	26 (21.0)	16 (17.2)	13 (20.3)	25 (25.8)	20 (15.6)	25 (21.7)	142 (19.2)
Other patients	17 (9.1)	23 (14.2)	11 (5.7)	12 (9.8)	12 (18.8)	24 (32.4)	23 (28.8)	122 (13.8)
Bacteremia incidence rate[b] (95% CI)								
Overall	9.2 (7.5–11.2)	14.4 (11.9–17.1)	7.4 (5.8–9.2)	7.4 (5.8–9.3)	15.2 (12.6–18.2)	15.4 (12.6–18.5)	19.8 (16.5–23.5)	12.0 (11.1–12.9)
AML patients	10.6 (8.2–13.5)	15.7 (12.3–19.7)	7.8 (5.7–10.4)	7.6 (5.6–10.0)	17.2 (13.6–21.4)	15.6 (12.0–20.0)	22.1 (17.5–27.5)	12.9 (11.7–14.1)
ALL patients	11.6 (7.0–18.1)	17.6 (11.8–25.5)	10.4 (6.2–16.5)	11.4 (6.3–19.0)	13.9 (9.2–20.3)	11.8 (7.4–18.0)	16.5 (10.9–24.0)	13.4 (11.3–15.7)
Other patients	5.6 (3.4–8.7)	9.8 (6.4–14.5)	4.5 (2.4–7.8)	5.0 (2.7–8.6)	9.8 (5.3–16.8)	19.4(12.7–28.4)	17.6(11.4–26.0)	8.7 (7.3–10.4)
Urinary tract infection, n (attack rate[a])								
Overall population	27 (4.4)	22 (4.0)	31 (5.7)	21 (4.8)	17 (4.3)	23 (5.6)	29 (7.2)	170 (5.1)
AML patients	11 (3.7)	11 (4.4)	18 (6.9)	11 (4.4)	11 (4.8)	11 (5.3)	14 (6.8)	87 (5.1)
ALL patients	8 (6.8)	6 (4.8)	5 (5.4)	5 (7.8)	1 (1.0)	5 (3.9)	7 (6.1)	37 (5.0)
Other patients	8 (4.3)	5 (3.1)	8 (4.1)	5 (4.1)	5 (7.8)	7 (9.5)	8 (10.0)	46 (5.2)
Urinary infection incidence rate[b] (95% CI)								
Overall	2.6 (1.8–3.8)	2.7 (1.7–4.0)	3.2 (2.2–4.5)	2.2 (1.4–3.3)	2.3 (1.4–3.6)	3.4 (2.2–5.0)	4.7 (3.2–6.6)	2.9 (2.5–3.4)
AML patients	1.9 (1.0–3.3)	2.5 (1.3–4.3)	3.2 (1.9–4.9)	1.8 (1.0–3.2)	2.5 (1.3–4.4)	2.9 (1.5–5.0)	4.1 (2.3–6.7)	2.6 (2.1–3.2)
ALL patients	5.4 (2.5–10.3)	4.1 (1.7–8.5)	3.3 (1.2–7.2)	4.4 (1.6–9.7)	0.6 (0.0–2.8)	3.0 (1.1–6.6)	4.6 (2.0–9.1)	3.5 (2.5–4.8)
Other patients	2.6 (1.2–5.0)	2.1 (0.8–4.7)	3.3 (1.5–6.2)	2.1 (0.8–4.7)	4.1 (1.5–9.1)	5.7 (2.5–11.2)	6.1 (2.8–11.6)	3.3 (2.4–4.4)

Notes: AML, acute myeloid leukaemia; ALL, acute lymphoid leukaemia; 95%CI, 95% confidence interval.
[a]number of diagnosed infection/100 patients;
[b]number of diagnosed infection/1000 patient-days at risk.

Between 2004 and 2010, variations in age ($P<0.001$), diagnosis of haematological disease ($P<0.001$), and reason for hospitalization ($P<0.001$) were observed but without linear trends. The proportions of patients with neutropenia or CVC exposure during hospital stay increased during the study period: from 66.9% of patients with neutropenia in 2004 to 74.9% in 2010 ($P<0.001$), and from 88.9% of patients with CVC in 2004 to 97.6% in 2010 ($P<0.001$).

HAI Incidence

In total, 1 055 (31.4%) patients had HAI: 191 (5.7%) had pneumonia, 694 (20.7%) had bacteraemia and 170 (5.1%) had UTI. Table 2 describes the incidence by site of infection, year and haematological disease. Figure 1 depicts trends of incidence over the years. The overall HAI attack rate was 31.4 per 100 patients and its incidence was 18.2 per 1000 patient-days at risk (95% confidence interval (95% CI): 17.1–19.3). The HA pneumonia attack rate was 5.7 per 100 patients and its incidence was 3.3 per 1000 patient-days at risk (95% CI: 2.8–3.8). The HA bacteraemia attack rate was 20.7 per 100 patients and its incidence was 12.0 per 1000 patient-days at risk (95% CI: 11.1–12.9). The HA UTI attack rate was 5.1 per 100 patients and its incidence was 2.9 per 1000 patient-days at risk (95% CI: 2.5–3.4). HA pneumonia incidence was higher among AML patients (incidence: 4.2‰ patient-days, 95% CI 3.5–4.9) compared to ALL patients (incidence: 1.8‰ patient-days, 95% CI 1.1–2.7). HA bacteremia incidence and UTI incidence were similar according to patient haematological diagnosis.

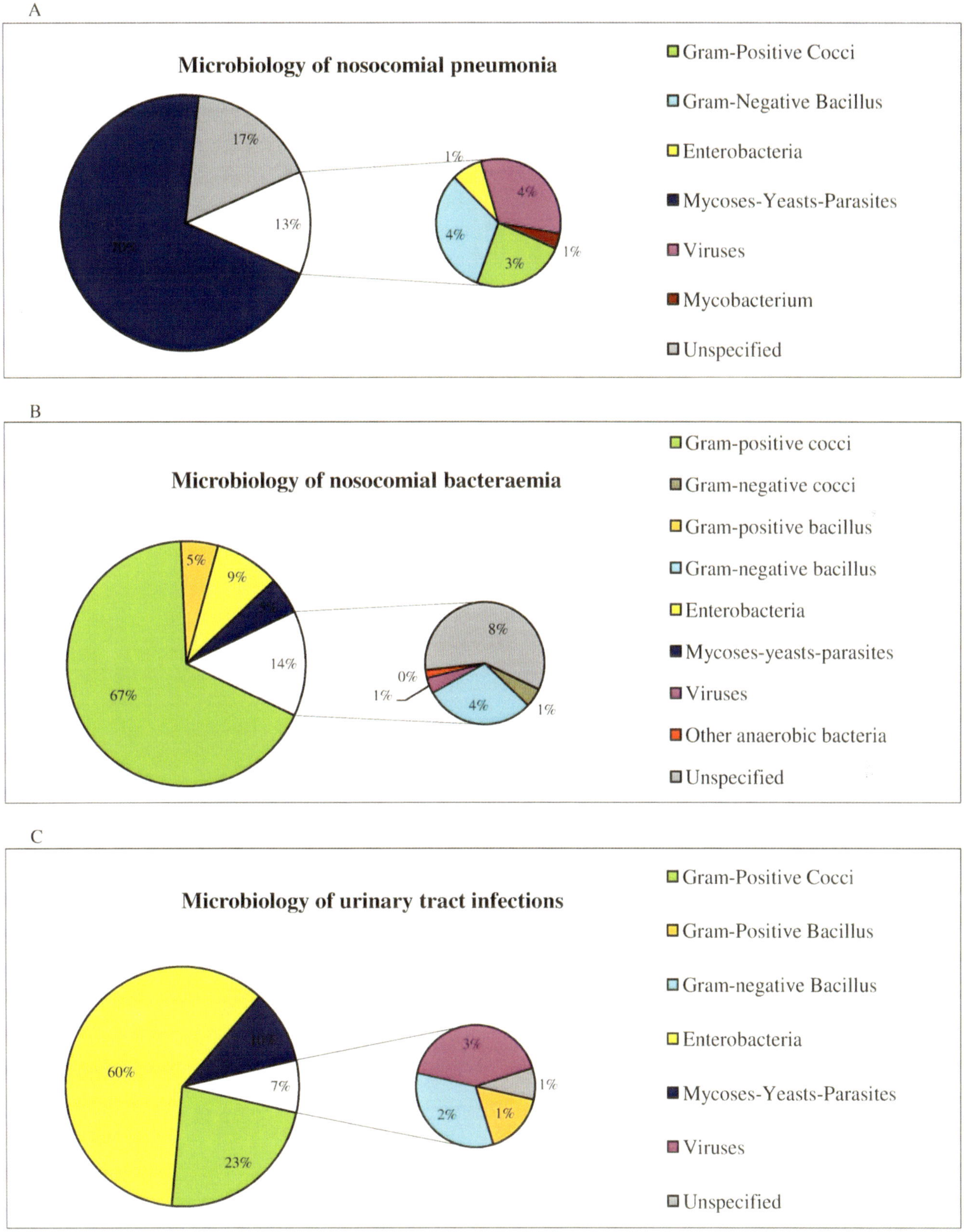

Figure 2. A. Distribution of the isolated pathogens in hospital-acquired pneumonia, Haematology Department, Edouard Herriot Hospital, Lyon (France) 2004–2010. B. Distribution of the isolated pathogens in hospital-acquired bacteraemia, Haematology Department, Edouard Herriot Hospital, Lyon (France) 2004–2010. C. Distribution of the isolated pathogens in hospital-acquired urinary tract infections, Haematology Department, Edouard Herriot Hospital, Lyon (France) 2004–2010.

Table 3. Comparison with other studies.

	Carlisle et al. 1993 [13]	Dettenkofer et al. 2003 [19]	Engelhart et al. 2002 [20]	Present study
Number of patients	920 neutropenic patients	351 patients	116 patients	3,355 patients
Study period	42 months	54 months	8 months	84 months
Pneumonia	5.5 per 100 neutropenic patients	22 per 100 patients	12.9 per 100 patients	5.7 per 100 patients
Incidence rate	–	5.4 per 1000 patient-days	9.7 per 1000 patient-days at risk	3.3 per 1000 patient-days at risk
Bacteraemia	13.5 per 100 neutropenic patients	24 per 100 patients	16.4 per 100 patients	20.7 per 100 patients
Incidence rate	–	6.0 per 1000 patient-days	11.2 per 1000 patient-days at risk	12.0 per 1000 patient-days at risk
Urinary tract infections	5.7 per 100 neutropenic patients	3.0 per 100 patients	6.0 per 100 patients	5.1 per 100 patients
Incidence rate	–	0.8 per 1000 patient-days	3.0 per 1000 patient-days at risk	2.9 per 1000 patient-days at risk

Univariate Poisson regression indicated that the incidence of HA pneumonia was stable between 2004 and 2010: −4% per year (95% CI: −11%, +3%, $P=0.23$). HA bacteraemia increased by 12% per year (95% CI: +8%, +16%, $P<0.001$). A trend for increased HA UTI was observed: +7% per year (95% CI: 0%, +16%, $P=0.08$).

Multivariate Poisson regression models after controlling for neutropenia and medical treatment showed a stable incidence rate for HA pneumonia over years: +5% per year (95% CI: −12%, +2%, $P=0.17$). Multivariate Poisson regression models after controlling for neutropenia, CVC and diagnosis of haematological disease showed an increase by 11% per year (95% CI: +6%, +15%, $P<0.001$). Multivariate Poisson regression models after controlling for patient gender showed a stable incidence rate for HA UTI: +6% per year (95% CI: −1%, +15%, $P=0.11$).

Microbiology

Figure 2 reports the distribution of microorganisms by infection site. The causative pathogens isolated most frequently in HA pneumonia were *Aspergillus spp.* (59.2%, n = 113) and *Candida* (7.8%, n = 15). Viral HA pneumonia affected 8 patients overall (4.2%). The causative pathogens isolated most frequently in HA bacteraemia were coagulase-negative *Staphylococcus* (44.2%, n = 307) and *Candida* (4.6%, n = 32). Hospital-acquired blood infection by a virus concerned 7 patients (1.0%). The causative pathogens isolated most frequently in HA UTI were enterobacteria (60%, n = 102). Viral HA UTI affected 5 patients (2.9%).

Discussion

The study's objective was to describe trends in HA pneumonia, bacteraemia and UTI incidence between 2004 and 2010 as they were the most frequent and lethal sites of infection in patients with haematological malignancies [17,20,22,28]. No significant trend was found in HA pneumonia and UTI incidence. HA bacteraemia incidence increased by 11% per year independently of neutropenia, CVC and patient's haematological disease. Table 3 compares our results with 3 previous surveillance studies about neutropenic cancer patients [13] and patients with haematological malignancies [19,20].

Engelhart et al. reported data on HAI and fever of unknown origin among adult haematology and oncology patients [20]. They discerned a higher pneumonia incidence (9.7 per 1000 patient-days), while most rooms in their department were not equipped with LAF or positive pressure isolation and HEPA filtration. Consequently, protection against *Aspergillus*, the most common pathogen in HA pneumonia in this patient group, would be less efficient [29,30]. In our study, the globally-stable incidence of HA pneumonia could be balanced by decreased invasive aspergillosis during the same period [31]. Consequently, it is not clear whether pneumonia of other origins was truly stable. However, we found a high rate of *Aspergillus* pneumonia (59.2% of the causative agents in pneumonia) although 56.9% of the patients were hospitalized in a protected room. *Aspergillosis* remained a large concern among our patients and *Aspergillus* pneumonia occurred mainly in immunosuppressed patients like AML or ALL patients [31,32]. Moreover, in our survey, incidence of HA-pneumonia appeared higher among AML patient compared with ALL patients or other patients.

The incidence of bacteraemia rose during the study period. Bacteraemia are mostly of endogenous origin, caused by pathogens or saprophytic cutaneous flora, such as *Staphyloccocus spp.* [33]. Over the years, we noted a higher proportion of patients with CVC, well-known to be a major risk factor for HA bloodstream infection [23]. The length and depth of the neutropenic phase, especially during chemotherapy, could also be related to incidence of bacteraemia. Nevertheless, the increased HA bacteraemia incidence was independent of CVC-exposure or neutropenia. Other factors could explain this increase, like more intense chemotherapy over the years, changes in antibiotic prophylaxis or hygiene practices. However, a previous study reported a protective impact of hygiene measures [34]. Then, the increase of incidence might be mostly related to the severity of patients or to their underlying diseases. Carlisle et al. recorded a lower HA bacteraemia rate than what we observed in our department [13]. They implemented 42-month surveillance and detected 13.5 bacteraemia per 100 neutropenic days. However, their study focused on neutropenic cancer patients and not on a specific population hospitalized with haematologic malignancies, the last population could have more severe immune system dysfunction related to their disease and not only chemotherapy. On the other hand, we found a similar incidence of bacteraemia as Engelhart et al. (11.2 per 1000 patient-days at risk) who investigated patients with haematological-oncologic diseases [20].

UTI incidence was stable. We encountered a similar incidence as Carlisle et al. (5.7 per 100 neutropenic patients) [13] and Engelhart et al. (6.0 per 100 patients) [20]. Dettenkofer et al. reported a much lower UTI rate (3.0 per 100 patients, 0.8 per 1,000 patient-days) in transplant patients [19], but all of them received antimicrobial prophylaxis, which could have reduced the risk of infection in prolonged neutropenia cases [35–37].

Our study had some limitations. First, the study population was mainly composed of AML and ALL patients. Our findings cannot be generalized to all haematological populations. Secondly, no post-discharge surveillance was undertaken, which could have led to underestimation of the incidence because infections with long incubation periods could have been missed. However, it did not affect trends because possible underestimation could be constant over the years. Furthermore, some potential risk factors for infection were not collected in our surveillance database, like length of CVC exposure, mechanical ventilation, type of stem-cell transplant (autologous or allogenous).

Its main strength was prospective data collection, with standardized case definitions. Ours was a single-centre study, which permitted us to compare trends and reinforced internal validity. Moreover, the true incidence was assessed because all patients were followed until their discharge. Few investigations have analyzed data over such a long time period and in such a large population, which increased the study's power calculation. Finally, major confounding factors were taken into account with multivariate analysis.

In summary, we observed that the incidence of HA pneumonia and HA UTI remained stable. This could be explained by improvement of infection control measures, and took account of patient exposure to more aggressive chemotherapies. The incidence of bacteraemia increased independently of CVC exposure or neutropenia, which are known risk factors of bacteraemia. Further etiological studies are needed to explore in depth the factors that could explain this trend.

Acknowledgments

We thank Ovid Da Silva for editing the manuscript. We thank all residents of the infection control unit who took part in case surveillance: Caroline Landelle, Silène Cronenberger, Maud Mandy-Bertin, Pauline Pluviaud, Guilaine Boursier, Valérie Paix, Pierre Cassier and Guillaume Debeurne. We acknowledge the nursing staff of the Infection Control Unit: Christine Chémorin, Monique Hulin, Sylvie Monier and Léone Monrandat. We are also indebted to the Microbiology and Virology Departments of Centre de biologie et pathologie Est (Bron, France) as well as the Parasitology and Mycology Laboratory of Groupement hospitalier Nord (Lyon, France). Finally, we appreciate the efforts of the nursing and medical staff of the Haematology Department at Edouard Herriot Hospital.

Author Contributions

Conceived and designed the experiments: PV M-CN MM TB. Analyzed the data: CH PV TB. Contributed reagents/materials/analysis tools: CH PV TB. Wrote the paper: CH PV M-CN MM TB.

References

1. Thirumala R, Ramaswamy M, Chawla S (2010) Diagnosis and management of infectious complications in critically ill patients with cancer. Crit Care Clin 26: 59–91.
2. Bailey LC, Reilly AF, Rheingold SR (2009) Infections in pediatric patients with hematologic malignancies. Semin Hematol 46: 313–24.
3. Wisplinghoff H, Cornely OA, Moser S, Bethe U, Stützer H, et al. (2003) Outcomes of nosocomial bloodstream infections in adult neutropenic patients: a prospective cohort and matched case-control study. Infect Control Hosp Epidemiol 24: 905–11.
4. Velasco E, Soares M, Byington R, Martins CA, Schirmer M, et al. (2004) Prospective evaluation of the epidemiology, microbiology, and outcome of bloodstream infections in adult surgical cancer patients. Eur J Clin Microbiol Infect Dis 23: 596–602.
5. Gonzales-Barca E, Fernandez-Sevilla A, Carratala J, Salar A, Peris J, et al. (1999) Prognostic factors influencing mortality in cancer patients with neutropenia and bacteremia. Eur J Clin Microbiol Infect Dis 18: 539–44.
6. Pannuti C, Gingrich R, Pfaller MA, Kao C, Wenzel RP (1992) Nosocomial pneumonia in patients having bone marrow transplant. Attributable mortality and risk factors. Cancer 69: 2653–62.
7. Pannuti C, Gingrich R, Pfaller MA, Wenzel RP (1991) Nosocomial pneumonia in adult patients undergoing bone marrow transplantation: a 9-year study. J Clin Oncol 9: 77–84.
8. Ewig S, Glasmacher A, Ulrich B, Wilhelm K, Schäfer H, et al. (1998) Pulmonary infiltrates in neutropenic patients with acute leukemia during chemotherapy: outcomes and prognostic factors. Chest 114: 444–51.
9. Gooley TA, Chien JW, Pergam SA, Hingorani S, Sorror ML, et al. (2010) Reduced mortality after allogeneic hematopoietic-cell transplantation. N Engl J Med 363: 2091–101.
10. Pulte D, Gondos A, Brenner H (2008) Trends in 5- and 10-year survival after diagnosis with childhood hematologic malignancies in the United States, 1990–2004. J Natl Cancer Inst 100: 1301–9.
11. Wayne AS, Reaman GH, Helman LJ (2008) Progress in the curative treatment of childhood hematologic malignancies. J Natl Cancer Inst 100: 1271–3.
12. Socié G, Stone JV, Wingard JR, Weisdorf D, Henslee-Downey PJ, et al. (1999) Long-term survival and late deaths after allogeneic bone marrow transplantation. Late Effects Working Committee of the International Bone Marrow Transplant Registry. N Engl J Med 341: 14–21.
13. Carlisle PS, Gucalp R, Wiernik PH (1993) Nosocomial infections in neutropenic cancer patients. Infect Control Hosp Epidemiol 14: 320–4.
14. Crawford J, Dale DC, Lyman GH (2004) Chemotherapy-induced neutropenia: risks, consequences, and new directions for its management. Cancer 100: 228–37.
15. De Angelis G, Murthy A, Beyersmann J, Harbarth S (2010) Estimating the impact of healthcare-associated infections on length of stay and costs. Clin Microbiol Infect 16: 1729–35.
16. Roberts RR, Scott RD 2nd, Hota B, Kampe LM, Abbasi F, et al. (2010) Cost attributable to healthcare-acquired infection in hospitalized adults and a comparison of economic methods. Med Care 48: 1026–35.
17. Dettenkofer M, Wenzler-Röttele S, Babikir R, Bertz H, Ebner W, et al. (2005) Surveillance of nosocomial sepsis and pneumonia in patients with a bone marrow or peripheral blood stem cell transplant: a multicenter project. Clin Infect Dis 40: 926–31.
18. Marena C, Zecca M, Carenini ML, Bruschi A, Bassi ML, et al. (2001) Incidence of, and risk factors for, nosocomial infections among hematopoietic stem cell transplantation recipients, with impact on procedure-related mortality. Infect Control Hosp Epidemiol 22: 510–7.
19. Dettenkofer M, Ebner W, Bertz H, Babikir R, Finke J, et al. (2003) Surveillance of nosocomial infections in adult recipients of allogeneic and autologous bone marrow and peripheral blood stem-cell transplantation. Bone Marrow Transplant 31: 795–801.
20. Engelhart S, Glasmacher A, Exner M, Kramer MH (2002) Surveillance for nosocomial infections and fever of unknown origin among adult hematology-oncology patients. Infect Control Hosp Epidemiol 23: 244–8.
21. Urrea M, Rives S, Cruz O, Navarro A, García JJ, et al. (2004) Nosocomial infections among pediatric hematology/oncology patients: results of a prospective incidence study. Am J Infect Control 32: 205–8.
22. Al-Tonbary YA, Soliman OE, Sarhan MM, Hegazi MA, El-Ashry RA, et al. (2011) Nosocomial infections and fever of unknown origin in pediatric hematology/oncology unit: a retrospective annual study. World J Pediatr 7: 60–4.
23. Wisplinghoff H, Seifert H, Wenzel RP, Edmond MB (2003) Current trends in the epidemiology of nosocomial bloodstream infections in patients with hematological malignancies and solid neoplasms in hospitals in the United States. Clin Infect Dis 36: 1103–10.
24. Saavedra S, Jarque I, Sanz GF, Moscardó F, Jiménez C, et al. (2002) Infectious complications in patients undergoing unrelated donor bone marrow transplantation: experience from a single institution. Clin Microbiol Infect 8: 725–33.
25. Saavedra S, Sanz GF, Jarque I, Moscardó F, Jiménez C, et al. (2002) Early infections in adult patients undergoing unrelated donor cord blood transplantation. Bone Marrow Transplant 30: 937–43.
26. Pottecher B, Herbrecht R, Blanc-Vincent MP, Bussy Malgrange V, Escande MC, et al. (2000) Standards, Options and Recommendations (SOR) for the surveillance and the prevention of cross infections in oncology. Fédération Nationale des Centres de Lutte Contre le Cancer. Bull Cancer 87 : 557–91.
27. Comité technique des infections nosocomiales (1999) 100 recommandations pour la surveillance et la prévention des infections nosocomiales. 2e éd. Ministère de l'Emploi et de la Solidarité, Secrétariat d'Etat à la Santé et à l'action sociale, Paris, France.
28. Velasco E, Thuler LC, Martins CA, Dias LM, Gonçalves VM (1997) Nosocomial infections in an oncology intensive care unit. Am J Infect Control 25: 458–62.
29. Bénet T, Nicolle MC, Thiebaut A, Piens MA, Nicolini FE, et al. (2007) Reduction of invasive aspergillosis incidence among immunocompromised patients after control of environmental exposure. Clin Infect Dis 45: 682–6.
30. Hahn T, Cummings KM, Michalek AM, Lipman BJ, Segal BH, et al. (2002) Efficacy of high-efficiency particulate air filtration in preventing aspergillosis in immunocompromised patients with hematologic malignancies. Infect Control Hosp Epidemiol 23: 525–31.
31. Nicolle MC, Bénet T, Thiebaut A, Bienvenu AL, Voirin N, et al. (2011) Invasive aspergillosis in patients with hematological malignancies: incidence and

description of 127 cases enrolled in a single institution prospective survey from 2004 to 2009. Haematologica 96: 1685–91.
32. Cornet M, Fleury L, Maslo C, Bernard JF, Brücker G, et al. (2002) Epidemiology of invasive aspergillosis in France: a six-year multicentric survey in the Greater Paris area. J Hosp Infect 51: 288–96.
33. Rupp ME (2004) Nosocomial bloodstream infections. In: Glen Mayhall C, editor. Hospital Epidemiology and Infection Control, 3rd edition. Lippincott Williams and Wilkins. 253–65.
34. Bénet T, Vanhems P (2009) Correlation of nosocomial bloodstream infection incidences: an ecological study. J Hosp Infect 73: 217–24.
35. Segal BH, Freifeld AG (2007) Antibacterial prophylaxis in patients with neutropenia. J Natl Compr Canc Netw 5: 235–42.
36. Leibovici L, Paul M, Cullen M, Bucaneve G, Gafter-Gvili A, et al. (2006) Antibiotic prophylaxis in neutropenic patients: new evidence, practical decisions. Cancer 107: 1743–51.
37. Cullen M, Baijal S (2009) Prevention of febrile neutropenia: use of prophylactic antibiotics. Br J Cancer 101: S11–4.

3

Human Alpha Defensin 5 Expression in the Human Kidney and Urinary Tract

John David Spencer[1,2]⁹, David S. Hains[2,3]⁹, Edith Porter[4], Charles L. Bevins[5], Julianne DiRosario[3], Brian Becknell[1,2], Huanyu Wang[3], Andrew L. Schwaderer[2,3]*⁹

1 Pediatric Nephrology Fellowship Program, Nationwide Children's Hospital, Columbus, Ohio, United States of America, **2** Division of Nephrology, Department of Pediatrics, Nationwide Children's Hospital, Columbus, Ohio, United States of America, **3** Center for Clinical and Translational Research, The Research Institute at Nationwide Children's Hospital, Columbus, Ohio, United States of America, **4** Department of Biological Sciences, California State University Los Angeles, Los Angeles, California, United States of America, **5** Department of Microbiology and Immunology, School of Medicine, University of California Davis, Davis, California, United States of America

Abstract

Background: The mechanisms that maintain sterility in the urinary tract are incompletely understood. Recent studies have implicated the importance of antimicrobial peptides (AMP) in protecting the urinary tract from infection. Here, we characterize the expression and relevance of the AMP human alpha-defensin 5 (HD5) in the human kidney and urinary tract in normal and infected subjects.

Methodology/Principal Findings: Using RNA isolated from human kidney, ureter, and bladder tissue, we performed quantitative real-time PCR to show that *DEFA5*, the gene encoding HD5, is constitutively expressed throughout the urinary tract. With pyelonephritis, *DEFA5* expression significantly increased in the kidney. Using immunoblot analysis, HD5 production also increased with pyelonephritis. Immunostaining localized HD5 to the urothelium of the bladder and ureter. In the kidney, HD5 was primarily produced in the distal nephron and collecting tubules. Using immunoblot and ELISA assays, HD5 was not routinely detected in non-infected human urine samples while mean urinary HD5 production increased with *E.coli* urinary tract infection.

Conclusions/Significance: *DEFA5* is expressed throughout the urinary tract in non-infected subjects. Specifically, HD5 is expressed throughout the urothelium of the lower urinary tract and in the collecting tubules of the kidney. With infection, HD5 expression increases in the kidney and levels become detectable in the urine. To our knowledge, our findings represent the first to quantitate HD5 expression and production in the human kidney. Moreover, this is the first report to detect the presence of HD5 in infected urine samples. Our results suggest that HD5 may have an important role in maintaining urinary tract sterility.

Editor: Daniela Flavia Hozbor, Universidad Nacional de La Plata., United States of America

Funding: JDS received intramural support from The Research Institute at Nationwide Children's Hospital. No current external funding sources for this study. The funders had no role in study design, data collection and analysis, decision to publish, or preparation of the manuscript.

Competing Interests: The authors have declared that no competing interests exist.

* E-mail: andrew.schwaderer@nationwidechildrens.org

⁹ These authors contributed equally to this work.

Introduction

The urinary tract, apart from the urethral meatus, is usually sterile despite its proximity with fecal flora. The precise mechanisms by which the urinary tract maintains its sterility are not well understood. Proposed mechanisms contributing to defense of the urinary tract include urine flow, alterations in urine pH and osmolarity, regular bladder emptying, chemical-defense components of the uroepithelium, and epithelial shedding/influx of effector immune cells with bacterial stimulation [1]. In addition, antimicrobial peptides (AMPs) have recently been shown to have an important role in maintaining urinary tract sterility [2].

AMPs, which serve as natural antibiotics produced by nearly all organisms, are a ubiquitous component of the innate immune system. AMPs are cationic molecules expressed by phagocytic white cells and epithelial cells. In humans and other mammals, defensins are a major family of AMPs. Defensins typically have broad-spectrum antimicrobial activity against gram-positive and gram-negative bacteria, viruses, fungi, and protozoa [2,3]. Defensins are initially synthesized as preproproteins and undergo processing to become mature, biologically active peptides [4]. In humans, defensins are classified into one of two families depending on their disulfide bridging pattern – the alpha-defensins or the beta-defensins [5].

In the urinary tract, the beta-defensins are widely expressed throughout the uroepithelium. Epithelial cells lining the kidney's loop of Henle, distal tubule, and collecting duct constitutively express human beta-defensin 1 (hBD1). Although urinary levels of hBD1 are insufficient to kill invading bacteria, hBD1 provides a fast-acting antimicrobial coating of tubular lumens and prevents infection by inhibiting bacterial attachment to the urothelium [6]. Recent studies indicate that the redox-state of hBD1 significantly affects antimicrobial potency, such that the reduced peptide is much more potent that the disulfide-linked oxidized form [7]. The significance of this at the urothelial surface has not been determined. Another defensin, human beta-defensin 2 (hBD2) is not constitutively expressed in healthy kidney tissue; however, hBD2 expression is induced by infection [8].

Unlike the beta-defensins, the role of epithelial-derived alpha-defensins is not well described in the urinary tract. The expression and function of alpha-defensin HD5 and HD6 have mostly been reported in the small intestine where they are secreted by Paneth cells into the intestinal crypts and contribute to the balance of intestinal microbiotica [9]. HD5 has also been localized in the male and female genital tracts, with evidence suggesting that it is inducible and important in eradicating infection [10,11,12]. Urinary HD5 has been detected in patients who have undergone ileal neobladder reconstruction and ileal conduit urinary diversion whereby the source of HD5 production was primarily credited to the ileal Paneth cells [13,14]. HD5 has antibacterial activity against common uropathogenic gram-positive bacteria and gram-negative bacteria [15]. HD5 also has antimicrobial activity against uropathogenic viruses like adenovirus and BK virus [16,17,18]. In this study, we provide the initial description and quantification of HD5 expression in the human kidney and further define its expression in the lower urinary tract during sterility and infection.

Results

DEFA5 mRNA is constitutively expressed in human bladder, ureter, and kidney

Quantitative real-time PCR demonstrates that all tested bladder, ureter, and kidney specimens without infection constitutively expressed *DEFA5*. *DEFA5* expression was significantly greater in the lower urinary tract than the upper urinary tract ($p = 0.014$). In the bladder ($n = 4$), mean *DEFA5* expression was 4,656±37 transcripts per 10 ng RNA and in the ureter ($n = 4$) mean *DEFA5* expression was 4,112±170 transcripts per 10 ng RNA (Figure 1A). In the kidney ($n = 6$), mean *DEFA5* expression was 2,937±274 transcripts per 10 ng RNA. *DEFA5* expression was analyzed separately in the renal cortex, medulla, and pelvis. *DEFA5* expression did not significantly vary by kidney region ($p = 0.45$).

DEFA5 expression and HD5 peptide expression increase with pyelonephritis

Quantitative real-time PCR analysis performed on kidney tissues with pyelonephritis demonstrated a significant increase in *DEFA5* expression compared to non-infected kidney tissues. With pyelonephritis ($n = 6$), mean *DEFA5* expression increased to 7,829±1,052 transcripts per 10 ng RNA ($p = 0.019$) (Figure 2A).

To further evaluate this increase in expression with pyelonephritis, we performed immunoblot analysis on the same kidney tissue used for real-time PCR analysis to evaluate for concurrent increases in HD5 peptide production (Figure 2B, middle panel). Immunoblot analysis, using polyclonal HD5 antisera, demonstrated significantly greater HD5 peptide production in kidney tissues with pyelonephritis ($n = 6$) compared to non-infected kidney tissues ($n = 6$). Non-infected kidney tissues expressed 300±25 ng HD5/gram wet tissue weight while kidney tissue with pyelonephritis expressed 600±21 ng HD5/gram wet tissue weight ($p < 0.0001$). Blots were re-probed with GAPDH to serve as a loading control (Figure 2B, middle panel) and a silver stain was also performed to confirm equal protein loading (Figure 2B, top panel).

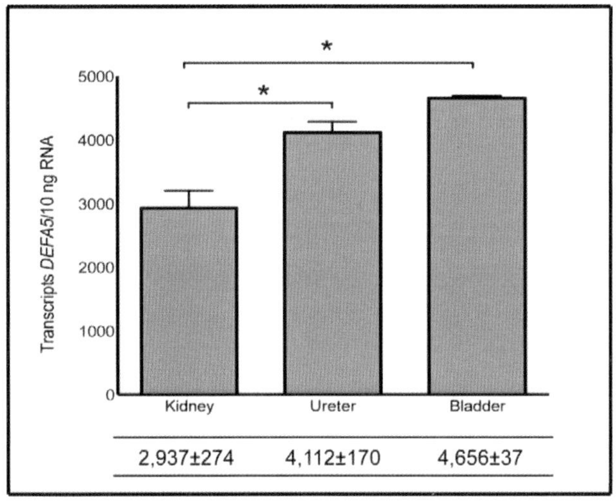

Figure 1. Expression of *DEFA5* in human kidney, ureter, and bladder. *DEFA5* mRNA transcript levels were quantified by real-time PCR in non-infected kidney, ureter, bladder. Shown are the results of three independent samples. In the table below, the mean transcript levels are shown with the SEM. *DEFA5* expression was significantly greater in the lower urinary tract ($p = 0.014$).

HD5 peptide is produced throughout the human kidney and urinary tract

Immunostaining was performed to localize HD5 production in the urinary tract. Immunohistochemistry (IHC) showed that HD5 immunoreactivity was present throughout the urothelium of the ureter and bladder of all investigated specimens ($n = 4$, Figure 3). IHC also showed that HD5 was produced in tubules of the renal cortex and medulla of all specimens ($n = 6$, Figure 4). Immunofluorescence (IF) demonstrated that HD5 expression was greatest in the distal nephron and the collecting tubules (Figure 5). The interstitium and glomeruli did not show HD5 immunoreactivity. The immunostaining shown in Figures 3, 4, and 5 was performed using a mouse monoclonal anti-HD5 antibody (8C8) that recognizes the HD5 propeptide (Abcam, Cambridge, MA). Results were similar when using rabbit polyclonal anti-HD5 antibody that recognizes the HD5 propeptide and mature peptide (data not shown) – suggesting that HD5 is stored as a propeptide.

With pyelonephritis, HD5 immunostaining markedly increased. HD5 immunoreactivity increased throughout the proximal nephron, the distal nephron, and the collecting tubules (Figure 4 and Figure 5). As in non-infected specimens, the glomeruli and interstitium showed no HD5 expression with infection. Negative controls showed no HD5 immunoreactivity.

Infected human urine contains measurable concentrations of HD5 peptide

Immunoblot analysis, using rabbit polyclonal antiserum that detects the precursor proHD5 and further processed forms identified measurable levels of HD5 in 13 of the 15 tested urine samples infected with uropathogenic *E.coli* (Figure 6A and B). When present, HD5 levels, normalized to urine creatinine, ranged from 299.8–669.7±30 ng HD5/mg urine Cr (110.67 ng/mL–276.67 ng/mL), which corresponds to 11.10–27.67 nmol/L. In non-infected urine samples ($n = 15$), HD5 was at or below the detection limit of (<50 ng). Enzyme linked immunosorbant assay (ELISA) on the same urine samples, using the mouse monoclonal antibody (8C8) that detects only the precursor proHD5, detected

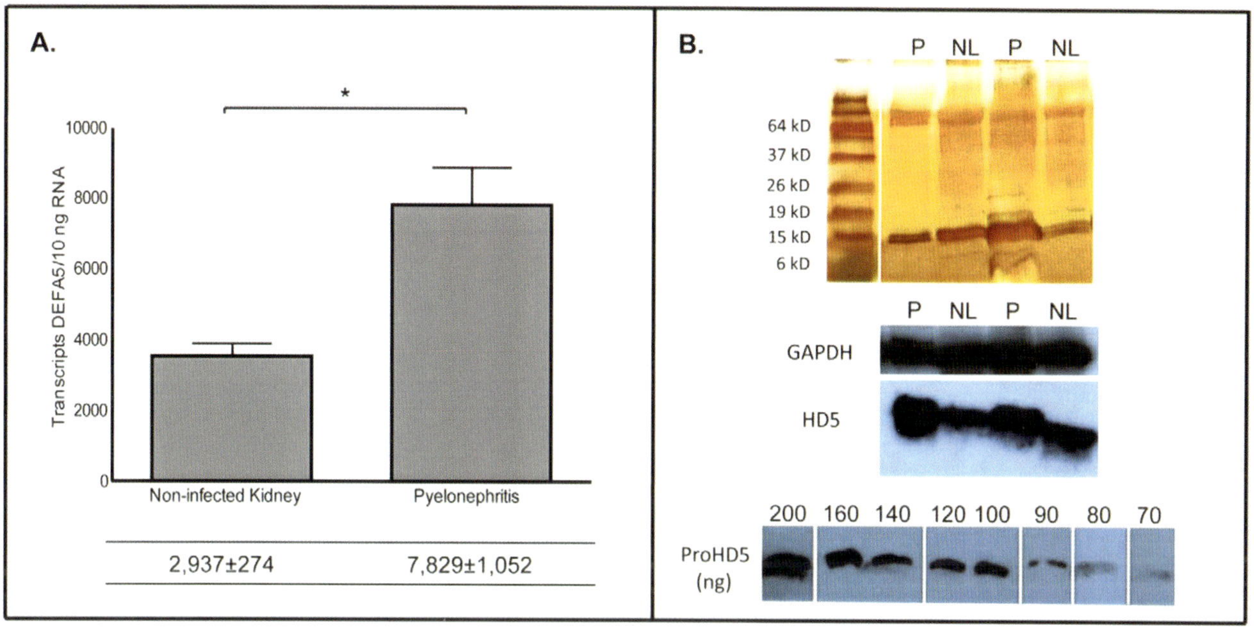

Figure 2. HD5 expression increases with pyelonephritis. (**A**) *DEFA5* mRNA transcript levels were quantified by real-time PCR in non-infected kidney tissue and in kidney tissue with pyelonephritis. Shown are the results for three independent samples. In the table below, the mean transcript levels are shown with the SEM. *DEFA5* expression was significantly greater with pyelonephritis ($p = 0.019$). (**B**) To confirm the increase in message is accompanied by an increase in HD5 protein production, cationic peptides from the same non-infected kidney tissues (NL) and kidney tissue with pyelonephritis (P) were subjected to SDS PAGE followed by Western immunoblot analysis. Each lane contained the equivalent of 800 µg of cationic protein. Silver stained PAGE gels (top panel) confirmed equal protein loading into each lane. Immunoblot analysis for GAPDH and HD5 (middle panel). Serial dilutions of proHD5 (200 ng–70 ng) were subjected to SDS PAGE followed by Western immunoblot analysis (bottom panel).

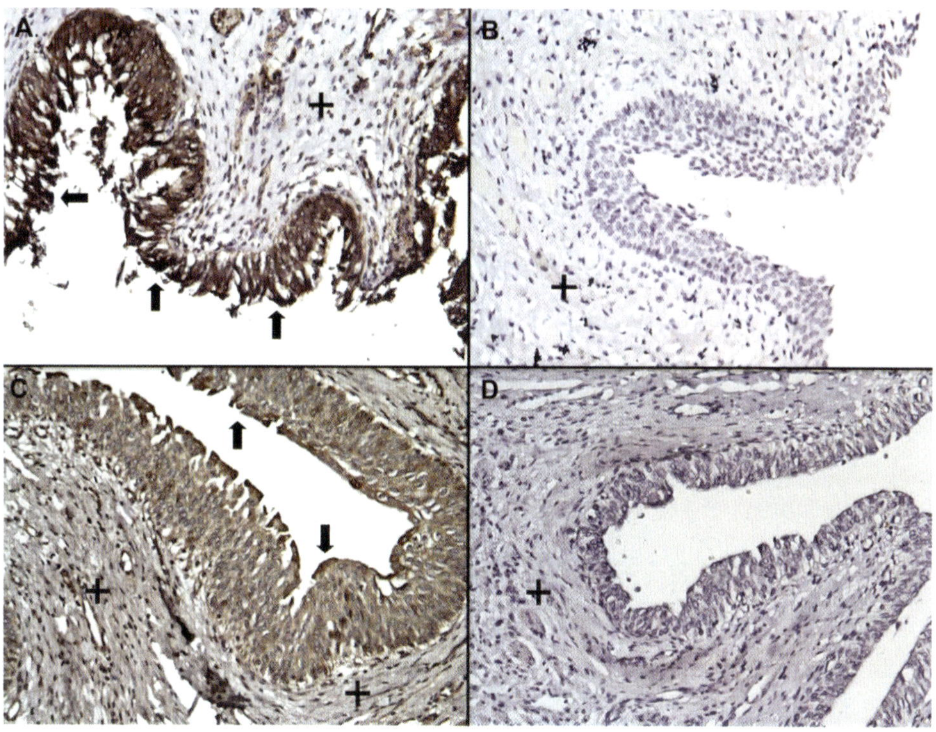

Figure 3. HD5 is expressed throughout the urothelium of the ureter and bladder. Immunohistochemistry demonstrates HD5 expression (brown/arrows) throughout the urothelium of the human bladder (**A**) and ureter (**C**). Immunostaining was most prominent in the luminal surfaces (brown/arrows). Immunostaining was not detected in the smooth muscle layers of the bladder or ureter (+). Negative control bladder (**B**) and ureter (**D**) showed no immunostaining. Magnification 20×.

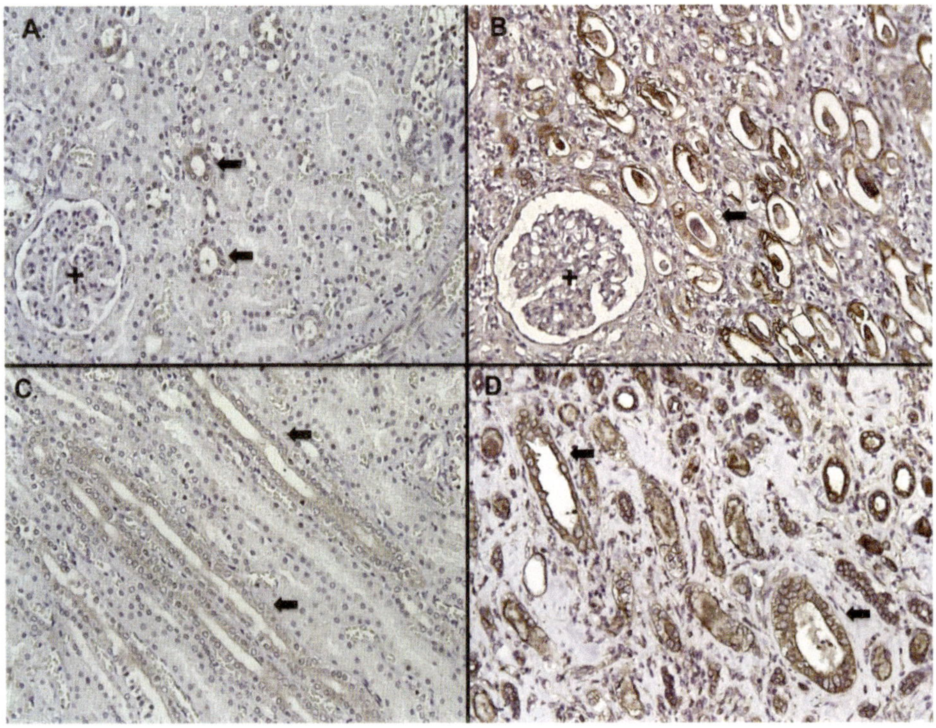

Figure 4. HD5 production in non-infected human kidney and kidney with pyelonephritis. Immunohistochemistry demonstrates HD5 production in isolated renal tubules (brown/arrows) in non-infected renal cortex (**A**) and medulla (**C**). With pyelonephritis, HD5 production increased in the renal tubules of the cortex (**B**) and medulla (**D**). The glomeruli (+) show no immunostaining in non-infected kidney samples and with pyelonephritis. Negative controls showed no immunostaining (not shown). Magnification 20×.

measurable levels of proHD5 in 13 of the 15 infected samples tested. Urinary proHD5 concentrations ranged from 122.78–490.0±0.03 ng HD5/mg urine Cr (30.02 ng/mL–200.5 ng/mL) when present (Figure 7).

Discussion

In this study, we provide the initial characterization HD5 in the human kidney, ureter, and bladder. HD5 has been shown to be an important AMP that prevents invasive infection in the intestine and is up-regulated in the genital tract during infection [11,18,19,20,21]. Epithelial derived AMPs, like HD5, have been shown to be important in maintaining sterility in the urinary tract [8,22,23,24]. Deficiencies in these innate mucosal defenses may result in acute and/or chronic infection [25,26].

Our quantitative real-time PCR results demonstrate that *DEFA5* is constitutively expressed in human kidney, ureter, and bladder. *DEFA5* expression increases from the upper urinary tract to the lower urinary tract – following the flow of the urinary stream and the increasing closeness to the microbiota's point of invasion. To our knowledge, this is the first study to quantify *DEFA5* expression in the human kidney and bladder. Recently, Townes *et al* demonstrated that normal distal ureter can express *DEFA5* [14]. Our results also suggest that *DEFA5* is constitutively expressed by the distal ureter. Although *DEFA5* expression in the urinary tract is nearly 100-fold lower than that found in gastrointestinal tissues, basal uroepithelial expression of *DEFA5* is comparable to the expression of previously described urinary tract AMPs like cathelicidin, hBD-1, hBD-2, and ribonuclease 7 [6,8,22,24,27].

In contrast to the mature gastrointestinal tract where *DEFA5* is expressed at high levels in both states of health and infection/inflammation, our quantitative real-time PCR data demonstrate that *DEFA5* expression in the kidney is significantly up-regulated with infection [27,28,29]. This inducible pattern of expression is analogous to *DEFA5* expression in the female reproductive tract where *DEFA5* expression increases with salpingitis [30]. In the urinary tract, Townes *et al* have shown a trend toward greater ureteral expression of *DEFA5* in patients with UTIs who have undergone ileal conduit urinary diversion [14].

Our immunoblot analysis complements the real-time PCR data by demonstrating that HD5 peptide production increases with pyelonephritis. This inducible pattern of HD5 production is similar to that seen in some members of the beta-defensin family. hBD2 shows an inducible pattern of production with infection of the urinary tract and/or chronic pyelonephritis [8,31,32]. HD5 peptide production has been shown to increase in the upper female genital tract and male urethra with inflammation [11,30].

Using immunostaining, we demonstrate that HD5 is uniformly produced throughout the urothelium of the ureter and bladder. Because the vast majority of UTIs result from fecal flora that ascend into the bladder, these results suggest that HD5 expression is present in locations where microbial exposure occurs most frequently [33]. Therefore, HD5 is ideally positioned to prevent an ascending microbial infection. In the kidney, HD5 is primarily produced in the distal nephron and collecting tubule. These findings suggest that HD5 is produced in locations where it will be positioned to have optimal antimicrobial activity. Previous studies have shown that the antimicrobial properties of defensins are dependent on salt concentration – with higher salt concentrations decreasing antimicrobial activity [23,34,35]. We speculate that the low salt concentrations of the distal nephron and collecting tubule provide a favorable milieu for HD5 antimicrobial activity.

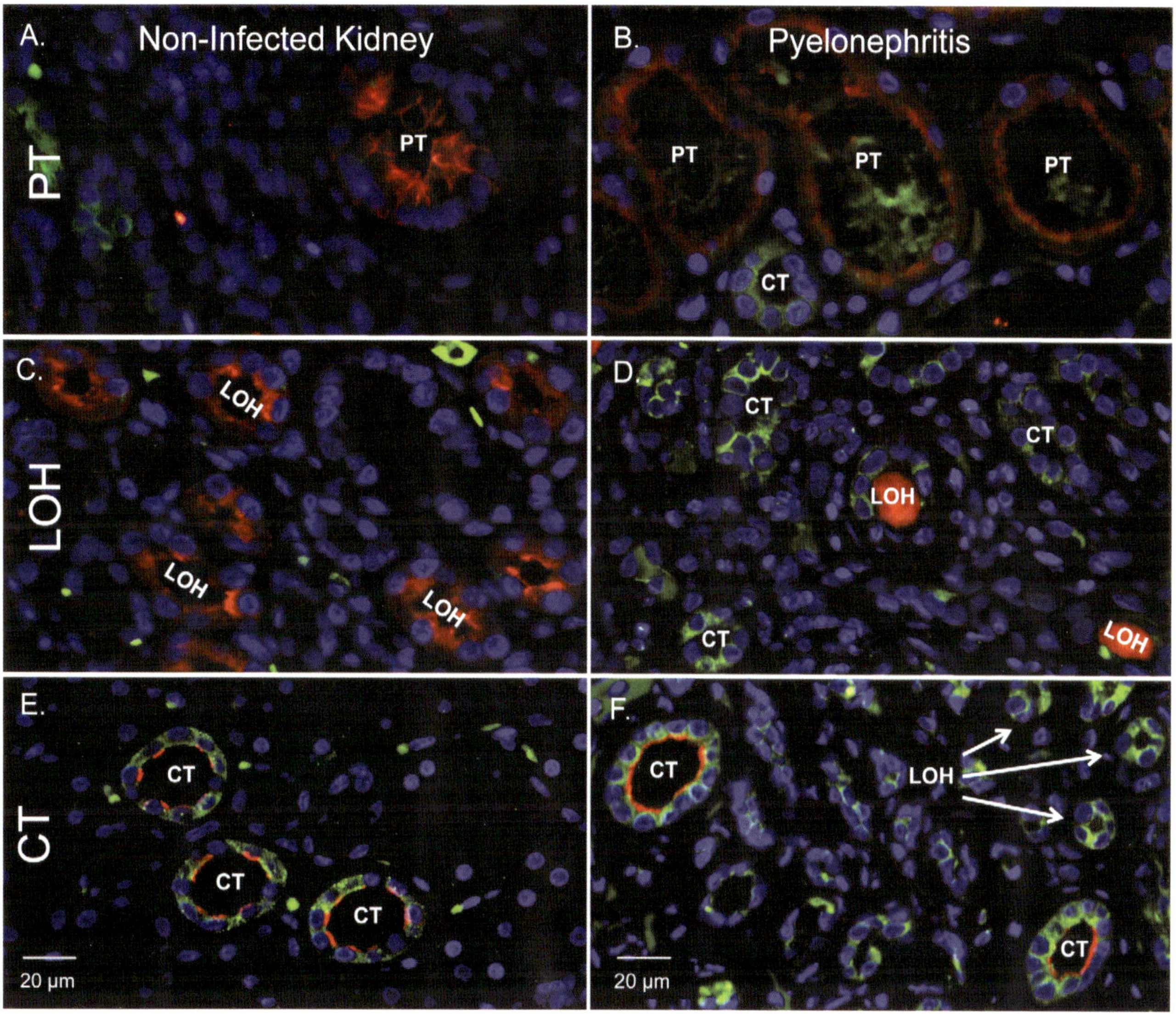

Figure 5. Tubular HD5 expression in states of sterility and infection. Human kidney labeled for HD5 (green), nuclei (blue) and nephron specific markers (red). Segment markers consisted of AQP-2 for collecting tubules (CT), THP for the loop of Henle (LOH), and AQP-1 for proximal tubules (PT). **A/B**: HD5 (green) was produced in the collecting tubules (red apical AQP-2 staining) of non-infected kidney tissue (A) and with pyelonephritis (B). Arrows indicate HD5 is produced in other nephron segments. **C/D**: HD5 (green) was expressed in the loops of Henle (red THP staining) in non-infected kidney tissue (C) and with pyelonephritis (D). **E/F**: HD5 (green) shows minimal production in the proximal tubules (red AQP-1 staining) of non-infected kidney tissue (E) and with pyelonephritis (F). Magnification 40×.

Immunoblot and ELISA analysis also demonstrates that HD5 is secreted into the urine at low levels. Given the size (8.1 kDa and 3.7 kDa) and positive charge of proHD5 and fully processed HD5, it is possible that some urinary HD5 peptide originates, at least in part, from plasma filtrate. Yet, there is little evidence suggesting that HD5 persists in the plasma [27]. Additionally, to appear in the urine, HD5 would need to escape the efficient peptide absorption mechanisms in the proximal tubule [6,36]. Finally, the urine samples used underwent centrifugation before the assays were performed, removing cellular sources of HD5.

At the detected concentrations, urinary HD5 is unlikely to be directly antimicrobial against uropathogenic microorganisms as fully processed HD5 has a minimal inhibitory concentration (MIC) between 6–10 μg/mL against common gram-negative uropathogenic bacteria [15]. However, mucosal surface concentrations are likely to be higher. Furthermore, immunoblot analysis demonstrates that HD5 concentrations are significantly greater in the kidney. These results suggest that HD5 is involved in mucosal defense of the urinary tract. An analogous pattern is seen with hBD1, where urinary concentrations of hBD1 are insufficient to exhibit antimicrobial activity but higher peptide concentrations are detected near the renal tubules [6,31].

Because IHC demonstrates that proHD5 is a major form of HD5 in the kidney and because both mature and proHD5 are detected in the urine, we speculate that HD5 is primarily secreted as a precursor molecule and then undergoes proteolytic processing to generate mature forms – similar to the gastrointestinal and genitourinary tracts [11,30,37]. In the small intestine, Paneth cells produce trypsin, which cleaves the HD5 propeptide so that the fully processed peptide is the predominant form in the intestinal lumen [37]. In the male urethra, the key processing and activating enzymes for HD5 are neutrophil proteases contributed by

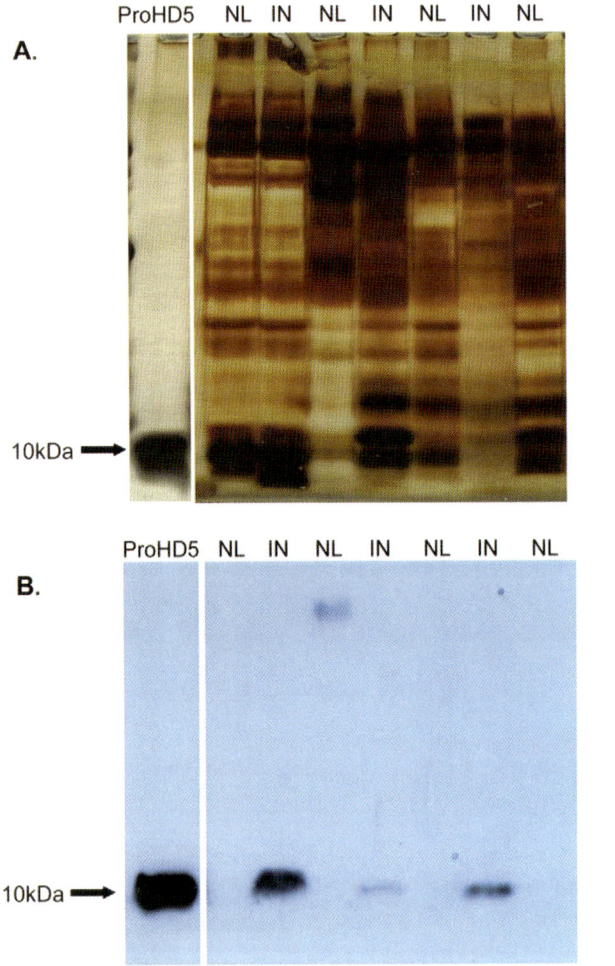

Figure 6. HD5 is present in infected urine samples. HD5 levels in sterile urine samples (n = 15) and urine samples infected with uropathogenic *E.coli* (*n* = 15). Cationic peptides from non-infected urine (NL) and infected urine (IN) were subjected to SDS PAGE followed by Western immunoblot analysis. Each lane contained the equivalent of 300 μg of urinary cationic protein. (**A**) Silver stained PAGE gels with 150 ng ProHD5 as standard to confirm equal protein loading into each lane. (**B**) Western blot analysis with 200 ng ProHD5 as standard.

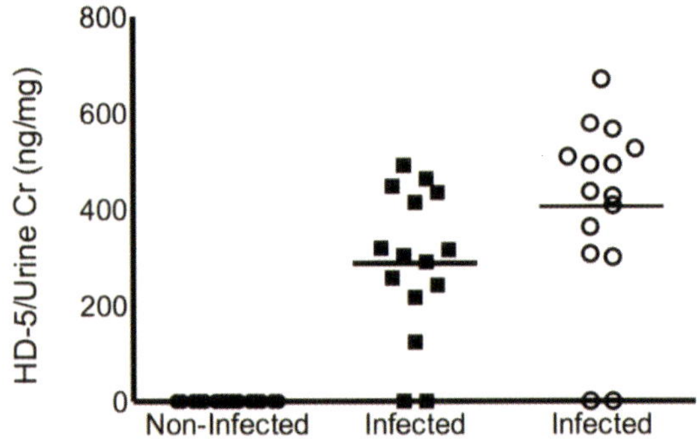

Figure 7. Urinary production of HD5 in infected urine samples. HD5 levels in sterile urine samples and urine samples infected with uropathogenic *E.coli*. The square boxes depict urinary proHD5 standardized to urine creatinine detected by ELISA assay using monoclonal antibody 8C8. The open circles depict urinary proHD5 and mature HD5 standardized to urine creatinine by immunoblot analysis. ProHD5 and mature HD5 were not detected in sterile urine samples using polyclonal HD5 antisera.

neutrophils recruited to the site of infection [11]. The contributions of epithelial trypsinogen, urinary trypsin, and/or neutrophil proteases on HD5 processing in the urinary tract during infection remain to be determined. Moreover, the effects of changes in the urinary environment on HD5 function (alterations in osmolarity, pH, and cationic concentrations) also remain to be determined.

In conclusion, this is the first study to identify and quantitate the expression and production of HD5 in the urinary tract. Our results suggest that HD5 is an epithelial-derived AMP that may play an important role in the innate immunity of the human uroepithelium preventing the translocation of invading pathogens into the circulation. Elucidation of the factors that regulate HD5 production may lend novel insight into the pathogenesis of UTIs in patients at risk for UTIs and patients with chronic infections.

Methods

Study approval

Informed written consent was obtained from all patients participating in this study. For subjects less than 18 year of age, written parental/guardian consent was obtained. The Nationwide Children's Hospital (NCH) Institutional Review Board approved this study along with the consent process and documents (IRB07-00383).

Human Tissue and Urine Samples

Non-infected distal ureter and bladder tissue (*n* = 4) was obtained from children undergoing ureteral re-implantation for reasons other than recurrent infection. Non-infected kidney samples (*n* = 6) were obtained from patients undergoing nephrectomy for renal tumors. Tissue samples were free of microscopic signs of disease or inflammation. Kidney tissue from patients with chronic pyelonephritis was provided by the Cooperative Human Tissue Network (*n* = 6) [38]. Two independent pathologists confirmed the histopathologic diagnosis of pyelonephritis. Tissue samples were snap-frozen or preserved as neutral formalin-fixed paraffin-embedded sections. Sections of non-infected kidney tissue were dissected into cortex, medulla, or renal pelvis before storage (*n* = 4).

Non-infected and infected urines samples were obtained from children presenting to the NCH emergency department or the nephrology clinic. The diagnosis of a UTI was made by a positive urine culture according to the American Academy of Pediatrics Guidelines [39]. All infected urine samples had $>10^6$ CFU/mL of *E.coli*. Urinary pH values ranged from 5.5 to 8.5 (mean urine pH 6.9). Urinary ionic composition was not measured. Urine samples were centrifuged to remove urine sediment, and protease inhibitor cocktail was added (Thermo Scientific, Rockford, IL, USA).

Ribonucleic Acid Isolation and Reverse Transcription

Total RNA was isolated from frozen tissue using the Promega Total RNA Isolation System (Promega, Madison, WI, USA). For cDNA synthesis, 4–8 μg of total RNA was reverse transcribed with Superscript III reverse transcriptase using an oligo-$(dT)_{12-18}$ primer according to the supplier's protocol (Invitrogen, Carlsbad, CA, USA).

Cloning of Gene Specific Plasmids for Standard Curves

The cDNA encoding *DEFA5* and *GAPDH* were cloned into a 4-Topo plasmid vector (Invitrogen) according to manufacturer's instructions. Plasmids were sequenced to confirm that the correct constructs were obtained. Serial dilutions of gene specific plasmids were quantitated (by spectrophotometric absorbance at 260 nm and ethidium bromide staining agarose gel electrophoresis) and used in real-time PCR to generate standard curves for each reaction.

Quantitative Real-time PCR

Quantitative real-time PCR was performed using single-stranded cDNA from human kidney, ureter, and bladder tissue with specific oligonucleotide primer pairs using the 7500 Real-Time PCR System (Applied Biosystems, Carlsbad, CA, USA). PCR exon junction spanning primers were designed and sequences were confirmed using DNAstar® Laser Gene SeqBuilder (*DEFA5* forward primer: 5′- TCC CTC CTG CAG GTG ACC CCA-3′ and *DEFA5* reverse primer 5′-GTG GCT CTT GCC TGA GAA CCT GA-3′).

Briefly, cDNA corresponding to 10 ng RNA served as a template in a 25 µl reaction containing 2.0 µM of each primer and 1× Light-Cycler-Fast Start DNA Master SYBR Green mix. The PCR conditions were: initial denaturation at 95°C for 10 minutes, followed by 40 cycles with each cycle consisting of denaturation at 94°C for 30 seconds, annealing at 64°C for 30 seconds, and extension at 72°C for 30 seconds. The cycle-to-cycle fluorescence emission was monitored at 530 nm and analyzed using 7500 Software V2.0.3 (Applied Biosystems). Gene specific plasmid standards were included with every set of reactions. As a positive control, terminal ileum RNA was included with each set of reactions and results were compared to previously published standards [27].

To confirm PCR amplification of the intended product, a representative sample was analyzed by electrophoresis on a 1.5% agarose gel. The products were visualized by ethidium bromide staining and compared to DNA size standards to confirm anticipated product size (not shown). In addition, a melting temperature profile curve of every PCR reaction was determined at the end of each reaction.

HD5 Antibodies

The HD5 propeptide (AA20-94) and partially processed forms (AA36-94 and 56–94) were identified using a commercially available mouse monoclonal (8C8) anti-HD5 antibody (Abcam). The HD5 propeptide and the mature peptide (AA63-94) were identified using previously described rabbit polyclonal antiserum [13,40].

Immunoblot

Sections of the same kidney specimens used for quantitative real time PCR analysis (3–6 mg wet weight) were pulverized using a mortar and pestle in liquid nitrogen and dissolved in RIPA buffer with protease inhibitors. Urinary proteins were extracted from urine samples using the Proteospin™ Urine Protein Concentration Micro Kit (Norgen Biotek Corporation, Thorold, ON, Canada). Kidney and urine protein concentrations were quantified using a modified Bradford Assay and confirmed using an $OD_{280\ nm}$ reading. Equal concentrations of kidney tissue or urinary protein were loaded onto 18% sodium dodecyl sulfate gradient gels and subjected to electrophoresis. To ensure equal protein loading, a silver stain was performed.

After electrophoretic separation, proteins were transferred onto a nitrocellulose membrane. After fixation with 0.05% glutaraldehyde in TBS, the membranes were blocked in 5% fat-free milk for 30 to 60 minutes and incubated in a 1:1,000 dilution of rabbit polyclonal HD5 antiserum overnight. After washing, the secondary antibody, an anti-rabbit horseradish peroxidase-conjugated anti-rabbit IgG diluted 1:10,000 (Cell Signaling Technology, Danvers, MA, USA), was applied for 1 hour at room temperature. Immunoblots from kidney tissues were also probed with anti-GAPDH antibody (Sigma Aldrich) for two hours at room temperature and then incubated with the secondary antibody described above. The proteins were visualized using and ECL detection system and chemiluminescence film according to the manufacturer's instructions (BioExpress, Kaysville, UT, USA).

HD5 was quantitated by comparing resulting band intensities with a serial dilution of recombinant standard proHD5 protein (Peptides International, Louisville, KY, USA). Kidney HD5 concentrations were standardized to wet tissue weight. Urinary HD 5 concentrations were divided by urine creatinine to establish standardized urine HD5-to-creatinine ratios (µg/mg) to account for urine dilution. Urine creatinine concentrations were determined using the Oxford Biomedical Research creatinine microplate assay (Rochester Hills, Michigan, USA).

Immunohistochemistry

Following deparaffinization, rehydration, and antigen retrieval, a biotin block and a serum-free protein block were performed (Superblock, ScyTek Laboratories, Logan, UT, USA). The slides were incubated overnight at 4°C with monoclonal mouse HD5 (8C8) antibody (1:200; Abcam) or rabbit polyclonal antiserum (1:500) followed by anti-polyvalent biotinylated antibody and UltraTek Streptavidin/HRP (ScyTek Laboratories). Sections were developed using 0.1% diaminobenzidine tetrachloride with 0.02% hydrogen peroxide and counterstained with hematoxylin. Negative controls sections were incubated with non-immune serum in place of HD5 antibody.

Immunofluorescence

Double-labeled immunofluorescence was performed to help localize HD5 expression in the kidney. The collecting duct was double-labeled for principal cells with goat polyclonal anti-human aquaporin-2 antibody (Santa Cruz Biotechnology, Santa Cruz, CA, USA) [41]. The loop of Henle was double-labeled with mouse polyclonal anti-human uromodulin antibody (Sigma-Aldrich) and the proximal tubule was double-labeled with goat polyclonal antihuman aquaporin-1 (Santa Cruz) [41,42]. Rhodamine donkey polyclonal anti-goat (Jackson ImmunoResearch Laboratories, West Grove, PA, USA), rhodamine goat anti-mouse (Jackson ImmunoResearch Laboratories), and FITC donkey polyclonal anti-rabbit (Santa Cruz) served as the secondary antibodies.

All sections were prepared as outlined above. They were incubated with a mixture of mouse antisera against HD5 (1:200) (Abcam), AQP-2 (1:500), uromodulin (1:500), AQP-1 (1:400) at room temperature for 90 minutes. The secondary antibody was applied for 90 minutes at room temperature and the sections were mounted using mounting media with DAPI. Non-immune serum was used as a negative control. The slides were examined with a Leica DM4000B microscope and digitally photographed using Spot RT camera/software (Diagnostic Instruments, Sterling Heights, MI, USA).

ELISA

96-well flat-bottomed plates (Maxisorb, Nunc™, Rochester, NY, USA) were coated overnight at 4°C with mouse monoclonal antibody to HD5 (3 µg/mL) (Abcam). After blocking with synthetic blocking buffer (Kem-En-Tec Diagnostics, Denmark), 100 µL standards and/or urine samples were added to the wells and incubated for 2 hours at room temperature. Serial dilutions of recombinant HD5 protein served as the standards (Novus Biologicals). Following incubation with a biotinylated (Lightning-

Link Biotin Antibody Labeling Kit, Novus Biologicals) mouse monoclonal antibody for 2 hours at room temperature, streptavidin-horse radish peroxidase (Biolegend, San Diego CA, USA) was added for 30 minutes. After incubation with TMB substrate solution for 15 minutes (Kem-En-Tec Diagnostics), the reaction was terminated with STOP solution (Cell Signaling Technology, Danvers, MA, USA) and read at a wavelength of 450 nm. HD5 concentrations from the ELISA assay were divided by urine creatinine to establish standardized urine HD5-to-creatinine ratios (μg/mg) to account for urine dilution as described above.

Acknowledgments

We acknowledge Dan Cohen and the NCH Emergency Department staff for providing us the infected urine samples. We would like to thank Peter Baker for reviewing the kidney pathology.

Author Contributions

Conceived and designed the experiments: JDS DH EP CB HW BB AS. Performed the experiments: JDS DH HW JD AS. Analyzed the data: JDS DH EP CB HW BB AS. Contributed reagents/materials/analysis tools: EP CB. Wrote the paper: JDS DH EP CB BB AS.

References

1. Weichhart T, Haidinger M, Horl WH, Saemann MD (2008) Current concepts of molecular defence mechanisms operative during urinary tract infection. European journal of clinical investigation 38 Suppl 2: 29–38.
2. Zasloff M (2007) Antimicrobial peptides, innate immunity, and the normally sterile urinary tract. J Am Soc Nephrol 18: 2810–2816.
3. Lehrer RI, Lichtenstein AK, Ganz T (1993) Defensins: antimicrobial and cytotoxic peptides of mammalian cells. Annu Rev Immunol 11: 105–128.
4. Valore EV, Ganz T (1992) Posttranslational processing of defensins in immature human myeloid cells. Blood 79: 1538–1544.
5. Liu L, Zhao C, Heng HH, Ganz T (1997) The human beta-defensin-1 and alpha-defensins are encoded by adjacent genes: two peptide families with differing disulfide topology share a common ancestry. Genomics 43: 316–320.
6. Valore EV, Park CH, Quayle AJ, Wiles KR, McCray PB, Jr., et al. (1998) Human beta-defensin-1: an antimicrobial peptide of urogenital tissues. J Clin Invest 101: 1633–1642.
7. Schroeder BO, Wu Z, Nuding S, Groscurth S, Marcinowski M, et al. (2011) Reduction of disulphide bonds unmasks potent antimicrobial activity of human beta-defensin 1. Nature 469: 419–423.
8. Lehmann J, Retz M, Harder J, Krams M, Kellner U, et al. (2002) Expression of human beta-defensins 1 and 2 in kidneys with chronic bacterial infection. BMC Infect Dis 2: 20.
9. Bevins CL (2006) Paneth cell defensins: key effector molecules of innate immunity. Biochemical Society transactions 34: 263–266.
10. Quayle AJ, Porter EM, Nussbaum AA, Wang YM, Brabec C, et al. (1998) Gene expression, immunolocalization, and secretion of human defensin-5 in human female reproductive tract. Am J Pathol 152: 1247–1258.
11. Porter E, Yang H, Yavagal S, Preza GC, Murillo O, et al. (2005) Distinct defensin profiles in Neisseria gonorrhoeae and Chlamydia trachomatis urethritis reveal novel epithelial cell-neutrophil interactions. Infect Immun 73: 4823–4833.
12. Com E, Bourgeon F, Evrard B, Ganz T, Colleu D, et al. (2003) Expression of antimicrobial defensins in the male reproductive tract of rats, mice, and humans. Biology of reproduction 68: 95–104.
13. Porter EM, Poles MA, Lee JS, Naitoh J, Bevins CL, et al. (1998) Isolation of human intestinal defensins from ileal neobladder urine. FEBS letters 434: 272–276.
14. Townes CL, Ali A, Robson W, Pickard R, Hall J (2011) Tolerance of bacteriuria after urinary diversion is linked to antimicrobial peptide activity. Urology 77: 509 e501–508.
15. Wang AP, Su YP, Wang S (2010) Antobacterial acitivity and mechanism of recombinant human alpha defensin 5 agains clinical antibiotic-resistant strains. Afr J Microbiol Res 4: 626–633.
16. Gropp R, Frye M, Wagner TO, Bargon J (1999) Epithelial defensins impair adenoviral infection: implication for adenovirus-mediated gene therapy. Human gene therapy 10: 957–964.
17. Smith JG, Nemerow GR (2008) Mechanism of adenovirus neutralization by Human alpha-defensins. Cell host & microbe 3: 11–19.
18. Dugan AS, Maginnis MS, Jordan JA, Gasparovic ML, Manley K, et al. (2008) Human alpha-defensins inhibit BK virus infection by aggregating virions and blocking binding to host cells. The Journal of biological chemistry 283: 31125–31132.
19. Zhang D, Liu ZH, Liao QP, Ma JM, Sun YF, et al. (2009) Study of local immunity of lower genital tract infections. Zhonghua fu chan ke za zhi 44: 13–15.
20. Quayle AJ (2002) The innate and early immune response to pathogen challenge in the female genital tract and the pivotal role of epithelial cells. Journal of reproductive immunology 57: 61–79.
21. Porter EM, van Dam E, Valore EV, Ganz T (1997) Broad-spectrum antimicrobial activity of human intestinal defensin 5. Infection and immunity 65: 2396–2401.
22. Chromek M, Slamova Z, Bergman P, Kovacs L, Podracka L, et al. (2006) The antimicrobial peptide cathelicidin protects the urinary tract against invasive bacterial infection. Nat Med 12: 636–641.
23. Nitschke M, Wiehl S, Baer PC, Kreft B (2002) Bactericidal activity of renal tubular cells: the putative role of human beta-defensins. Experimental nephrology 10: 332–337.
24. Spencer JD, Schwaderer AL, Dirosario JD, McHugh KM, McGillivary G, et al. (2011) Ribonuclease 7 is a potent antimicrobial peptide within the human urinary tract. Kidney Int.
25. Ganz T (2001) Defensins in the urinary tract and other tissues. J Infect Dis 183 Suppl 1: S41–42.
26. Ganz T (2001) Antimicrobial proteins and peptides in host defense. Semin Respir Infect 16: 4–10.
27. Wehkamp J, Chu H, Shen B, Feathers RW, Kays RJ, et al. (2006) Paneth cell antimicrobial peptides: topographical distribution and quantification in human gastrointestinal tissues. FEBS Lett 580: 5344–5350.
28. Cunliffe RN (2003) Alpha-defensins in the gastrointestinal tract. Molecular immunology 40: 463–467.
29. Wehkamp J, Salzman NH, Porter E, Nuding S, Weichenthal M, et al. (2005) Reduced Paneth cell alpha-defensins in ileal Crohn's disease. Proceedings of the National Academy of Sciences of the United States of America 102: 18129–18134.
30. Quayle AJ, Porter EM, Nussbaum AA, Wang YM, Brabec C, et al. (1998) Gene expression, immunolocalization, and secretion of human defensin-5 in human female reproductive tract. The American journal of pathology 152: 1247–1258.
31. Hiratsuka T, Nakazato M, Ihi T, Minematsu T, Chino N, et al. (2000) Structural analysis of human beta-defensin-1 and its significance in urinary tract infection. Nephron 85: 34–40.
32. Tikhonov I, Rebenok A, Chyzh A (1997) A study of interleukin-8 and defensins in urine and plasma of patients with pyelonephritis and glomerulonephritis. Nephrology, dialysis, transplantation: official publication of the European Dialysis and Transplant Association - European Renal Association 12: 2557–2561.
33. Chon CH, Lai FC, Shortliffe LM (2001) Pediatric urinary tract infections. Pediatric clinics of North America 48: 1441–1459.
34. Goldman MJ, Anderson GM, Stolzenberg ED, Kari UP, Zasloff M, et al. (1997) Human beta-defensin-1 is a salt-sensitive antibiotic in lung that is inactivated in cystic fibrosis. Cell 88: 553–560.
35. Bals R, Wang X, Wu Z, Freeman T, Bafna V, et al. (1998) Human beta-defensin 2 is a salt-sensitive peptide antibiotic expressed in human lung. The Journal of clinical investigation 102: 874–880.
36. Carone FA, Peterson DR, Flouret G (1982) Renal tubular processing of small peptide hormones. The Journal of laboratory and clinical medicine 100: 1–14.
37. Ghosh D, Porter E, Shen B, Lee SK, Wilk D, et al. (2002) Paneth cell trypsin is the processing enzyme for human defensin-5. Nature immunology 3: 583–590.
38. LiVolsi VA, Clausen KP, Grizzle W, Newton W, Pretlow TG, 2nd, et al. (1993) The Cooperative Human Tissue Network. An update. Cancer 71: 1391–1394.
39. Shai Y (1999) Mechanism of the binding, insertion and destabilization of phospholipid bilayer membranes by alpha-helical antimicrobial and cell non-selective membrane-lytic peptides. Biochim Biophys Acta 1462: 55–70.
40. Shen B, Porter EM, Reynoso E, Shen C, Ghosh D, et al. (2005) Human defensin 5 expression in intestinal metaplasia of the upper gastrointestinal tract. Journal of clinical pathology 58: 687–694.
41. Nielsen S, Frokiaer J, Marples D, Kwon TH, Agre P, et al. (2002) Aquaporins in the kidney: from molecules to medicine. Physiological reviews 82: 205–244.
42. Malagolini N, Cavallone D, Serafini-Cessi F (1997) Intracellular transport, cell-surface exposure and release of recombinant Tamm-Horsfall glycoprotein. Kidney international 52: 1340–1350.

Association of Toll-Like Receptor 4 Gene Polymorphism and Expression with Urinary Tract Infection Types in Adults

Xiaolin Yin[1], Tianwen Hou[2], Ying Liu[1], Jing Chen[2], Zhiyan Yao[1], Cuiqing Ma[1], Lijuan Yang[1], Lin Wei[1]*

1 Department of Immunology, Hebei Medical University, Shijiazhuan, China, **2** Department of Laboratory Medicine, Bethune International Peace Hospital, Shijiazhuan, China

Abstract

Background: Innate immunity of which Toll-like receptor (TLR) 4 and CXCR1 are key elements plays a central role in the development of urinary tract infection (UTI). Although the relation between the genetics of TLR4 and CXCR1 and UTI is investigated partly, the polymorphisms and expression of TLR4 and CXCR1 in different types of UTI in adults are not extremely clear.

Methodology/Principal Findings: This study investigates the presence of TLR4 A (896) G and CXCR1 G (2608) C polymorphisms in 129 UTI patients using RFLP-PCR. Gene and allelic prevalence were compared with 248 healthy controls. Flow cytometry was used to detect TLR4 and CXCR1 expression in the monocytes of UTI patients and healthy controls. TLR4 (896) AG genotype and TLR4 (896) G allele had higher prevalence in UTI (especially in acute cystitis and urethritis) patients, whereas CXCR1 (2608) GC genotype and CXCR1 (2608) C allele had lower prevalence in UTI patients than controls. TLR4 expression was significantly lower in chronic UTI patients than in acute pyelonephritis or healthy controls. CXCR1 expression was similar in both controls and patients. TLR4 expression in chronic UTI patients after astragalus treatment was higher than pre-treatment.

Conclusions: The results indicate the relationship between the carrier status of TLR4 (896) G alleles and the development of UTI, especially acute cystitis and urethritis, in adults. TLR4 expression levels are correlated with chronic UTI.

Editor: Ludovic Tailleux, Institut Pasteur, France

Funding: The authors have no support or funding to report.

Competing Interests: The authors have declared that no competing interests exist.

* E-mail: weilin_212603@yahoo.com

Introduction

Urinary tract infections (UTIs) are common infectious diseases,and the non-complex UTI cases show no obvious behavioral, functional, and structural risk factors. The early response against UTI is provided by innate immune response, in which, TLR4 plays an important role in activating innate immune response, and its recognized ligands, such as lipopolysaccharide, have been demonstrated to initiate anti-UTI responses [1]. TLR4 actions in bladder cells include promotion of IL-6 and IL-8 secretion by activation of MyD88-dependent or cAMP-dependent signaling pathways, and inhibition of bacterial invasion and promotion of bacterial expulsion in bladder epithelial cells [2–6]. In addition, neutrophil chemokine receptors, such as CXCR1, are necessary for neutrophil migration to infected sites [7]and are involved in innate immune response. CXCR1 is closely correlated with neutrophil quantity and extent of inflammatory reaction in the urinary tract.

The individual's response to UTI is variable and the susceptibility to the infection is inheritable. Lundstedt et al. found in a family study, 15% of the relatives of pyelonephritis-prone children had UTI history, whereas the value was 3% in the controls [8]. A evaluation of a familal predisposition about women with recurrent UTI described that 65.5% of mothers, 60.7% of daughters, and 48.6% of sisters of the women had a similar history [9]. Many studies discovered that genitic variations of TLR4 and CXCR1 are association with susceptibility to different type of UTIs. And TLR4(896)AG genotype and TLR4(896)G alleles could increase the risk for UTI in childhood [10,11], CXCR1 G (2608) C gene polymorphism and expression are strong linked to acute pyelonephritis in children [12]. Reduced expression levels of CXCR1 and TLR4 in neutrophils are associated with pyelonephritis, recurrent cystitis, and asymptomatic bacteriuria in children and premenopausal women [13–15]. Although these studies suggest the association of gene polymorphisms and expression of TLR4 and CXCR1 to UTIs, whether the variants are associated with UTI in Chinese adults is still unknown, TLR4 and CXCR1 expression levels in different type UTIs is also not clear.

Astragalus is a Chinese herbal medicine, and Astragalus polysaccharide (APS) is its main compoents. Our previous study demonstrated that APS could induce enhancement of expression of TLR4 on bladder epithilial cells [16]. So we hope that astragalus also increases the TLR4 expression on monocytes in UTI patients.

Table 1. Genotypic frequencies at the TLR4 A(896)G andCXCR1G(2608)C polymorphisms in patients suffering UTI compared with healthy reference populations.

Group	No.	TLR4A(896)G			CXCR1G(2608)C		
		AA	AG	GG	GG	GC	CC
healthy controls	248	227(91.5%)	21(8.5%)	0(0%)	196(79%)	50(20.2%)	2(0.8%)
UTI patients total	129	109(84.5%)	20*(15.5%)	0(0%)	111(86.1%)	15#(11.6%)	3(2.3%)
Patients with acute pyelonephritis	32	29(90.6%)	3(9.4%)	0(0%)	28(87.5%)	3(9.4%)	1(3.1%)
Patients with Chronical UTI	38	32(84.2%)	6(15.8%)	0(0%)	37(97.4%)	1†(2.6%)	0(0%)
Patients with Acute cystitis and urethritis	59	48(81.4%)	11**(18.6%)	0(0%)	46(78%)	11‡(18.6%)	2(3.4%)

*p = 0.03vs healthy controls;
**p = 0.024vs healthy controls;
#p = 0.024vs healthy controls;
†p = 0.003vs healthy controls;
‡p = 0.016 vs chronical UTIs.

In this study, we summarize the results of a case-control study examing whether polymorphisms and expression in TLR4 and CXCR1 are associated with susceptibility to acute pyelonephritis, chronic UTI, and acute cystitis and urethritis in UTI patients in China, and evaluating whether astragalus can boost innate immnue respons against UTI through enhancing TLR4 expression.

Results

1. Clinical data

Urinary bacterial strains were identified as follows: *E. coli* in 109 patients (84.5%); *Klebsiella pneumoniae* in 5 patients (3.9%); *Proteus mirabilis* in 2 patients (1.55%); *Morganella morganii* in 2 patients (1.55%); *Enterobacter aerogenes* in 2 patients (1.55%); *Staphylococcus aureus* in 2 patients (1.55%); *Enterococcus faecalis* in 2 patients (1.55%); *Enterococcus faecium* in 3 patients (2.32%); *Monilia albicans* in 1 patient (0.78%); and *Candida glabrata* in 1 patient (0.78%).

2. Genotype distribution of TLR4 A (896) G and CXCR1 G (2608) C

The gene polymorphisms of TLR4 A (896) G and CXCR1G (2608) C are shown in Table 1. The genotype of TLR4 (896) AG had higher prevalence among UTI patients than in healthy controls (p = 0.03), and especially TLR4 (896) AG genotype tended to occur more frequently in acute cystitis and urethritis patients than in controls (p = 0.02). Interestingly the genotype of CXCR1 (2608) GC had lower prevalence among UTI patients than in healthy controls (p = 0.024). Compared to controls and acute cystitis and urethritis patients, the genotype of CXCR1 (2608) GC in chronic UTI patients were also lower than the two groups (p = 0.003; 0.016).

3.Allele frequencies of TLR4 (896) G and CXCR1 (2608) C

The prevalence of TLR4 (896) G alleles showed higher in UTI patients than that in the controls (p = 0.034), and the alleles trended to show more frequently in acute cystitis and urethritis patients than in the controls (p = 0.028). While CXCR1 (2608) C alleles had lower prevalence in chronic UTI than in the controls (p = 0.003). Compared to acute cystitis and urethritis patients, chronic UTI patients also had lower CXCR1 (2608)C allele prevalence (p = 0.003) (Table 2).

4. TLR4 expression levels in monocytes in different types of UTI

The percentage of TLR4 expression in healthy controls, chronic UTI patients, and acute pyelonephritis patients was 8.57±2.88, 5.1±3.11 and 9.4±3.1%, respectively. TLR4 expression in monocytes in patients with chronic UTI was significantly lower

Table 2. Allelic frequencies at the TLR4 A(896)G andCXCR1G(2608)C polymorphisms in patients suffering UTI compared with healthy reference populations.

Group	No.	TLR4A(896)G		CXCR1G(2608)C	
		A	G	G	C
healthy controls	248	475(96%)	21(4%)	442(89%)	54(11%)
UTI patients total	129	238(92%)	20*(8%)	237(92%)	21 (8%)
Patients with acute pyelonephritis	32	61(95%)	3(5%)	59(92%)	5(8%)
Patients with Chronical UTI	38	70(92%)	6(8%)	75(99%)	1† (1%)
Patients acute cystitis and urethritis	59	107(91%)	11** (9%)	103(87%)	15‡ (13%)

*p = 0.034vs healthy controls;
**p = 0.028 vs healthy controls;
†p = 0.003 vs healthy controls;
‡p = 0.003 vs chronical UTIs.

than in healthy controls and in patients with acute pyelonephritis (p = 0.03; 0.03) (Fig. 1).

5. CXCR1 expression levels in neutrophils in different types of UTI

The percentage of CXCR1 expression in healthy controls, chronic UTI patients, and acute pyelonephritis patients was 96±1.75, 97±2.4 and 97±1.7%, respectively. There were no significant differences among these groups ($p > 0.05$) (Fig. 2, Fig. 3).

6. TLR4 expression levels in monocytes before and after astralagus treatment

The percentage of TLR4 expression in chronic UTI patients before astralagus treatment (4.1±2.2%) significantly increased to 17.4±5.6% post-treatment (p = 0.001) (Fig. 4).

Discussion

The relationship between function, expression and gene mutation of the TLR4 gene and the occurrence of UTI has interested many researchers. C3H/HeJ mice without response to LPS (TLR4 mutant mice) couldn't clear the urinary tract infection. The reason lay in that they couldn't make adequate regulation on pathogens. Maybe this defection was related to TLR4 gene mutation [17,18,19]Reported studies on children with urinary tract infection showed that TLR4 gene polymorphism test indicated gene carrier statuses at TLR4A(896)G allele were obviously related to recurrent urinary tract infection in children, while it had no relation with other kidney diseases [11]. Hawn etc. also carried out polymorphism test of several TLRs of adult women with 18–49 years old, and found that TLR4A (896) G

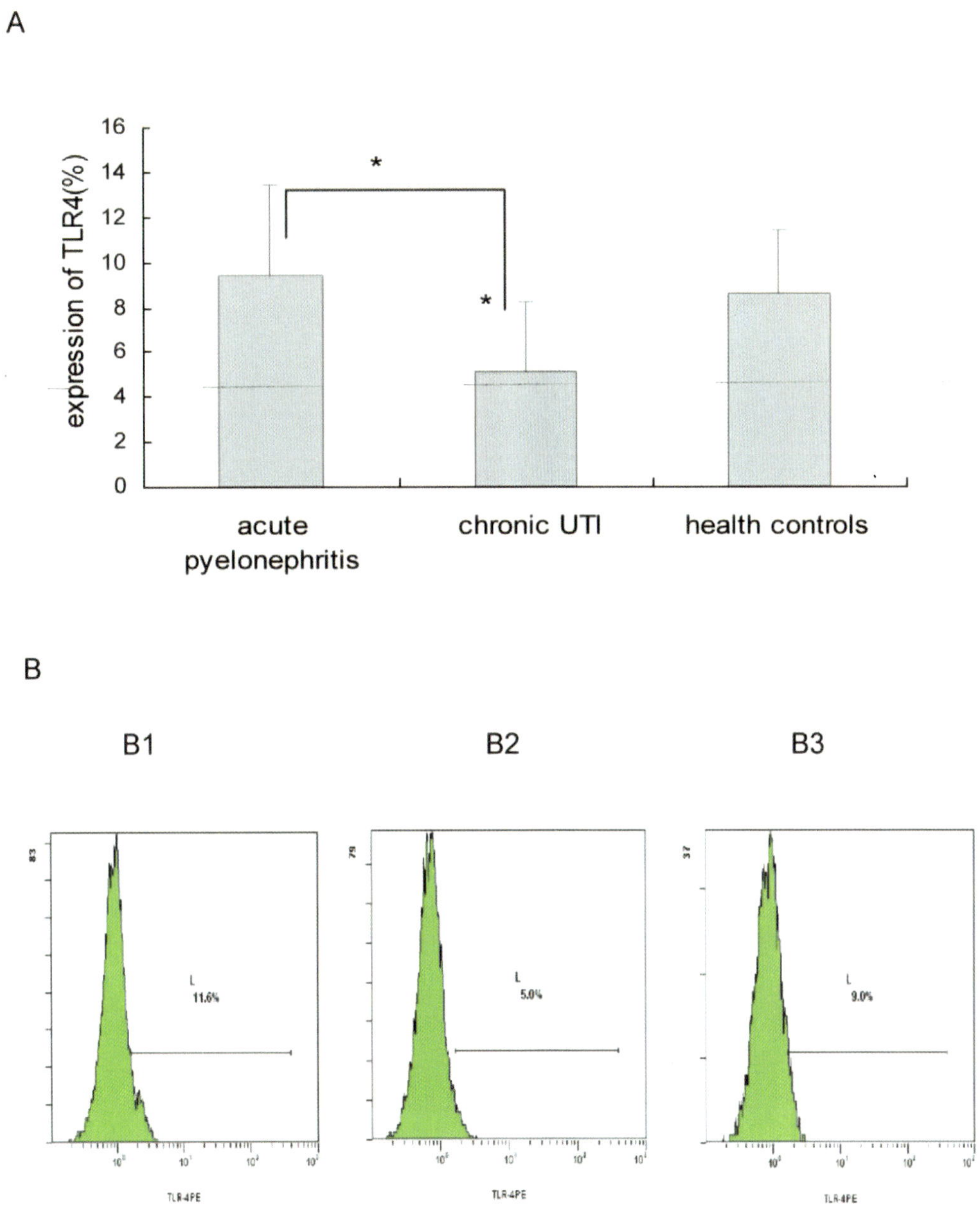

Figure 1. The expression levels of TLR4 on monocytes in different types of UTIs. A: Comparation of percent of TLR4 expression in different types of UTIs. B: The drawing of TLR4 detected by FCM on monocytes of UTI patients. B1: acute pyelonephritis; B2: chronical UTI; B3: health controls.

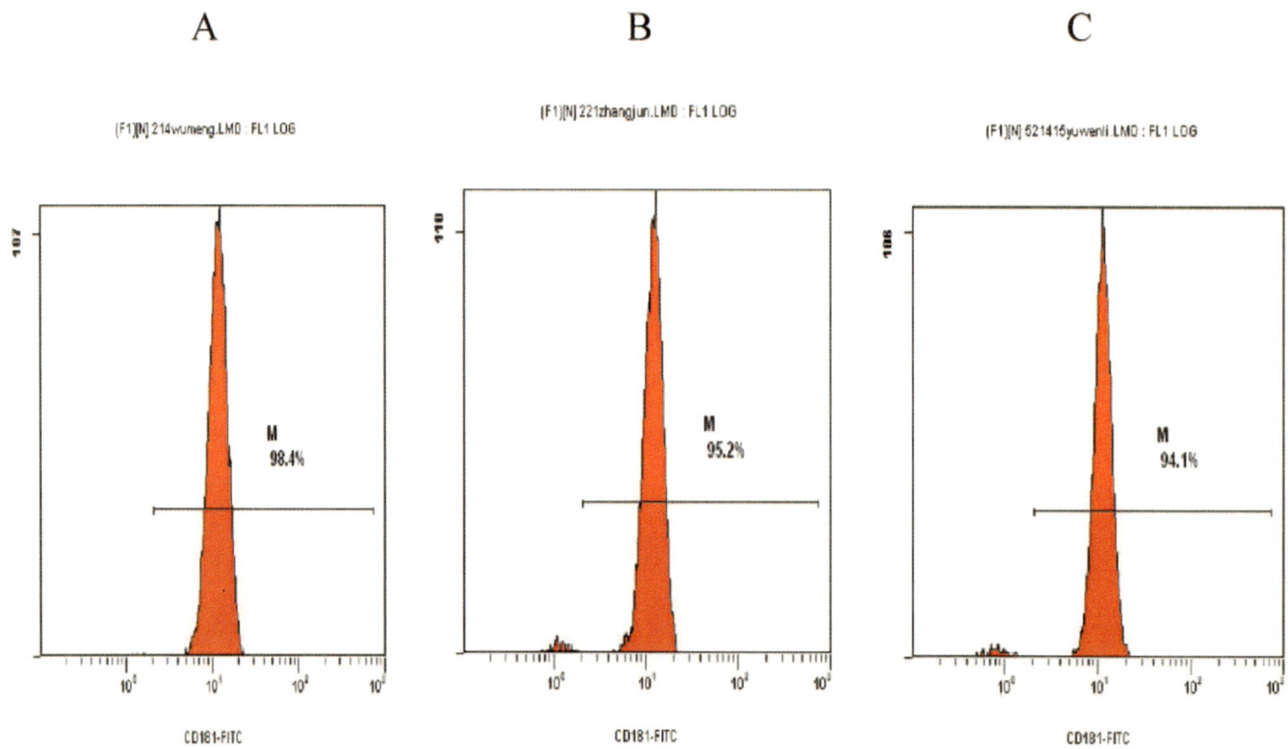

Figure 2. The drawing of CXCR1 detected by FCM on neutrophils of UTI patients. A:health controls; B:acute pyelonephritis; C:chronical UTI.

polymorphism was related to UTI protection, but not related to pyelonephritis [20]. The results of this study show that the gene prevalence of TLR4 (896) AG and TLR4 (896) G alleles in UTI patients is higher than that in the control group, and the gene prevalence of TLR4 (896) AG and TLR4 (896) G alleles in patients with acute cystitis and urethritis is higher than that in the healthy control and acute pyelonephritis groups. These results indicate that TLR4A(896)G mutation is associated with increased risk of UTI in adults, especially with acute cystitis and urethritis, but is not associated with acute pyelonephritis and chronic UTI. Our data are in line with previous studies, which revealed similar occurrence of TLR4(896)AG genotype in rUTI in children [11]. But the previous also revealed that TLR4A(896)G polymorphism was associated with protection from rUTI, but not pyelonephritis

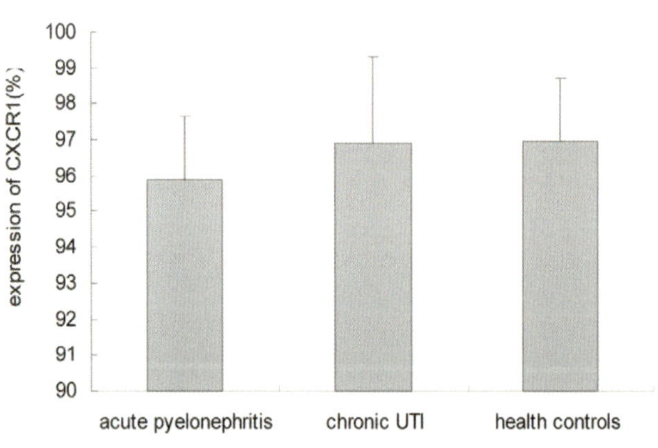

Figure 3. Expression of CXCR1 on monocytes of different type of UTI.

in women 18–49 years old [20]. Obviously, TLR4A(896)G gene polymorphism are associated with adult susceptibility to UTIs, but this relationship could vary in different populations and disease types. Further surveys of more cases and different races are needed to make conclusive statements.

Acute pyelonephritis and asymptomatic bacteriuria (ABU) represent the two extremes of UTI respectively. Studies have shown that TLR4−/− and C3H/HeJ mice lost the function of TLR4 and could not clear effectively infection, acquired ABU status, suggesting that the absence of TLR4 signals can make an infected host appear asymptomatic [18,21]. TLR5 and TLR11 had equal characters [22,23]. But the extreme status was not exist almost in people. Then their susceptibility to UTI were also associated with TLR4 expression except polymorphism. Thus, the relationship between TLR4 expression level and the type of UTI has become a subject of interest. A survey of ABU children showed that compared with the healthy group, TLR4 expression level in the patient group is lower. Furthermore, TLR4 expression levels in children with primary ABU is lower than in children with secondary ABU [13]. However, there is still a lack of information on the relationship of TLR4 expression and other types of UTI. The results of this study show that TLR4 expression in patients with chronic UTI is significantly lower than that in the control and acute pyelonephritis groups, suggesting that chronic UTI can be the result of reduced TLR4 expression, thereby effectively inducing innate immune response.

TLR4 determines the efficiency of bacteria identification, but chemokine receptors are the ones that affect clearing of bacteria [24]. Defects in expression of IL-8 receptors CXCR1 and CXCR2 have been associated with many infectious diseases, particularly acute pyelonephritis. Mice lacking the CXCR1 homologue Mcxcr 2 frequently have acute pyelonephritis with bladder infection. As bacteria numbers increase, bacteremia prevalence and mortality

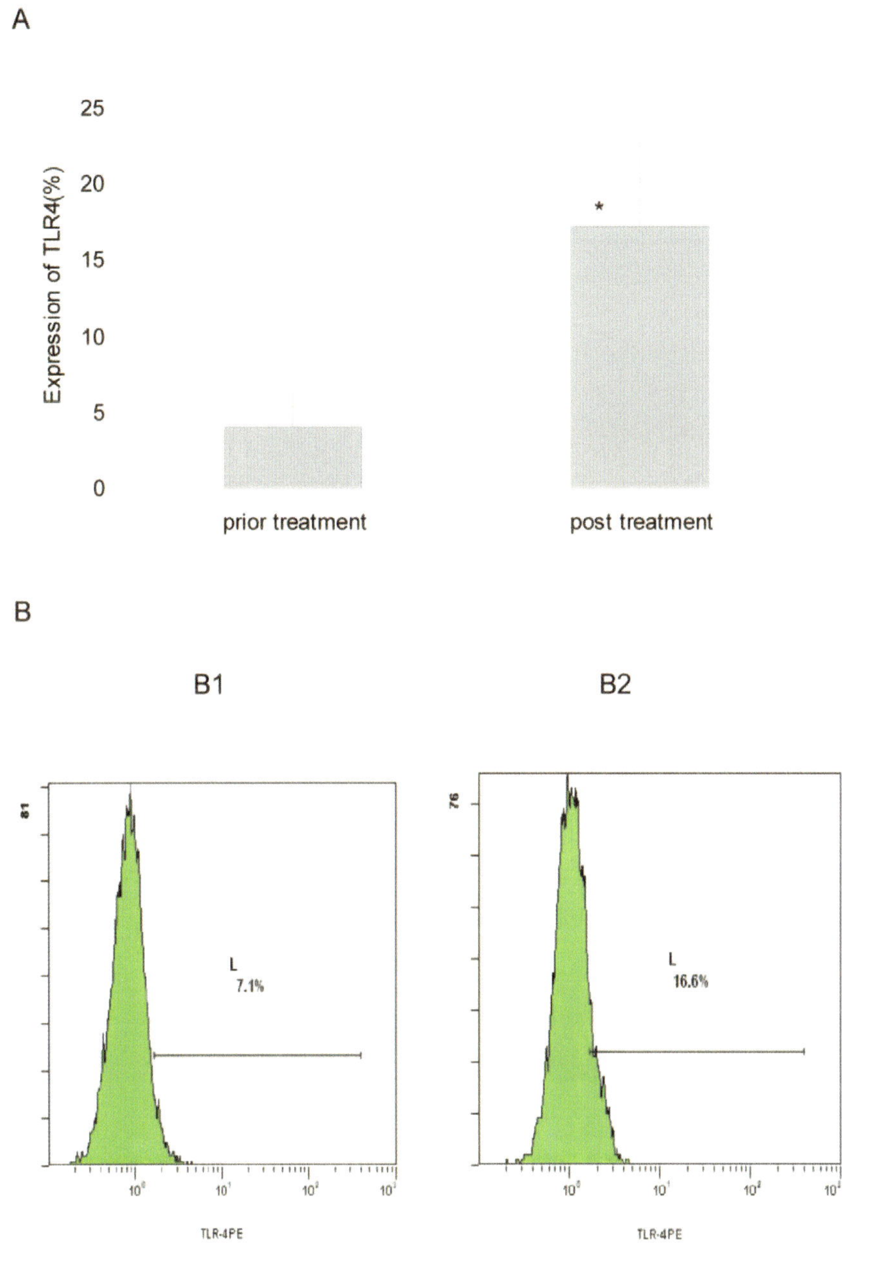

Figure 4. Expression of TLR4 on monocytes of pre-or post-treatment of chronic UTI. A: The percent of TLR4 expression on monocytes of pre-or post-treatment of chronic UTI. **B**: The drawing of TLR4 detected by FCM on monocytes of pre-or post-treatment of chronic UTI. **B1**: Pre-treatment by astralagus; B2: post-treatment by astralagus.

rate increase to 50% [14]. Lundstedt et al. showed that CXCR1 expression in pyelonephritis-prone children is lower than that in the control group, and CXCR1 expression level in children with UTI is significantly lower than that in the control group [8,14]. The results of this study show that the prevalence frequencies of CXCR1 (2608) GC and CXCR1 (2608) C in UTI patients and patients with chronic UTI are lower than those in the healthy and acute cystitis groups, but expression levels of CXCR1 in neutrophils were not different. These results indicate polymorphism of CXCR1 G(2608)C was associated with protection from UTIs in adults, especialy from chronical UTIs.

The over use of broad spectrum antibiotics has led to the emergence of antibiotic resistant bacteria. As a consequence, the treatment of UTIs especially chronic UTIs becomes a very difficult clinical problem. Modulating the powerful innate and adaptive immune systems of the urinary tract would have important therapeutic and prophylactic implications for the treatment of UTIs, particularly treatment of antibiotics alone is ineffective. Since the lining of the urinary tract is highly enrichedin TLR4 molecules, administering TLR4 specific ligands directly to the urinary tract could trigger TLR4 mediated innate immune responses thereby enhancing local reactivity and resistance to infection [24]. In present many immunomodulator were used in clinical treatment of UTI or animal experemen, such as thymosin, astragalus and ligands of TLR4. Although we have not known the mechanism, their use benefit in the urinary tract. APS is an agonist for TLR4 receptor, and it is antagonistic in a case of coexistence of LPS [25]. And we have demonstrated that APS was effective in inducing TLR4 expression and enhancing the anti-bacterial activity of bladder epithelial cells(BECs) [16]. In this study, we applicated astragalus injection and antibiotics simultaneously to treat chronic UTI patients, the TLR4 expression levels on monocytes in the patients increased after recovery. Thus we think that astragalus as an immunomodulator enhanced TLR4 expression and thereby increased the innate immune capability of patients with chronic UTI and promoted clearance of infection.

In conclusion, the TLR4A (896) G genotype was found to be associated with adult UTi, especially acute urethritis. TLR4 expression in the mononuclear cells of patients with chronic UTI was significantly reduced. Thus, TLR4 gene and expression tests can be used as auxiliary indicators for the diagnosis and treatment of UTI. With the increase of antibiotic resistance, the therapy of UTI patients can be supplemented with immunomodulators for improved results. The results of this study could provide reliable clinical evidence for the development and research of drugs targeting TLR4 for UTI treatment.

Materials and Methods

Patients

The study protocols were approved by Ethics committiee of Bthune International Peace Hospital Shijiazhuang City, Heibei Province, China. The different types of UTI included in this study are acute pyelonephritis (32 cases), chronic UTI (38 cases), and acute cystitis and urethritis (59 cases). Acute pyelonephritis were defined as a febrile infection ($\geq 38.5°C$) with significant bacteriuria, Creactive protein >20 mg/l and lack of symptoms of other infections. Acute cystitis and urethritis subjects were defined that patients appeared obvious irritative symptoms of bladder with bacteriuria or blood urine. Chronic UTI subjects were defined as a UTI episode within a 12-month time frame or 2 UTIs within 6 months. After obtaining their consent, blood samples were collected from 129 patients (104 women/25 men, age: 19–80y) with UTI at the Department of Nephrology, Bethune International Peace Hospital.

Healthy controls

Health controls were enrolled and came from Bethune International Peace Hospital and verified to have no infectious disease history. There were 248 health controls (202women/46men) aged 20–70 years. After gaining their consent, blood samples were drawn for the tests.

Samples and genotyping

Genomic DNA was extracted from whole blood samples using blood DNA extraction kit (Qiangen) according to the manufacturer's instructions. TLR4 A (896) G and CXCR1 G (2608) C genotypes were detected by RFLP-PCR as previously described [10,26].

Astragalus treatment of chronic UTI patients

Astragalus injection was purchased from Shanghai Fuda Pharmaceuticals Company. 20 patients with chronic UTI were selected to receive parenteral astralagus treatment. Each patient received 500 mg/kg/d astralagus intravenously for 1 or 2 weeks. At the same time they were injected antibiotics by same approachs. Antibiotics used included cefoperazone/sulbactarm(4 cases), cefotiam(6 cases), cefuroxime(4 cases), mezlocillin/sulbactarm(5 cases) and imipenem(1 case). Their TLR4 expression levels on monocytes were detected before and after treatment.

Flow cytometry

TLR4 and CXCR1 protein expression was detected by flow cytometry. Three groups were detected: acute pyelonephritis patients, chronic UTI and health controls. There are 20 cases in each group. Monocytes and neutrophils were incubated for 30 min with PE- and FITC-labeled monoclonal antibodies against human TLR4 and CXCR1 (CD181) (BioLegend, USA), respectively. After washing with PBS, the stained cells were run on a flow cytometer (Beckman Coulter, USA). The percentage of TLR4 and CXCR1 was counted.

Statistical analysis

Data were analyzed using SPSS13.0 software. Statistical significance was calculated by X^2 test and t-test. Significance was set at $p<0.05$.

Author Contributions

Conceived and designed the experiments: XY LW. Performed the experiments: XY TH YL JC. Analyzed the data: XY CM. Contributed reagents/materials/analysis tools: ZY LY. Wrote the paper: XY.

References

1. Takeda K, Kaisho T, Akira S (2003) Toll-like receptors. Annu Rev Immunol 21: 335–376.
2. Bishop BL, Duncan MJ, Song J, Li G, Zaas D, et al. (2007) Cyclic AMP-regulated exocytosis of Escherichia coli from infected bladder epithelial cells. Nat Med 13: 625–630.
3. Song J, Bishop BL, Li G, Duncan MJ, Abraham SN (2007) TLR4 initiated and cAMP mediated abrogation of bacterial invasion of the bladder. Cell Host Microbe 1: 287–298.
4. Song J, Bishop BL, Li G, Grady R, Stapleton A, et al. (2009) TLR4-mediated expulsion of bacteria from infected bladder epithelial cells. Proc Natl Acad Sci 106: 14966–14971.
5. Miyazaki J, Kawai K, Oikawa T, Johraku A, Hattori K, et al. (2006) Uroepithelial cells can directly respond to Mycobacterium bovis bacillus Calmette-Guerin through Toll like receptor signaling. BJU Int 97: 860–864.
6. Schilling JD, Martin SM, Hunstad DA, Patel KP, Mulvey MA, et al. (2003) CD14- and Toll-like receptor-dependent activation of bladder epithelial cells by lipopolysaccharide and type 1 piliated Escherichia coli. Infect Immun 71: 1470–1480.
7. Godaly G, Hang L, Frendeus B, Svanborg C (2000) Transepithelial neutrophil migration is CXCR1 dependent in vitro and is defective in IL-8 receptor knockout mice. J Immunol 165: 5287–5294.
8. Lundstedt AC, Leijonhufvud I, Ragnarsdottir B, Karpman D, Andersson B, et al. (2007) Inherited susceptibility to acute pyelonephritis: a family study of urinary tract infection. J Infect Dis 195: 1227–34.
9. Hopkins WJ, Uehling DT, Wargowski DS (1999) Evaluation of a familial predisposition to recurrent urinary tract infections in women. Am J Med Genet 83: 22–424.
10. Lundstedt AC, McCarthy S, Gustafsson MC, Godaly G, Jodal U, et al. (2007) A genetic basis of susceptibility to acute pyelonephritis. PLoS ONE 9: e825.
11. Karoly E, Fekete A, Banki NF, Szebeni B, Vannay A, et al. (2007) Heat shock protein 72 (HSPA1B) gene polymorphism and Toll-like receptor (TLR) 4 mutation are associated with increased risk of urinary tract infection in children. Pediatr Res 61: 371–374.
12. Artifoni L, Negrisolo S, Montini G, Zucchetta P, Molinari PP, et al. (2007) Interleukin-8 and CXCR1 receptor functional polymorphisms and susceptibility to acute pyelonephritis. J Urol 177: 1102–1106.
13. Ragnarsdottir B, Samuelsson M, Gustafsson MC, Leijonhufvud I, Karpman D, et al. (2007) Reduced toll-like receptor 4 expression in children with asymptomatic bacteriuria. J Infect Dis 196: 475–484.
14. Frendeus B, Godaly G, Hang L, Karpman D, Lundstedt AC, et al. (2000) Interleukin 8 receptor deficiency confers susceptibility to acute experimental pyelonephritis and may have a human counterpart. J Exp Med 192: 881–890.
15. Smithson A, Sarrias MR, Barcelo J, Suarez B, Horcajada JP, et al. (2005) Expression of interleukin-8 receptors (CXCR1 and CXCR2) in premenopausal women with recurrent urinary tract infections. Clin Diagn Lab Immunol 12: 1358–1363.
16. XiaolinYin, LeiChen, YingLiu, JianlingYang, CuiqingMa, ZhiyanYao, et al. (2010) Enhancement of the innate immune response of bladder epithelial cells by

Astragalus polysaccharides through upregulation of TLR4 expression. BBRC 397: 232–238.
17. Hagberg L, Hull R, Hull S, McGhee JR, Michalek SM, et al. (1984) Difference in susceptibility to gram-negative urinary tract infection between C3H/HeJ and C3H/HeN mice. Infect Immun 46: 839–844.
18. Shahin RD, Engberg I, Hagberg L, Svanborg EC (1987) Neutrophil recruitment and bacterial clearance correlated with LPS responsiveness in local gram-negative infection. J Immunol 138: 3475–3480.
19. Song J, Abraham SN (2008) Innate and adaptive immune responses in the urinary tract. Eur J Clin Invest 38(S2): 21–28.
20. Hawn TR, Scholes D, Li SS, Wang HW, Yang Y, et al. (2009) Toll-Like Receptor Polymorphisms and Susceptibility to Urinary Tract Infections in Adult Women. PLOS ONE 4: e5990.
21. Poltorak A, He X, Smirnova I, Liu MY, Van Huffel C, et al. (1998) Defective LPS signaling in C3H/HeJ and C57BL/10ScCr mice:mutations in Tlr4 gene. Science 282: 2085–2088.
22. Andersen-Nissen E, Hawn TR, Smith KD, Nachman A, Lampano AE, et al. (2007) Cutting edge: Tlr5-/- mice are more susceptible to Escherichia coli urinary tract infection. J Immunol 178: 4717–4720.
23. Zhang D, Zhang G, Hayden MS, Greenblatt MB, Bussey C, et al. (2004) A toll-like receptor that prevents infection by uropathogenic bacteria. Science 303: 1522–1526.
24. Song J, Abraham SN (2008) TLR-mediated immune responses in the urinary tract. Current opininon microbiology 11: 66–73.
25. Bao-Mei Shao, Wen Xu, Hui Dai, Pengfei Tu, Zhongjun Li, Xiao-Ming Gao (2004) A study on the immune receptors for polysaccharides from the roots of Astragalus membranaceus, a Chinese medicinal herb, BBRC 320: 1103–1111.
26. Szebeni B, Szekeres R, Rusai K, Vannay A, Veres G, et al. (2006) Genetic polymorphism of CD14, Toll-like receptor 4 and caspase recruitment domain 15 are not associated with necrotizing enterocolitis in very low birth weight infants. J Pediatr Gastroenterol Nutr 42: 27–31.

5

Genetic Polymorphisms in Toll-Like Receptors among Pediatric Patients with Renal Parenchymal Infections of Different Clinical Severities

Chi-Hui Cheng[1,2]*, Yun-Shien Lee[3,4], Chee-Jen Chang[5], Tzou-Yien Lin[2,6]

1 Division of Pediatric Nephrology, Department of Pediatrics, Chang Gung Children's Hospital, Chang Gung Memorial Hospital, Taoyuan, Taiwan, **2** College of Medicine, Chang Gung University, Taoyuan, Taiwan, **3** Genomic Medicine Research Core Laboratory (GMRCL), Chang Gung Memorial Hospital, Taoyuan, Taiwan, **4** Department of Biotechnology, Ming-Chuan University, Taoyuan, Taiwan, **5** Statistical Center for Clinical Research, Chang Gung Memorial Hospital, Taoyuan, Taiwan, **6** Division of Pediatric Infectious Diseases, Department of Pediatrics, Chang Gung Children's Hospital, Chang Gung Memorial Hospital, Taoyuan, Taiwan

Abstract

Background: Although several studies have suggested single gene defects or variations in the genes associated with host immune response could confer differences in susceptibility to urinary pathogen invasion, no studies have examined the genetic polymorphisms in various toll-like receptors (TLRs) that activate innate immune responses in pediatric renal parenchymal infections of different clinical severities, namely acute pyelonephritis and the clinically more severe disease, acute lobar nephronia.

Methodology: Patients who fulfilled the diagnostic criteria for acute pyelonephritis (APN) and acute lobar nephronia (ALN) without underlying diseases or structural anomalies, except for vesicoureteral reflux (VUR), were enrolled. Genotyping of the single nucleotide polymorphisms (SNPs) in the genes encoding TLR-1, TLR-2, TLR-4, TLR-5, and TLR-6 was performed by matrix-assisted laser desorption/ionization time-of-flight-based mini-sequencing analysis.

Principal Findings: A total of 16 SNPs were selected for genotyping. Analysis of 96 normal and 48 patients' samples revealed that only four SNPs had heterozygosity rates >0.01. These SNPs were selected for further investigation. Hardy-Weinberg equilibrium was satisfied for the observed genotype frequencies. Statistically significant differences in the genotype frequency of *TLR-2* (rs3804100, T1350C) between controls and ALN or (APN+ALN) combined group were identified using the recessive model with the correction for multiple-SNP testing. Further genotype pattern frequency analysis in *TLR-2* SNPs (rs3804099 and rs3804100) showed significantly reduced occurrence of the rare allele homozygote (CC+CC) in the no-VUR subgroup of APN and ALN cases.

Conclusions: As the inflammatory responses in ALN patients are more severe than those in APN patients (higher CRP levels, longer duration of fever after antibiotic treatment), these findings suggest that the genetic variant in *TLR-2* (rs3804100, T1350C) may protect the host from severe urinary tract infections as ALN.

Editor: Ashok Kumar, Wayne State University School of Medicine, United States of America

Funding: Financial support was provided by the National Science Council of Taiwan (98-2314-B-182A-007-MY3) and Chang Gung Memorial Hospital (CMRPG 470033, 4A0111). The funders had no role in study design, data collection and analysis, decision to publish, or preparation of the manuscript.

Competing Interests: The authors have declared that no competing interests exist.

* E-mail: pedneph.cheng@msa.hinet.net

Introduction

Urinary tract infections (UTIs) are among the most prevalent infectious bacterial diseases in infants and children. The morbidity risk was estimated to be approximately 3% in prepubertal girls, 1% in prepubertal boys, and 8% in girls [1]. The clinical severity of UTIs ranges from uncomplicated lower urinary tract infections to frank abscess formation. Among the UTIs, acute lobar nephronia (ALN), also known as acute focal bacterial nephritis, presents as a localized nonliquefactive inflammatory renal bacterial infection and has previously been identified as a complicated form of acute renal infection, representing progression of the inflammatory process of acute pyelonephritis (APN) [2]. ALN may also represent a relatively early stage in renal abscess development [3]. It is generally accepted that renal parenchymal infections, including APN, ALN, and intrarenal abscess formation, are the more serious forms of UTI and have a longer duration of antibiotic treatment. Moreover, in some cases, surgical procedures are recommended for proper management [2,4,5].

Complex host-pathogen interactions determine patient susceptibility to UTIs and clinical severity. A number of studies have demonstrated that certain virulence factors associated with the uropathogenic bacterium Escherichia coli, a common clinical isolate, are more prevalent in specific UTIs [4,6]. Nevertheless, intra-individual variation in clinical presentation has been noted among UTI patients. This indicates that host factors such as mechanistic dysfunction [e.g., vesicoureteral reflux (VUR)] and

Table 1. Primers used for the amplification and mini-sequencing analysis of the SNPs.

Position	Primer sequence (5′→3′)	PCR product size	Mini-sequencing primer sequence (5′→3′)	Molecular weight of mini-sequencing product
TLR-1 (rs4833095), C>T	Sense: tccagctgaccctgtagctt	157 bp	caatgttgtttaaggtaaga	Primer: 6,195.06
	Anti-sense: ttctggcgaaacttcaaaca			T allele: 6,483.25
				C allele: 6,772.43
TLR-2 (rs3804099), C>T	Sense: tgctggacttaccttccttga	182 bp	agtttgaagtcaattcagaa	Primer: 6,164.05
	Anti-sense: ctcgcagttccaaacattcc			T allele: 6,781.45
				C allele: 6,437.23
TLR-2 (rs3804100), T>C	Sense: aaccggagagactttgctca	226 bp	agcacacgaatacacag	Primer: 5,181.42
	Anti-sense: gagttgcggcaaattcaaag			C allele: 5,454.60
				T allele: 5,798.82
TLR-5 (rs5744168), C>T	Sense: acggacttgacaacctccaa	223 bp	tacagaccttggatctc	Primer: 5,145.36
	Anti-sense: tcgggtatgcttggaataaaa			T allele: 5,762.76
				C allele: 5,418.55

genetic variation in the susceptibility to bacterial invasion and infection should not be overlooked [7–9].

The innate immune system has been recognized as the first line of defense against invading pathogens and plays a primary role in acute host defense [10]. Variations in genes that modulate innate immune responses may result in distinct clinical presentations in UTIs. Among these genes are those encoding Toll-like receptors (TLRs), which recognize pathogen-associated molecular patterns (PAMPs), and those encoding chemokines and chemokine receptors, which facilitate the migration of neutrophils to the infected urinary tract. Single gene defects or variations in these genes could confer differences in susceptibility to urinary pathogen invasion [7–9,11–13].

Escherichia coli, the most common uropathogen in renal parenchymal infections [4,5], is recognized by various TLRs, including TLR-1, TLR-2, TLR-4, TLR-5, TLR-6 (in humans and mice), and TLR-11 (in mice) [7,11,14,15]. Previous studies have shown that single nucleotide polymorphisms (SNPs) in the TLR-2 and TLR-4 genes can affect host susceptibility to UTIs [7,11,13,16–19]. In contrast, we did not observe this association for TLR-4 in APN and ALN [12].

To extend our previous analysis of genetic polymorphisms in pediatric patients with renal parenchymal infections [12], this study explored the correlations between polymorphisms in UTI-related TLR genes (TLR-1, TLR-2, TLR-4, TLR-5, and TLR-6) and clinical severity among pediatric patients with UTIs of different severities (APN and the clinically more severe disease, ALN). In addition, as VUR is a well-known risk factor for severe parenchymal infectious disease [8,20], a subgroup of APN and ALN patients without VUR was also examined to exclude the possible effects of VUR.

Materials and Methods

Ethics Statement

This investigation was approved by the Institutional Review Board of Chang Gung Memorial Hospital, and following a full explanation of the study, written informed consent was obtained from the parents of all patients.

Study Setting and Patient Selection Criteria

This study is a part of our continuing analyses of the pathogenic host and bacterial urovirulence factors related to APN and ALN [4,5,12]. The participating patients were admitted to Chang Gung Children's Hospital, a tertiary medical center located in a suburb of Taipei in northern Taiwan, between January 2004 and December 2008. Patients who fulfilled the diagnostic criteria for APN and ALN caused by *E. coli* while lacking any of the exclusion

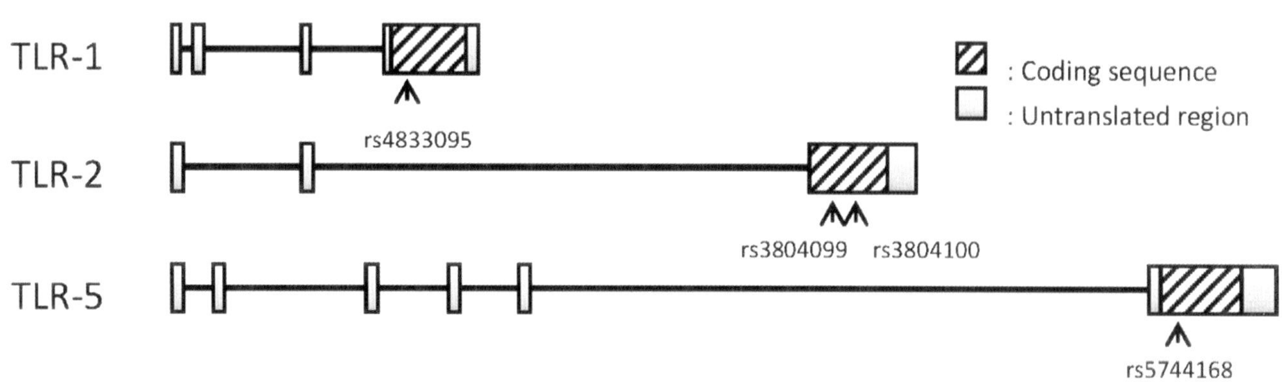

Figure 1. Position of the four SNPs that had heterozygosity rates >0.01 in each TLR sequence.

criteria were enrolled in the study. The controls were pediatric patients who presented to the outpatient clinic for reasons other than a UTI or severe infection and were interviewed to ensure that they did not have a history of UTI or severe infections as well as not having positive urine culture.

The diagnostic scheme for patients suspected of having APN or ALN was as described previously [2,4,5,12]. In brief, all patients with a suspected UTI because of the presence of pyuria (>5 white blood cells/high-power field) and fever with symptoms and signs related to UTIs (*e.g.*, pain, dysuria, and frequency of urination) or without focus underwent renal ultrasonography on the first or second day after admission. Computed tomography (CT) was performed immediately when the initial ultrasonographic findings met either of two criteria: evidence of unilateral or bilateral nephromegaly or a focal renal mass. For children who presented with borderline nephromegaly on ultrasonography, CT was performed when the child remained febrile for 72 h after the commencement of antibiotic therapy. A diagnosis of ALN was made on the basis of positive CT findings. Technetium 99m-dimercaptosuccinic acid scintigraphy (^{99m}Tc-DMSA) was performed within 3–7 days of admission in patients suspected of having a febrile UTI who did not satisfy the sonographic criteria for ALN. APN was defined as focal or diffuse areas of decreased ^{99m}Tc-DMSA uptake without evidence of cortical loss.

Patients with evidence of an underlying disease, including diabetes and immunodeficiency, or structural anomalies such as neurogenic bladder, posterior urethral valve, urinary diversion, bladder diverticulum, ureterocele, or urinary tract obstruction other than VUR were excluded.

Genotyping by Matrix-assisted Laser Desorption/ionization Time-of-flight (MALDI-TOF)-based Mini-sequencing Analysis

SNPs in the genes encoding TLR-1, TLR-2, TLR-4, TLR-5, and TLR-6, as well as in their respective promoter regions, were identified in the NCBI dbSNP database [21]. A total of 16 SNPs (rs4833095, rs5743611, and rs5743618 for *TLR-1*; rs3804099, rs3804100, rs5743704, and rs5743708 for *TLR-2*; zA11547G, rs2149356, and rs5030710 for *TLR-4*; rs2072493, rs5744168, and rs5744174 for *TLR-5* and rs3821985, rs5743810 and rs5743815 for *TLR-6*) were selected for genotyping based on previous studies on Toll-like receptors polymorphisms on APN adult patients [7,11]. Analysis of 96 normal and 48 patients' samples revealed that only four SNPs had heterozygosity rates >0.01. These SNPs (Table 1, Figure 1) were used to analyze the control and patient genotypes by a MALDI-TOF-based mini-sequencing genotyping method.

Genomic DNA was extracted from peripheral blood lymphocytes using a Nucleospin® blood kit (Macherey-Nagel, Düren,

Table 2. Genotypic analysis of the SNPs.

SNP	Group	Genotype, *n* (%)			Log-additive model		Dominant model		Recessive model	
		00	01	11			(01, 11 *vs.* 00)		(11 *vs.* 00, 01)	
		CC	CT	TT	OR (95% CI)	*P*[a]	OR (95% CI)	*P*[a]	OR (95% CI)	*P*[a]
TLR-1	Control	75 (34.1)	113 (51.4)	32 (14.5)			1.00		1.00	
(rs4833095)	APN	44 (40.7)	51 (47.2)	13 (12.0)	0.81 (0.57, 1.15)	0.243	0.75 (0.47, 1.21)	0.241	0.80 (0.40, 1.69)	0.531
	ALN	59 (35.1)	81 (48.2)	28 (16.7)	1.02 (0.76, 1.37)	0.876	0.96 (0.63, 1.46)	0.833	1.17 (0.68, 2.04)	0.568
	Combined[b]	103 (37.3)	132 (47.8)	41 (14.9)	0.94 (0.72, 1.22)	0.635	0.87 (0.60, 1.26)	0.456	1.02 (0.62, 1.69)	0.923
		TT	TC	CC	OR (95% CI)	*P*	OR (95% CI)	*P*	OR (95% CI)	*P*
TLR-2	Control	102 (46.8)	97 (44.5)	19 (8.7)			1.00		1.00	
(rs3804099)	APN	47 (43.5)	57 (52.8)	4 (3.7)	0.95 (0.66, 1.39)	0.810	1.14 (0.72, 1.82)	0.577	0.40 (0.13, 1.22)	0.080
	ALN	72 (43.4)	81 (48.8)	13 (7.8)	1.07 (0.77, 1.47)	0.698	1.15 (0.76, 1.72)	0.505	0.89 (0.43, 1.86)	0.756
	Combined	119 (43.4)	138 (50.4)	17 (6.2)	1.02 (0.77, 1.36)	0.880	1.15 (0.80, 1.64)	0.457	0.69 (0.35, 1.37)	0.290
		TT	TC	CC	OR (95% CI)	*P*	OR (95% CI)	*P*	OR (95% CI)	*P*
TLR-2	Control	112 (50.9)	92 (41.8)	16 (7.3)			1.00		1.00	
(rs3804100)	APN	53 (48.6)	54 (49.5)	2 (1.8)	0.91 (0.62, 1.35)	0.652	1.10 (0.69, 1.73)	0.696	0.24 (0.05, 1.06)	**0.026**
	ALN	83 (50.0)	80 (48.2)	3 (1.8)	0.88 (0.62, 1.24)	0.451	1.04 (0.69, 1.55)	0.860	0.23 (0.07, 0.82)	**0.009**[c]
	Combined	136 (49.5)	134 (48.7)	5 (1.8)	0.89 (0.65, 1.21)	0.444	1.06 (0.74, 1.51)	0.748	0.24 (0.09, 0.66)	**0.003**[c]
		CC	CT	TT	OR (95% CI)	*P*	OR (95% CI)	*P*	OR (95% CI)	*P*
TLR-5	Control	210 (95.5)	10 (4.5)	0 (0.0)						
(rs5744168)	APN	100 (92.6)	8 (7.4)	0 (0.0)	1.68 (0.64, 4.39)	0.296				
	ALN	153 (93.9)	10 (6.1)	0 (0.0)	1.37 (0.56, 3.38)	0.492				
	Combined	253 (93.4)	18 (6.6)	0 (0.0)	1.49 (0.68, 3.31)	0.315				

[a]*P* values <0.05 are shown in bold.
[b]APN+ALN.
[c]Statistical significance with correction for multiple-SNP testing (*P*<0.0125).

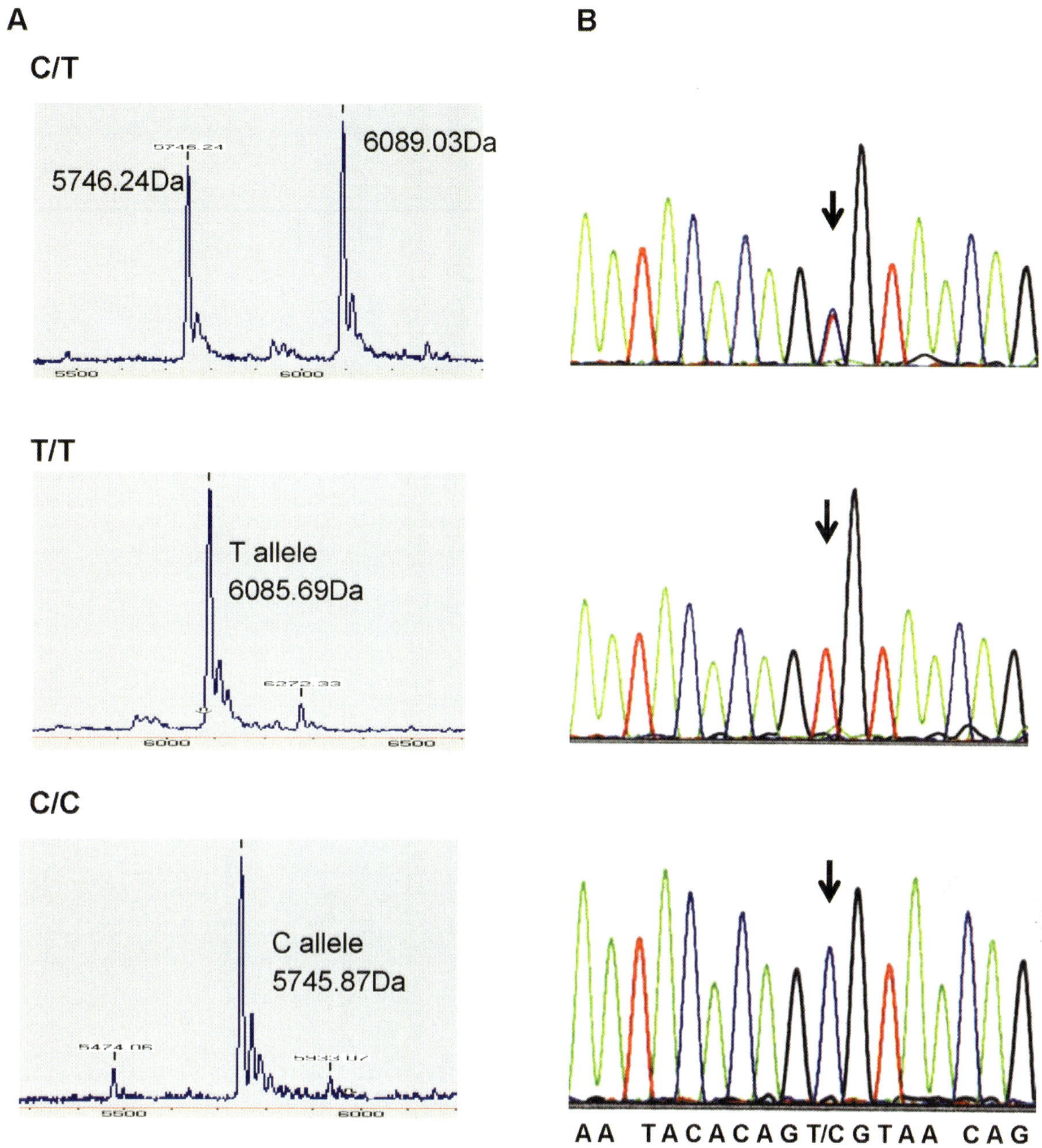

Figure 2. MALDI-TOF mass spectra from the genotyping of *TLR-2* (rs3804100) PCR product and its sequencing results. (A) The SNPs were genotyped by MALDI-TOF MS based on the molecular weights of the mini-sequencing products listed in Table 1. (B) Sequencing results for each of the PCR products from the C/T, T/T, and C/C genotypes of rs3804100. The SNPs are indicated by arrowheads.

Germany) according to the manufacturer's recommendations. The SNPs were genotyped as described previously [12] using the primers listed in Table 1. Briefly, PCR was performed in a total volume of 25 μL containing 200 ng of genomic DNA, primers (25 pM each), dNTPs (0.2 mM), 1× Fast-Start PCR buffer (50 mM Tris-HCl, 10 mM KCl, 5 mM $[NH_4]_2SO_4$, 2mM $MgCl_2$; pH 8.3), 1 M betaine, and 1 U of Fast-Start Taq Polymerase (Roche Diagnostics, Basel, Switzerland). The reaction comprised initiation at 95°C for 5 min, followed by 40 cycles of 95°C for 45 s, 50°C for 45 s, and 60°C for 45 s, with a final extension at 52°C for 10 min. Unincorporated dNTPs and primers were removed automatically by MAPIIA (GenePure PCR Purification System; Bruker, Bremen, Germany). The purified products were collected and mini-sequencing reactions were run using individual mini-sequencing primers (Table 1) in 20 μL of a solution containing 50 ng of the PCR product, 1 μL (10 pmol) of mini-sequencing primer, 0.5 μL of 1 mM ddNTP/dNTP mixture (for *TLR-1* rs4833095, dC ddT; for *TLR-2* rs3804099, dT ddC ddG; for *TLR-2* rs3804100, dT ddC ddG; and for *TLR-5* rs5744168, dT ddC ddG), 0.5 U of Thermo Sequenase DNA Polymerase (Amersham Biosciences, Piscataway, NJ), and 2 μL of the reaction buffer provided by the manufacturer. The reactions were carried out in a multiblock thermal cycler (Thermo Hybaid, Waltham, MA) with initial denaturation

Table 3. Allele frequency analysis of the SNPs using the logistic regression model.

SNP	T allele frequency (%)				APN *vs.* control		ALN *vs.* control		Combined[a] *vs.* control	
	Control	APN	ALN	Combined[a]	OR (95% CI)	*P*	OR (95% CI)	*P*	OR (95% CI)	*P*
TLR-1 (rs4833095)	40.23	35.65	40.77	38.77	0.82 (0.59, 1.15)	0.257	1.02 (0.77, 1.37)	0.878	0.94 (0.73, 1.22)	0.640
TLR-2 (rs3804099)	69.04	69.91	67.77	68.61	1.04 (0.73, 1.49)	0.820	0.94 (0.69, 1.28)	0.709	0.98 (0.75, 1.29)	0.887
TLR-2 (rs3804100)	71.82	73.39	74.10	73.82	1.08 (0.75, 1.56)	0.670	1.12 (0.81, 1.55)	0.481	1.11 (0.83, 1.47)	0.482
TLR-5 (rs5744168)	2.27	3.70	3.07	3.32	1.65 (0.64, 4.25)	0.303	1.36 (0.56, 3.31)	0.500	1.48 (0.67, 3.23)	0.322

[a]APN+ALN.

at 96°C for 1 min, followed by 50 cycles of 96°C for 15 s, 50°C for 15 s, 60°C for 100 s, and 96°C for 30 s. The reaction products were purified automatically by MAPIIA (Single-Strand DNA Binding Beads; Bruker) and analyzed by MALDI-TOF mass spectrometry (MS).

The samples were then mixed with 0.5 μL of matrix solution (50 mg/mL 3-hydropicolinic acid in a 4:5:1 mixture of water, acetonitrile, and 50 mg/mL diammonium citrate) and spotted onto 384-well Teflon sample plates (PerSeptive Biosystems, Framingham, MA). MALDI-TOF mass spectra were acquired with a Bruker Autoflex MALDI-TOF mass spectrometer (Bruker) and AutoXecute software (Bruker) to validate the genotype data. To confirm the MALDI-TOF analysis results, 10% of the PCR products were randomly selected for auto-sequencing analysis using an ABI 3730 autosequencer (Applied Biosystems, Foster City, CA).

Statistical Analysis

Hardy-Weinberg equilibrium was tested for goodness-of-fit using a χ^2 test with one degree of freedom, to compare the observed and expected genotype frequencies among the study subjects. The association of case-control status (outcome) and SNP genotype was analyzed using log-additive (or allelic-trend test), recessive, and dominant models [7,11]. In the log-additive model, common homozygous genotypes (00) were assigned a value of 0; heterozygotes (01), a value of 1; and minor homozygous genotypes (11), a value of 2. For the dominant model, the genotypes 01 and 11 were combined and compared with genotype 00. In a similar manner, the genotypes 00 and 01 were combined and compared with genotype 11 for recessive model analysis. Odds ratios and significance levels were assessed using a logistic regression model. Statistical comparisons of categorical variables or binominal results (*e.g.*, allele frequency) among the control, APN, and ALN groups were performed by χ^2 analysis or two-sided Fisher's exact test, as appropriate. Genotype pattern frequency analysis for the SNPs with heterozygosity rates >0.01 in *TLR-2* (i.e. rs3804099, rs3804100) was also performed using a similar method as described by Ragnarsdóttir et al [17]. All statistical analyses were performed using SPSS software (Version 16.0, IBM SPSS Statistics) or otherwise, the website tools as stated.

At first, 96 cases (48 APN and 48 ALN) and 96 control samples were analyzed for *TLR-2* (rs3804100) SNP. The prior data (192 samples) indicated that the probability of exposure among controls is 0.10417. With the recessive model, if the true odds ratio for disease in exposed subjects relative to unexposed subjects is 0.182979 as we noted among these 192 samples, we will need to study 154 patients and 154 control patients to be able to reject the null hypothesis that this odds ratio equals 1 with probability (power) of 0.8. The Type I error probability associated with this test of this null hypothesis is 0.05. The samples size estimate was performed with PS Power and Sample Size Calculations Version 3.0 (http://biostat.mc.vanderbilt.edu/PowerSampleSize) [22].

The demographic and clinical characteristics of the patients enrolled were described in a previous publication [12]. All cases are Taiwanese. The gender ratio and age were not significantly different ($p>0.05$) among the control patients ($n = 222$), APN patients ($n = 113$), and ALN patients ($n = 172$). In addition, patients with ALN (the clinically more severe UTI) presented with a significantly higher C-reactive protein (CRP) level than the APN patients. Moreover, the durations of fever prior to admission and after antibiotic treatment were longer in the ALN patients than in the APN patients. However, no statistically significant difference in white blood cell count was noted.

Results

Hardy-Weinberg equilibrium was satisfied in the observed genotype frequencies for all groups (Table 2). Auto-sequencing of randomly selected PCR products, for example, *TLR-2* (rs3804100) for three enrolled individuals, gave results that were identical to those derived from the MALDI-TOF mass spectra (Figure 2). This indicates the MALDI-TOF method was able to precisely determine the DNA sequences of the SNPs.

Statistical analyses revealed that only the *TLR-2* (rs3804100) SNP showed a significant difference in genotype frequency between the control group and the APN and ALN groups (and a combined APN+ALN group) using the recessive model [OR (95% CI): APN *vs.* control, 0.24 (0.05, 1.06); ALN *vs.* control, 0.23 (0.07, 0.82); APN+ALN *vs.* control, 0.24 (0.09, 0.66)] (Table 2). After correction for multiple-SNP testing (4 SNPs examined here), only ALN and (APN+ALN) groups showed significant difference *vs.* control in recessive model ($P<0.0125$). There were no statistically significant differences in the allele frequencies of the SNPs we examined (Table 3).

Because VUR has been suggested to be a significant host risk factor for upper UTIs [8,20], further genetic analysis was conducted in subgroups of APN and ALN patients with no VUR (APN, 50 patients; ALN, 108 patients). As a voiding cystourethrography was not medically indicated in the control patients, the number of patients with VUR in the control group was calculated based on a reported prevalence rate [23]. Given a 0.3% prevalence rate of VUR at the mean age of the control group (2.91±3.01 years), the number of individuals with VUR among the 222 control cases was assumed to be zero. The age and gender ratios remained not significantly different ($p>0.05$) between the control group and the APN and ALN subgroups with no VUR.

In comparison with the *TLR-2* (rs3804100) TT and TC genotype frequencies, the CC genotype frequency was significantly

Table 4. Genotypic analysis of the SNPs in the no-VUR patient subgroup.

SNP	Group	Genotype, *n* (%)			Log-additive model		Dominant model		Recessive model	
		00	01	11			(01, 11 *vs.* 00)		(11 *vs.* 00, 01)	
		CC	CT	TT	OR (95% CI)	*P*[a]	OR (95% CI)	*P*[a]	OR (95% CI)	*P*[a]
TLR-1	Control	75 (34.1)	113 (51.4)	32 (14.5)			1.00		1.00	
(rs4833095)	APN	21 (42.0)	24 (48.0)	5 (10.0)	0.75 (0.47, 1.20)	0.230	0.71 (0.38, 1.34)	0.296	0.65 (0.24, 1.77)	0.383
	ALN	33 (30.6)	55 (50.9)	20 (18.5)	1.18 (0.84, 1.65)	0.346	1.18 (0.72, 1.93)	0.521	1.34 (0.72, 2.47)	0.360
	Combined[b]	54 (34.2)	79 (50.0)	25 (15.8)	1.03 (0.76, 1.39)	0.866	1.00 (0.65, 1.53)	0.986	1.10 (0.63, 1.95)	0.733
		TT	TC	CC	OR (95% CI)	*P*	OR (95% CI)	*P*	OR (95% CI)	*P*
TLR-2	Control	102 (46.8)	97 (44.5)	19 (8.7)			1.00		1.00	
(rs3804099)	APN	21 (42.0)	27 (54.0)	2 (4.0)	1.00 (0.61, 1.64)	0.994	1.21 (0.65, 2.26)	0.539	0.44 (0.10, 1.94)	0.228
	ALN	46 (42.6)	56 (51.9)	6 (5.6)	1.03 (0.71, 1.49)	0.888	1.19 (0.74, 1.89)	0.473	0.62 (0.24, 1.59)	0.300
	Combined	67 (42.4)	83 (52.5)	8 (5.1)	1.02 (0.73, 1.42)	0.909	1.19 (0.79, 1.80)	0.399	0.56 (0.24, 1.31)	0.168
		TT	TC	CC	OR (95% CI)	*P*	OR (95% CI)	*P*	OR (95% CI)	*P*
TLR-2	Control	112 (50.9)	92 (41.8)	16 (7.3)			1.00		1.00	
(rs3804100)	APN	25 (50.0)	23 (46.0)	2 (4.0)	0.94 (0.57, 1.55)	0.806	1.04 (0.56, 1.92)	0.908	0.53 (0.12, 2.39)	0.375
	ALN	54 (50.0)	52 (48.1)	2 (1.9)	0.88 (0.60, 1.30)	0.519	1.04 (0.65, 1.64)	0.877	0.24 (0.05, 1.07)	**0.027**[c]
	Combined	79 (50.0)	75 (47.5)	4 (2.5)	0.90 (0.64, 1.27)	0.536	1.04 (0.69, 1.56)	0.862	0.33 (0.11, 1.01)	**0.034**[c]
		CC	CT	TT	OR (95% CI)	*P*	OR (95% CI)	*P*	OR (95% CI)	*P*
TLR-5	Control	210 (95.5)	10 (4.5)	0 (0.0)						
(rs5744168)	APN	45 (93.8)	3 (6.2)	0 (0.0)	1.40 (0.37, 5.29)	0.630				
	ALN	99 (94.3)	6 (5.7)	0 (0.0)	1.27 (0.45, 3.60)	0.653				
	Combined	144 (94.1)	9 (5.9)	0 (0.0)	1.31 (0.52, 3.31)	0.566				

[a]*P* values <0.05 are shown in bold.
[b]APN+ALN.
[c]Statistical non-significance with correction for multiple-SNP testing (*P*>0.0125).

lower in the no-VUR ALN and APN+ALN patient subgroups [recessive model, OR (95% CI): ALN *vs.* control, 0.24 (0.05, 1.07); APN+ALN *vs.* control, 0.33 (0.11, 1.01)] (Table 4). With correction for multiple-SNP testing, no significant difference was noted between the control and the no-VUR disease subgroups. The allele frequency analyses showed no significant difference between the control group and the no-VUR APN, ALN, or APN+ALN patient subgroup (Table 5).

Genotype patterns in *TLR-2* were assigned by combining multiple SNPs that had heterozygosity rates >0.01 (i.e. rs3804099, rs3804100) in each individual (Figure 3) [17]. The frequency of genotype pattern IV (CC+CC) was significantly reduced in the APN+ALN combined group (Table 6). After the elimination of cases with VUR, genotype pattern IV can not even be noted in the no-VUR subgroup of APN and ALN (Table 7).

Discussion

Successful defense against bacterial infection requires well-integrated host innate and adaptive immune responses. The initial pathogen recognition process is mediated by the coordinated actions of various TLRs, which are located on the cell surface or

Table 5. Allele frequency analysis of the SNPs in the no-VUR patient subgroup using the logistic regression model.

SNP	T allele frequency (%)				APN *vs.* control		ALN *vs.* control		Combined[a] *vs.* control	
	Control	APN	ALN	Combined[a]	OR (95% CI)	*P*	OR (95% CI)	*P*	OR (95% CI)	*P*
TLR-1 (rs4833095)	40.23	34.00	43.98	40.82	0.77 (0.49, 1.21)	0.246	1.17 (0.84, 1.62)	0.360	1.03 (0.76, 1.38)	0.869
TLR-2 (rs3804099)	69.04	69.00	68.52	68.67	1.00 (0.62, 1.60)	0.994	0.98 (0.69, 1.39)	0.893	0.98 (0.72, 1.34)	0.915
TLR-2 (rs3804100)	71.82	73.00	74.07	73.73	1.06 (0.65, 1.73)	0.812	1.12 (0.78, 1.62)	0.542	1.10 (0.80, 1.53)	0.560
TLR-5 (rs5744168)	2.27	3.13	2.86	2.94	1.39 (0.37, 5.14)	0.634	1.26 (0.45, 3.53)	0.657	1.30 (0.52, 3.25)	0.571

[a]APN+ALN.

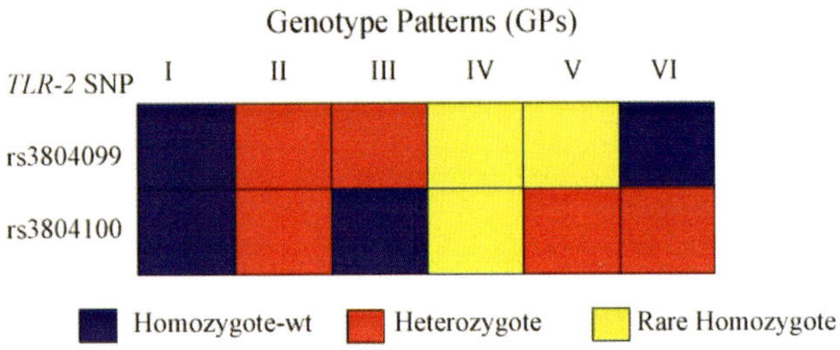

Figure 3. *TLR-2* genotype patterns of the SNPs with heterozygosity rates >0.01. Each column represents a genotype pattern and each row a SNP in *TLR-2*. Common allele homozygote (blue), heterozygote (red) and rare allele homozygote (yellow) are shown.

within organelles such as phagosomes, and PAMPs, including bacterial flagellin, lipopolysaccharide, and bacterial lipopeptides [7,10–12]. Following this microbe-sensing step, sequential activation of the immune system leads to cytokine release, recruitment of neutrophils to the site of infection, phagocytosis, and the release of free radicals [16]. The cytokines that are released play essential roles in the host innate immune response and activation of the adaptive immune system [24]. These responses determine the balance between health and disease severity [8]. Defective signal transmission in the immune response due to, for example, genetic polymorphisms in receptors and cytokines, influences an individual's risk for infectious diseases [7,9,11,12,16,19].

TLRs are crucial for the recognition of microbes by the innate immune system and for bridging the innate and acquired immune responses [16]. In addition to acting as critical sensors of microbial attack, TLRs also serve as effectors of TLR-dependent innate defense, which enables the host to eliminate pathogens that would otherwise cause disease morbidity or mortality [17]. Many studies have suggested that SNPs in TLR genes can affect an individual's ability to respond to TLR ligands, leading to altered susceptibility to infections or inflammation [25]. This altered susceptibility can be either a reduced inflammatory response, as occurs in asymptomatic bacteriuria, protection against pyelonephritis, and recurrent UTIs [11,17,19], or an exaggerated immune response that results in a severe infection, as occurs in tuberculosis and severe atopic dermatitis [26,27].

The APN and ALN patients in this study had a lower TLR-2 (rs3804100) CC genotype frequency compared with the controls. No differences in the other TLR SNPs examined were noted among the APN, ALN, and control groups. Furthermore, after the elimination of patients with VUR, a well-known risk factor for severe UTI, from the analysis, patients with ALN, but not those with APN, had a lower TLR-2 (rs3804100) CC genotype frequency. With the correction for multiple-SNP testing, only the ALN and (APN+ALN) combined group that include VUR diagnosis showed significant reduced TLR-2 (rs3804100) CC genotype frequency compared with the controls. Further, the genotype pattern frequency analysis for the TLR-2 has shown the genotype pattern of CC+CC (rs3804099+rs3804100) was not even noted in the no-VUR subgroup of patients with APN and ALN. As the inflammatory responses in ALN patients are more severe than those in APN patients (higher CRP levels, longer fever duration after antibiotic treatment), these findings suggest that the genetic variant in TLR-2 (rs3804100, T1350C) may protect the host from severe urinary tract infections as ALN.

Among the TLRs that have been described, TLR-2 was the first human TLR to be described in host defense against gram-negative bacteria [28] but subsequent studies have demonstrated that TLR-4 is the receptor for lipopolysaccharide [16,29]. TLR-2 polymorphisms have also been linked to various severe infections, including tuberculosis, leprosy, and septic shock [10,30,31]. A few studies have reported associations between UTIs and TLR-2 polymorphism at the TLR-2 (rs5743708; G2258A; Arg753Gln) site [11,16]. The current study found that another TLR-2 genetic variant, TLR-2 (rs3804100; T1350C; Ser450Ser), can also change the host risk to severe UTIs (APN vs. ALN).

The TLR-2 (rs3804100; T1350C; Ser450Ser) SNP described here did not induce an amino acid change, and the molecular mechanism by which this synonymous polymorphism affects host susceptibility to severe UTIs is not fully understood. Many studies have provided evidence that synonymous SNPs lead to changes in protein amount, structure, and/or function via alterations in mRNA structure and stability, kinetics of translation, and alternative splicing. Moreover, synonymous SNPs may be proxies for other polymorphisms that have not been examined [32]. Further investigations of phenotypes or functional assessment of synonymous SNPs, such as using the luciferase reporter assay or gene knock-out mice [9,17,19], are warranted to properly determine their effects on TLR-2 expression.

Table 6. Genotype pattern frequency analysis of the SNPs in *TLR-2* (rs3804099 and rs3804100) using the two-tailed Fisher's Exact Test[#].

Genotype pattern	Genotype pattern frequency (*n*)			APN *vs.* control	ALN *vs.* control	Combined[b] *vs.* Control
	Control (218)	**APN (107)**	**ALN (166)**	***P*** [a]	***P*** [a]	***P*** [a]
I (TT+TT)	99	43	70	0.406	0.535	0.409
II (TC+TC)	83	49	70	0.189	0.462	0.231
III (TC+TT)	12	8	11	0.624	0.669	0.578
IV (CC+CC)	12	2	3	0.156	0.108	**0.044**
V (CC+TC)	7	2	8	0.723	0.438	0.810
VI (TT+TC)	1	3	2	0.106	0.581	0.234
Others	4	0	2	0.307	0.702	0.414

[a]*P* values <0.05 are shown in bold.
[b]APN+ALN.
[#]2×2 contingency table, http://www.vassarstats.net/tab2×2.html.

Table 7. Genotype pattern frequency analysis of the SNPs in *TLR-2* (rs3804099 and rs3804100) in the no-VUR patient subgroup using the two-tailed Fisher's Exact Test[#].

Genotype pattern	Genotype pattern frequency (*n*)			APN *vs.* control	ALN *vs.* control	Combined[b] *vs.* Control
	Control (218)	APN (50)	ALN (108)	*P* [a]	*P* [a]	*P* [a]
I (TT+TT)	99	19	42	0.350	0.286	0.206
II (TC+TC)	83	20	47	0.872	0.400	0.455
III (TC+TT)	12	6	9	0.116	0.344	0.159
IV (CC+CC)	12	0	0	0.131	**0.023**	**0.002**
V (CC+TC)	7	2	3	1.000	1.000	1.000
VI (TT+TC)	1	1	2	0.339	0.256	0.314
Others	4	2	5	0.597	0.164	0.214

[a]*P* values <0.05 are shown in bold.
[b]APN+ALN.
[#]2×2 contingency table, http://www.vassarstats.net/tab2×2.html.

As the statistical power to detect significant associations with rare genetic variants is determined based on sample size, the major limitation of this study is the small population of individuals with the CC genotype of TLR-2 (rs3804100, T1350C). A large cohort study is recommended to replicate and validate the associations of SNPs with the severe UTIs, APN and ALN.

Acknowledgments

The authors thank Mr. Yu-Jr Lin for his assistance with the statistical analyses.

Author Contributions

Conceived and designed the experiments: CHC YSL TYL. Performed the experiments: CHC YSL. Analyzed the data: CHC YSL CJC. Contributed reagents/materials/analysis tools: CHC YSL CJC. Wrote the paper: CHC.

References

1. Ma JF, Shortliffe LM (2004) Urinary tract infection in children: etiology and epidemiology. Urologic Clinics of North America 31: 517–526.
2. Cheng CH, Tsau YK, Lin TY (2006) Effective duration of antimicrobial therapy for the treatment of acute lobar nephronia. Pediatrics 117: e84–89.
3. Cheng CH, Tsau YK, Lin TY (2010) Is acute lobar nephronia the midpoint in the spectrum of upper urinary tract infections between acute pyelonephritis and renal abscess? Journal of Pediatrics 156: 82–86.
4. Cheng CH, Tsau YK, Su LH, Lin CL, Lin TY (2007) Comparison of urovirulence factors and genotypes for bacteria causing acute lobar nephronia and acute pyelonephritis. Pediatric Infectious Disease Journal 26: 228–232.
5. Cheng CH, Tsau YK, Kuo CY, Su LH, Lin TY (2010) Comparison of extended virulence genotypes for bacteria isolated from pediatric patients with urosepsis, acute pyelonephritis, and acute lobar nephronia. Pediatric Infectious Disease Journal 29: 736–740.
6. Tseng CC, Wu JJ, Liu HL, Sung JM, Huang JJ (2002) Roles of host and bacterial virulence factors in the development of upper urinary tract infection caused by Escherichia coli. Am J Kidney Dis 39: 744–752.
7. Hawn TR, Scholes D, Li SS, Wang H, Yang Y, et al. (2009) Toll-like receptor polymorphisms and susceptibility to urinary tract infections in adult women. PLoS ONE [Electronic Resource] 4: e5990.
8. Artifoni L, Negrisolo S, Montini G, Zucchetta P, Molinari PP, et al. (2007) Interleukin-8 and CXCR1 receptor functional polymorphisms and susceptibility to acute pyelonephritis. Journal of Urology 177: 1102–1106.
9. Lundstedt AC, McCarthy S, Gustafsson MC, Godaly G, Jodal U, et al. (2007) A genetic basis of susceptibility to acute pyelonephritis. PLoS ONE [Electronic Resource] 2: e825.
10. Texereau J, Chiche J-D, Taylor W, Choukroun G, Comba B, et al. (2005) The importance of Toll-like receptor 2 polymorphisms in severe infections. Clinical Infectious Diseases 41 Suppl 7: S408–415.
11. Hawn TR, Scholes D, Wang H, Li SS, Stapleton AE, et al. (2009) Genetic variation of the human urinary tract innate immune response and asymptomatic bacteriuria in women. PLoS ONE [Electronic Resource] 4: e8300.
12. Cheng CH, Lee YS, Tsau YK, Lin TY (2011) Genetic polymorphisms and susceptibility to parenchymal renal infection among pediatric patients. Pediatric Infectious Disease Journal 30: 309–314.
13. Yin X, Hou T, Liu Y, Chen J, Yao Z, et al. (2010) Association of Toll-like receptor 4 gene polymorphism and expression with urinary tract infection types in adults. PLoS ONE [Electronic Resource] 5: e14223.
14. Medzhitov R (2007) Recognition of microorganisms and activation of the immune response. Nature 449: 819–826.
15. Beutler B, Jiang Z, Georgel P, Crozat K, Croker B, et al. (2006) Genetic analysis of host resistance: Toll-like receptor signaling and immunity at large. Annual Review of Immunology 24: 353–389.
16. Tabel Y, Berdeli A, Mir S (2007) Association of TLR2 gene Arg753Gln polymorphism with urinary tract infection in children. International Journal of Immunogenetics 34: 399–405.
17. Ragnarsdottir B, Jonsson K, Urbano A, Gronberg-Hernandez J, Lutay N, et al. (2010) Toll-like receptor 4 promoter polymorphisms: common TLR4 variants may protect against severe urinary tract infection. PLoS ONE [Electronic Resource] 5: e10734.
18. Karoly E, Fekete A, Banki NF, Szebeni B, Vannay A, et al. (2007) Heat shock protein 72 (HSPA1B) gene polymorphism and Toll-like receptor (TLR) 4 mutation are associated with increased risk of urinary tract infection in children. Pediatr Res 61: 371–374.
19. Ragnarsdottir B, Lutay N, Gronberg-Hernandez J, Koves B, Svanborg C (2011) Genetics of innate immunity and UTI susceptibility. Nature Reviews Urology 8: 449–468.
20. Orellana P, Baquedano P, Rangarajan V, Zhao JH, Eng ND, et al. (2004) Relationship between acute pyelonephritis, renal scarring, and vesicoureteral reflux. Results of a coordinated research project. Pediatric Nephrology 19: 1122–1126.
21. Sayers EW, Barrett T, Benson DA, Bolton E, Bryant SH, et al. (2010) Database resources of the National Center for Biotechnology Information. Nucleic Acids Research 38: D5–16.
22. Dupont WD, Plummer WD Jr (1998) Power and sample size calculations for studies involving linear regression. Controlled Clinical Trials 19: 589–601.
23. American Academy of Pediatrics, Committee on Quality Improvement, Subcommittee on Urinary Tract Infection (1999) Practice parameter: the diagnosis, treatment, and evaluation of the initial urinary tract infection in febrile infants and young children. Pediatrics 103: 843–852.
24. Bochud P-Y, Hawn TR, Siddiqui MR, Saunderson P, Britton S, et al. (2008) Toll-like receptor 2 (TLR2) polymorphisms are associated with reversal reaction in leprosy. Journal of Infectious Diseases 197: 253–261.
25. Netea MG, Wijmenga C, O'Neill LA (2012) Genetic variation in Toll-like receptors and disease susceptibility. Nat Immunol 13: 535–542.
26. Ogus AC, Yoldas B, Ozdemir T, Uguz A, Olcen S, et al. (2004) The Arg753GLn polymorphism of the human toll-like receptor 2 gene in tuberculosis disease. European Respiratory Journal 23: 219–223.
27. Ahmad-Nejad P, Mrabet-Dahbi S, Breuer K, Klotz M, Werfel T, et al. (2004) The toll-like receptor 2 R753Q polymorphism defines a subgroup of patients

with atopic dermatitis having severe phenotype. Journal of Allergy & Clinical Immunology 113: 565–567.
28. Kirschning CJ, Wesche H, Merrill Ayres T, Rothe M (1998) Human toll-like receptor 2 confers responsiveness to bacterial lipopolysaccharide. Journal of Experimental Medicine 188: 2091–2097.
29. Beutler B, Du X, Poltorak A (2001) Identification of Toll-like receptor 4 (Tlr4) as the sole conduit for LPS signal transduction: genetic and evolutionary studies. Journal of Endotoxin Research 7: 277–280.
30. Abu-Maziad A, Schaa K, Bell EF, Dagle JM, Cooper M, et al. (2010) Role of polymorphic variants as genetic modulators of infection in neonatal sepsis. Pediatric Research 68: 323–329.
31. Chen Y-C, Hsiao C-C, Chen C-J, Chin C-H, Liu S-F, et al. (2010) Toll-like receptor 2 gene polymorphisms, pulmonary tuberculosis, and natural killer cell counts. BMC Medical Genetics 11: 17.
32. Junpee A, Tencomnao T, Sanprasert V, Nuchprayoon S (2010) Association between Toll-like receptor 2 (TLR2) polymorphisms and asymptomatic bancroftian filariasis. Parasitology Research 107: 807–816.

6

The Importance of Gender-Stratified Antibiotic Resistance Surveillance of Unselected Uropathogens: A Dutch Nationwide Extramural Surveillance Study

Casper D. J. den Heijer[1], John Penders[1], Gé A. Donker[2], Cathrien A. Bruggeman[1], Ellen E. Stobberingh[1]*

1 Department of Medical Microbiology, Maastricht University Medical Centre/Care and Public Health Research Institute, Maastricht, The Netherlands, **2** NIVEL, The Netherlands Institute for Health Services Research, Utrecht, The Netherlands

Abstract

Few studies have been performed on urinary tract infections (UTIs) in men. In the present study, general practitioners (n = 42) from the Dutch Sentinel General Practice Network collected urinary samples from 560 male patients (≥18 years) suspected of UTI and recorded prescribed antibiotic treatment. In this way, the antibiotic susceptibility of Gram-negative uropathogens, including extended-spectrum beta-lactamase (ESBL-) producing *Escherichia coli* could be determined. In addition, *E. coli* susceptibility and antibiotic prescriptions were compared with data from a similar UTI study among women and with data collected 7 years earlier. Of 367 uropathogens (66%) identified (≥10^3 cfu/mL), most were Gram-negative (83%) and *E. coli* being isolated most frequently (51%). Antibiotic susceptibility to ciprofloxacin, norfloxacin and nitrofurantoin was 94%, 92% and 88%, respectively, whereas co-amoxiclav (76%) and co-trimoxazole (80%) showed lower susceptibilities. One ESBL (0.5%) was found. A significantly higher proportion of female UTIs was caused by *E. coli* compared with men (72% versus 51%, $P<0.05$). *E. coli* susceptibility tended to be lower in men compared with women, although not reaching statistical significance. No changes in *E. coli* susceptibility were observed over time (all $P>0.05$). Co-amoxiclav and nitrofurantoin prescriptions increased over time (11% versus 28% and 16% versus 23% respectively, both $P<0.05$), whereas co-trimoxazole prescriptions decreased (24% versus 14%, $P<0.05$). In conclusion, given the observed gender differences in uropathogen distribution and (tendency in) *E. coli* antibiotic susceptibility, empirical male UTI treatment options should be based on surveillance studies including men only. When awaiting the culture result is clinically not possible, fluoroquinolones are advised as first-choice antibiotics for male UTIs in Dutch general practices based on current antibiotic susceptibility data. The prevalence of ESBL-producers was low and no differences were observed in antibiotic susceptibility over a 7-year period. In addition, antibiotic prescriptions changed in accordance with national guidelines during this time period.

Editor: Praveen Thumbikat, Northwestern University, United States of America

Funding: This work was supported by the Dutch Foundation of the Working Party on Antibiotic Policy (SWAB). The Dutch Sentinel GP network is supported by a grant from the Ministry of Health, Welfare and Sports (the Netherlands). The funders had no role in study design, data collection and analysis, decision to publish, or preparation of the manuscript.

Competing Interests: The authors have declared that no competing interests exist.

* E-mail: e.stobberingh@mumc.nl

Introduction

Most studies of urinary tract infections (UTIs) focus on female patients because of the higher incidence in women than in men. For this reason, most UTI guidelines are based on studies performed among women, despite the obvious genito-urinary differences [1]. Even so, it was estimated that in 2010 128,000 episodes of UTI were experienced by men in the Dutch general practice setting, representing 16 per 1000 male patients [2].

Several authors have stressed the importance that gender-stratified UTI surveillance studies should be performed, because of observed differences in antimicrobial susceptibility [3,4]. However, these studies were biased by the inclusion of selected isolates, probably after initial treatment failure leading to an overestimation of resistance [3,5].

In the Netherlands, regular surveillance studies are performed on unselected urinary isolates of both men and women to evaluate empirical treatment options in general practice, from which the female data have recently been reported [6]. With this data, we were able to assess the actual difference in *E. coli* susceptibility between male and female patients.

Furthermore, the current treatment options for male UTIs could be evaluated as stated in the guidelines of the Dutch College of General Practitioners (NHG). These are based on the presence of symptoms of tissue invasion (i.e. high fever (>38°C), chills, malaise, flank or perineal pain) with nitrofurantoin as first-choice agent and trimethoprim as second option for men without these symptoms. Male UTI with symptoms of tissue invasion should preferably be treated with co-amoxiclav followed by fluoroquinolones and co-trimoxazole as shared second-choice [7].

Also, the prevalence of extended-spectrum beta-lactamase (ESBL-) producing *E. coli* was assessed, as male gender has been identified as a risk factor for ESBL-producing Enterobacteriaceae [8].

Finally, differences in antibiotic susceptibility results over time could be determined for men, because a similar UTI surveillance study was performed between January 2003 and December 2004 [9].

Methods

Ethics statement

All data in this study were analyzed anonymously, only diagnostic specimens sent for diagnostic investigations and clinical data were used. Therefore, no consent was required from the patient and the ethics committee did not have to be approached. This is in agreement with the Medical Research Involving Human Subjects Act, the code for proper use of human tissue as formulated by the Dutch Federation of Medical Scientific Societies and the policy of the Medical Ethics Committee of the Maastricht University Medical Centre.

Patients and antibiotic prescriptions

General practices (n = 42) from the Dutch NIVEL Sentinel General Practice Network were used for the recruitment of patients. The patient population of this network is nationally representative by age, gender, region and population density [10].

From January 2009 to June 2011, GPs included male general practice patients (≥18 years of age) with symptoms of UTI, i.e. dysuria, urinary frequency and/or urgency. Catheterized patients and patients suspected of having a sexually transmitted disease were excluded. With the exception of benign prostate hypertrophy, patients were also excluded when having urological or nephrological co-morbidity, diabetes mellitus or other immunocompromising diseases.

For all eligible patients, GPs filled in a patient form including age, symptoms of tissue invasion (fever (>38°C), flank pain) (yes/no) and empirical antibiotic treatment prescribed during the patient's visit (yes/no and if yes the prescribed agent was specified).

Urine collection and processing

Patients provided a fresh-voided (midstream) urine sample, which was used to prepare a dipslide (Uriline, 56508, Biomérieux, Plainview, NY, USA) according to the manufacturer's instructions. For incubation and further microbiological analysis, dipslides were sent to the microbiological laboratory of Maastricht University Medical Centre, The Netherlands.

Bacterial growth was determined on the day of arrival and was considered positive at $\geq 10^3$ cfu/mL [11]. If no growth was observed, dipslides were incubated overnight at 37°C and assessed again. Standard microbiological methods were used for the identification of the uropathogens [12]. When more than one bacterium was cultured, only the predominant one was included in the final analysis. After isolation and identification, all bacterial strains were kept at −20°C in peptone/glycerol (30% w/v) for further testing.

Antibiotic susceptibility testing

The susceptibility of Gram-negative isolates was determined using the microdilution method for the following antibiotics: amoxicillin, co-amoxiclav, trimethoprim, co-trimoxazole, norfloxacin, ciprofloxacin and nitrofurantoin. *E. coli* ATCC 35218 and ATCC 25922 were used as control strains. Methods and susceptibility breakpoints were in accordance with the EUCAST guidelines [13].

Putative ESBL-producing *E. coli* strains were selected on the basis of resistance to co-amoxiclav [6], and confirmed by means of a combination disc diffusion test (Neo Sensitabs, Rosco Diagnostica, Denmark) with ceftazidime, cefepime and cefotaxime with and without clavulanic acid, following the guidelines of the Dutch Society of Medical Microbiology (NVMM) [14].

Comparison of E. coli susceptibility between men and women

From January 2009 to July 2009, a similar surveillance study among women suspected of UTI was performed [6]. This study was conducted by the same research group as the present study and patients were also recruited by GPs from the Dutch NIVEL Sentinel General Practice Network.

Comparison between 2004 and 2011 data

The chosen categories (uropathogens and antibiotics) and all methods, including the network of the participating GPs, were the same in both studies, except for the guidelines used for the *E. coli* susceptibility breakpoints, i.e. CLSI (2004) and EUCAST (2011). Since both studies were performed by the same research group, the original MIC values from the 2004 study were available and 2004 susceptibility data could be recalculated according to the EUCAST guidelines.

Statistical methods

For the comparison of two groups, a Pearson's Chi-square test was used for categorical variables and an independent-samples t-test for continuous variables when parametric assumptions were met. The Mantel-Haenszel extension test for trend was used to determine a trend between more than two categorical variables. The programme PSAW 18.0 for Windows was used for statistical analyses and $P<0.05$ was considered statistically significant.

Results

Patients and culture results

In total, 603 men were included with a median age of 65 years (range 18–97 years). Patients were considered eligible for analyses when data from the patient form were complete (560/603, 93%). The median age of population with complete data did not differ from the full patient population. Of these 560 patients, 137 (24%) had symptoms of tissue invasion. The median age of the populations with and without signs of tissue invasion was similar (66 years versus 64 years, respectively, $P>0.05$).

A positive culture result was found in 367 (66%) men, of whom 100 (27%) had symptoms of tissue invasion. The probability of a culture being positive increased with age, with men aged 70+ having a 3-times higher chance of a positive culture than men below the age of 50 years (Table 1).

Of all isolated uropathogens, 83% was Gram-negative with *E. coli* being most commonly found (51% of all uropathogens). Differences in uropathogen distribution per age category were not observed (Table 2).

Prevalence of antibiotic susceptibility

With respect to the preferred agents for men without signs of tissue invasion according to NHG, Gram-negatives showed a high overall susceptibility to nitrofurantoin (88%), whereas a lower susceptibility was found to trimethoprim (75%). Co-amoxiclav, the first-choice agent for men with signs of tissue invasion according to NHG, showed a relatively low antibiotic susceptibility (76%), as well as co-trimoxazole (80%). On the other hand, the fluoroquinolones (i.e. norfloxacin and ciprofloxacin) had a high susceptibility to the Gram negatives (92% and 94% respectively) (Table 3). When these Gram-negative susceptibility data were stratified according to the age categories mentioned earlier, i.e. 18–50, 51–70 and 70+ years, no differences were observed per antibiotic with age (all $P>0.05$, data not shown).

Table 1. Relationship between patient's age and culture result.

	Culture result[a]			
Age categories (years)	**Bacteriuria[b] (n = 367)**	**No bacteriuria[b] (n = 193)**	**OR (95% CI)**	**P for trend[c]**
18–50	58	56	1.0 (reference)	
51–70	152	87	1.9 (1.2–2.9)	<0.001
>70	157	44	3.8 (2.3–6.2)	

NOTE. OR = odds ratio; 95% CI = 95% confidence interval. Values are given in numbers.
[a]Culture results per age category are given in numbers.
[b]Bacteriuria is defined as the presence of $\geq 10^3$ cfu/mL on the urine dipslide.
[c]P for trend was calculated using the Mantel extension test for trend.

Antibiotic use

Empirical antibiotic treatment was prescribed to 359 patients (64%), of whom 284 (79%) were later confirmed as being culture positive. 70+ year old men had a 2-times higher chance to receive antibiotic treatment empirically compared with 18-50 year old men (OR: 2.0, 95% confidence interval: 1.2–3.2, P for trend <0.001). Fluoroquinolones showed the highest prevalence of prescription (29%), followed by co-amoxiclav (28%), nitrofurantoin (23%) and co-trimoxazole (14%).

In Figure 1 a flow chart is given based on the presence or absence of signs of tissue invasion, empirical therapy and a positive culture result. In the group with signs of tissue invasion (n = 137), co-amoxiclav was prescribed more frequently and nitrofurantoin less frequently compared with the prescriptions of the population without signs of tissue invasion (39% versus 24%, P = 0.004, and 11% versus 27%, P = 0.002, respectively).

Comparison of E. coli susceptibility between men and women

In women, *E. coli* accounted for 72% of the total isolates, compared with 51% in men (P<0.001). Except for nitrofurantoin, *E. coli* susceptibilities tended to be lower in men compared with women: amoxicillin (65% versus 66%), co-amoxiclav (84% versus 87%), trimethoprim (77% versus 81%), co-trimoxazole (78% versus 84%), fluoroquinolones (94% versus 97%) and nitrofurantoin (both 100%), without being significant for the antibiotics tested (all P>0.05).

Table 2. Distribution of isolated uropathogens per age category.

	Age category (years)			
	18–50	**51–70**	**>70**	**Total**
	(n = 58)	**(n = 152)**	**(n = 157)**	**(n = 367)**
E. coli	57	52	48	51
P. mirabilis	3	3	8	5
Klebsiella species	12	5	4	6
Non-fermenters[a]	10	9	11	10
Other Gram-negatives[b]	7	8	15	11
Enterococcus species	3	6	4	5
Other Gram-positives[c]	7	17	10	12

NOTE. Values are given in percentages.
[a]Consist of Pseudomonas and Acinetobacter species.
[b]Consist of Morganella, Citrobacter, Serratia, Pasteurella, Providentia and Enterobacter species.
[c]Consist of *Staphylococcus saprophyticus, Staphylococcus aureus* and Streptococcus species
No trends with age were observed for the given uropathogens (all P>0.05).

Comparison of 2004 and 2011 data

No differences were observed between *E. coli* antibiotic susceptibilities in the 2004 and 2011 studies (Table 4). This also applied to the prevalence of extended-spectrum beta-lactamases (ESBLs), as no ESBL-producing *E. coli* were found in 2004 and one (0.5%) in 2011 (P = 0.44).

No significant differences in *E. coli* susceptibilities (EUCAST) were observed between 2004 and 2011 study (all P>0.05)When comparing the antibiotic prescriptions between 2004 and 2011, GPs prescribed more co-amoxiclav and nitrofurantoin (11% versus 28%, P<0.001, and 16% versus 23%, P = 0.023, respectively) and less co-trimoxazole (24% versus 14%, P = 0.002) in 2011. For fluoroquinolones, amoxicillin and trimethoprim the prevalence of prescription was similar in the two studies (33% versus 29%, 2% versus 3% and 2% versus 1% respectively).

Discussion

In this study of UTIs in Dutch general practice, differences were observed between men and women regarding the distribution of uropathogens, and uropathogenic *E. coli* susceptibilities tended to be lower among men compared with women. For male UTIs, fluoroquinolones showed the highest prevalence of susceptibility to isolated Gram-negative uropathogens, followed by nitrofurantoin. ESBL-producing *E. coli* prevalence was low and no differences in *E. coli* susceptibility were observed over a 7-year period.

The important feature of this study is the participation of general practices from the NIVEL Sentinel General Practice Network. This network has a nationally representative patient population, making it possible to generalize our conclusions to the whole Dutch outpatient population. Moreover, to our knowledge, no other study has been able to include over 600 unselected urinary samples from men suspected of UTI in an outpatient setting.

The fact that no susceptibilities were determined for Gram-positive bacteria could be seen as a limitation. However, empirical treatment for uncomplicated female UTIs is often primarily based on *E. coli* susceptibilities, covering 75–95% of the total spectrum of uropathogens in female UTIs [15]. The proportion of Gram-negatives in the present study is within this range, as also described by Lipski [16], thereby supporting an evidence-based empirical antibiotic choice for UTI in men.

Also, our study population could be regarded as heterogeneous with the inclusion of men aged 18+, because pathophysiology of

Table 3. Antibiotic susceptibility of Gram-negative uropathogens.

	Total (n)	Antibiotic susceptibility (%)						
Uropathogens		**AMOX**	**AMC**	**TMP**	**SXT**	**NOR**	**CIP**	**NIT**
Escherichia coli	188	65	84	77	78	93	94	100
Proteus mirabilis	18	82	100	82	88	100	100	41
Klebsiella species	21	0	83	94	100	100	100	94
Non-fermenters[a]	38	42	52	35	38	81	84	55
Other Gram-negatives[b]	39	20	49	83	89	89	97	86
All Gram-negative uropathogens	304	53	76	75	80	92	94	88

NOTE. AMOX = amoxicillin; AMC = co-amoxiclav; TMP = trimethoprim; SXT = co-trimoxazole; NOR = norfloxacin; CIP = ciprofloxacin; NIT = nitrofurantoin.[a]Consist of Pseudomonas and Acinetobacter species.[b]Consist of Morganella, Citrobacter, Serratia, Pasteurella, Providentia and Enterobacter species.

male UTI differs with age [16]. We have tried to circumvent this problem by using strict in- and exclusion criteria, in order to obtain a homogeneous sample of men suspected of UTI. Moreover, stratification of antibiotic susceptibility results showed no differences by age.

UTI in men has also been studied by Hummers-Pradier et al. and they used 10^2 and 10^5 cfu/mL as cut-off values to determine a UTI [17]. However, their prevalence of UTI (60%), using 10^2 cfu/mL as cut-off, was still lower than our prevalence. The fact that only 36% of the patients included were prescribed an antibiotic in that study and that GPs suspected a UTI in just over 50% of the included patients, suggests that their patient population was at lower risk of UTI than our population with a prescription rate of 64%. In addition, their results were derived from a relatively small patient population (n = 79), resulting in estimates with large confidence intervals. Our choice to use 10^3 cfu/mL as cut-off value for the diagnosis of male UTI was based on the European urinalysis guidelines and is supported by Lipsky et al. [11,18].

The prevalence of positive culture (66%) we found was also slightly higher than the one reported in the 2004 study (56%) [9]. The higher median age in the present study (65 versus 58 years) could explain this difference, because it is known that UTI incidence increases with age, and especially in men, due to the higher frequency of prostatic hypertrophy [16]. In the present study we could confirm this age-dependent trend for positive cultures.

Only 51% of the uropathogens causing male UTI was *E. coli* versus 72% of the UTIs in women. Moreover, uropathogenic *E. coli* susceptibilities tended to be lower in men in women, although no statistical significance was reached. The difference in these important characteristics for determining optimal empirical treatment, show that men with UTI should be considered as a specific patient category.

Given the more heterogeneous population of uropathogens that causes a UTI in men compared with women, empirical treatment should best be avoided for male UTI. When immediate treatment is necessary based on clinical judgement, our data can be used for the optimal choice of empirical treatment. Our recommendations can be applied to all men aged 18+ suspected of UTI in the Dutch GP setting, because no differences in uropathogen distribution and antibiotic susceptibility per age category were observed.

We found that fluoroquinolones showed a higher prevalence of susceptibility than co-amoxiclav, the current first-choice for men with symptoms of tissue invasion [7], and the former agents possess specific pharmacokinetic properties leading to high prostate tissue concentrations, which co-amoxiclav lacks [19–21].

The choice for EUCAST instead of CLSI guidelines had an impact on the *E. coli* susceptibility to co-amoxiclav. Using EUCAST breakpoints, the *E. coli* susceptibility to co-amoxiclav

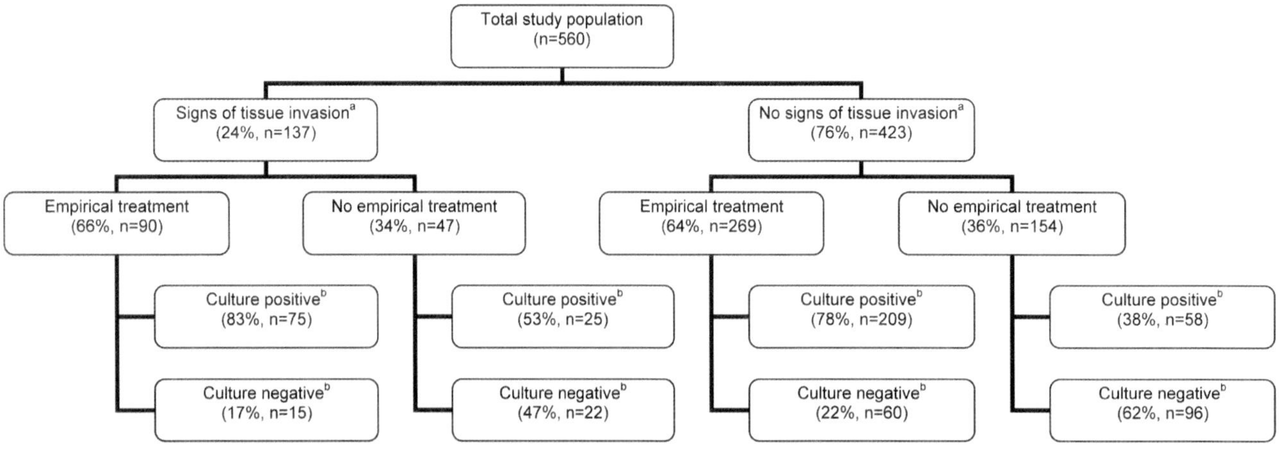

Figure 1. Patient population flow diagram based on signs of tissue invasion, empirical therapy and culture result. The denominator of the given percentage per box was derived from the number given in the box one level up.[a]Consisted of fever (>38°C) and flank pain.[b]Based on the presence of $\geq 10^3$ cfu/mL uropathogens on the urine dipslide.

Table 4. *Escherichia coli* antibiotic susceptibility between 2004 and 2011 studies according to guidelines used for susceptibility breakpoints.

	Study year		
	2004 (n = 113)		2011 (n = 188)
	CLSI	EUCAST	EUCAST
Amoxicillin	75	72	65
Co-amoxiclav	100	89	84
Trimethoprim	81	78	77
Co-trimoxazole	81	81	78
Norfloxacin	97	95	93
Ciprofloxacin	97	96	94
Nitrofurantoin	97	97	100

NOTE. Values are given in percentages.
No significant differences in *E. coli* susceptiblilities (EUCAST) were observed between 2004 and 2011 study (all P>0.05)

in 2004 decreased from 100% to 89%. The current prevalence of susceptibility of Gram-negatives to co-amoxiclav (77%) is below the proposed threshold (80%) for antibiotics to still be effective as empirical treatment for UTI [22].

Based on these findings, fluoroquinolones may be regarded as the current preferred treatment in men with tissue invasion. However, in addition to antibiotic resistance data, side effects of the drugs related to age, financial consequences and patient characteristics should be included in the choice of the preferred antibiotics.

Except for *Proteus* species and non-fermenters, high antibiotic susceptibilities (≥87%) to Gram-negatives were also found for nitrofurantoin. Similar results were described by Guay [23]. Despite this high prevalence of susceptibility, clinical trials on the effectiveness of nitrofurantoin for male UTIs are currently lacking. Since nitrofurantoin does not reach therapeutic concentrations in prostatic tissue [21], differentiation between cystitis with and without prostatitis is important. So far, no symptoms have been found that allow a conclusive differentiation between these two conditions [24]. The Dutch GP guidelines have based their treatment choices on the presence or absence of so-called 'symptoms of tissue invasion', although no reference was given. Results from future trials would support evidence-based treatment of UTI in men and could help to restrict the use of fluoroquinolones, thereby limiting the chance of the development of antibiotic resistance to this antibiotic group. In this perspective, also the value of fosfomycin for male UTIs needs exploration [25].

For male UTIs, second-choice agents (i.e. fluoroquinolones) were still prescribed most, although overall compliance with national guidelines improved in comparison with prescription data from 2004. This was shown by an increase in co-amoxiclav and nitrofurantoin prescriptions, the first-choice agents for men with and without symptoms of tissue invasion respectively.

In the surveillance study on female UTIs in Dutch general practices, *E. coli* susceptibilities from 2004 and 2009 were compared, and also no differences in time trend were observed [6]. Several other studies, including urinary samples from men and women, have reported an increased resistance over time among isolates from an outpatient setting [26,27]. Our regular surveillance studies, the results of which are implemented in clinical practice by including them in the update of the national GP guidelines, appear to have contributed to the control of antibiotic resistance in Dutch general practices. The low prevalence of ESBL-producing *E. coli* is in accordance with these findings.

In conclusion, among unselected *E. coli* originating from Dutch male GP patients suspected of UTI, the prevalence of ESBL-producers was low and no differences were observed in antibiotic susceptibility over a 7-year period. In addition, antibiotic prescriptions changed in accordance with national guidelines during this time period. For male UTIs in Dutch general practice, fluoroquinolones may be regarded as the best treatment option on the basis of current susceptibility data. Differences in uropathogen distribution, together with the tendency of a lower *E. coli* antibiotic susceptibility in men versus women, make it necessary to base male UTI treatment recommendations on UTI studies performed among men only.

Acknowledgments

We thank all participating GPs and their patients. Without their help this study could not have been conducted. In addition, we would like to acknowledge Christel Driessen, Mayk Lucchesi, Jacqueline Maes and Jacqueline Peeters for their excellent help with the performance of the microbiological analyses.

Author Contributions

Conceived and designed the experiments: GD ES. Performed the experiments: CH. Analyzed the data: CH JP. Wrote the paper: CH JP GD CB ES.

References

1. Koeijers JJ, Kessels AG, Nys S, Bartelds A, Donker G, et al. (2007) Evaluation of the nitrite and leukocyte esterase activity tests for the diagnosis of acute symptomatic urinary tract infection in men. Clin Infect Dis 45: 894–896.
2. Donker GA Continuous Morbidity Registration Sentinel General Practice Network. Annual Report 2010. NIVEL, , Utrecht. Available: www.nivel.nl/peilstations.
3. Rocha JL, Tuon FF, Johnson JR (2012) Sex, drugs, bugs, and age: rational selection of empirical therapy for outpatient urinary tract infection in an era of extensive antimicrobial resistance. Braz J Infect Dis 16: 115–121.
4. Bean DC, Krahe D, Wareham DW (2008) Antimicrobial resistance in community and nosocomial Escherichia coli urinary tract isolates, London 2005–2006. Ann Clin Microbiol Antimicrob 7: 13.
5. Critchley IA, Karlowsky JA (2004) Optimal use of antibiotic resistance surveillance systems. Clin Microbiol Infect 10: 502–511.
6. den Heijer CD, Donker GA, Maes J, Stobberingh EE (2010) Antibiotic susceptibility of unselected uropathogenic Escherichia coli from female Dutch general practice patients: a comparison of two surveys with a 5 year interval. J Antimicrob Chemother 65: 2128–2133.
7. van Pinxteren B, van Vliet SM, Wiersma TJ, Goudswaard AN (2006) [Summary of the practice guideline 'Urinary-tract infections' (second revision) from the Dutch College of General Practitioners]. Ned Tijdschr Geneeskd 150: 718–722.
8. Ben-Ami R, Rodriguez-Bano J, Arslan H, Pitout JD, Quentin C, et al. (2009) A multinational survey of risk factors for infection with extended-spectrum beta-lactamase-producing enterobacteriaceae in nonhospitalized patients. Clin Infect Dis 49: 682–690.
9. Koeijers JJ, Verbon A, Kessels AG, Bartelds A, Donkers G, et al. (2010) Urinary tract infection in male general practice patients: uropathogens and antibiotic susceptibility. Urology 76: 336–340.
10. Donker GA (2010) Continuous morbidity registration at Dutch sentinel stations, 2008. Utrecht: Netherlands Institute for Health Services Research (NIVEL).
11. Lipsky BA, Ireton RC, Fihn SD, Hackett R, Berger RE (1987) Diagnosis of bacteriuria in men: specimen collection and culture interpretation. J Infect Dis 155: 847–854.
12. Isenberg HD (1998) Essential procedures for clinical microbiology. Washington, D.C.: ASM Press. xv, 838 p. p.
13. European Committee for Antimicrobial Susceptibility Testing (EUCAST) of the European Society of Clinical Microbiology and Infectious Diseases (ESCMID)

(2000) EUCAST Definitive Document E.DEF 3.1, June 2000: Determination of minimum inhibitory concentrations (MICs) of antibacterial agents by agar dilution. Clin Microbiol Infect 6: 509-515.
14. NVMM *NVMM-richtlijn voor screening en confirmatie van extended-spectrum beta-lactamases(ESBL's) in Enterobacteriaceae*. Kwaliteitskoepel website. Available: http://www.kwaliteitskoepel.nl/assets/structured-files/NVMM/SCREENING+EN+CONFIRMATIE+VAN+EXTENDEDSPECTRUM+BETA-LACTAMASES+ESBLs+IN+ENTEROBACTERIACEAE.pdf Accessed: 2013 Jan 28.
15. Gupta K, Hooton TM, Naber KG, Wullt B, Colgan R, et al. (2011) International clinical practice guidelines for the treatment of acute uncomplicated cystitis and pyelonephritis in women: A 2010 update by the Infectious Diseases Society of America and the European Society for Microbiology and Infectious Diseases. Clin Infect Dis 52: e103-120.
16. Lipsky BA (1999) Prostatitis and urinary tract infection in men: what's new; what's true? Am J Med 106: 327-334.
17. Hummers-Pradier E, Ohse AM, Koch M, Heizmann WR, Kochen MM (2004) Urinary tract infection in men. Int J Clin Pharmacol Ther 42: 360-366.
18. European Confederation of Laboratory Medicine (2000) European urinalysis guidelines. Scand J Clin Lab Invest Suppl 60: 231-296.
19. Wagenlehner FM, Weidner W, Naber KG (2007) Therapy for prostatitis, with emphasis on bacterial prostatitis. Expert Opin Pharmacother 8: 1667-1674.
20. Wagenlehner FM, Naber KG (2006) Current challenges in the treatment of complicated urinary tract infections and prostatitis. Clin Microbiol Infect 12 Suppl 3: 67-80.
21. Charalabopoulos K, Karachalios G, Baltogiannis D, Charalabopoulos A, Giannakopoulos X, et al. (2003) Penetration of antimicrobial agents into the prostate. Chemotherapy 49: 269-279.
22. Gupta K, Hooton TM, Stamm WE (2001) Increasing antimicrobial resistance and the management of uncomplicated community-acquired urinary tract infections. Ann Intern Med 135: 41-50.
23. Guay DR (2001) An update on the role of nitrofurans in the management of urinary tract infections. Drugs 61: 353-364.
24. Etienne M, Chavanet P, Sibert L, Michel F, Levesque H, et al. (2008) Acute bacterial prostatitis: heterogeneity in diagnostic criteria and management. Retrospective multicentric analysis of 371 patients diagnosed with acute prostatitis. BMC Infect Dis 8: 12.
25. Falagas ME, Vouloumanou EK, Togias AG, Karadima M, Kapaskelis AM, et al. (2010) Fosfomycin versus other antibiotics for the treatment of cystitis: a meta-analysis of randomized controlled trials. J Antimicrob Chemother 65: 1862-1877.
26. Yilmaz N, Agus N, Yurtsever SG, Pullukcu H, Gulay Z, et al. (2009) Prevalence and antimicrobial susceptibility of Escherichia coli in outpatient urinary isolates in Izmir, Turkey. Med Sci Monit 15: PI61-65.
27. Zhanel GG, Hisanaga TL, Laing NM, DeCorby MR, Nichol KA, et al. (2005) Antibiotic resistance in outpatient urinary isolates: final results from the North American Urinary Tract Infection Collaborative Alliance (NAUTICA). Int J Antimicrob Agents 26: 380-388.

7

The CTX-M-15-Producing *Escherichia coli* Clone O25b: H4-ST131 Has High Intestine Colonization and Urinary Tract Infection Abilities

Sophie Vimont[1,2]*, Anders Boyd[2,3], Alexandre Bleibtreu[4,5], Marcelle Bens[4,6], Jean-Michel Goujon[7], Louis Garry[4,5], Olivier Clermont[4,5], Erick Denamur[4,5], Guillaume Arlet[1,2], Alain Vandewalle[4,6]

1 AP-HP, Hôpitaux Universitaires Est Parisien - site Tenon, Service de Bactériologie, Paris, France, **2** Université Paris 6 - Pierre et Marie Curie, Paris, France, **3** INSERM U707, Paris, France, **4** Université Paris Diderot, Sorbonne Paris Cité, Paris, France, **5** INSERM U722, Paris, France, **6** INSERM U773, Paris, France, **7** Unité de Pathologie Ultrastructurale et Expérimentale, Centre Hospitalier et Université de Poitiers; Université de Poitiers, Poitiers, France

Abstract

Increasing numbers of pyelonephritis-associated uropathogenic *Escherichia coli* (UPEC) are exhibiting high resistance to antibiotic therapy. They include a particular clonal group, the CTX-M-15-producing O25b:H4-ST131 clone, which has been shown to have a high dissemination potential. Here we show that a representative isolate of this *E. coli* clone, referred to as TN03, has enhanced metabolic capacities, acts as a potent intestine- colonizing strain, and displays the typical features of UPEC strains. In a modified streptomycin-treated mouse model of intestinal colonization where streptomycin was stopped 5 days before inoculation, we show that TN03 outcompetes the commensal *E. coli* strains K-12 MG1655, IAI1, and ED1a at days 1 and 7. Using an experimental model of ascending UTI in C3H/HeN mice, we then show that TN03 colonized the urinary tract. One week after the transurethral inoculation of the TN03 isolates, the bacterial loads in the bladder and kidneys were significantly greater than those of two other UPEC strains (CFT073 and HT7) belonging to the same B2 phylogenetic group. The differences in bacterial loads did not seem to be directly linked to differences in the inflammatory response, since the intrarenal expression of chemokines and cytokines and the number of polymorphonuclear neutrophils attracted to the site of inflammation was the same in kidneys colonized by TN03, CFT073, or HT7. Lastly, we show that *in vitro* TN03 has a high maximum growth rate in both complex (Luria-Bertani and human urine) and minimum media. In conclusion, our findings indicate that TN03 is a potent UPEC strain that colonizes the intestinal tract and may persist in the kidneys of infected hosts.

Editor: Ulrich Dobrindt, University of Würzburg, Germany

Funding: This work was funded in part by a grant from the French National Research Agency under reference ANR-08-MIE-030 (to GA, and AV). AV was in receipt of a "Contrat Hospitalier de Recherche Translationnelle" (CHRP, INSERM-APHP, 2010). A.B. was supported by a "Bourse Médico-Scientifique" from the "Fondation pour la Recherche Médicale". The funders had no role in study design, data collection and analysis, decision to publish, or preparation of the manuscript.

Competing Interests: The authors have declared that no competing interests exist.

* E-mail: sophie.vimont@tnn.aphp.fr

Introduction

Urinary tract infections (UTIs) are one of the bacterial infections that most often affect children, young adults, and also renal transplanted patients. UTIs are mainly due to uropathogenic *Escherichia coli* (UPEC), which are becoming more resistant, thus hampering the therapeutic management of UTI.

E. coli is a ubiquitous human pathogen responsible for both community- and hospital-acquired infections. Over the past five decades, scientists have witnessed increasing antimicrobial resistance in the community setting. Initially, resistance was previously limited to certain specific antibiotics, such as ampicillin or trimethoprim [1], but recently the horizon of resistance has expanded, with the emergence of broad resistance to large families agents. In particular, plasmid-mediated extended-spectrum ß-lactamases (ESBLs), have become prominent in the community [2][3]. Unfortunately, in addition to being resistant to most-ß-lactam antibiotics, ESBL producers are also often resistant to aminoglycosides and fluoroquinolones. Over the last decade, the CTX-M enzymes, have gradually replaced the classical TEM and SHV-type ESBLs in many countries [4,5] and have gained worldwide attention. In 2008, two research groups, analyzing the population of *E. coli* ESBL-producing strains, described a particular CTX-M-15-producing clonal group. This clone occurred in both in-patients and out-patients worldwide, strongly suggesting that it is widely disseminated [6,7], which constitutes a major health problem [8,9]. Indeed, such bacterial resistance frequently delays the establishment of appropriate therapy [10], leading to higher costs and increased use of the "last resort" antimicrobials (i.e. carbapenems) [5]. This clone, which exhibits an O25b:H4 serotype, belongs to phylogenetic group B2 and sequence type (ST) 131 [7,11]. Interestingly, several studies have confirmed the worldwide prevalence of this *E. coli* with the ST131 sequence type harboring a broad range of resistance genes on a transferable plasmid, mostly from the CTX-M family, and virulence genes [12]. This ST131 sequence type has also been detected in companion animals, non-companion animals, and food [12].

The clinical spectrum of disease induced by ST131 *E. coli* is similar to that for other *E. coli*. UTIs predominate, ranging from uncomplicated cystitis to life threatening sepsis. As this clone is mainly isolated from UTI, we determined the ability of a representative isolate of the O25b:H4 ST131 CTX-M-15 *E. coli* clone, known as the TN03 strain [11,13,14], first to colonize the intestine and then to infect the kidney using experimental mouse models in order to gain insights into its evolutionary success.

Results and Discussion

The TN03 strain is a potent colonizer of the intestine

Infection of the urinary tract presumably begins with the colonization of the bowel by a uropathogenic strain [15], as suggested by the fact that the UPEC isolates present in infected urine are almost always detectable in the host's fecal flora at the time of presentation [16]. We therefore determined the ability of *E. coli* strain TN03 to colonize the gut using a mouse model of competition for intestinal colonization. A classical streptomycin-treated mouse model is usually used [17], because *E. coli* colonization cannot be studied experimentally in conventional animals due to colonization resistance. Streptomycin is used in this case to eliminate the natural coliform intestinal population and allows *E. coli* to colonize. Indeed, such experiments require an animal model with open niches where *E. coli* can colonize in relatively high numbers, but must also have a dense and diverse anaerobic community that matches the native microbiota of the conventional animal as closely as possible. In our case, however, the TN03 strain is resistant to streptomycin in contrast to all its other experimental competitors. Although, *in-vitro* streptomycin competitor mutants could have been used, these mutations could have been a burden on the fitness of the strains, which would have introduced bias into the experiment. We decided to modify slightly the classical protocol. Six-week-old CD1 female mice were pre-treated with streptomycin (5 g/liter) during five days in order to create the appropriate conditions for colonization. Streptomycin administration was then stopped five days before inoculation, thus avoiding bias linked to antibiotic pressure. Natural coliform removal efficiency was checked just before bacterial inoculation. The absence of residual streptomycin in the stools was assessed by a microbiological assay (data not shown). Mice were given 10^6 of each *E. coli* strain *per os*: the TN03 bacteria, or one of three commensal strains, belonging to different phylogenetic groups: the K-12 MG1655 [18], IAI1 and ED1a strains [19] from phylogenetic groups A, B1 and B2, respectively (Table 1), to check the individual capacities of each strain to colonize the mouse intestinal tract. The sizes of bacterial populations in the intestine were evaluated at days 1 and 7 following administration. All individual strains colonized the mouse intestine at levels ranging from 10^4 to 10^9 bacteria/g feces at day 1, and from 10^3 to 10^9 bacteria/g feces at day 7, with no difference being found between the strains (data not shown). The observed intra-strain variability can be attributed to the variability of the natural mouse microbiota in the absence of streptomycin treatment. To circumvent this variability, we decided to evaluate the competition capacities of the pathogenic *E. coli* TN03 isolate. To do this, the bacteria were mixed in a 1:1 ratio of TN03 with commensal *E. coli* K-12 MG1655, IAI1, or ED1a bacteria. 10^6 of this bacterial mix was then administered *per os* to the mice as described above, The sizes of the bacterial populations in the intestine were evaluated at days 1, 2, 4 and 7 following inoculation. They tended to decrease slowly over time (data not shown). A competitive index (CI) which could be used to compare the colonization success of the different strains was calculated as previously described [20]. Analysis of the CI showed that the TN03 *E. coli* strain had outcompeted all of the commensal *E. coli* strains. Significant differences between TN03 with K-12 MG1655 or ED1a as a competitor ($CI_{MG\text{-}D1} = 7.87$, $p = 0.007$, $CI_{ED\text{-}D1} = 2.86$, $p = 0.03$) were already detected day 1 post-bacterial administration, and persisted between TN03 with K-12 MG1655 ($CI_{MG\text{-}D7} = 7.25$, $p = 0.005$) at day 7 post-bacterial administration (Fig. 1). It is worth noting that all the competitors did not react equally strongly, and that it was easier for TN03 to compete with K-12 MG1655 or ED1a than with IAI1, although TN03 was always the most effective. These data attested that the TN03 strain has a high capability to colonize the intestine rapidly, for a period of at least one week, despite the presence of competitors.

Metabolic capacities of the TN03 strain

In order to better understand the capacity of this strain to colonize the intestinal tract, we first checked for potential production of bacteriocins by TN03. These antimicrobial peptides are widespread among the Bacteria and Archaea and are active against other bacteria, whether of the same species or across genera [21]. TN03 strain of *E. coli* was spotted onto a layer of *E. coli* K-12 MG1655 spread on a mitomycin plate and incubated for 18 h at 37°C. No halo was visible around the spot, indicating that no colicin (or phage) was present. Moreover, TN03 appears to be devoid of the *iroN* gene [11] (Table 1), which is associated with the main microcin genes (*micH47* and *micV*) [22]. Given these negative results, we then checked whether the TN03 strain had better metabolic capacities than the other strains. This experiment was based on the hypothesis that *E. coli* is probably a highly successful competitor in the mammalian colon, because it exploits its ability to utilize the available nutrients more efficiently than other resident species [15]. We therefore studied the bacterial metabolic capacities of the TN03 strain by measuring its maximal growth rate (MGR) under three culture conditions using Luria Bertani (LB) broth, a rich medium, and two minimum media: a minimum medium containing gluconate (MMGluconate), as gluconate has been reported to be a major carbon source in the intestine [23], and a minimum medium containing glucose (MMGlc). Indeed, in addition to the capacity of TN03 to colonize the bowel, the question arises as to whether the TN03 strains exhibit better metabolic capacities than other UPEC strains. We therefore compared the metabolic capacity of TN03 to that of the non-pathogenic K-12 MG1655 strain and two B2-UPEC strains, *i.e.* CFT073 [24] and HT7 [25]. All the strains studied were precultured in the corresponding medium for 24 h with constant stirring. They were each then inoculated into the appropriate medium into plates containing 96 flat-bottomed wells. OD_{600} was measured every 5 minutes in order to determine the growth over a period of 24 hours. Interestingly, the TN03 strain exhibited high *in-vitro* growth capacity in all three media tested (Fig. 2). TN03 had a greater MGR than CFT073 in LB (1.58 *vs* 1.43, p = 0.01), or MMGluconate (0.65 *vs* 0.47 $p<0.01$). TN03 also exhibited a higher MGR that the other three strains (TN03-K-12 MG1655 0.64 vs 0.55 p = 0.01; TN03-HT7 0.64 vs 0.06 p<0.01; TN03-CFT073 0.64 vs 0.31 p<0.01) when grown in MMGlc. Taken together, these data suggest that TN03 has high metabolic potential, facilitating its adaptation to different environments, and probably an enhanced ability to establish and maintain intestinal colonization, the first step of uropathogenicity. These data support the hypothesis suggested by Johnson *et al* [26] that ST131 strains may have enhanced fitness for upstream steps, including colonization.

The TN03 strain is able to infect the urinary tract for at least 7 days

After having colonized the intestinal bowel, UPEC are then able to colonize the periurethral area, and secondly colonize the lower

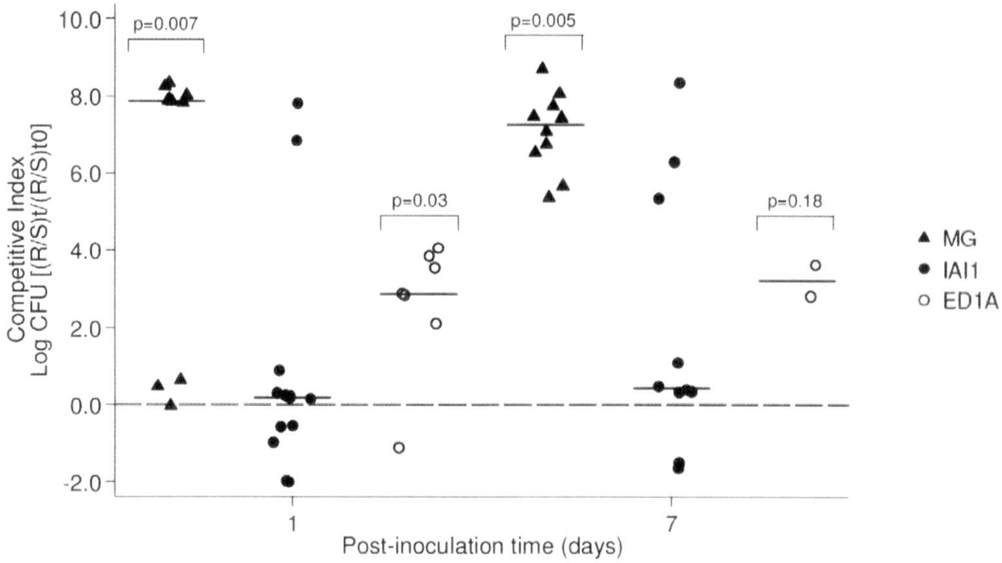

Figure 1. Intestinal colonization. Intestinal competition tests were performed in streptomycin-pre-treated CD1 mice. Competitive indexes (CIs) are given for day 1 and day 7 post-inoculation. The CI index is a ratio of ratios, in which the ratio between resistant (TN03) and sensitive (K-12 MG1655, IAI1 or ED1a) strains at post-inoculation time points is divided by this same ratio at the initial inoculation time. Horizontal bars represent median $\log_{10}$ CI ratios and compared to a ratio of null effect (0, that is $\log_{10}$ 1.0) using a Wilcoxon signed-rank test.

(*i.e.* the bladder) and the upper (*i.e.* kidneys) urinary tract. To better understand the uropathogenic abilities of the *E. coli* TN03 strain, experiments were then performed using an experimental model of ascending UTI as previously described [25,27]. Renal retrograde urinary tract infection was carried out on C3H/HeN (Lps^n) mice, which were then sacrificed at days 1, 2, and 7 post bacterial inoculation. Median $\log_{10}$ bacterial counts per bladder or per kidney were calculated and compared in the different strains at each of the post-infection time-points (days 1, 2, and 7) using a Kruskal-Wallis equality-of-populations rank test. Murine models of UTI have been established in different strains of mice with different genetic backgrounds, such as C57BL/6, CBA, FVB/NJ or different strains of C3H mice (for review see [28]). However, these strains exhibit large differences in the levels of bacterial loads in the lower and upper urinary tract and in the degree of host inflammatory response. Whereas C57BL/6 mice produce a more robust inflammatory response and resolve acute infection and bacteriuria more rapidly than the other strains, C3H background mouse strains have been reported to develop chronic UTI for up to 2 weeks post-infection [29–31]. Studies using CH3/HeN (LPS^n) mice exhibiting functional Toll-like receptor 4 (TLR4), and C3H/HeJ (LPS^d) mice exhibiting an inactivating mutation in the *tlr4* gene have demonstrated the importance of the UPEC-mediated TLR4 signaling pathway (reviewed in [32]). We also showed that different UPEC strains colonize the kidneys of C3H/HeN mice [25]. C3H/HeN mice were therefore used as a model of chronic infection to study the outcome of the early and delayed kinetics of renal colonization and renal inflammatory response caused by TN03, which were compared, as controls, to the same two B2-UPEC strains used above: CFT073 and HT7. These strains belong to B2 subgroups II (ST73) and IX (ST95), respectively, whereas TN03 belongs to subgroup I (ST131) (Table 1) [33]. As CFT073 is cytotoxic for renal tubule epithelial cells, whereas HT7 is not [25], mice were infected either with the TN03 strain or with the CFT073 or the HT7 strains. Like the UPEC CFT073 and HT7 strains [34,35], the *E. coli* TN03 strain colonized the bladder and the kidneys 24 h after retrograde inoculation. One and two days after the inoculation of UPEC, the bacterial burdens were significantly greater in the bladders from CFT073-infected mice than those from HT7- or TN03-infected mice, but no significant difference was observed in the bacterial loads at days 1 and 2 in the kidneys (Fig. 3 A and B). However, at day 7, the median value of CFU in the bladder was greater for TN03 than for HT7 (1480 *vs* 283 CFU/bladder, $p = 0.01$), and to a lesser extent, for CFT073 (Fig. 3A). In the kidneys, the median value of CFU at day 7 was significantly higher for TN03 than for HT7 (1170 *vs* 175 CFU/kidney, $p = 0.02$) or CFT073 (1170 *vs* 50 CFU/kidney, $p = 0.0009$) isolates (Fig. 3B). These data, which highlighted the better capacities of this strain to persist in the kidneys, led us to check its metabolic capacities in the urinary tract. We therefore compared the MGR of the TN03 strain, the CFT073 and HT7 UPEC strains and the K-12 MG1655 strain in urine from healthy volunteers as described above. Interestingly, the TN03 strain grew better than K-12 MG1655 (0.98 *vs* 0.81, $p = 0.03$), and to a lesser extent, better than the other UPEC strains analyzed (Fig. 2). Collectively, these findings suggest that the TN03 strain is indeed an UPEC strain, in agreement with the study of Totsika *et al.* [36] on ST131 *E. coli* strains. We showed, in addition, that the TN03 UPEC strain invades the bladder less rapidly than the CFT073 strain, but persists at higher level in the bladder and kidneys than the UPEC CFT073 and HT7 strains, one week after bacterial inoculation.

TN03 induces a low renal host inflammatory response

We next investigated the host's inflammatory response following urinary tract infection caused by TN03. For this purpose, we analyzed the levels of mRNA expression of the TNF-α cytokine and 6 pro-inflammatory cytokines, such as MIP-2, KC, IL-1β, RANTES, IL-6, and MCP-1, by real-time PCR as previously described [25] in kidneys from mice infected with TN03 using CFT073 UPEC as a control. Among the proinflammatory mediators tested, only MIP-2/CXCL2, which is a chemoattractant chemokine playing a key role in the migration of polymorphonuclear neutrophils to the site of inflammation [37,38], showed

Table 1. Main characteristics of the *E. coli* isolates used in this study.

Strain ID	K-12 MG1655	IAI1	ED1a	TN03	HT7	CFT073
Origin	Feces	Feces	Feces	Urine	Urine	Blood
Pathogenicity	Commensal	Commensal	Commensal	UTI	UTI	Urosepsis
Phylogenetic group[1]	A	B1	B2	B2	B2	B2
ST Achtman[2]	98	1128	452	131	95	73
B2 sub-group[3]	/	/	VIII	I	IX	II
O-type	O16	O8w	O81	O25b	O1	O6
Virulence factors						
Adhesins						
fimH	+	+	+	+	+	+
papC	–	–	–	–	+	+
papG	–	–	–	–	II	II
sfa/foc	–	–	–	–	–	+
hra	–	–	–	–	–	–
iha	–	–	+	+	–	+
ibeA	–	–	–	–	–	–
Toxins						
hly	–	–	–	–	–	+
sat	–	+	–	+	–	+
cnf1	–	–	–	–	–	–
Siderophores						
iroN	–	–	–	–	+	+
aer (iucC)	–	–	+	+	+	+
fyuA	–	–	+	+	+	+
irp2	–	–	+	+	+	+
ireA	–	–	+	–	+	+
Capsule						
neuC-K1	–	–	–	–	+	–
Miscellaneous						
usp	–	–	+	+	+	+
ompT	+	–	+	+	+	+
traT	–	–	–	+	+	–

[1]Determined by the triplex PCR method of Clermont *et al.* [53].
[2]According to Wirth *et al.* [55].
[3]According to Le Gall *et al.* [33].

a significantly higher level in the day-2 TN03 than day-2 CFT073 post-infected kidneys (Fig. 4). The expression level of KC/CXCL1 which also plays a key role in the neutrophils chemoattraction and the expression levels of the other pro-inflammatory mediators tested (Fig. 4), as well as the number of Ly6-G-positive neutrophils attracted to the kidneys, did not differ significantly either in the day 2 post TN03-infection kidneys versus the CFT073-infected kidneys nor in those for day 7 (data not shown). These findings suggest that TN03 causes quite similar inflammatory response compared to that induced by CFT073. Colonization of the urinary tract by UPEC induces the rapid (within the first 6–12 h) activation of proinflammatory mediators and the recruitment of the neutrophils for the efficient phagocytic killing of bacteria. Thereafter, the increase in pro-inflammatory mediators tends to return to normal levels. Given that all measurements were performed 48 h after the inoculation of UPEC, no direct conclusions could be drawn concerning the possibility that TN03 alters the inflammatory response and subsequent recruitment of neutrophils to the site of inflammation. Bacterial attachment to mucosal bladder and renal epithelial cells by fimbrial adhesins constitutes the initial step in UPEC pathogenicity. Pyelonephritis-associated UPEC strains usually express P-fimbriae, such as PapGII, which preferentially binds to the globoseries glycosphingolipids that are abundantly expressed on the surface of renal epithelial cells (see for review [39]). The attachment of fimbriated UPEC to renal epithelial cells triggers the innate host response, mediated in part by TLR4, which recognizes lipopolysaccharide [27,40–42]. The activation of TLR4 signaling stimulates the production of pro-inflammatory mediators leading to the recruitment of neutrophils and macrophages to the site of inflammation for the efficient killing of bacteria. The fact that TN03 does not express PapGII (Table 1), could suggest that the low binding capacity of TN03 to epithelial cells may favor the persistence of long-lived bacteria within the kidneys. The ability of

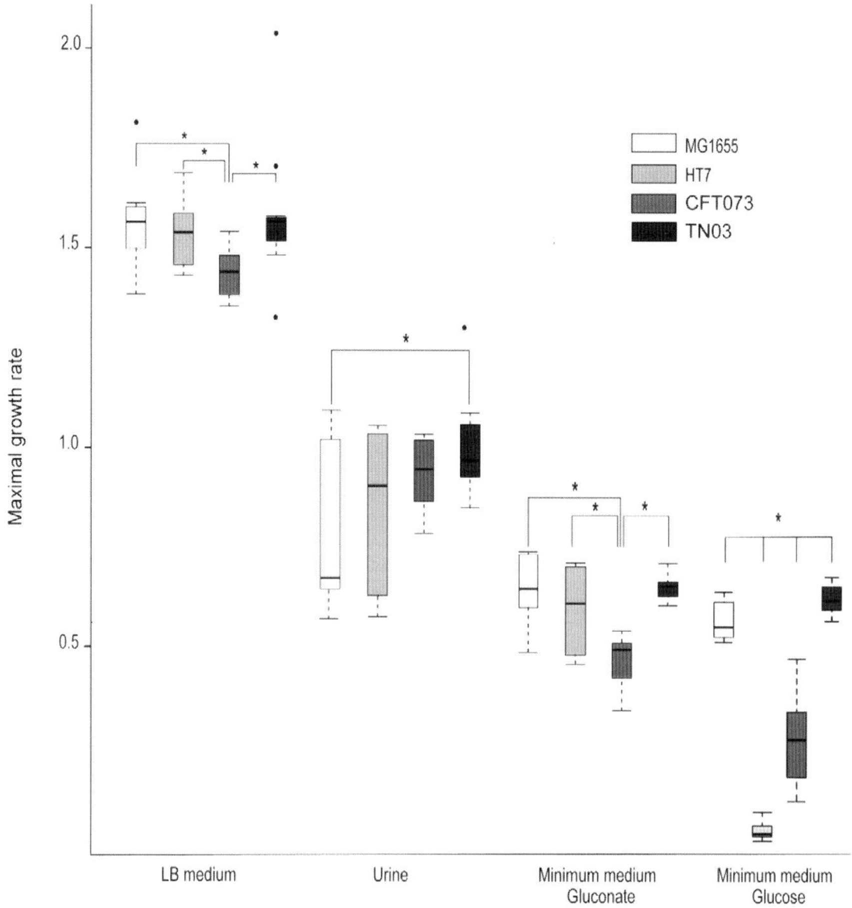

Figure 2. Maximum growth rate in four media. Four *E. coli* strains: K-12 MG1655 (white), HT7 (light grey), CFT073 (grey) and TN03 (dark grey) were grown in four different media: Luria Bertani (LB), urine, minimum medium with gluconate and minimum medium with glucose. Boxplots represent distribution of maximal growth rates (MGRs) calculated during the three repetitions of culture assays with the smooth spline function from R network. Black bars inside each boxplot represent medians. Dots located far from the box represent outliers. Links between boxplots with asterisks represent significant differences between two strains tested by Welch test for observed mean comparison. * $p<0.05$.

the UPEC TN03 strain to limit the inflammatory response and the subsequent clearance of bacteria, and to persist in the upper urinary tract without activating a significant inflammatory response calls for further studies.

Concluding remarks

Special pathogenicity traits and the prevalence of the *E. coli* strain in the fecal microbiota are both important features required for the occurrence of UTI [16]. Virulence traits and group B2 status were shown to be closely associated with the fecal abundance and dominance of *E. coli* strains and their pauciclonality – *i.e.* the fact that no more than 4 different *E. coli* clones coexist concurrently. Collectively, these various different factors contribute jointly to UTI pathogenesis, in association with other still-unidentified virulence factors and other group B2-associated characteristics. This latter may promote intestinal dominance [33], thereby increasing the probability that the subsequent steps in pathogenesis will occur. Johnson *et al* [26] also suggest that the epidemiological success of ST131 may reflect the fact that it displays greater fitness during the upstream steps involved in pathogenesis, colonization or in transmission. In this study, we suggest that the TN03 strain has higher metabolic capacities, and that these may explain its enhanced capacities to colonize and subsequently to cause infectious disease. Indeed, epidemiological studies both during UTI in 2003 [43] and on stools of healthy subjects in 2006 [44] have reported a high prevalence of the ST131 clone of *E. coli* (3% and 7%, respectively). Rogers *et al* [12] and Johnson *et al* [45] also confirmed the worldwide prevalence of ST131 harboring a broad range of virulence and resistance genes. Undoubtedly, the increasing prevalence of the ESBL not only at the hospital, but also in the community setting, suggests that this particular clone harboring ESBL is also increasing. However, further investigations are needed to define the current prevalence of this clone more precisely.

The spectrum of clinical infections caused by the ST131 clone appears broadly similar to that of other strains of *E. coli*. The urinary tract is the most common site of human infection at which *E. coli* predominates. Pitout *et al* [46] identified a greater propensity for urinary sepsis above other sites of infection in ST131 than in non-ST131 *E. coli* bacteriemia. The results from the present work suggest that the specific TN03 ST131 strain expressing CTX-M is a potent uropathogenic strain that can efficiently colonize the intestine, as a result of its greater metabolic capacities or other still-unknown factors, and subsequently infect the urinary tract, conferring on it an intrinsic evolutionary success, regardless of its selection as a result of antibiotic pressure. This TN03 clone possesses a number of virulence factors (Table 1), including the pathogenicity island HPI (*fyuA*, *irp2*), siderophores (*iutA*, *iha*), the

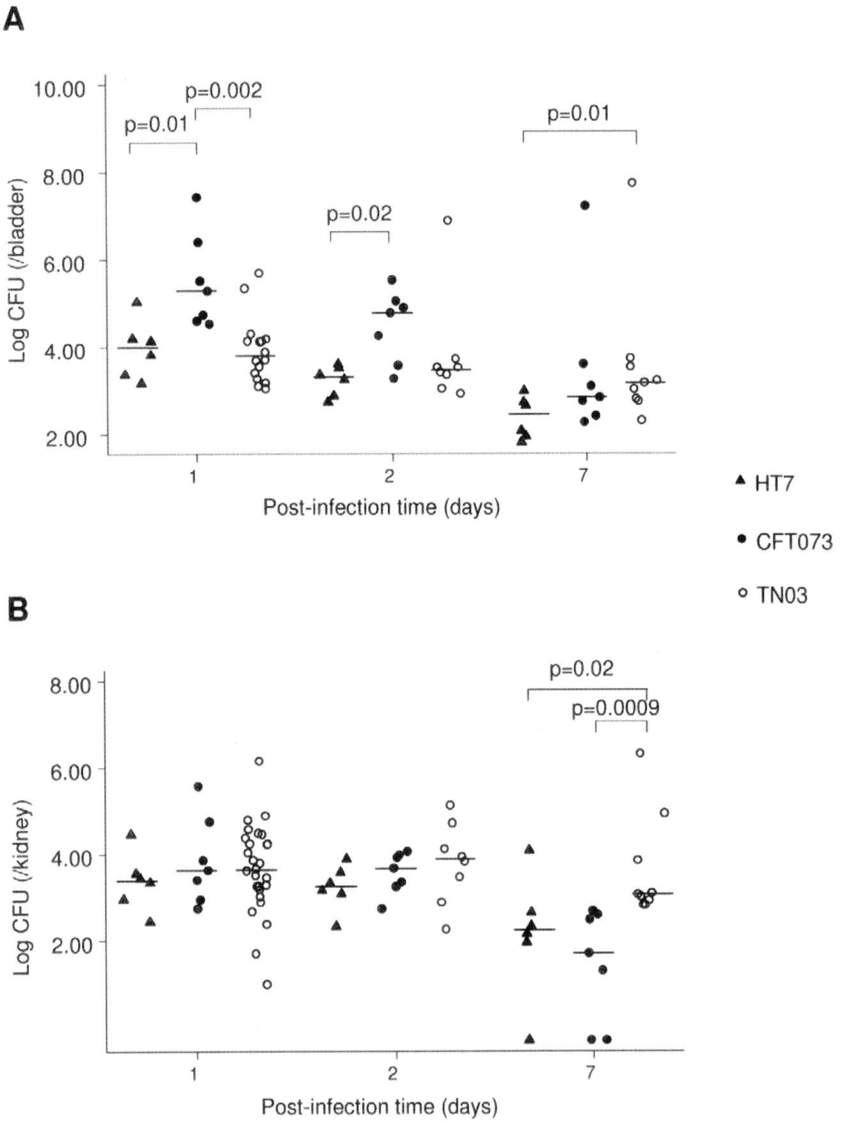

Figure 3. Experimental model of UTI. C3H/HeN mice were infected with the HT7, CFT073, or TN03 strains directly by transurethral inoculation of the bacteria (10^8 cfu in 50 µl sterile PBS). At day 1, day 2 and day 7 post infection, bladders (A) and kidneys (B) were harvested and their bacterial burdens determined. Horizontal bars represent median $\log_{10}$ bacterial counts. Statistical differences between strains at each post-infection time point were performed using the Kruskal-Wallis equality-of-populations rank test.

capacity for serum resistance (*traT*) and a capsule (*kpsE*) [47], but it does not possess the classical extraintestinal PAIs (PAI_{CFT073}, PAI II_{J96} and PAI III_{536}), which may limit the inflammatory host response and the subsequent clearance of bacteria. The group of Frimodt-Møller showed that some B2 *E. coli* strains, with a higher aggregate virulence factor genes score, are associated with persistence or relapse in recurrent UTI [48]. In this line, TN03 also has the ability to form a biofilm [11], a property which may contribute to its long-term persistence in various environments and to its resistance to antimicrobial agents or disinfectants [49].

However, our data should be balanced by the fact that we have studied only one isolate representing the ST131 clone, *i.e.* TN03, and that high genetic [45,50,51] and intrinsic virulence [26] polymorphism has been reported within isolates of this clone. More isolates clearly need to be studied.

Given the rapid emergence of the ST131 CTX-M-15 *E. coli* clone, particular attention should be paid to this particular uropathogenic strain, which expresses resistance to classical antibiotic therapy and constitutes a major health problem [8]. Our experimental data on a representative strain of the emerging O25b ST131 clone support the link between the B2 group, intestinal colonization, virulence determinants, and UTI. Further studies will be required to identify the additional factor(s) responsible for intestinal colonization and the ability of the TN03 strain to invade the urinary tract system.

Materials and Methods

Bacterial strains and growth conditions

Experiments were carried out using several different *E. coli* strains: the TN03 strain, which is a representative isolate of the O25b:H4-ST131 CTX-M-15 *E. coli* clone [11], two UPEC strains belonging to phylogenetic group B2: the CFT073 strain [24] and the HT7 strain, which was isolated from the infected urine of a

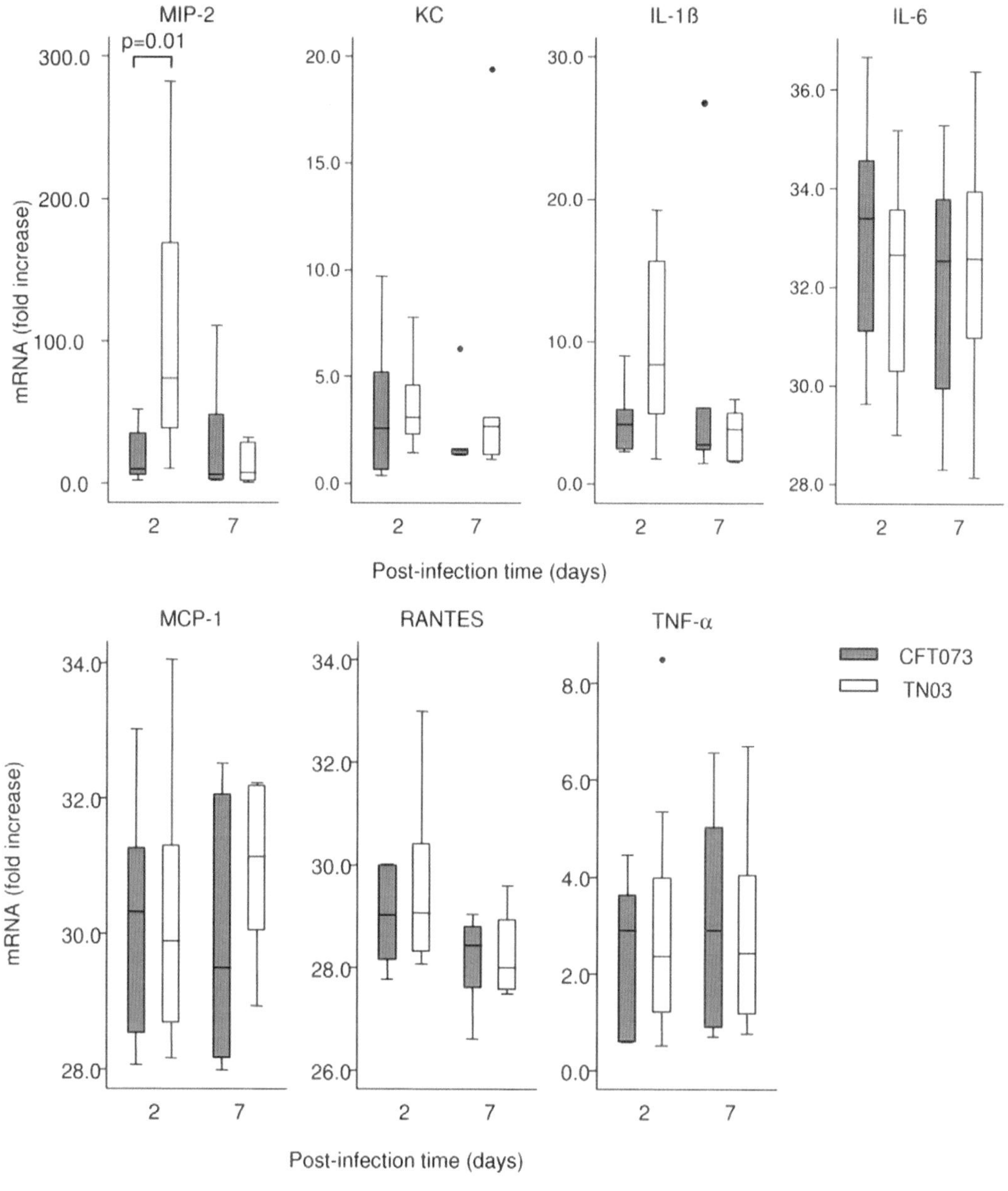

Figure 4. Expression of pro-inflammatory mediators in kidneys infected by UPEC. Expression of MIP-2, KC, IL-1ß, IL-6, MCP-1, RANTES and TNF-α in the day 2 and day 7 post-infection kidneys following the transurethral inoculation of the CFT073 and TN03 UPEC isolates. mRNA expression of each inflammatory marker was calculated using the $-\Delta\Delta CT$ method. Values are expressed as the relative fold increase in kidneys of each mRNA level of proinflammatory mediator in comparison with that measured in naive mice. Horizontal bars represent the median values. Statistical differences between the strains were determined at each time point using the Kruskal-Wallis equality-of-populations rank test.

young woman hospitalized following an episode of pyelonephritis at the Tenon hospital (Paris, France) [27,35], two commensal *E. coli* strains: IAI1 and ED1a, one from phylogenetic group B1 and the other from phylogenetic group B2, and the non-pathogenic laboratory strain *E. coli* K-12 MG1655 [18] (Table 1). When not otherwise indicated, bacteria were grown in LB broth with shaking for 18 h at 37°C.

For the comparative growth assays, strains were grown at 37°C in four different media: LB (tryptone 10 g, yeast extract 5 g, NaCl 10 g/L), minimum medium with glucose (MMGlc) 20 mM [NaH_2PO_4,1 H_2O 4.69 g, Na_2HPO_4 11.15 g/L, $(NH_4)_2SO_4$ 2.65 g/L, $MgSO_4$ 7 H_2O 0.075 g/L, KCl 3 g/L, $FeCl_3$ 0.2 ml Molar Solution 0.1%, glucose 20 mM/L], minimum medium with gluconate (MMGluconate) 20 mM (the same as the minimum medium, but with glucose instead of gluconate), and urine. Urine was collected from ten healthy male volunteers who were not taking any medication, pooled, filtered, and stored at −20°C before use. LB and urine are complex media, whereas MMGlc and MMGluconate are minimal media with only one source of carbon. The MMGluconate is used, as this sugar has been reported to be a major source of carbon in the intestine [23]. All the strains studied were grown overnight (O/N) in the three media in flasks at 37°C with constant stirring at 280 rpm. O/N cultures were prediluted at 1/100 in PBS and strains were inoculated in twelve different wells each at 1/100 in a Costar® 96 flat-bottomed well plate. Growth was recorded by an Infinite 200 Tecan®, which measured the OD_{600} in each well every 5 minutes at 37°C, while stirring for 24 hours. Growth assays were repeated 3 times. The MGR was calculated from growth curves obtained by Tecan®. OD_{600} in nm were collected and Log-transformed. Curves were calculated from a smoothed spline function. The MGR was defined as the time point at which the maximum value of the derivative of the smoothed function was observed. All MGRs were compared by strain and by medium using a Welch test.

Intestinal colonization

Six-week-old female mice (Charles River CD-1) pretreated with streptomycin were used to monitor the ability of *E. coli* strains to colonize the intestine of a mammalian host. The mice were isolated and had free access to sterile food and drinking water supplemented with streptomycin sulfate (5 g/liter) for 5 days. The mice did not receive streptomycin for 5 days before bacterial inoculation. This modification of the classical streptomycin-treated mouse colonization assay [17] permits the subsequent colonization of the mouse intestine by streptomycin-sensitive strains. The effectiveness of the antibiotic treatment against the coliform intestinal population was checked by plating a pure suspension of feces on Drigalski's selective agar medium. The absence of streptomycin was also confirmed by assaying the antibiotic in the stools. The day of inoculation, 10^6 *E. coli* bacteria were then administered in 200 µl of PBS by oral route to mice free of coliform flora, either alone or mixed at a ratio of 1:1. On days 1, 2, 4 and 7 after bacterial administration, the sizes of bacterial populations in the intestine of mice were evaluated by plating dilutions of weighed fresh feces on Drigalski's agar with or without 2 µg/ml cefotaxime. At least four mice were used in three independent experiments. As previously described [20], a competitive index (CI) was calculated. The CI index is a ratio of ratios, in which the ratio between resistant and sensitive strains at post-inoculation time points is divided by the same ratio at the initial inoculation time. All experiments were performed in accordance with the recommendations of the French Ministry of Agriculture and approved by the French Veterinary Services (accreditation number A 75-18-05).

Production of colicins and phages

Colicins and phages were detected as previously described [52]. Briefly, they were detected using an overnight (O/N) preculture suspension of *E. coli* K-12 MG1655 as a sensitive strain. K-12 MG1655 bacteria were plated on a LB agar medium containing mitomycin (25 µm/L). Then, 10 µl of an O/N culture in LB medium of each strain were spotted. After an O/N culture at 37°C, the presence of colicin (or phage) were detected for the strains surrounded by a halo reflecting an inhibition of the culture of the *E. coli* K-12 strain.

Bacterial determinants

As previously described, the strains were assigned to 1 of the 4 main *E. coli* phylogenetic groups, i.e., groups A, B1, B2, and D, using triplex PCR developed previously by Clermont et al [53]. MLST was performed by gene amplification and sequencing as in [54] and/or [55]. The B2 subgroup O-type was determined as described by Le Gall *et al* [33]. The presence of 19 virulence factors representative of identified *E. coli* extraintestinal virulence determinants were tested by PCR [56].

Murine model of ascending urinary tract infection

Renal retrograde urinary tract infection was carried out on 8-week-old female C3H/HeN (Lps^n) mice (Janvier Breeding Center, Le Genest St Isle, France), which were caged individually. Mice subjected to water restriction for 12 h were anesthetized, and then infected with various *E. coli* strains introduced (10^8 bacteria diluted in 50 µ l sterile PBS) *via* the transurethral route into the bladder as described previously [27,35]. Once the mice had recovered from anesthesia, they were provided with water for the 7 days following the bacterial inoculation. Mice were then sacrificed at days 1, 2, and 7 after bacterial inoculation, and the kidneys and bladder were aseptically removed. Two halves of one kidney were fixed or quickly frozen in liquid nitrogen, and the contralateral kidney was homogenized, diluted in sterile PBS, and plated on LB agar plates to count the number of colony forming units (CFUs). Kidney sections were stained using an anti-Ly6-G antibody (BD Biosciences France SA) to quantify the number of infiltrating neutrophils. Mice were infected either with the TN03 strain or with either the UPEC CFT073 or HT7 strain belonging to phylogenetic group B2. At least ten mice were used for each condition. The experiments were performed in accordance with the guidelines of the French Agriculture Ministry (see above).

Quantitative real time PCR

Total RNA was extracted from kidneys using the RNABle kit (Eurobio, Courtaboeuf, France), and reverse-transcribed using Moloney Murine Leukemia Virus reverse transcriptase (Invitrogen, Cergy-Pontoise, France). cDNA was subjected to real-time PCR, using a Chromo IV sequence detector (MJ Research, Waltham, MA) using mouse primers and TaqMan probes used for 6 different proinflammatory cytokines: chemokine (C-X-C motif) ligand 2 (CXCL2) also called macrophage inflammatory protein 2 α (MIP-2α), chemokine (C-X-C motif) ligand 1 (CXCL1) also called keratinocyte-derived chemokine (KC), Interleukin-1β (IL-1β), Interleukin-6 (IL-6), chemokine (C-C motif) ligand 2 (CCL2) also known as monocyte chemoattractant protein-1 (MCP-1), chemokine (C-C motif) ligand 5 (CCL5) also known as regulated upon activation normal T cell expressed and secreted (RANTES); the tumor necrosis factor-α (TNF-α) cytokine, and ß-actin as previously described earlier [25]. PCR data were reported as the relative increase, after infection, in mRNA transcripts *versus* non infected kidneys, and corrected by the levels of ß-actin mRNA, used as the internal standard. Values are the means of 6–8 separate determinations.

Statistical analysis

The values are given as medians (IQR) and, unless specified otherwise, comparisons between strains were performed using either the Wilcoxon signed-rank test or the Kruskal-Wallis equality-of-populations rank test. All statistics were computed using STATA (v10.0, College Station, TX, USA) or R (R Development Core Team, 2009, Vienna, Austria) and statistical significance was determined at a p-value of less than 0.05.

Acknowledgments

We would like to thank M.D. Kitzis for assaying the residual rate of streptomycin in the stools of the mice.

Author Contributions

Conceived and designed the experiments: SV ED GA AV. Performed the experiments: SV A. Bleibtreu MB JMG LG OC. Analyzed the data: SV A. Boyd A. Bleibtreu JMG OC ED GA AV. Contributed reagents/materials/analysis tools: MB JMG LG OC ED GA AV. Wrote the paper: SV A. Boyd JMG ED GA AV.

References

1. Gupta K, Scholes D, Stamm WE (1999) Increasing prevalence of antimicrobial resistance among uropathogens causing acute uncomplicated cystitis in women. Jama 281: 736–738.
2. Pitout JD, Nordmann P, Laupland KB, Poirel L (2005) Emergence of Enterobacteriaceae producing extended-spectrum beta-lactamases (ESBLs) in the community. J Antimicrob Chemother 56: 52–59.
3. Rodriguez-Bano J, Paterson DL (2006) A change in the epidemiology of infections due to extended-spectrum beta-lactamase-producing organisms. Clin Infect Dis 42: 935–937.
4. Paterson DL, Bonomo RA (2005) Extended-spectrum beta-lactamases: a clinical update. Clin Microbiol Rev 18: 657–686.
5. Pitout JD, Laupland KB (2008) Extended-spectrum beta-lactamase-producing Enterobacteriaceae: an emerging public-health concern. Lancet Infect Dis 8: 159–166.
6. Coque TM, Novais A, Carattoli A, Poirel L, Pitout J, et al. (2008) Dissemination of clonally related *Escherichia coli* strains expressing extended-spectrum beta-lactamase CTX-M-15. Emerg Infect Dis 14: 195–200.
7. Nicolas-Chanoine MH, Blanco J, Leflon-Guibout V, Demarty R, Alonso M P, et al. (2008) Intercontinental emergence of *Escherichia coli* clone O25:H4-ST131 producing CTX-M-15. J Antimicrob Chemother 61: 273–281.
8. Johnson JR, Johnston B, Clabots C, Kuskowski MA, Castanheira M, et al. (2010) *Escherichia coli* sequence type ST131 as the major cause of serious multidrug-resistant *E. coli* infections in the United States. Clin Infect Dis 51: 286–294.
9. Peirano G, Pitout JD (2010) Molecular epidemiology of *Escherichia coli* producing CTX-M beta-lactamases: the worldwide emergence of clone ST131 O25:H4. Int J Antimicrob Agents 35: 316–321.
10. Owens RC Jr, Johnson JR, Stogsdill P, Yarmus L, Lolans K, et al. (2011) Community Transmission in the United States of a CTX-M-15-Producing Sequence Type ST131 *Escherichia coli* Strain Resulting in Death. J Clin Microbiol 49: 3406–3408.
11. Clermont O, Lavollay M, Vimont S, Deschamps C, Forestier C, et al. (2008) The CTX-M-15-producing *Escherichia coli* diffusing clone belongs to a highly virulent B2 phylogenetic subgroup. J Antimicrob Chemother 61: 1024–1028.
12. Rogers BA, Sidjabat HE, Paterson DL (2011) *Escherichia coli* O25b-ST131: a pandemic, multiresistant, community-associated strain. J Antimicrob Chemother 66: 1–14.
13. Eckert C, Gautier V, Saladin-Allard M, Hidri N, Verdet C, et al. (2004) Dissemination of CTX-M-type beta-lactamases among clinical isolates of Enterobacteriaceae in Paris, France. Antimicrob Agents Chemother 48: 1249–1255.
14. Lavollay M, Mamlouk K, Frank T, Akpabie A, Burghoffer B, et al. (2006) Clonal dissemination of a CTX-M-15 beta-lactamase-producing *Escherichia coli* strain in the Paris area, Tunis, and Bangui. Antimicrob Agents Chemother 50: 2433–2438.
15. Kaper JB, Nataro JP, Mobley HL (2004) Pathogenic *Escherichia coli*. Nat Rev Microbiol 2: 123–140.
16. Moreno E, Andreu A, Pigrau C, Kuskowski MA, Johnson JR, et al. (2008) Relationship between *Escherichia coli* strains causing acute cystitis in women and the fecal E. coli population of the host. J Clin Microbiol 46(8): 2529–2534.
17. Myhal ML, Laux DC, Cohen PS (1982) Relative colonizing abilities of human fecal and K 12 strains of *Escherichia coli* in the large intestines of streptomycin-treated mice. Eur J Clin Microbiol 1: 186–192.
18. Blattner FR, Plunkett G3rd, Bloch CA, Perna NT, Burland V, et al. (1997) The complete genome sequence of *Escherichia coli* K-12. Science 277: 1453–1474.
19. Touchon M, Hoede C, Tenaillon O, Barbe V, Baeriswyl S, et al (2009) Organised genome dynamics in the *Escherichia coli* species results in highly diverse adaptive paths. PLoS Genet 5: e1000344.
20. Diard M, Garry L, Selva M, Mosser T, Denamur E, et al. (2010) Pathogenicity-associated islands in extraintestinal pathogenic *Escherichia coli* are fitness elements involved in intestinal colonization. J Bacteriol 192: 4885–4893.
21. Riley MA, Wertz JE (2002) Bacteriocins: evolution, ecology, and application. Annu Rev Microbiol 56: 117–137.
22. Waters VL, Crosa JH (1991) Colicin V virulence plasmids. Microbiol Rev 55: 437–450.
23. Chang DE, Smalley DJ, Tucker DL, Leatham MP, Norris WE, et al. (2004) Carbon nutrition of *Escherichia coli* in the mouse intestine. Proc Natl Acad Sci U S A 101: 7427–7432.
24. Welch RA, Burland V, Plunkett G3rd, Redford P, Roesch P, et al. (2002) Extensive mosaic structure revealed by the complete genome sequence of uropathogenic *Escherichia coli*. Proc Natl Acad Sci U S A 99: 17020–17024. Epub 2002 Dec 05.
25. Chassin C, Vimont S, Cluzeaud F, Bens M, Goujon JM, et al. (2008) TLR4 facilitates translocation of bacteria across renal collecting duct cells. J Am Soc Nephrol 19: 2364–2374.
26. Johnson JR, Porter SB, Zhanel G, Kuskowski MA, Denamur E (2012) Virulence of *Escherichia coli* clinical isolates in a murine sepsis model in relation to sequence type ST131 status, fluoroquinolone resistance, and virulence genotype. Infect Immun 80: 1554–1562.
27. Chassin C, Goujon JM, Darche S, du Merle L, Bens M, et al. (2006) Renal collecting duct epithelial cells react to pyelonephritis-associated *Escherichia coli* by activating distinct TLR4-dependent and -independent inflammatory pathways. J Immunol 177: 4773–4784.
28. Hung CS, Dodson KW, Hultgren SJ (2009) A murine model of urinary tract infection. Nat Protoc 4: 1230–1243.
29. Hopkins WJ, Gendron-Fitzpatrick A, Balish E, Uehling DT (1998) Time course and host responses to *Escherichia coli* urinary tract infection in genetically distinct mouse strains. Infect Immun 66: 2798–2802.
30. Schilling JD, Lorenz RG, Hultgren SJ (2002) Effect of trimethoprim-sulfamethoxazole on recurrent bacteriuria and bacterial persistence in mice infected with uropathogenic *Escherichia coli*. Infect Immun 70: 7042–7049.
31. Hannan TJ, Mysorekar IU, Hung CS, Isaacson-Schmid ML, Hultgren SJ (2010) Early severe inflammatory responses to uropathogenic *E. coli* predispose to chronic and recurrent urinary tract infection. PLoS Pathog 6: e1001042.
32. Song J, Abraham SN (2008) Innate and adaptive immune responses in the urinary tract. Eur J Clin Invest 38 Suppl 2: 21–28.
33. Le Gall T, Clermont O, Gouriou S, Picard B, Nassif X, et al. (2007) Extraintestinal virulence is a coincidental by-product of commensalism in B2 phylogenetic group *Escherichia coli* strains. Mol Biol Evol 24: 2373–2384.
34. Lane MC, Alteri CJ, Smith SN, Mobley HL (2007) Expression of flagella is coincident with uropathogenic *Escherichia coli* ascension to the upper urinary tract. Proc Natl Acad Sci U S A 104: 16669–16674.
35. Chassin C, Hornef MW, Bens M, Lotz M, Goujon JM, et al. (2007) Hormonal control of the renal immune response and antibacterial host defense by arginine vasopressin. J Exp Med 204: 2837–2852.
36. Totsika M, Beatson SA, Sarkar S, Phan MD, Petty NK, et al. (2011) Insights into a multidrug resistant *Escherichia coli* pathogen of the globally disseminated ST131 lineage: genome analysis and virulence mechanisms. PLoS One 6: e26578.
37. Hang L, Haraoka M, Agace WW, Leffler H, Burdick M, et al. (1999) Macrophage inflammatory protein-2 is required for neutrophil passage across the epithelial barrier of the infected urinary tract. J Immunol 162: 3037–3044.
38. Frendeus B, Godaly G, Hang L, Karpman D, Lundstedt AC, et al. (2000) Interleukin 8 receptor deficiency confers susceptibility to acute experimental pyelonephritis and may have a human counterpart. J Exp Med 192: 881–890.
39. Lane MC, Mobley HL (2007) Role of P-fimbrial-mediated adherence in pyelonephritis and persistence of uropathogenic *Escherichia coli* (UPEC) in the mammalian kidney. Kidney Int 72: 19–25.
40. Schilling JD, Martin SM, Hung CS, Lorenz RG, Hultgren SJ (2003) Toll-like receptor 4 on stromal and hematopoietic cells mediates innate resistance to uropathogenic *Escherichia coli*. Proc Natl Acad Sci U S A 100: 4203–4208.
41. Song J, Duncan MJ, Li G, Chan C, Grady R, et al. (2007) A novel TLR4-mediated signaling pathway leading to IL-6 responses in human bladder epithelial cells. PLoS Pathog 3: e60.
42. Hagberg L, Hull R, Hull S, McGhee JR, Michalek SM, et al. (1984) Difference in susceptibility to gram-negative urinary tract infection between C3H/HeJ and C3H/HeN mice. Infect Immun 46: 839–844.
43. Clermont O, Dhanji H, Upton M, Gibreel T, Fox A, et al. (2009) Rapid detection of the O25b-ST131 clone of *Escherichia coli* encompassing the CTX-M-15-producing strains. J Antimicrob Chemother 64: 274–277.
44. Leflon-Guibout V, Blanco J, Amaqdouf K, Mora A, Guize L, et al. (2008) Absence of CTX-M enzymes but high prevalence of clones, including clone ST131, among fecal *Escherichia coli* isolates from healthy subjects living in the area of Paris, France. J Clin Microbiol 46: 3900–3905.
45. Johnson JR, Nicolas-Chanoine MH, DebRoy C, Castanheira M, Robicsek A, et al. (2012) Comparison of *Escherichia coli* ST131 pulsotypes, by epidemiologic traits, 1967–2009. Emerg Infect Dis 18: 598–607.
46. Pitout JD, Gregson DB, Campbell L, Laupland KB (2009) Molecular characteristics of extended-spectrum-beta-lactamase-producing *Escherichia coli* isolates causing bacteremia in the Calgary Health Region from 2000 to 2007: emergence of clone ST131 as a cause of community-acquired infections. Antimicrob Agents Chemother 53: 2846–2851.
47. Clermont O, Olier M, Hoede C, Diancourt L, Brisse S, et al. (2011) Animal and human pathogenic *Escherichia coli* strains share common genetic backgrounds. Infect Genet Evol 11: 654–662.
48. Ejrnaes K, Stegger M, Reisner A, Ferry S, Monsen T, et al. (2011) Characteristics of *Escherichia coli* causing persistence or relapse of urinary tract infections: phylogenetic groups, virulence factors and biofilm formation. Virulence 2: 528–537.
49. Ghigo JM (2001) Natural conjugative plasmids induce bacterial biofilm development. Nature 412: 442–445.
50. Johnson JR, Urban C, Weissman SJ, Jorgensen JH, Lewis JS2nd, et al. (2012) Molecular epidemiological analysis of *Escherichia coli* sequence type ST131 (O25:H4) and blaCTX-M-15 among extended-spectrum-beta-lactamase-producing E. coli from the United States, 2000 to 2009. Antimicrob Agents Chemother 56: 2364–2370.
51. Coelho A, Mora A, Mamani R, Lopez C, Gonzalez-Lopez JJ, et al. (2011) Spread of *Escherichia coli* O25b:H4-B2-ST131 producing CTX-M-15 and SHV-12 with high virulence gene content in Barcelona (Spain). J Antimicrob Chemother 66: 517–526.
52. Lescat M, Clermont O, Woerther PL, Glodt J, Dion S, et al. (2012) Commensal *Escherichia coli* strains in Guiana reveal a high genetic diversity with host-dependant population structure. Submitted.

8

Frequent Detection of Human Adenovirus from the Lower Gastrointestinal Tract in Men Who Have Sex with Men

Marcel E. Curlin[1,2*], Meei-Li Huang[2], Xiaoyan Lu[8], Connie L. Celum[2,4,5], Jorge Sanchez[6], Stacy Selke[2], Jared M. Baeten[2,5], Richard A. Zuckerman[7], Dean D. Erdman[8], Lawrence Corey[1,2,3]

1 Fred Hutchinson Cancer Research Center, Seattle, Washington, United States of America, **2** Department of Medicine, University of Washington, Seattle, Washington, United States of America, **3** Department of Laboratory Medicine, University of Washington, Seattle, Washington, United States of America, **4** Department of Epidemiology, University of Washington, Seattle, Washington, United States of America, **5** Department of Global Health, University of Washington, Seattle, Washington, United States of America, **6** Asociación Civil Impacta Salud y Educación, Lima, Peru, **7** Division of Infectious Diseases, Dartmouth-Hitchcock Medical Center, Lebanon, New Hampshire, United States of America, **8** Centers for Disease Control and Prevention, Atlanta, Georgia, United States of America

Abstract

Background: The association between baseline seropositivity to human adenovirus (HAdV) type 5 and increased HIV acquisition in the Step HIV Vaccine Study has raised questions concerning frequency of acquired and/or persistent Adenovirus infections among adults at high risk of HIV-1 infection.

Methodology: To evaluate the frequency and pattern of HAdV shedding from the lower GI tract, we retrospectively tested rectal swabs for HAdVs in a cohort of 20 HSV-2 positive HIV-positive Peruvian men who have sex with men (MSM) undergoing rectal swabbing three times/week for 18 consecutive weeks, in a prospective study of HSV-2 suppression in HIV infection. Viral DNA was extracted and amplified using a sensitive multiplex PCR assay that detects all currently recognized HAdV types. Molecular typing of viruses was performed on selected samples by hexon gene sequencing. Baseline neutralizing antibody titers to HAdVs −5, −26, −35 and −48 were also assessed.

Principal Findings: 15/20 individuals had HAdV detected during follow up. The median frequency of HAdV detection was 30% of samples (range 2.0% to 64.7%). HAdV shedding typically occurred on consecutive days in clustered episodes lasting a median of 4 days (range 1 to 9 days) separated by periods without shedding, suggesting frequent new infections or reactivation of latent infections over time. 8 of the 15 shedders had more than one type detected in follow-up. 20 HAdV types from species B, C, and D were identified, including HAdV-5, −26 and −48, HAdV types under development as potential vaccine candidates. 14/20 subjects were seropositive for HAdV-5; 15/20 for HAdV-26; 3/20 for HAdV-35; and 2/20 for HAdV-48. HAdV shedding did not correlate with CD4 count, plasma HIV-1 viral load, or titers to HAdV-5 or HAdV-35. The sole individual with HAdV-5 shedding was HAdV-5 seropositive.

Conclusions: HAdV shedding was highly prevalent and diverse, including types presently under consideration as HIV vaccine vectors. Subclinical HAdV infection of the GI tract is common among MSM in Peru; the prevalence of HAdV in the enteric tract should be evaluated in other populations. The association between ongoing recent enteric HAdV and the immune response to recombinant HAdV vaccines should be evaluated.

Editor: Esper Georges Kallas, University of Sao Paulo, Brazil

Funding: This study was supported by a research grant from GlaxoSmithKline and NIH CFAR Clinical Research and Laboratory Core Grants AI-27757 & AI-38858, R37 AI-42528 and NIAID Grant AI-30731. The funders had no role in study design, data collection and analysis, decision to publish, or preparation of the manuscript.

Competing Interests: One author has received past research support from Glaxo-Smith Kline. The funders had no role in study design, data collection and analysis, decision to publish, or preparation of the manuscript.

* E-mail: cemarcel@u.washington.edu

Introduction

Human adenoviruses (HAdVs) are non-enveloped, moderate-sized DNA viruses that cause asymptomatic infection and clinical syndromes, including upper respiratory tract infection, conjunctivitis, gastroenteritis, infections of the urinary tract, and serious systemic infections in immunocompromised individuals [1,2]. HAdVs are grouped into seven species, A–G, and further subdivided into at least 52 known types. HAdV shedding from the lower GI tract may occur in healthy adults [3,4,5], but is more common in children (where it may represent a primary infection) [6,7,8,9], immunocompromised individuals [2], and persons with HIV infection, particularly those with symptomatic infection and low CD4 counts [3,10,11,12]. In HIV-infected individuals, HAdV shedding has been associated with lower gastrointestinal symptoms such as diarrhea and proctitis in some [3,13,14] but not all studies

[5,10,12]. However, in many cases other copathogens are also present, and it remains unclear to what extent HAdVs other than HAdV-40/41 cause symptomatic infection in the lower GI tract.

HAdVs have been widely explored as vector systems for the delivery of therapeutic and immunogenic gene products because of their ability to infect a range of mammalian host cells, their capacity to accommodate substantial genetic inserts, and their generally favorable safety profile. HAdV type 5 (HAd-5) has been most extensively investigated for applications in gene therapy. In the past ten years, recombinant HAdVs, including type 5, have also been used as vectors in the development of vaccines against several human pathogens, including human immunodeficiency virus (HIV)[15], malaria [16], influenza [17], tuberculosis [18], and Ebola virus [19].

Recent studies have indicated that pre-existing humoral immunity to HAdV-5 is associated with reduced immunogenicity to vaccination with recombinant Ad5 vaccines. In the Step Vaccine Study, a phase II test-of-concept study trial of the Merck HIV-1 gag/pol/nef vaccine, men who have sex with men (MSM) with previous exposure to HAdV-5 through natural infection appear to have had at least transiently increased risk of acquiring HIV after vaccination [15,20]. The mechanism(s) underlying this observation remain unknown, and may include a spurious association because of the small sample size of the trial, or true biological phenomena such as upregulation of HIV-susceptible target cells within mucosal tissues, and interactions between HAdV-5 immune complexes and dendritic cells resulting in enhanced T cell infection [21]. Recent studies also have demonstrated cross-reactive T cell responses to many human adenoviruses [22] (and unpublished data). These observations draw attention to the potentially important role of natural adenovirus infections in influencing responses to recombinant Ad vector vaccines, and highlight the need to more clearly define the epidemiology and virology of natural human adenovirus infections.

Several HAdV types, including HAdV-5, −26, −35 and −48 are presently under active investigation for use as novel HIV, malaria and TB vaccine vectors [16,23,24,25,26]. To evaluate whether natural HAdV infections are common in MSM at risk for HIV infection, we examined patterns of HAdV shedding from the genital and lower gastrointestinal tract and tested for preexisting neutralizing antibodies to several proposed HAdV vaccine vectors among HIV-infected MSM undergoing intensive longitudinal mucosal sampling.

Methods

Ethics Statement

The human experimentation guidelines of the US Department of Health and Human Services and the individual institutions were followed in the conduct of the clinical research. The institutional review boards of the University of Washington and the Asociación Civil Impacta Salud y Educación approved the protocol. Participants provided written informed consent and were compensated for travel and related expenses.

Study Subjects

We retrospectively examined genital and anoscopy swab samples obtained from a cohort study of twenty HIV positive MSM in Lima, Peru participating in a prospective randomized, placebo-controlled cross-over study to determine the effect of HSV-2 suppression with acyclovir (40 orally BID) on plasma HIV levels [27]. Study subjects were greater than 18 years of age, with no previous anti-retroviral history and peripheral CD4 counts >200 cells/uL. This cohort offered several advantages for the study of HAdVs; the lengthy observation period and frequent sampling of both the anal and genital areas permitted sensitive detection of short episodes of subclinical infection, and a determination of whether adenovirus infection of the genital tract was present. Because acyclovir has no known antiviral activity against HAdVs [28,29], the clinical interventions in this cohort allowed an unconfounded study of the prevalence and diversity of adenoviruses infections over time in each participant.

Clinical visits and procedures

Study subjects returned to the clinic 3 times per week for a total of 18 weeks. Swabbing of the anal and genital regions for viral pathogens was performed by two methods. Rectal mucosal swabbing was performed via anoscopy by placing a sterile Dacron-tipped plastic applicator (Puritan Medical Products, Guilford, ME) against the rectal mucosa 3 to 4 cm above the squamocolumnar junction and rotating for approximately 20 seconds. Surface swabbing of the anogenital region was performed by rubbing the swab over the glans and full length of the penis, the scrotum, perianal skin and completed by inserting the swab in the anus and rotating once (360 degrees). Rectal and anogenital swabbing was performed at each clinic visit. To characterize viral shedding between visits, anogenital swabbing was also self-performed by participants at home. Applicator tips were placed in vials containing 1.0 ml proteinase K digestion buffer (100 mM KCl, 25 mM EDTA, 10 mM Tris-HCl pH 8.0, 1% IGEPAL) and stored at −20°C until processing by the laboratory. Home swabs were maintained at room temperature until the nearest clinic visit and then stored as above.

DNA extraction and real-time PCR

DNA was extracted from 200 uL of proteinase K digestion buffer using the QIAamp 96 DNA Blood Kit (Qiagen, Inc., Valencia, CA) according to manufacturer instructions and eluted in a total of 100 uL AE buffer. Ten uL of the extract was used to amplify adenoviral DNA using a multiplex PCR assay previously validated to detect 51 recognized HAdV types [30]. The PCR assays were performed on blinded samples at the University of Washington Clinical Virology Laboratories.

Table 1. Cohort demographics and clinical data.

Demographic data	N
Median Age (range)	31 (22,44)
Gender–male (percent)	20 (100)
Median numbers of sex partners in the last month (range)	1 (0,10)
Median numbers of sex partners in the last 6 months (range)	4 (1,40)
Clinical data	**N**
Number of rectal swabs	969
Median number of rectal swabs per person (range)	49 (33,51)
Median number of positive swabs per person (range)	11 (0,33)
Median percent of positive swabs per person (range)	22.8 (0,64.7)
Median per person mean Log10 Ad copies/ml (range)	3.9 (2.5,5.1)
Baseline HIV viral load (range)	4.3 (3.4,5.1)
Median CD4/mm3 at screen (range)	406 (232, 869)
Number of patients who shed adenovirus at least once	15

Demographic, clinical and virologic data obtained from 20 MSM providing rectal swabs over 18 weeks. "Positive swabs" indicate swabs in which adenovirus was detected by real-time PCR. Baseline HIV viral load provided as $\log_{10}$ copies/ml plasma on day 1.

HAdV typing

An aliquot of DNA from all episodes of HAdV was designated for molecular typing based on nested PCR amplification and sequencing of a partial region of the HAdV hexon gene [31,32]; 116 such samples were submitted to the Centers for Disease Control and Prevention laboratory performing these assays. Predicted amino acid sequences of the hexon hypervariable regions 1–6 (corresponding to amino acid position 192–332 of HAdV type 1 [accession number AP_000512]) were aligned with HAdV prototype sequences (accession numbers DQ115407-DQ115457) using Clustal X ver. 1.83 implemented in BioEdit ver. 7.0.9.0 [33]. Phylogenetic trees were constructed using

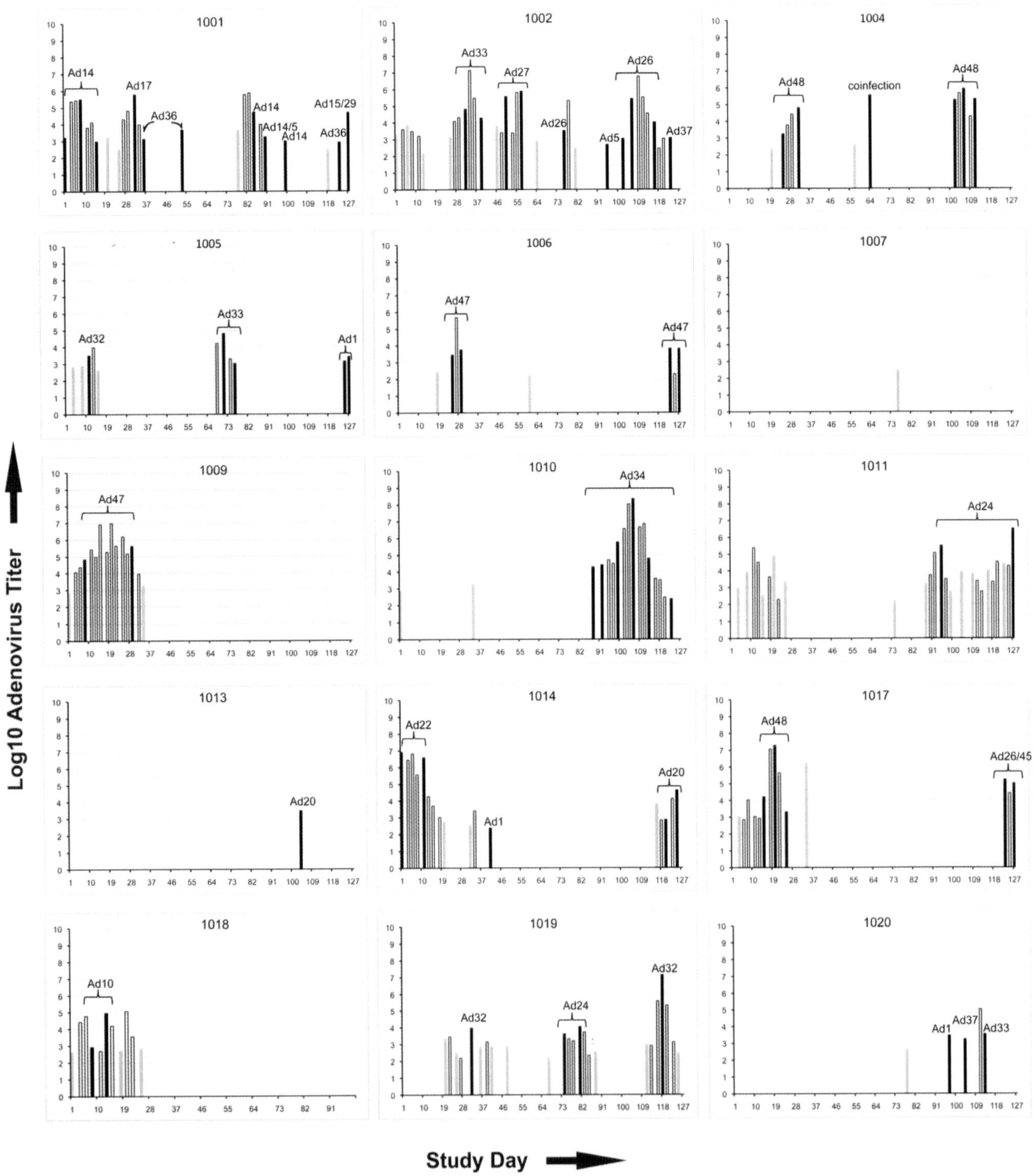

Figure 1. Adenoviral shedding by study day. Pattern of HAdV shedding from the lower gastrointestinal tract by study day. Y axis: Log_{10} HAdV titers from rectal swab material. X-axis: study day. Outlined bars: no typing attempted. Black bars: sequence-based HAdV typing performed. Gray bars: serotyping unsuccessful.

Table 2. Hexon sequence identity with nearest reference strain.

Patient ID	Study Day	Best matching Ref. strain	% aa identity score	2nd best match Ref. Strain	% aa identity score
1001	8/8/03	Ad14	91.4	Ad50	84.3
1001	8/15/03	Ad14	91.4	Ad50	84.3
1001	8/22/03	Ad14	91.4	Ad50	84.3
1001	9/8/03	Ad17	99.3	Ad26	81.6
1001	9/12/03	(Ad36)	81.8	Ad33	76.2
1001	9/29/03	(Ad36)	81.8	Ad33	76.2
1001	10/31/03	Ad14	91.4	Ad50	84.3
1001	11/5/03	Ad5	95.6	Ad6	62.5
1001	11/14/03	Ad14	91.4	Ad50	84.3
1001	12/8/03	(Ad36)	81.8	Ad33	76.2
1001	12/12/03	(Ad15/Ad29)	80.6	Ad17	80.2
1002	9/8/03	Ad33	100	Ad43	81.1
1002	9/15/03	Ad33	100	Ad43	81.1
1002	9/26/03	Ad27	99.2	Ad28	83.9
1002	10/3/03	Ad27	99.2	Ad28	83.9
1002	10/22/03	Ad26	92.5	Ad17	81.5
1002	11/10/03	Ad5	95.6	Ad6	62.5
1002	11/17/03	Ad26	92.5	Ad17	81.5
1002	11/21/03	Ad26	92.5	Ad17	81.5
1002	12/1/03	Ad26	92.5	Ad17	81.5
1002	12/8/03	Ad37	100	Ad13	94.8
1004	9/1/03	Ad48	95.3	Ad47	82.5
1004	9/8/03	Ad48	95.3	Ad47	82.5
1004	11/17/03	Ad48	100	Ad47	84.5
1004	11/21/03	Ad48	100	Ad47	84.5
1004	11/26/03	Ad48	100	Ad47	84.5
1005	8/18/03	Ad32	95.8	Ad9	72.3
1005	10/17/03	(Ad33)	83.9	Ad36	81.8
1005	10/22/03	(Ad33)	83.9	Ad36	81.8
1005	12/10/03	Ad1	100	Ad6	71.5
1005	12/12/03	Ad1	100	Ad6	71.5
1006	11/17/03	Ad47	90.6	Ad38	77.9
1006	11/21/03	Ad47	90.6	Ad38	77.9
1006	2/23/04	Ad47	90.6	Ad38	77.9
1006	2/27/04	Ad47	90.6	Ad38	77.9
1009	10/31/03	Ad47	90.6	Ad38	77.9
1009	11/21/03	Ad47	90.6	Ad38	77.9
1010	1/19/04	Ad34	100	Ad14	81.9
1010	1/23/04	Ad34	100	Ad14	81.9
1010	1/30/04	Ad34	100	Ad14	81.9
1010	2/6/04	Ad34	100	Ad14	81.9
1010	2/13/04	Ad34	100	Ad14	81.9
1010	2/23/04	Ad34	100	Ad14	81.9
1011	4/26/04	Ad24	97.9	Ad38	80.4
1011	5/28/04	Ad24	97.9	Ad38	80.4
1013	5/5/04	Ad20	95.1	Ad42	80.4
1014	1/23/04	Ad22	100	Ad48	73.8

Table 2. Cont.

Patient ID	Study Day	Best matching	% aa identity	2nd best match	% aa identity
		Ref. strain	score	Ref. Strain	score
1014	2/2/04	Ad22	100	Ad48	73.8
1014	3/3/04	Ad1	100	Ad6	71.5
1014	5/21/04	Ad20	100	Ad42	79.7
1017	3/26/04	Ad48	95.9	Ad47	82.5
1017	3/31/04	Ad48	95.9	Ad47	82.5
1017	4/5/04	Ad48	95.9	Ad47	82.5
1017	7/12/04	(Ad26)	87.7	Ad45	83.7
1017	7/16/04	(Ad26)	87.7	Ad45	83.7
1018	3/19/04	Ad10	93.2	Ad25	81.2
1018	3/24/04	Ad10	93.2	Ad25	81.2
1019	4/12/04	Ad32	95.8	Ad9	72.3
1019	5/24/04	Ad24	97.2	Ad38	80.4
1019	5/31/04	Ad24	97.2	Ad38	80.4
1019	7/7/04	Ad32	95.8	Ad9	72.3
1020	6/16/04	Ad1	100	Ad6	71.5
1020	6/23/04	Ad37	100	Ad13	94.8
1020	7/2/04	Ad33	100	Ad39/Ad43	81.1

Predicted partial-length hexon amino acid sequence identity with nearest and second nearest reference sequences, by subject ID and sample collection day for all samples with available sequence data. Sequence relatedness to reference strains is calculated based the percentage of shared amino acids at each position in an alignment of sequences. Samples with no closely matching reference strain (< 90% sequence identity to known adenoviral types) are denoted by "()", indicating possible new viral types.

neighbor-joining method in MEGA version 4.0.2 [34] and midpoint-rooted using minimum F-value optimization. Evolutionary distances were computed using the JTT matrix-based method with all positions containing alignment gaps and missing data eliminated in pair-wise sequence comparisons. For the purpose of this study, HAdVs were typed based on the reference prototype strain that showed the highest sequence identity score at ≥90% and phylogenetic association with ≥90% bootstrap support. HAdV sequences with identity scores <90% were classified by species, but not assigned a type [32,35]. Sequence submission to GenBank pending manuscript acceptance.

Serum neutralization

Neutralizing antibody titers for prototype HAdVs −5, −26, −35 and −48 were determined using a modified microneutralization assay [36]. Briefly, 50 µl of heat-inactivated serum (56°C for 30 min) was diluted 1:10 and then serially 2-fold (Eagle's minimal essential medium with 10% fetal calf serum) in 4-fold replicates in a 96-well microtiter plate. Four $TCID_{50}$ units of pretitered virus in 50 µl was added to each well and incubated for 1 h at room temperature after gentle agitation. Fifty µl of A549 cell suspension (400,000 cells/ml) was then added to each well and mixed thoroughly. After incubation for 5 days at 37°C in 5% CO2, the plate was stained with crystal violet. The neutralization titer was defined as the highest serum dilution that fully inhibited 4 $TCID_{50}$ units of virus.

Results

A total of 969 rectal swabs were obtained (Table 1). HAdV was detected in 218 samples (22.5%), and 15 of 20 (75%) individuals had HAdV detected at one or more timepoints. For 932 of the rectal samples collected, a concomitant anogenital swab was performed, and HAdV was detected in 97/932 (10.4%) of these samples. In 84/97 (86.6%) of the HAdV-positive anogenital swabs, HAdV was also detected in the corresponding rectal swab collected on the same day. Rectal swabs were also positive on 121 of the days in which no HAdV was detected in the anogenital swab. These data suggested that the source of the adenovirus was invariably the enteric tract, and therefore all further analyses were restricted to samples obtained by anoscopy.

HAdV shedding in the rectal mucosa occurred on 21.1% of days sampled (range 2.6–52.5). Mean $\log_{10}$ HAdV concentration was 4.1/ml buffer (range 2.2–8.3). The pattern of HAdV shedding in all 15 persons in whom virus shedding was detected is shown in Figure 1. Enteric infection was characterized by frequent clusters or "bursts" of shedding. HAdV concentrations in rectal swabs varied by episode, but were generally bell-shaped over each "cluster" period. Sequential infections of multiple types were documented in 9 of the 15 shedders. Median CD4 count was 406 cells/µl (range 232–869) and mean plasma HIV-1 level was 4.3 $\log_{10}$ copies/ml. CD4 count and plasma HIV-1 load did not differ between participants with and without HAdV shedding (Mann-Whitney, $p = 0.349$ and $p = 0.497$, resp.). HAdV shedding patterns did not correlate with shedding of HSV2 or cytomegalovirus (CMV), nor with use of oral acyclovir (data not shown).

Molecular typing was attempted on a representative subset of samples from each shedder, selected to cover all observed shedding episodes in this cohort (N = 116 samples). Fifty samples could not be definitively assigned to a known HAdV type due to insufficient amplified DNA for sequencing, the presence of a mixed virus infection that could not be resolved or, in a few cases, to significant differences between the sequenced strain and known reference sequences. Among the 56 positive samples successfully sequenced, numerous HAdV types distributed among species B, C, and D

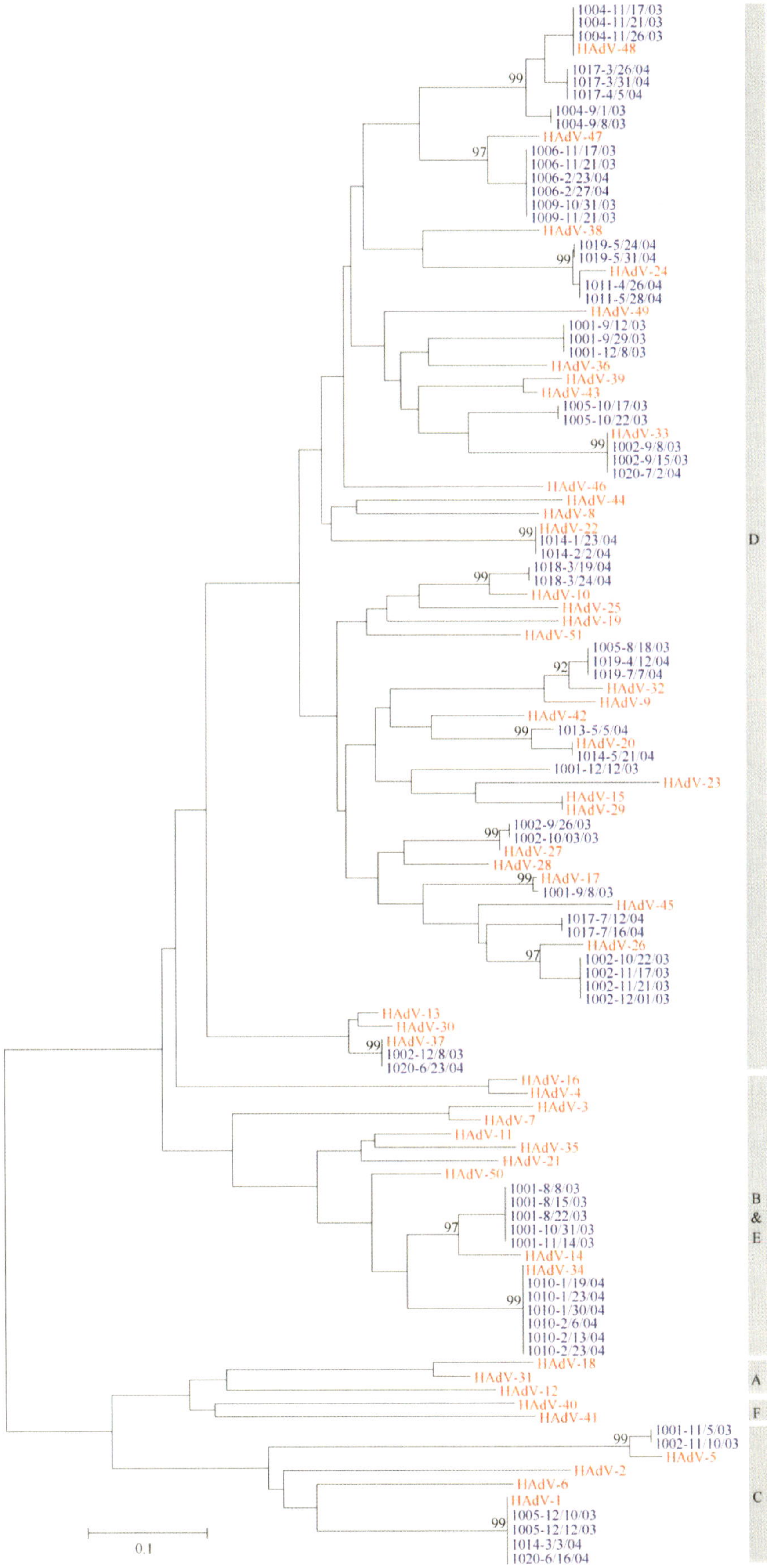
1004-11/17/03
1004-11/21/03
1004-11/26/03
HAdV-48
1017-3/26/04
1017-3/31/04
1017-4/5/04
1004-9/1/03
1004-9/8/03
HAdV-47
1006-11/17/03
1006-11/21/03
1006-2/23/04
1006-2/27/04
1009-10/31/03
1009-11/21/03
HAdV-38
1019-5/24/04
1019-5/31/04
HAdV-24
1011-4/26/04
1011-5/28/04
HAdV-49
1001-9/12/03
1001-9/29/03
1001-12/8/03
HAdV-36
HAdV-39
HAdV-43
1005-10/17/03
1005-10/22/03
HAdV-33
1002-9/8/03
1002-9/15/03
1020-7/2/04
HAdV-46
HAdV-44
HAdV-8
HAdV-22
1014-1/23/04
1014-2/2/04
1018-3/19/04
1018-3/24/04
HAdV-10
HAdV-25
HAdV-19
HAdV-51
1005-8/18/03
1019-4/12/04
1019-7/7/04
HAdV-32
HAdV-9
HAdV-42
1013-5/5/04
HAdV-20
1014-5/21/04
1001-12/12/03
HAdV-23
HAdV-15
HAdV-29
1002-9/26/03
1002-10/03/03
HAdV-27
HAdV-28
HAdV-17
1001-9/8/03
HAdV-45
1017-7/12/04
1017-7/16/04
HAdV-26
1002-10/22/03
1002-11/17/03
1002-11/21/03
1002-12/01/03
HAdV-13
HAdV-30
HAdV-37
1002-12/8/03
1020-6/23/04
HAdV-16
HAdV-4
HAdV-3
HAdV-7
HAdV-11
HAdV-35
HAdV-21
HAdV-50
1001-8/8/03
1001-8/15/03
1001-8/22/03
1001-10/31/03
1001-11/14/03
HAdV-14
HAdV-34
1010-1/19/04
1010-1/23/04
1010-1/30/04
1010-2/6/04
1010-2/13/04
1010-2/23/04
HAdV-18
HAdV-31
HAdV-12
HAdV-40
HAdV-41
1001-11/5/03
1002-11/10/03
HAdV-5
HAdV-2
HAdV-6
HAdV-1
1005-12/10/03
1005-12/12/03
1014-3/3/04
1020-6/16/04
99
97
99
99
92
99
99
99
99
97
97
99
99
99
D
B & E
A
F
C
0.1

Figure 2. Phylogenetic tree of hexon sequences and reference strains. Neighbor-joining phylogenetic tree of partial length HAdV hexon gene sequences obtained from 64 clinical samples (blue) and reference strains (red).

were identified (Table 2; Figure 2). Multiple HAdV types were detected in eight subjects, while only a single type was observed in the remaining seven individuals shedding virus. Four genetically distinct viruses were identified that had <90% predicted amino acid sequence identity with the prototype viruses, and may therefore represent new types. Three unique genetic variants of HAdV-48 were identified in two study subjects; subject 1004 shed one variant in September followed by a second variant in November, 2003 (Figure 2). The most prevalent types were HAdV-1 and −33, which were seen in three individuals. The remaining types were each seen in one or two individuals among the 15 shedders.

Baseline serum neutralizing antibodies to HAdV-5, −26, −35 and −48 were assessed in all study participants. Fourteen of 20 individuals (70%) were seropositive for HAdV-5; 15 of 20 (75%) for HAdV-26; three of 20 (15%) for HAdV-35; and 2 of 20 (10%) for HAdV-48 (Table 3).

Discussion

In this study, we examined the prevalence and shedding patterns of HAdV from the lower gastrointestinal tract of HIV-positive Peruvian MSM through intensive longitudinal sampling over 18 weeks. We observed viral shedding in 75% of study participants, who collectively yielded at least 20 different HAdV types including four potentially new types and two additional variants of type 48. Several previous studies have examined the prevalence of enteric viruses in a variety of populations [2,3,4,5,6,7,8,10,11,12,13,14,37,38,39,40,41,42,43,44]. While HAdV infections in otherwise healthy individuals generally manifest as transient infections with complete resolution, numerous studies have demonstrated the potential for these viruses to establish prolonged and/or latent infection in a variety of sites including adenoidal tissue [45], peripherally circulating mononuclear cells [46], the urinary tract [44], the conjunctiva [47], and the GI tract [9,11].

One striking difference between this report and prior studies is the remarkably high prevalence of HAdV shedding observed in our study. Earlier work has suggested shedding rates ranging from 0–4% in healthy adults and from 0–28% in selected individuals with HIV infection. In contrast, we observed shedding in 75% of study subjects. This large disparity is likely due to the detection methods employed. Few studies have utilized sensitive molecular methods and the frequent sampling entailed in this protocol; past studies have generally relied on electron microscopy, enzyme immunoassays and cytopathogenicity assays for detection of HAdVs, and employed relatively sparse sampling. In our study, HAdV shedding was episodic, occurring on only 30% of days sampled among those excreting virus at any time. It is therefore likely that many instances of viral shedding were missed in studies relying on limited sampling, due to the short duration of viral shedding episodes. We also note that in this study, we have examined HIV-positive persons who might also manifest more frequent or prolonged HAdV reactivity [11,48]. Additionally, we observed that the prevalence of positive neutralizing antibody titers to HAdV-5, HAdV-35 and HAdV-48 were consistent with several previously published reports [24,49,50,51]. However, in this cohort, the baseline seroprevalence to HAdV-26 was considerably higher than in most earlier studies, with the exception of one study reporting seroprevalence rates ranging from 12%–88% depending on the geographic region studied [51].

In this study, we have defined several previously underappreciated aspects of enteric HAdV infection, including an extremely high prevalence of viral shedding, a high rate of serological immunity to "rare" serotypes, the frequent occurrence of mixed infections, and several new adenoviral serotypes. The methods used in this study do not permit us to conclusively distinguish between incident infection, persistent infection with intermittent viral reactivation, and passive shedding of viral nucleic acids associated with latently infected cells in the absence of viral replication. However, in several subjects, the presence of discrete shedding episodes with rising and falling viral loads is highly suggestive of active replication. PCR detection of adenovirus from the enteric tract has been shown to correlate with presence of infectious virus in non-human primates and humans [52], and thus the shedding we have observed in our study is likely reflect the presence of infectious virus. Whether intermittent shedding of the same type of HAdV in several subjects over time indicates low-grade persistent infection or episodic reactivation of latent infection is unclear. We also note that individuals 1002, 1004 and 1017 shed viruses for which the corresponding baseline serologies were negative (HAdV-26, −48 and −48, respectively), suggesting that these episodes were new infections. Sequence-based typing of mixed infections is likely to only identify the predominant genotype present, and novel genetic variants are

Table 3. Baseline serum neutralizing antibody titers by subject.

Subject ID	Ad5 titer	Ad26 titer	Ad35 titer	Ad48 titer
1001	>1:80	>1:80	Neg	1:10
1002	>1:80	Neg	Neg	Neg
1003	1:80	Neg	Neg	Neg
1004	>1:80	1:20	Neg	Neg
1005	Neg	1:10	Neg	Neg
1006	>1:80	>1:80	Neg	Neg
1007	>1:80	>1:80	Neg	Neg
1008	Neg	>1:80	1:10	Neg
1009	1:80	1:10	Neg	Neg
1010	Neg	>1:80	Neg	Neg
1011	Neg	Neg	Neg	Neg
1012	1:10	>1:80	1:20	>1:80
1013	1:20	1:20	Neg	Neg
1014	Neg	>1:80	Neg	Neg
1015	1:40	Neg	Neg	Neg
1016	Neg	Neg	Neg	Neg
1017	1:20	1:40	>1:80	Neg
1018	1:40	1:40	Neg	Neg
1019	1:80	1:20	Neg	Neg
1020	1:20	1:40	Neg	Neg
% positive	70%	75%	15%	10%

Serum neutralizing antibody titers to HAdV-35, −5, −26 and −48 in each subject at beginning of study.

difficult to identify by the methods used. It is therefore likely that the true diversity of HAdV types present has been underestimated in this study.

This study is limited by modest cohort size, relatively narrow geographical sampling and by the limited serological data presently available. However, our serology results suggest that infection with "rare" HAdVs with and/or without persistent shedding may be more prevalent than previously thought [24,49,50] among certain HIV+ MSM populations, and highlight the need to further investigate the prevalence and transmission of HAdVs in sexually active MSM and other populations at high risk of acquiring sexually transmitted diseases. It is presently unknown to what extent the presence of natural adenoviral infections may interact with vaccines based on similar strains. These results must therefore also be considered in the context of vaccine development and immunization efforts using adenoviral vaccine vectors.

Acknowledgments

We thank Anya Luke-Killam for her technical editing work, and Rachel Tompa for her editorial review of the manuscript; we also gratefully acknowledge the generous contribution of the clinical staff and volunteers at the Asociación Civil Impacta Salud y Educación, Lima, Peru, without whom this study would not have been possible.

Author Contributions

Conceived and designed the experiments: MEC CC RZ DDE LC. Performed the experiments: MLH XL JS. Analyzed the data: MEC XL CC JS SS JB DDE. Wrote the paper: MEC CC JB RZ DDE LC.

References

1. Echavarria M (2008) Adenoviruses in immunocompromised hosts. Clin Microbiol Rev 21: 704–715.
2. Hierholzer JC (1992) Adenoviruses in the immunocompromised host. Clin Microbiol Rev 5: 262–274.
3. Cunningham AL, Grohman GS, Harkness J, Law C, Marriott D, et al. (1988) Gastrointestinal viral infections in homosexual men who were symptomatic and seropositive for human immunodeficiency virus. J Infect Dis 158: 386–391.
4. Buimovici-Klein E, Lange M, Ong KR, Grieco MH, Cooper LZ (1988) Virus isolation and immune studies in a cohort of homosexual men. J Med Virol 25: 371–385.
5. Durepaire N, Ranger-Rogez S, Gandji JA, Weinbreck P, Rogez JP, et al. (1995) Enteric prevalence of adenovirus in human immunodeficiency virus seropositive patients. J Med Virol 45: 56–60.
6. Cinek O, Witso E, Jeansson S, Rasmussen T, Drevinek P, et al. (2006) Longitudinal observation of enterovirus and adenovirus in stool samples from Norwegian infants with the highest genetic risk of type 1 diabetes. J Clin Virol 35: 33–40.
7. (1993) Intestinal malabsorption of HIV-infected children: relationship to diarrhoea, failure to thrive, enteric micro-organisms and immune impairment. The Italian Paediatric Intestinal/HIV Study Group. AIDS 7: 1435–1440.
8. Lew JF, Moe CL, Monroe SS, Allen JR, Harrison BM, et al. (1991) Astrovirus and adenovirus associated with diarrhea in children in day care settings. J Infect Dis 164: 673–678.
9. Hillis WD, Cooper MR, Bang FB (1973) Adenovirus infections in West Bengal. I. Persistence of viruses in infants and young children. Indian J Med Res 61: 980–988.
10. Kaljot KT, Ling JP, Gold JW, Laughon BE, Bartlett JG, et al. (1989) Prevalence of acute enteric viral pathogens in acquired immunodeficiency syndrome patients with diarrhea. Gastroenterology 97: 1031–1032.
11. Khoo SH, Bailey AS, de Jong JC, Mandal BK (1995) Adenovirus infections in human immunodeficiency virus-positive patients: clinical features and molecular epidemiology. J Infect Dis 172: 629–637.
12. Gonzalez GG, Pujol FH, Liprandi F, Deibis L, Ludert JE (1998) Prevalence of enteric viruses in human immunodeficiency virus seropositive patients in Venezuela. J Med Virol 55: 288–292.
13. Grohmann GS, Glass RI, Pereira HG, Monroe SS, Hightower AW, et al. (1993) Enteric viruses and diarrhea in HIV-infected patients. Enteric Opportunistic Infections Working Group. N Engl J Med 329: 14–20.
14. Schmidt W, Schneider T, Heise W, Weinke T, pple HJ, et al. (1996) Stool viruses, coinfections, and diarrhea in HIV-infected patients. Berlin Diarrhea/Wasting Syndrome Study Group. J Acquir Immune Defic Syndr Hum Retrovirol 13: 33–38.
15. Buchbinder SP, Mehrotra DV, Duerr A, Fitzgerald DW, Mogg R, et al. (2008) Efficacy assessment of a cell-mediated immunity HIV-1 vaccine (the Step Study): a double-blind, randomised, placebo-controlled, test-of-concept trial. Lancet 372: 1881–1893.
16. Rodriguez A, Goudsmit J, Companjen A, Mintardjo R, Gillissen G, et al. (2008) Impact of recombinant adenovirus serotype 35 priming versus boosting of a Plasmodium falciparum protein: characterization of T- and B-cell responses to liver-stage antigen 1. Infect Immun 76: 1709–1718.
17. Hoelscher MA, Garg S, Bangari DS, Belser JA, Lu X, et al. (2006) Development of adenoviral-vector-based pandemic influenza vaccine against antigenically distinct human H5N1 strains in mice. Lancet 367: 475–481.
18. Wang J, Thorson L, Stokes RW, Santosuosso M, Huygen K, et al. (2004) Single mucosal, but not parenteral, immunization with recombinant adenoviral-based vaccine provides potent protection from pulmonary tuberculosis. J Immunol 173: 6357–6365.
19. Sullivan NJ, Sanchez A, Rollin PE, Yang ZY, Nabel GJ (2000) Development of a preventive vaccine for Ebola virus infection in primates. Nature 408: 605–609.
20. Robb ML (2008) Failure of the Merck HIV vaccine: an uncertain step forward. Lancet 372: 1857–1858.
21. Perreau M, Pantaleo G, Kremer EJ (2008) Activation of a dendritic cell-T cell axis by Ad5 immune complexes creates an improved environment for replication of HIV in T cells. J Exp Med 205: 2717–2725.
22. Leen AM, Sili U, Vanin EF, Jewell AM, Xie W, et al. (2004) Conserved CTL epitopes on the adenovirus hexon protein expand subgroup cross-reactive and subgroup-specific CD8+ T cells. Blood 104: 2432–2440.
23. Lemckert AA, Sumida SM, Holterman L, Vogels R, Truitt DM, et al. (2005) Immunogenicity of heterologous prime-boost regimens involving recombinant adenovirus serotype 11 (Ad11) and Ad35 vaccine vectors in the presence of anti-ad5 immunity. J Virol 79: 9694–9701.
24. Vogels R, Zuijdgeest D, van Rijnsoever R, Hartkoorn E, Damen I, et al. (2003) Replication-deficient human adenovirus type 35 vectors for gene transfer and vaccination: efficient human cell infection and bypass of preexisting adenovirus immunity. J Virol 77: 8263–8271.
25. Radosevic K, Wieland CW, Rodriguez A, Weverling GJ, Mintardjo R, et al. (2007) Protective immune responses to a recombinant adenovirus type 35 tuberculosis vaccine in two mouse strains: CD4 and CD8 T-cell epitope mapping and role of gamma interferon. Infect Immun 75: 4105–4115.
26. Baden L, Dolin R, O'Brien K, Abbink P, La Porte A, et al. (2009) OA05-06 LB. First-in-human Phase 1 safety and immunigenicity of an adenovirus serotype 26 HIV-1 vaccine vector. Retrovirology 6: O36.
27. Zuckerman RA, Lucchetti A, Whittington WL, Sanchez J, Coombs RW, et al. (2007) Herpes simplex virus (HSV) suppression with valacyclovir reduces rectal and blood plasma HIV-1 levels in HIV-1/HSV-2-seropositive men: a randomized, double-blind, placebo-controlled crossover trial. J Infect Dis 196: 1500–1508.
28. Kurosaki K, Miwa N, Yoshida Y, Kurokawa M, Kurimoto M, et al. (2004) Therapeutic basis of vidarabine on adenovirus-induced haemorrhagic cystitis. Antivir Chem Chemother 15: 281–285.
29. Naesens L, Lenaerts L, Andrei G, Snoeck R, Van Beers D, et al. (2005) Antiadenovirus activities of several classes of nucleoside and nucleotide analogues. Antimicrob Agents Chemother 49: 1010–1016.
30. Huang ML, Nguy L, Ferrenberg J, Boeckh M, Cent A, et al. (2008) Development of multiplexed real-time quantitative polymerase chain reaction assay for detecting human adenoviruses. Diagn Microbiol Infect Dis 62: 263–271.
31. Gray GC, McCarthy T, Lebeck MG, Schnurr DP, Russell KL, et al. (2007) Genotype prevalence and risk factors for severe clinical adenovirus infection, United States 2004-2006. Clin Infect Dis 45: 1120–1131.
32. Lu X, Erdman DD (2006) Molecular typing of human adenoviruses by PCR and sequencing of a partial region of the hexon gene. Arch Virol 151: 1587–1602.
33. Hall T (1999) Bioedit: a user-friendly biological sequence alignment editor and analysis program for Windows 95/98/NT. Nucleic Acids Symposium series. pp 95–98.
34. Tamura K, Dudley J, Nei M, Kumar S (2007) MEGA4: Molecular Evolutionary Genetics Analysis (MEGA) software version 4.0. Mol Biol Evol 24: 1596–1599.
35. Ebner K, Pinsker W, Lion T (2005) Comparative sequence analysis of the hexon gene in the entire spectrum of human adenovirus serotypes: phylogenetic, taxonomic, and clinical implications. J Virol 79: 12635–12642.
36. Hierholzer JC, Bingham PG (1978) Vero microcultures for adenovirus neutralization tests. J Clin Microbiol 7: 499–506.
37. Laughon BE, Druckman DA, Vernon A, Quinn TC, Polk BF, et al. (1988) Prevalence of enteric pathogens in homosexual men with and without acquired immunodeficiency syndrome. Gastroenterology 94: 984–993.
38. Saulsbury FT, Winkelstein JA, Yolken RH (1980) Chronic rotavirus infection in immunodeficiency. J Pediatr 97: 61–65.
39. Gray JR, Rabeneck L (1989) Atypical mycobacterial infection of the gastrointestinal tract in AIDS patients. Am J Gastroenterol 84: 1521–1524.
40. Thea DM, Glass R, Grohmann GS, Perriens J, Ngoy B, et al. (1993) Prevalence of enteric viruses among hospital patients with AIDS in Kinshasa, Zaire. Trans R Soc Trop Med Hyg 87: 263–266.

41. Rodriguez-Baez N, O'Brien R, Qiu SQ, Bass DM (2002) Astrovirus, adenovirus, and rotavirus in hospitalized children: prevalence and association with gastroenteritis. J Pediatr Gastroenterol Nutr 35: 64–68.
42. Thomas PD, Pollok RC, Gazzard BG (1999) Enteric viral infections as a cause of diarrhoea in the acquired immunodeficiency syndrome. HIV Med 1: 19–24.
43. Albrecht H, Stellbrink HJ, Fenske S, Ermer M, Raedler A, et al. (1993) Rotavirus antigen detection in patients with HIV infection and diarrhea. Scand J Gastroenterol 28: 307–310.
44. Horwitz MS, Valderrama G, Hatcher V, Korn R, deJong P, et al. (1984) Characterization of adenovirus isolates from AIDS patients. Ann N Y Acad Sci 437: 161–174.
45. Evans AS (1958) Latent adenovirus infections of the human respiratory tract. Am J Hyg 67: 256–266.
46. Horvath J, Palkonyay L, Weber J (1986) Group C adenovirus DNA sequences in human lymphoid cells. J Virol 59: 189–192.
47. Kaye SB, Lloyd M, Williams H, Yuen C, Scott JA, et al. (2005) Evidence for persistence of adenovirus in the tear film a decade following conjunctivitis. J Med Virol 77: 227–231.
48. Hierholzer JC, Wigand R, Anderson LJ, Adrian T, Gold JW (1988) Adenoviruses from patients with AIDS: a plethora of serotypes and a description of five new serotypes of subgenus D (types 43-47). J Infect Dis 158: 804–813.
49. Abbink P, Lemckert AA, Ewald BA, Lynch DM, Denholtz M, et al. (2007) Comparative seroprevalence and immunogenicity of six rare serotype recombinant adenovirus vaccine vectors from subgroups B and D. J Virol 81: 4654–4663.
50. Thorner AR, Vogels R, Kaspers J, Weverling GJ, Holterman L, et al. (2006) Age dependence of adenovirus-specific neutralizing antibody titers in individuals from sub-Saharan Africa. J Clin Microbiol 44: 3781–3783.
51. Mast TC, Kierstead L, Gupta SB, Nikas AA, Kallas EG, et al. (2009) International epidemiology of human pre-existing adenovirus (Ad) type-5, type-6, type-26 and type-36 neutralizing antibodies: Correlates of high Ad5 titers and implications for potential HIV vaccine trials. Vaccine.
52. Roy S, Vandenberghe LH, Kryazhimskiy S, Grant R, Calcedo R, et al. (2009) Isolation and characterization of adenoviruses persistently shed from the gastrointestinal tract of non-human primates. PLoS Pathog 5: e1000503.

Copeptin, Procalcitonin and Routine Inflammatory Markers–Predictors of Infection after Stroke

Felix Fluri[1,2]*, Nils G. Morgenthaler[3], Beat Mueller[4], Mirjam Christ-Crain[5], Mira Katan[2,6]

1 Department of Neurology, University Hospital Basel, Basel, Switzerland, **2** Department of Neurology, University Hospital Zürich, Zürich, Switzerland, **3** Institut für Experimentelle Endokrinologie, Charité, Berlin, Germany, **4** Medical University Clinic, Cantonal Hospital Aarau, Aarau, Switzerland, **5** Department of Endocrinology, University Hospital Basel, Basel, Switzerland, **6** Columbia University, Department of Neurology, Division of Stroke, New York, New York, United States of America

Abstract

Background: Early predictors for the development of stroke-associated infection may identify patients at high risk and reduce post-stroke infection and mortality.

Methods: In 383 prospectively enrolled acute stroke patients we assessed time point and type of post-stroke infections (i.e. pneumonia, urinary tract infection (UTI) other infection (OI)). Blood samples were collected on admission, and days 1, and 3 to assess white blood cells (WBC), monocytes, C-reactive protein (CRP), procalcitonin (PCT), and copeptin. To determine the magnitude of association with the development of infections, odds ratios (OR) were calculated for each prognostic blood marker. The discriminatory ability of different predictors was assessed, by calculating area under the receiver operating characteristic curves (AUC). Prognostic models including the three parameters with the best performance were identified.

Results: Of 383 patients, 66 (17.2%) developed an infection after onset of stroke. WBC, CRP, copeptin and PCT were all independent predictors of any infection, pneumonia and UTI developed at least 24 hours after measurements. The combination of the biomarkers WBC, CRP and copeptin (AUC: 0.92) and WBC, CRP and PCT (AUC: 0.90) showed a better predictive accuracy concerning the development of pneumonia during hospitalization compared to each marker by itself (p-Wald <0.0001).

Conclusion: Among ischemic stroke patients, copeptin, PCT, WBC and CRP measured on admission were predictors of infection in general, and specifically for pneumonia and UTI within 5 days after stroke. The combination of these biomarkers improved the prediction of patients who developed an infection.

Editor: Thiruma V. Arumugam, University of Queensland, Australia

Funding: This work was supported by the Swiss National Science Foundation (PBZHP3-130982, to MK) and the Fondation Leducq (career development grant, to MK). The funding institutions had no role in study design, data collection, analysis decision to publish, or preparation of the manuscript.

Competing Interests: FF reports no disclosures. NM was employed by B.R.A.H.M.S., the manufacturer of the copeptin and procalcitonin-assays. BM, MCC and MK received payments from B.R.A.H.M.S. unrelated to this study.

* E-mail: ffluri@gmx.ch

Introduction

Infection during the first days after ischemic stroke (IS) occurs in 25–65% of patients [1,2]. Pneumonia and urinary tract infection (UTI) are the most common infectious complications after IS [3]. It has been suggested that the predominance of infections during the acute phase of stroke [1] is due to stroke-induced immunosuppression (SIS) [4]. The central nervous system modulates the activity of the immune system through complex pathways that include the hypothalamic pituitary adrenal axis (HPAA), the vagus nerve, and the sympathetic nervous system [5,6]. Several studies found an independent association between stroke-associated infections (SAI) and poor functional outcome after IS [7–9].

Therefore, early initiation of antibiotic treatments is recommended if infection is present [10]. However, gold-standard clinical diagnostics are time-consuming and delay early antibiotic therapy. Thus, accurate and simply available prognostic markers for optimal risk stratification are needed. We therefore selected C-reactive protein (CRP), white blood cells (WBC), monocytes (Mcyt), as they represent the most commonly measured and well-established inflammatory markers in clinical routine. Procalcitonin (PCT) was selected to better discriminate infections from general inflammation [11,12]. Copeptin, a reliable stress marker [13] was selected because SIS may be mediated by changes in the neuroendocrine system. All these biomarkers are available immediately due to rapid analytic procedure.

We hypothesize that these blood markers are predictive for the development of post-stroke infections. First we planned to evaluate the prognostic value of each blood biomarker to predict infections in the acute phase of IS. Second, we aimed to identify the best prognostic model consisting of a batch of the best prognostic biomarkers. Thereafter, the prognostic value of this batch was compared to that of each prognostic biomarker alone.

Patients and Methods

Ethics Statement

The study has been approved by the local Ethics Committee at the University Hospital of Basel. All participants or their representative gave written informed consent for the study.

Study Population

We performed a post-hoc analysis of a prospective cohort study [14]. All patients with IS within 72 hours before admission at the Emergency Department, University Hospital of Basel, were eligible and prospectively enrolled (11/2006–11/2007). IS was confirmed by CT and/or MRI on admission. Neurological deficits were measured at presentation with the National Institutes of Health Stroke Scale (NIHSS) score.

Definition of Stroke-associated Infections

SAI was defined as any infection occurring within the first 5 days of hospital admission [13]. Infections were diagnosed according to the criteria of the U.S. Centers for Disease Control and Prevention (CDC) [15]. We distinguished between pneumonia, urinary tract infection (UTI) and "other infections" (OI). Pneumonia was diagnosed when at least one of each of the first and latter criteria was fulfilled: i) abnormal respiratory examination, pulmonary infiltrates in chest x-rays; ii) productive cough with purulent sputum, positive microbiological cultures from lower respiratory tract or blood cultures. Diagnosis of UTI was based on two of the following criteria: fever (≥38.0°C), urine sample positive for nitrite, leukocyturia (>40/μL), or significant bacteriuria ($\geq 10^4$/mL of an uropathogen). OI was defined if temperature was ≥38.0°C, white blood cell count was ≥11000/mL or CRP≥10 mg/L and an infectious manifestation was present. Diagnosis of infection was done by the treating physician during hospitalization and was then validated post-hoc using charts, both diagnosis by treating physicians as well as secondary validation was blinded to biomarker levels with the exception of WBC and CRP for the diagnosis of (OI). Time point of diagnosis was referred to the beginning of clinical symptoms, which lead to diagnostic work-up and resulted in the diagnosis of infection.

In order to exclude acute infections preceding stroke, patients with admission temperature ≥38°C, or patients reporting an infection lasting up to 3 days before onset of stroke or patients who required mechanical intubation were not included in the study.

Laboratory Methods

Blood samples were collected on admission (baseline) within 72 hours from symptom onset, and 1, and 3 days after admission to assess WBC and Mcyt count, CRP level, PCT and copeptin. PCT serum concentration was measured using a commercially available time-resolved amplified cryptate emission technology assay (Kryptor PCT, Brahms, Hennigsdorf, Germany) [16]. Measurement of copeptin was performed in a single batch with a commercial sandwich immunoluminometric assay (LUMItest CT-proAVP, B.R.A.H.M.S, Hennigsdorf/Berlin, Germany) [17]. In patients who died within 5 days after admission, or in patients who were discharged before day 5, only data from admission or until the day of discharge were collected.

Statistical Analysis

Descriptive statistics were expressed as means ± standard deviations, medians and quartiles or absolute and relative frequencies depending on their distribution. Group differences were assessed using the Kruskal-Wallis test or Chi 2-test. Logarithmic transformation was performed to obtain an approximately normal distribution for all parameters except temperature and Mcyt.

First, the association of the biomarkers measured at admission with the presences of infections developed within 5 days was assessed using simple logistic regression.

Second we calculated pooled logistic regression considering patients to be at risk until the manifestation of an infection or until day 5 whichever occurred first. Each of these models had one time dependent predictor variable, i.e., the measurement of a given blood parameter 1 or 2 days before the respective day of diagnosis of infection. To adjust for potential clustering of data within subjects, robust standard errors were computed using the method of Huber-White. Odds ratios (OR) and associated 95% confidence intervals (95%CI) refer to an increase of the respective parameter from the lowest to the highest quartile.

Third, we compared the discriminatory ability of different predictors by calculating receiver operating characteristic (ROC) analysis. Bootstrap methods were used to derive 95%CIs for AUCs, index of Youden and optimal cutpoints to statistically compare AUC's of different predictors.

Forth, to assess the prognostic independence from age, NIHSS score (as indicator of stroke severity) and Charlson index (as indicator of comorbidity burden) as well as infratentorial and supratentorial infarct localization, we performed bivariate logistic regression (to avoid over-fitting) with these potential confounders.

Finally, we calculated 2 prediction models (batch 1 and 2) by including established inflammatory parameters (WBC and CRP) and either Copeptin or PCT, the 2 new makers. Since robust precision estimates were used, model comparisons could not be done using likelihood ratio tests but were based on Wald p-values.

P-values less than 0.05 were considered to indicate statistical significance. All calculations were performed using SAS software, version 9.2 (SAS Institute Inc., Cary, NC, USA).

Results

Baseline Data

Of 383 patients with stroke, 66 (17.2%) developed an infection within 5 days after onset of stroke. Twenty (5.2%) patients suffered from pneumonia, 25 (6.5%) patients had UTI and 21 (5.5%) patients an OI (sepsis: 7 patients; phlebitis: 6 patients; gastroenteritis: 4 patients, erysipelas: 1 patient; panniculitis: 1 patient, colpitis: 2 patients). Baseline data are summarized in table 1.

Blood Biomarkers as Predictors of Post-stroke Infections

Copeptin, PCT, WBC and CRP-levels on admission predicted any infection, pneumonia and UTI in the acute phase of stroke. ORs and AUCs for each marker measured on admission (i.e. day 0) are provided in table 2. ORs to predict infections associated with nearest predictor measurements over time (i.e. performed 1 or 2 days prior to the onset of infection) are presented in table 3. After adjusting for either age, NIHSS, CI or infarct localization (infra−/supratentorial) in a bivariate model all biomarkers remained significant predictors (table 4).

Copeptin as a new prognostic marker for SAI was a strong predictor of any infection, pneumonia and UTI (table 3). Copeptin had the same prognostic accuracy compared to WBC, CRP, and the only statistical significant difference in AUCs was found when comparing WBC and copeptin regarding the outcome of OI ($p = 0.02$) (table 5).

Predictive Models for Post-stroke Infections

We defined two batches of the three parameters with highest AUC values for any infection, pneumonia, UTI and OI by

Table 1. Baseline Data.

	All patients	Patients without infection	Patients with any infection	Pneumonia	UTI	Other infections
N	383	317	66	20	25	21
Age						
Median (±SD)	71.4±13.7	70.5±14.1	75.6±10.6	77.0±10.5	77.3±10.8	74.4
Gender (male)						
% (n)	57.7 (221)	60.8 (192)	43.3 (29)	45.0 (9)	32.0 (8)	50 (13)
Laboratory Findings on admission						
CRP (mg/ml)						
median	3.0	3.0	5.1	5.6	4.9	4.5
(IQR)	(3.0–6.7)	(3.0–5.8)	(3.0–15.8)	(3.0–19.7)	(3.0–24.3)	(3.0–8.8)
WBC (10^9/l)						
median	8.0	7.8	9.7	9.8	9.9	9.2
(IQR)	(6.6–9.8)	(6.5–9.4)	(7.5–11.4)	(7.5–13.5)	(8.3–11.2)	(7.4–11.3)
Monocyte (10^9/l)						
Mean (±SD)	0.410±0.167	0.398±0.143	0.463±0.243	0.557±0.357	0.471±0.277	0.413±0.152
Procalcitonin (μg/l)						
median	0.017	0.016	0.018	0.022	0.017	0.027
(IQR)	(0.01–0.02)	(0.01–0.02)	(0.01–0.03)	(0.02–0.03)	(0.01–0.04)	(0.01–0.03)
Copeptin (pmol/l)						
median	8.19	7.68	19.6	24.1	24.5	15.0
(IQR)	(4.4–31.4)	(4.2–16.5)	(6.2–61.9)	(8.6–42.4)	(5.2–73.5)	(5.7–62.3)
Temperature (°C)						
Mean (±SD)	37.0±0.6	37.0±0.6	36.9±0.7	37.0±0.9	36.8±0.7	37.0±0.7
Risk factors % (n)						
Heart failure	13.4 (48/357)	11.6 (34/293)	21.9 (14/64)	25.0 (5/20)	17.4 (4/23)	20.0 (5/25)
AH	80.0 (286/358)	77.7 (227/292)	89.4 (59/66)	85.0 (17/20)	91.7 (22/24)	88.5 (23/26)
PAD	8.3 (30/363)	8.4 (25/298)	7.7 (5/65)	10.0 (2/20)	4.3 (1/23)	7.7 (2/26)
Diabetes mellitus	19.3 (71/367)	18.9 (57/301)	21.2 (14/66)	35.0 (7/20)	25.0 (6/24)	7.7 (2/26)
CHD	21.0 (76/363)	21.2 (63/297)	19.7 (13/66)	25.0 (5/20)	16.7 (4/24)	19.2 (5/26)
Atrial fibrillation	19.4 (69/355)	15.9 (46/289)	34.8 (23/66)	45.0 (9/20)	25.0 (6/24)	38.5 (10/26)
Hyperchol	29.2 (99/339)	29.1 (82/282)	29.8 (17/57)	41.2 (7/17)	25.0 (5/20)	21.7 (5/23)
Family history of stroke	30.1 (106/352)	31.3 (90/288)	25.0 (16/64)	25.0 (5/20)	24.0 (6/25)	21.7 (5/23)
NIHSS						
Median	5	4	11	12	9	11
(IQR)	(2–10)	(2–7)	(5–18)	(5–19)	(3–15.5)	(5.5–19)
Charlson Index						
Median	1	0	1	1.5	1	0.5
(IQR)	(0–2)	(0–2)	(0–2)	(0–2.5)	(0–2)	(0–2)
BP on admission						
Systolic BP						
Mean (±SD)	160±29	161±34	158±34	153±36	158±36	159±34
Diastolic BP						
Mean (±SD)	86±21	85±20	92±23	103±30	89±22	92±18

UTI: urinary tract infection; CRP: C-reactive protein; WBC: white blood cells; NIHSS: National Institutes of Health Stroke Scale; BP: blood pressure; IQR: interquartile range (log transformed), AH: arterial hypertension; PAD: peripheral artery disease; CHD: coronary heart disease; Hyperchol: Hypercholestrolemia.

combining WBC, CRP and copeptin (batch 1) as well as WBC, CRP and PCT (batch 2).

Batch 1 (WBC, CRP, copeptin) better predicted any infection (Wald-p$<$0.001) and pneumonia (Wald-p$<$0.001) than the best single predictor alone. However, batch 1 was not a better predictor of UTI (Wald-p = 0.058) and OI (Wald-p = 0.25) than WBC (table 6).

Table 2. OR/AUC to predict infections (measurements on admission (day 0)).

Univariate analyses variables	Odds Ratio	CI (95%)	p-value	AUC
Any Infection (n = 66)				
Temperature	0.88	0.59–1.33	0.055	0.51
PCT	1.91	1.38–2.63	<.001	0.68
CRP	1.50	1.22–1.84	<.001	0.65
WBC	3.35	2.14–5.23	<.001	0.74
Mcyt	1.43	1.03–2.00	0.035	0.56
Copeptin	2.51	1.68–3.75	<.001	0.73
Pneumonia (n = 20)				
Temperature	0.90	0.48–1.69	0.75	0.49
PCT	1.96	1.34–2.86	<.001	0.69
CRP	1.67	1.25–2.24	<.001	0.77
WBC	3.38	1.85–6.20	<.001	0.76
Mcyt	2.00	1.28–3.11	0.002	0.63
Copeptin	2.35	1.29–4.28	0.005	0.75
Urinary Tract Infection (n = 25)				
Temperature	0.77	0.40–1.48	0.43	0.56
PCT	1.90	1.30–2.78	<.001	0.70
CRP	1.61	1.20–2.16	0.002	0.65
WBC	3.23	1.75–5.96	<.001	0.77
Mcyt	1.46	0.89–2.40	0.14	0.54
Copeptin	2.99	1.60–5.60	<.001	0.77
Other Infection (n = 21)				
Temperature	0.99	0.48–2.04	0.97	0.46
PCT	1.48	0.96–2.28	0.08	0.66
CRP	1.36	0.96–1.91	0.08	0.60
WBC	4.14	2.13–8.02	<.001	0.78
Mcyt	1.72	1.07–2.76	0.02	0.71
Copeptin	1.70	0.86–3.37	0.13	0.67

OR referred to an increment to predict values from the 1st to the 3th interquartile range (IQR). IQRs for the parameters are given in Table 1. PCT: procalcitonin; CRP: C-reactive protein; WBC: white blood cells; Mcyt: monocytes.

Table 3. Odds ratios/AUC to predict infections associated with nearest predictor measurements*.

Univariate analyses variables	Odds Ratio	CI (95%)	p-value	AUC
Any Infection				
Temperature	2.30	1.46–3.63	0.0003	0.64
PCT	1.69	1.30–2.20	<.0001	0.67
CRP	2.28	1.75–2.96	<.0001	0.74
WBC	4.91	3.38–7.14	<.0001	0.82
Mcyt	1.72	1.40–2.11	<.0001	0.65
Copeptin	2.40	1.81–3.20	<.0001	0.75
Pneumonia				
Temperature	3.00	1.22–7.37	0.02	0.67
PCT	1.95	1.36–2.79	0.0003	0.71
CRP	2.65	1.83–3.84	<.0001	0.80
WBC	4.29	2.52–7.31	<.0001	0.81
Mcyt	2.17	1.71–2.77	<.0001	0.72
Copeptin	3.32	2.32–4.76	<.0001	0.86
Urinary Tract Infection				
Temperature	1.64	0.77–3.48	0.20	0.57
PCT	1.61	1.18–2.20	0.003	0.63
CRP	2.26	1.52–3.37	<.0001	0.74
WBC	4.65	2.85–7.58	<.0001	0.83
Mcyt	2.04	1.60–2.60	<.0001	0.69
Copeptin	2.09	1.39–3.13	0.0004	0.71
Other Infection				
Temperature	6.82	2.34–19.89	0.0004	0.80
PCT	1.33	0.95–1.85	0.09	0.58
CRP	2.31	1.50–3.55	0.0001	0.74
WBC	5.69	3.44–9.39	<.0001	0.84
Mcyt	1.32	0.93–1.87	0.12	0.61
Copeptin	2.22	1.39–3.55	0.0008	0.75

OR referred to an increment to predict values from the 1st to the 3th interquartile range (IQR). IQRs for the parameters are given in Table 1. PCT: procalcitonin; CRP: C-reactive protein; WBC: white blood cells; Mcyt: monocytes performed 1 or 2 days prior to the onset of infection.

Batch 2 (WBC, CRP, PCT) better predicted any infection (Wald-p<0.001), pneumonia (Wald-p<0.001) and UTI (Wald-p = 0.014) than the best single predictor alone. However, batch 2 was not better in predicting OI compared to the best single predictor (Wald-p = 0.25) (table 6).

Discussion

The value of rapidly available blood markers as predictors for SAI has not been studied extensively, although WBC, CRP and Mcyt are routinely measured within the first hours of admission. Copeptin and PCT measured on admission were good predictors of any infection, pneumonia and UTI in the present cohort. They showed a similar predictive value for future infection compared to WBC and CRP. In a recent study neither WBC, CRP, Mcyt nor PCT measured on admission were sensitive enough to reliably be associated with SAI [18]. In another study, WBC and Mcyt count on admission did not differ between infected and non-infected stroke patients [19]. Only on day 1 after stroke onset, body temperature [18] and WBC [18,19] became significantly associated with infections after stroke. However, in these studies the time point of diagnosis in relation to biomarker measurements was not taken into account. Therefore, they could not really establish the predictive value of these markers but rather their diagnostic accuracy at the time of infection. Moreover the sample size was somewhat small and associations might have been missed due to lack of power. To our knowledge our study is the first to assess the predictive value of these markers taking into account the time point of measurements as well as diagnosis.

In the present study, each laboratory parameter remained a strong predictor after adjusting for NIHSS, age and CI and infarct localization. This is an unexpected finding because age and stroke severity may also contribute to SIS and thus infection after acute ischemic stroke [20–22]. However, these biomarkers seem to add prognostic information beyond age, stroke severity and a higher CI as well as infarct localization.

Copeptin was a strong predictor for SAI on admission and during the acute phase of stroke. The predictive value of copeptin

Table 4. OR to predict infections associated with nearest predictor measurements adjusted for age, NIHSS and CI as well as supra- or infratentorial infarct localization.

	OR (95%CI) adjusted for age	OR (95%CI) adjusted for NIHSS	OR (95%CI) adjusted for CI	OR (95%CI) adjusted for supra–/ infratentorial infarctions
Any Infection				
Temperature	2.36 (1.48–3.75)	2.10 (1.35–3.28)	2.82 (1.46–3.56)	2.30 (1.45–3.65)
PCT	1.64 (1.27–2.12)	1.62 (1.26–2.07)	1.81 (1.37–2.40)	1.69 (1.30–2.20)
CRP	2.23 (1.72–2.90)	1.96 (1.47–2.60)	2.22 (1.70–2.90)	2.28 (1.75–2.96)
WBC	4.97 (3.42–7.21)	4.22 (2.86–6.21)	4.90 (3.34–7.20)	4.80 (3.33–6.91)
Mcyt	1.69 (1.37–2.07)	1.70 (1.37–2.10)	1.68 (1.37–2.06)	1.72 (1.40–2.11)
Copeptin	2.22 (1.64–3.02)	1.84 (1.21–2.79)	2.30 (1.72–3.70)	2.43 (1.81–3.25)
Pneumonia				
Temperature	3.11 (1.23–7.86)	2.64 (1.11–6.29)	2.95 (1.23–7.09)	2.95 (1.24–7.00)
PCT	1.89 (1.33–2.67)	1.88 (1.33–2.65)	2.15 (1.40–3.32)	1.95 (1.37–2.79)
CRP	2.58 (1.79–3.71)	2.25 (1.48–3.42)	2.60 (1.77–3.80)	2.67(1.86–3.82)
WBC	4.17 (2.41–7.22)	3.73 (2.17–6.41)	4.32 (2.58–7.23)	4.30 (2.55–7.28)
Mcyt	2.09 (1.63–2.67)	2.13 (1.65–2.75)	2.15 (1.71–2.71)	2.19 (1.72–2.79)
Copeptin	3.07 (2.08–4.53)	2.95 (1.70–5.11)	3.28 (2.24–4.81)	3.37 (2.28–4.98)
Urinary Tract Infection				
Temperature	1.66 (0.78–3.55)	1.48 (0.76–2.88)	1.61 (0.76–3.42)	1.63 (0.78–3.42)
PCT	1.56 (1.16–2.10)	1.54 (1.12–2.11)	1.74 (1.19–2.53)	1.67 (1.21–2.29)
CRP	2.21 (1.49–3.29)	1.98 (1.31–3.00)	2.21 (1.45–3.36)	2.46 (1.64–3.69)
WBC	4.50 (2.82–7.18)	4.18 (2.48–7.06)	4.76 (2.75–8.25)	4.86 (2.99–7.92)
Mcyt	1.97 (1.56–2.49)	1.99 (1.56–2.53)	2.02 (1.48–2.77)	2.08 (1.63–2.67)
Copeptin	1.86 (1.20–2.89)	1.65 (0.85–3.20)	1.92 (1.19–3.09)	2.02 (1.32–3.10)
Other Infection				
Temperature	6.94 (2.52–19.12)	5.75 (2.10–15.71)	6.57 (2.50–17.29)	6.52 (2.23–19.06)
PCT	1.29 (0.93–1.78)	1.24 (0.87–1.77)	1.37 (0.97–1.92)	1.36 0.99–1.88)
CRP	2.25 (1.50–3.37)	1.91 (1.16–3.14)	2.30 (1.53–3.44)	2.44 (1.56–3.81)
WBC	5.54 (3.49–8.78)	5.01 (2.93–8.56)	5.62 (3.48–9.08)	6.08 (3.75–9.88)
Mcyt	1.32 (0.96–1.82)	1.30 (0.95–1.79)	1.33 (0.95–1.84)	1.34 (0.95–1.91)
Copeptin	2.28 (1.36–3.79)	1.60 (0.75–3.42)	2.37 (1.50–3.74)	2.17 (1.31–3.59)

PCT: procalcitonin; CRP: C-reactive protein; WBC: white blood cells; Mcyt: monocytes.

in respect of SAI was similar to that of established biomarkers of infection (i.e. WBC, CRP). This finding might be due to the association of copeptin with the activation of the HPAA: increased copeptin-levels probably indicate a high degree of stress and SIS, which means a higher susceptibility to develop an infection. The prognostic value of PCT was also in the range of WBC and CRP. In the literature PCT is a superior diagnostic marker in pneumonia and other bacterial infections when compared to WBC and CRP [23]. However, the prognostic accuracy of a single PCT valueis limited [24]. PCT might be rather a specific than a sensitive prognostic marker in predicting infections.

The combination of established inflammatory makers (WBC, CRP) combined with a biomarker of stress, i.e. copeptin or a biomarker of bacterial infection, i.e. PCT [16] improves prediction of SAI compared to the strongest prognostic marker alone. The combination of biomarkers probably reflects better the complexity of an infection than one biomarker alone and may lead to a more accurate prediction of a beginning but not yet clinically apparent infection.

The investigated biomarkers seem to detect infections before clinical or paraclinical signs prompt further diagnostic work-up leading to the diagnosis of infection. Thus, these markers may help in risk stratification and may select high-risk patients for intervention studies.

We are aware of the following limitations: First, our results are based ona single cohort and our findings need to be validated in an independent and larger cohort. Second, the sample size was relatively small when assessing subgroups of infection. The bivariate analysis may have a limited statistical power and validity underestimating possible effects of biomarkers and other potential predictors. Third, although WBC and CRP was not a criterion for making the diagnosis of pneumonia, any infection and UTI, one must take into account that WBC was one of three criteria for the diagnosis of the subgroup of OI. Therefore, the good predictive value of WBC - in the case of OI - is most probably due to incorporation bias. This, on the other hand, strengthens the predictive value of copeptin that might be underestimated compared to WBC in this study. Fourth, we are not able to proof causalities or provide more insights into pathomechanisms, to explain why these markers are good predictors of infections even before clinical signs occur. But even if these markers are only surrogates of underlying processes which predispose patients for

Table 5. Comparison of AUCs for developing infection between the predictors WBC, Mcyt, CRP and Copeptin.

Variables	AUC	p-value
Any Infection		
WBC vs Mcyt	0.82 vs 0.65	<.001
WBC vs CRP	0.82 vs 0.74	0.16
WBC vs Copeptin	0.82 vs 0.75	0.07
CRP vs Copeptin	0.74 vs 0.75	0.75
CRP vs Mcyt	0.74 vs 0.65	0.04
Copeptin vs Mcyt	0.75 vs 0.65	0.05
Pneumonia		
WBC vs Mcyt	0.81 vs 0.72	0.13
WBC vs CRP	0.81 vs 0.80	0.78
WBC vs Copeptin	0.81 vs 0.86	0.72
CRP vs Copeptin	0.80 vs 0.86	0.98
CRP vs Mcyt	0.80 vs 0.72	0.36
Copeptin vs Mcyt	0.86 vs 0.72	0.28
Urinary Tract Infection		
WBC vs Mcyt	0.83 vs 0.69	0.09
WBC vs CRP	0.83 vs 0.74	0.24
WBC vs Copeptin	0.83 vs 0.71	0.14
CRP vs Copeptin	0.74 vs 0.71	0.86
CRP vs Mcyt	0.74 vs 0.69	0.64
Copeptin vs Mcyt	0.71 vs 0.69	0.68
Other Infection		
WBC vs Mcyt	0.84 vs 0.61	0.008
WBC vs CRP	0.84 vs 0.74	0.10
WBC vs Copeptin	0.84 vs 0.75	0.02
CRP vs Copeptin	0.74 vs 0.75	0.80
CRP vs Mcyt	0.74 vs 0.61	0.28
Copeptin vs Mcyt	0.75 vs 0.61	0.30

PCT: procalcitonin; CRP: C-reactive protein; WBC: white blood cells; Mcyt: monocytes.

infections, from a clinical standpoint we belief that the observed associations are very interesting since we identified accurate prognostic markers for risk stratification. Finally, the distinction between prediction and early diagnosis of infection is difficult. We are not able to differentiate whether the biomarkers investigated in this study might rather detect infections at an early state or predict vulnerability for future post-stroke infections, although we excluded patients with possible infection prior to the onset of stroke.

In summary, copeptin, PCT, WBC and CRP were good predictors of the development of any infection, pneumonia and UTI. The combination of the 3 biomarkers even improved the prognostic value by accurately separating patients with and without future infections already on admission. If validated in larger prospective studies the combination of these 3 biomarkers with best AUC values may add significant information for the early identification of high-risk patients. Future intervention studies could select patients with high-risk profiles according to these biomarker levels and these high-risk patients may proof to benefit from prophylactic antibiotic treatment.

Table 6. Comparison of batches with best predictors of specific type of infection alone.

	Adjusted OR*	CI (95%)	p-value	AUC	Wald-p**
Batches 1: WBC+CRP+Copeptin					
Any infection					
WBC	3.70	2.26–6.08	<0.001	0.86	<0.001
CRP	1.66	1.24–2.21	<0.001		
Copeptin	1.53	1.07–2.18	0.019		
Pneumonia					
WBC	4.12	1.63–10.39	0.003	0.92	<0.001
CRP	1.92	1.30–2.84	0.001		
Copeptin	2.06	1.19–3.57	0.010		
Urinary Tract infection					
WBC	3.11	1.55–6.24	0.001	0.85	0.058
CRP	1.62	1.01–2.61	0.047		
Copeptin	1.26	0.73–2.19	0.411		
Other Infections					
WBC	6.84	3.00–15.60	<0.001	0.90	0.43
CRP	1.29	0.87–1.93	0.208		
Copeptin	1.18	0.69–2.03	0.550		
Batch 2: WBC+CRP+PCT					
Any infection					
WBC	3.67	2.42–5.58	<0.001	0.84	<0.001
CRP	1.56	1.16–2.11	0.003		
PCT	1.25	0.99–1.57	0.064		
Pneumonia					
WBC	4.25	2.27–7.97	<0.001	0.90	<0.001
CRP	1.87	1.39–2.52	<0.001		
PCT	1.36	1.00–1.85	0.052		
Urinary Tract Infection					
WBC	2.89	1.69–4.95	<0.001	0.82	0.014
CRP	1.59	0.90–2.81	0.114		
PCT	1.19	0.82–1.70	0.359		
Other Infections					
WBC	5.74	3.33–9.87	<0.001	0.89	0.25
CRP	1.53	0.92–2.55	0.103		
PCT	0.85	0.59–1.24	0.407		

WBC: white blood cells; CRP: C-reactive protein; PCT: procalcitonin. AUC: Area under the curve to predict infection using the combined model of all predictors.g.
*adjusted for all predictors in the respective model.
**Wald-p: refers to the comparison of the combined model with the model of the strongest predictor, alone which always was WBC.

Acknowledgments

We thank Dr. C. Schindler for statistical analyses and Prof. M. S. Elkind for his time and the appreciated comments as an expert in the field of inflammation and infection in stroke.

Author Contributions

Conceived and designed the experiments: FF MK. Performed the experiments: FF MK. Analyzed the data: FF MK BM MCC. Contributed reagents/materials/analysis tools: BM MCC NGM. Wrote the paper: FF

MK. assay development and measurement of copeptin and procalcitonin levels: NGM Supervision of the writing of the report: MCC, BM.

References

1. Chamorro A, Horcajada JP, Obach V, Vargas M, Revilla M, et al. (2005) The Early Systemic Prophylaxis of Infection After Stroke study: a randomized clinical trial. Stroke 36: 1495–1500.
2. Vargas M, Horcajada JP, Obach V, Revilla M, Cervera A, et al. (2006) Clinical consequences of infection in patients with acute stroke: is it prime time for further antibiotic trials? Stroke 37: 461–465.
3. Weimar C, Roth MP, Zillessen G, Glahn J, Wimmer MLJ, et al. (2002) Complications following acute ischemic stroke. Eur Neurol 48: 133–140.
4. Chamorro A, Urra X, Planas AM (2007) Infection after acute ischemic stroke: a manifestation of brain-induced immunodepression. Stroke 38: 1097–1103.
5. Elenkov IJ, Wilder RL, Chrousos GP, Vizi ES (2000) The sympathetic nerve–an integrative interface between two supersystems: the brain and the immune system. Pharmacol Rev 52: 595–638.
6. Harms H, Reimnitz P, Bohner G, Werich T, Klingebiel R, et al. (2011) Influence of stroke localization on autonomic activation, immunodepression, and post-stroke infection. Cerebrovasc Dis 32: 552–560.
7. Aslanyan S, Weir CJ, Diener H-C, Kaste M, Lees KR (2004) Pneumonia and urinary tract infection after acute ischaemic stroke: a tertiary analysis of the GAIN International trial. Eur J Neurol 11: 49–53.
8. Vermeij FH, Scholte op Reimer WJM, de Man P, van Oostenbrugge RJ, Franke CL, et al. (2009) Stroke-associated infection is an independent risk factor for poor outcome after acute ischemic stroke: data from the Netherlands Stroke Survey. Cerebrovasc Dis 27: 465–471.
9. Salat D, Delgado P, Alonso S, Ribó M, Santamarina E, et al. (2011) Ischemic stroke outcome and early infection: its deleterious effect seems to operate also among tissue plasminogen activator-treated patients. Eur Neurol 65: 82–87.
10. Emsley HCA, Smith CJ, Tyrrell PJ, Hopkins SJ (2008) Inflammation in acute ischemic stroke and its relevance to stroke critical care. Neurocrit Care 9: 125–138.
11. Sakr Y, Sponholz C, Tuche F, Brunkhorst F, Reinhart K (2008) The role of procalcitonin in febrile neutropenic patients: review of the literature. Infection 36: 396–407.
12. Kofoed K, Andersen O, Kronborg G, Tvede M, Petersen J, et al. (2007) Use of plasma C-reactive protein, procalcitonin, neutrophils, macrophage migration inhibitory factor, soluble urokinase-type plasminogen activator receptor, and soluble triggering receptor expressed on myeloid cells-1 in combination to diagnose infections: a prospective study. Crit Care 11: R38.
13. Katan M, Morgenthaler N, Widmer I, Puder JJ, König C, et al. (2008) Copeptin, a stable peptide derived from the vasopressin precursor, correlates with the individual stress level. Neuro Endocrinol Lett 29: 341–346.
14. Katan M, Fluri F, Morgenthaler NG, Schuetz P, Zweifel C, et al. (2009) Copeptin: a novel, independent prognostic marker in patients with ischemic stroke. Ann Neurol 66: 799–808.
15. Garner JS, Jarvis WR, Emori TG, Horan TC, Hughes JM (1988) CDC definitions for nosocomial infections, 1988. Am J Infect Control 16: 128–140.
16. Christ-Crain M, Jaccard-Stolz D, Bingisser R, Gencay MM, Huber PR, et al. (2004) Effect of procalcitonin-guided treatment on antibiotic use and outcome in lower respiratory tract infections: cluster-randomised, single-blinded intervention trial. Lancet 363: 600–607.
17. Morgenthaler NG, Struck J, Alonso C, Bergmann A (2006) Assay for the measurement of copeptin, a stable peptide derived from the precursor of vasopressin. Clin Chem 52: 112–119.
18. Wartenberg KE, Stoll A, Funk A, Meyer A, Schmidt JM, et al. (2011) Infection after acute ischemic stroke: risk factors, biomarkers, and outcome. Stroke Res Treat 2011: 830614.
19. Vogelgesang A, Grunwald U, Langner S, Jack R, Bröker BM, et al. (2008) Analysis of lymphocyte subsets in patients with stroke and their influence on infection after stroke. Stroke 39: 237–241.
20. Haeusler KG, Schmidt WUH, Föhring F, Meisel C, Helms T, et al. (2008) Cellular immunodepression preceding infectious complications after acute ischemic stroke in humans. Cerebrovasc Dis 25: 50–58.
21. Chamorro A, Amaro S, Vargas M, Obach V, Cervera A, et al. (2006) Interleukin 10, monocytes and increased risk of early infection in ischaemic stroke. J Neurol Neurosurg Psychiatr 77: 1279–1281.
22. Chamorro A, Amaro S, Vargas M, Obach V, Cervera A, et al. (2007) Catecholamines, infection, and death in acute ischemic stroke. J Neurol Sci 252: 29–35.
23. Simon L, Gauvin F, Amre DK, Saint-Louis P, Lacroix J (2004) Serum procalcitonin and C-reactive protein levels as markers of bacterial infection: a systematic review and meta-analysis. Clin Infect Dis 39: 206–217.
24. Schuetz P, Suter-Widmer I, Chaudri A, Christ-Crain M, Zimmerli W, et al. (2011) Prognostic value of procalcitonin in community-acquired pneumonia. Eur Respir J 37: 384–392.

Virulence Characteristics and Genetic Affinities of Multiple Drug Resistant Uropathogenic *Escherichia coli* from a Semi Urban Locality in India

Savita Jadhav[1]¶, Arif Hussain[2]¶, Savita Devi[2]¶, Ashutosh Kumar[2], Sana Parveen[2], Nageshwari Gandham[1], Lothar H. Wieler[3], Christa Ewers[3], Niyaz Ahmed[2,4,5]*

1 Department of Microbiology, Dr. D. Y. Patil Medical College and Hospital, Pimpri, Pune, India, **2** Pathogen Biology Laboratory, Department of Biotechnology, School of Life Sciences, University of Hyderabad, Hyderabad, India, **3** Veterinary Faculty, Institute for Microbiology and Epizootics, Freie Universitaet Berlin, Berlin, Germany, **4** Institute of Biological Sciences, University of Malaya, Kuala Lumpur, Malaysia, **5** Institute of Life Sciences, University of Hyderabad Campus, Hyderabad, India

Abstract

Extraintestinal pathogenic *Escherichia coli* (ExPEC) are of significant health concern. The emergence of drug resistant *E. coli* with high virulence potential is alarming. Lack of sufficient data on transmission dynamics, virulence spectrum and antimicrobial resistance of certain pathogens such as the uropathogenic *E. coli* (UPEC) from countries with high infection burden, such as India, hinders the infection control and management efforts. In this study, we extensively genotyped and phenotyped a collection of 150 UPEC obtained from patients belonging to a semi-urban, industrialized setting near Pune, India. The isolates representing different clinical categories were analyzed in comparison with 50 commensal *E. coli* isolates from India as well as 50 ExPEC strains from Germany. Virulent strains were identified based on hemolysis, haemagglutination, cell surface hydrophobicity, serum bactericidal activity as well as with the help of O serotyping. We generated antimicrobial resistance profiles for all the clinical isolates and carried out phylogenetic analysis based on repetitive extragenic palindromic (rep)-PCR. *E. coli* from urinary tract infection cases expressed higher percentages of type I (45%) and P fimbriae (40%) when compared to fecal isolates (25% and 8% respectively). Hemolytic group comprised of 60% of UPEC and only 2% of *E. coli* from feces. Additionally, we found that serum resistance and cell surface hydrophobicity were not significantly ($p = 0.16/p = 0.51$) associated with UPEC from clinical cases. Moreover, clinical isolates exhibited highest resistance against amoxicillin (67.3%) and least against nitrofurantoin (57.3%). We also observed that 31.3% of UPEC were extended-spectrum beta-lactamase (ESBL) producers belonging to serotype O25, of which four were also positive for O25b subgroup that is linked to B2-O25b-ST131-CTX-M-15 virulent/multiresistant type. Furthermore, isolates from India and Germany (as well as global sources) were found to be genetically distinct with no evidence to espouse expansion of *E. coli* from India to the west or *vice-versa*.

Editor: Ramy Aziz, Cairo University, Egypt

Funding: This study was funded by the University of Hyderabad through intramural, startup grants to Niyaz Ahmed and was carried out as part of the Indo-German Research Training Group - Internationales Graduiertenkolleg (GRK1673) - Functional Molecular Infection Epidemiology, an initiative of the German Research Foundation (DFG) and the University of Hyderabad (India), of which Niyaz Ahmed and Lothar Wieler are Speakers. The funders had no role in study design, data collection and analysis, decision to publish, or preparation of the manuscript.

* E-mail: niyazSL@uohyd.ernet.in

¶ These authors contributed equally to this work.

Introduction

Urinary tract infections (UTI) are the second most common human infections and are mainly caused by uropathogenic *E. coli*. The severity of UTI depends both on the virulence of the bacteria and the susceptibility of the host [1]. UPEC harbor numerous virulence factors including alpha-hemolysin, cytotoxic necrotizing factor, adhesins and iron acquisition systems. These factors support their ability to adhere to uroepethelial cells, help resist the bactericidal effect of serum and augment cell surface hydrophobicity thereby leading ultimately to tissue damage [2,3,4,5].

Adherence to the urinary tract mucosa might protect bacteria from urinary lavage and in turn augment their ability to survive and invade renal tissues [6]. Specific adhesion is mediated by certain adhesins which can be differentiated based on their receptor binding specificity.

P fimbriae that are encoded by the *E. coli pap* (pyelonephritis-associated pilus) operon are the most important mannose-resistant adhesins, although they are expressed by only a limited number of *E. coli* serotypes. The most rampant P-fimbriated serotypes of the UPEC strains revealed one of the six O groups O1, O2, O4, O6, O7, and O18 [6,7,8].

Hemolysin production is another important virulence property of UPEC. Hemolysins inflict direct cytotoxic effects on renal epithelium resulting in scaring. Alpha-hemolysin is described to be a lethal factor with dermonecrotic effects and is antigenic in nature. Also, hemolysins are toxic to a series of host tissues and cells including RBCs, leucocytes, epithelial and endothelial cells. The frequency of isolation of hemolytic *E. coli* significantly associates with the severity of the infection [7,8].

The importance of cell surface hydrophobicity as a virulence attribute (that facilitates bacterial adherence to mammalian cells) is known for nearly a century now, thanks to the pioneering studies of Mudd and Mudd [4]. It is an important factor helping *E. coli* to adhere to various surfaces for colonization. Bacteria are lysed by normal serum due to the activity of the complement system. The alternate pathway of complement activation is potentially important than the classical pathway. Bacterial resistance to killing by serum results from individual or combined effects of capsular polysaccharides, lipopolysaccharides and surface proteins [4]. Given this generic virulence 'arsenal' of UPEC, strains from different geographical regions pose different disease severity and should be genetically different.

To screen for the above mentioned virulence attributes and to find the most predominant serotypes among UPEC in the western Indian region, we analyzed 150 human clinical isolates. We intended to classify them epidemiologically into different serotypes and to obtain virulence marker profiles of UPEC (which have different frequencies in different disease conditions ranging from asymptomatic bacteriuria to chronic pyelonephritis). In addition, increasing antimicrobial resistance in bacterial pathogens is of major concern as it can vary according to geographical and regional situations [9,10,11,12]. It is very relevant to ensure the appropriate therapy based on full knowledge of the organisms that cause UTI and their antibiotic susceptibility profiles. Therefore, it is necessary to do bacteriological testing also with reference to extended-spectrum beta-lactamase (ESBL) producers with resistance to beta-lactam antibiotics, including third generation cephalosporins such as cefotaxime, ceftriaxone and ceftazidime. Not much information on ESBL producing organisms causing UTI is available from India.

The present work was essentially carried out as an important precursor of a larger study aimed at understanding the transmission dynamics, population genetic structure and virulence mechanisms of UPEC from India. Herein, we present a much needed snapshot comprising of the virulence characteristics and antimicrobial resistance patterns of the available UPEC strains from western India representing the clinical conditions such as symptomatic UTI, bacteriuria, pyelonephritis, cystitis, prostatitis, septicemia and pyrexia of unknown origin (PUO). We sought to define the clinical correlates of different virulence factors and their association with various biological and life-style related factors of the host. In addition, we used rep-PCR based DNA profiling to know the genetic affinities of our isolates and to explore if this simple PCR based genetic analysis helps in understanding their spread patterns indicative of their diverse or clonal relationships. Also, we attempted to use this technique to know whether the bacterial isolates have any geographic inclination and how similar or different they are when compared to some of the well characterized isolates from western countries such as Germany.

Materials and Methods

Ethics statement

Written informed consents were obtained from all patients and healthy controls for the use of their strains which were cultured as part of compulsory diagnostic screening. Study protocols were approved by the institutional ethics committee of Dr. D. Y. Patil Medical College, Pune and by the Institutional Biosafety Committee of the School of Life Sciences of the University of Hyderabad, India.

Study population and strains

One hundred and fifty *E. coli* isolates were obtained from urine samples of human patients in cell counts of 10^5/ml. Fifty fecal *E. coli* isolates (that were used as controls), were isolated from the feces of healthy individuals who had reported for routine health checkup between January 2009–March 2010 at Dr. D. Y. Patil Medical College and Hospital, Pimpri, Pune, India. Patient background and provisional diagnosis of the infection were obtained from hospital records (Table S1). Identification of isolates was done using standard microbiological techniques [13,14,15]. All strains were stored on 15% glycerol-supplemented Luria-Bertani medium at $-80°C$.

DNA samples

DNA samples of fifty ExPEC isolates from Germany and from global sources [16] were obtained; these represented various animal and human specimens, including 17 UPEC and archetypical newborn meningitis strain RS218 from humans, two UPEC from dogs and 31 avian pathogenic *E. coli* (APEC) from different birds. These strains were used for repetitive extragenic palindromic (rep) PCR together with the aforementioned human clinical isolates.

Antimicrobial susceptibility test

The antimicrobial susceptibility testing was carried out on Mueller Hinton agar by disc diffusion method using the following antimicrobial substances [17]: amoxicillin (10 µg), ceftazidime (30 µg), ciprofloxacin (10 µg), co-trimoxazole (25 µg), gentamicin (10 µg), nitrofurantoin (300 µg), nalidixic acid (30 µg), and tetracycline (30 µg). Multi-drug resistant (MDR) strains were defined as those which showed resistance to three or more antimicrobial substances. Extended-spectrum beta-lactamase (ESBL) production was detected by the double-disk synergy (DDS) test as recommended by the Clinical and Laboratory Standards Institute (CLSI, 2006). Its presence was assayed using the antibiotic disks comprising of ceftazidime and ceftazidime/clavulanic acid (30/10 µg). An isolate was graded ESBL producer when its zone of inhibition varied by $\geq$5 mm among at least one of the combination disks and its coordinate comprising of standard antibiotic disk. *E. coli* ATCC 25922 was used as a negative control while *K. pneumoniae* ssp. *pneumoniae* ATCC 700603 served as positive control [18,19].

Phenotypic assays to determine virulence factors

a) Alpha-hemolysin production. The detection of alpha-hemolysin was performed by analysing the hemolytic zone observed after overnight growth at 37°C on sheep blood (5%) agar [20].

b) Haemagglutination. A suspension of human A +ve blood and PBS was mixed on a VDRL (venereal diseases research laboratory - test) cavity slide with a single colony of *E. coli*. After incubation on rotor at room temperature for some minutes, agglutination was seen. Similarly, haemagglutination was carried out in the presence of D-mannose. An ATCC *E. coli* 25922 strain was used as a negative control for mannose sensitive haemagglutination assay and a known strain of *E. coli* repeatedly giving positive was taken as control for the assay [21].

c) Cell Surface Hydrophobicity. Bacteria were tested for their hydrophobic property by using different molar concentrations of ammonium sulphate in VDRL tile; 40 µl of bacterial suspension in PBS was added in each of the wells containing 1 M, 1.4 M and 2 M ammonium sulphate. Clumps were seen by naked eyes. Strains were considered hydrophobic, if they aggregated in the PBS concentration of $\leq$1.4 M [21].

d) Serum Bactericidal Assay. Bacteria were diluted in Hank's balanced salt solution to get appropriate dilutions and mixed with human serum in a sterile tube and incubated in a water bath at 37°C and inoculated on nutrient agar plates at 0 hr, 1 hr, 2 hr of incubation in water bath. Growth at 0 hr was taken as control. *E. coli* was considered sensitive if count dropped to 1% and was considered resistant if >90% of the organisms survived after 2 hrs of incubation. An *E. coli* isolate that was consistently serum resistant and a one which was consistently sensitive were used as positive and negative controls respectively [22].

Serotyping

Typing of somatic antigens was performed at the National Salmonella and *Escherichia* Centre, Central Research Institute, Kasauli, India, using antisera against O antigens - O1 to O173. O25 positive *E. coli* strains were further subjected to genotyping by a recent method based on allele-specific PCR targeting the *rfb*O25b subgroup gene locus [23].

Repetive extragenic palindromic PCR

DNA sequences of primers used for Rep - fingerprinting were as follows: Forward Rep2a2: 5′-ACGGCTTATCGGGCCTA-3′, Reverse Rep1Ra1:5′-GCGACGGCATCAGGC-3′. PCR amplification was carried out in 20 µl reaction mixture consisting of 10× Taq buffer, 25 mM $MgCl_2$, 10 mM dNTP, 100% DMSO, 100 pM of each primer and 2 U of Taq DNA polymerase and 5 µl of template. The PCR conditions were 95°C for 7 min, followed by 30 cycles of DNA amplification consisting of 45 s at 95°C, 1 min at 40°C and 8 min at 65°C followed by 16 min incubation at 65°C. The amplicons were run on 1.5% agarose gels and were analyzed by Bionumerics® software [24,25].

Detection of O25b subgroup strain by PCR

The newly described O25b O type *E. coli* were detected by using the following primers gndbis.f (5′ATACCGACGACGCCGATCTG-3′) and rfbO25b.r (5′TGCTATTCATTATGCGCAGC-3′). Annealing temperature of 60°C was used to generate a PCR product of 300 bp with the conditions as previously described [23].

Statistical Analysis

Chi square test was used to compare the occurrence of virulence markers in cases and controls. P values less than 0.05 was considered significant.

Results and Discussion

Incidence of UTI in relationship with gender and socioeconomic status

In this study we observed a higher proportion of UTI in females (64%) than in males (36%). This is understandable due to the anatomy and is a consistent trend worldwide. Peak in the incidence of UTI was observed in the age groups 11–21 and 60–71 years. Among these, elderly patients are likely predisposed to conditions such as urinary tract obstruction, poor bladder emptying, and diabetes mellitus, etc. These factors favor colonization of bacteria and play an important role in UTI. Other studies have also reported similar findings [26,27]. India has a large infection burden and the genito-urinary infections are very prominent. This may be due to a less affordable personal/ community hygiene for some of the economically backword populations. We targeted these groups and analyzed strains obtained from such communities who reported for the UTI in periurban Pune. As such there is not much information available from India on the genetic and phenotypic diversity of UPEC. This information should therefore be construed as the first systematic analysis performed on a diverse type of patients/samples.

Virulence characteristics of UPEC from India

a) Type 1 (MSHA) and P fimbriae (MRHA). In the present study, 45% of the UTI isolates and 25% of fecal isolates showed the presence of type 1 (Mannose sensitive hemagglutination - MSHA) fimbriae. Thus the difference among UTI and fecal isolates was not statistically significant. It was found that 40% of UTI isolates and 8% of *E. coli* isolates from the controls exhibited P fimbriae (Mannose resistant hemagglutination -MRHA). The difference was statistically significant (P = 0.0002). Expression of type 1 fimbriae was more discerned in isolates from the cases of simple UTI and cystitis. In our observation, maximum P fimbriae positive isolates were highly associated with simple UTI, while only 10% of such isolates caused pyelonephritis. As such there is no relation among the occurrence or severity of symptoms/the site of infection and fimbrial expression (of P or type1) in case of bacterial isolates from urine [28].

Our observation was in agreement with another study [29], wherein the presence of type 1 fimbriae was seen in 71% of isolates of *E. coli* from UTI and in 60% of isolates of *E. coli* from the control fecal flora. Taken together, UTI associated isolates did not show any significant expression of MSHA compared to controls; however, Najar *et al.* (2007) [29] showed an overall higher expression of type 1 fimbriae in both the UTI isolates and controls. Many studies have demonstrated the presence of P fimbriae as maximum in UTI isolates than in fecal isolates of healthy persons [29,30].

Although, since we looked only at phenotypes of the isolates *in vitro*, it is difficult to dwell upon the real significance of the fimbrial expression patterns *vis a vis* the niche tropism (upper or lower UTI) and its impact on different outcomes of infection – these are largely the phenomena due to microbial mechanisms operating *in vivo*. Normally, the expression of P fimbriae is increased among isolates associated with lower urinary tract infections, basically resembling an '*in vivo*' situation as there is an interplay between type1-fimbriae and P-fimbriae expression ("switch-off" of Type 1 fimbriae leads to increased motility of bacteria and finally to binding of P-fimbrial adhesin to receptors on kidney epithelial cells). The higher or lower expression itself might therefore only give an idea about the quantitative occurrence of P fimbriae, but not about the different adhesion subunits which would be more relevant with respect to upper/lower UTI infections.

b) Hemolysin. Production of alpha hemolysin was observed in 60% of UPEC from the cases while only 2% of *E. coli* isolates from feces produced alpha hemolysin (P = 0.0001). Other studies have also reported similar findings [31]. In our observation, hemolysin was highest in pyelonephritis, lower in cystitis and least in asymptomatic bacteriuria.

c) Serum resistance and cell surface hydrophobicity. Serum resistance and cell surface hydrophobicity markers were not significantly present in *E. coli* isolates from patients compared to control fecal isolates: 55% and 76% of urinary *E. coli* isolates showed serum resistance and cell surface hydrophobicity respectively and the control isolates showed 40% and 70% for serum resistance and cell surface hydrophobicity respectively.

The difference in both the cases was not statistically significant (p = 0.16/p = 0.51). This trend has been reported earlier and our study confirmed the same for Indian isolates [32].

Occurrence of virulence factors in UPEC strains confirms the association of UPEC with urinary pathogenicity. It was interesting

Table 1. Occurrence of virulence phenotypes in *E. coli* isolates from cases and controls.

Virulence phenotypes	Number of isolates from cases (%) total cases = 150	Number of isolates from controls (%) total controls = 50	P-value
MRHA	60 (40.0)	4 (8.0)	0.0002
MSHA	68 (45.3)	12 (24.0)	0.406
Hemolysin	90 (60.0)	1 (2.0)	0.00001
SR	83 (55.3)	20 (40.0)	0.16
CSH	120 (80.0)	35 (70.0)	0.51

to note that UPEC with virulence factors were significantly more prevalent in patient groups than in controls (Table 1). Such a significant difference was noticed earlier, indicating that several virulence factors act synergistically to cause infection of the urinary tract [33]. Nevertheless, it was interesting that 8% of the isolates (12/150) from infection cases did not reveal any virulence markers under investigation. These were the isolates from complicated UTI. It appears that these isolates, though devoid of any virulence factors as probed by us, were able to localize in the deeper tissues of a compromised urinary tract where scarcely any drug reaches in therapeutic quantum. It may also be due to the reason that they might possess virulence markers/mechanisms other than those tested by us.

We screened 19 mucoid UPEC isolates by phenotypic and biochemical characterization and found that all were from patient groups and were capsulated. Out of the 19 mucoid UPEC, 11 were capsulated and serum resistant. Capsule confers serum and phagocyte resistance and this could be attributed to sialic acid residues that subvert the ability of bacterial surface to activate complement by alternative pathway thereby augmenting the virulence potential of such pathogens. However, eight of the mucoid strains were susceptible to serum, perhaps due to the non capsular factors and this might have a role in serum resistance.

Antimicrobial susceptibility profiles of UPEC

Antimicrobial susceptibility testing was carried out on all the clinical isolates. The majority of isolates were sensitive to nitrofurantoin - 86 (57.3%) followed by ciprofloxacin - 78 (52%) and nalidixic acid - 74 (49%). This study showed high resistance to amoxicillin - 101 (67.3%), tetracycline - 92 (61.3%), and cefotaxime - 68 (45.3%) (Figure 1). Upon testing for ESBL, we found that 32 (21.3%) were ESBL producers. A high proportion (31.3%) of these ESBL-producing isolates was belonging to the serotype O25. Four of these were positively tested for the subgroup O25b (Figure 2), which has been linked to a clonally related group of highly virulent, multiresistant *E. coli* strains (B2-O25b-ST131-CTX-M-15) that are emerging among humans and animals worldwide [34,35]. Further studies, i.e. multi locus sequence typing (MLST), macrorestriction analysis, and determination of beta-lactamase enzymes are needed to unravel the phylogenetic

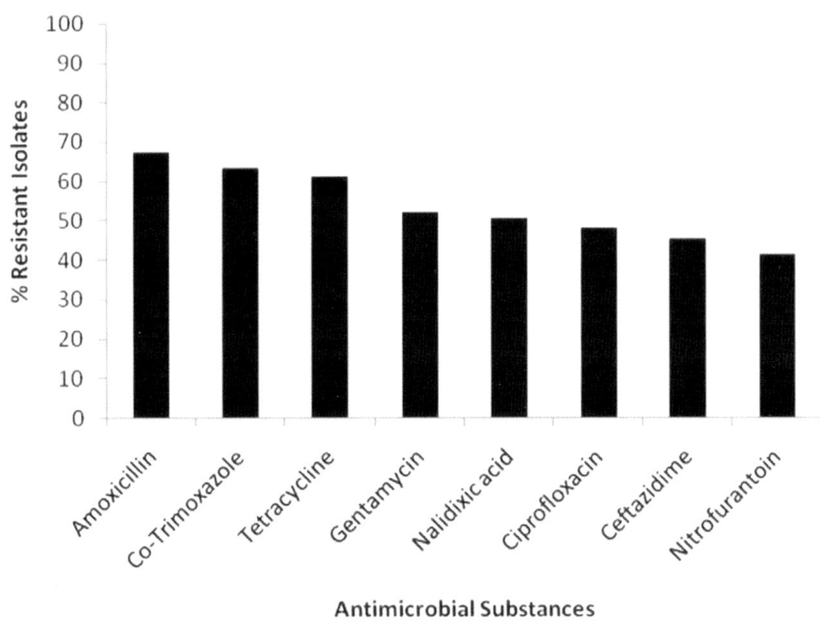

Figure 1. The antimicrobial susceptibility and resistance pattern of 150 UTI isolates from India. Nitrofurantoin was consistently the most active (59%) of the systemically active antimicrobials, with ceftazidime, giving similar results (54.7%). These were followed by ciprofloxacin (52%), nalidixic acid (49%) and gentamicin (48%), but sensitivity to amoxicillin was found to be low (32.7%). Sensivity profiles of Co-trimoxazole (36.7%) and tetracycline (38.7%) were quite similar.

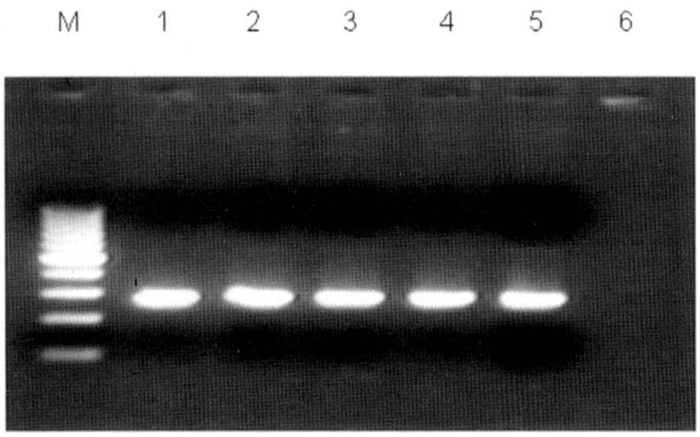

Figure 2. PCR based detection of O25b subgroup that is linked to the B2-O25b-ST131-CTX-M-15 clonal group of strains. Among 32 ESBL producers in our collection (n = 150) four were positive for O25b subgroup (Lanes 1 to 4); lane 5, positive (strain showing consistently positive); lane 6, negative; M, 100 bp DNA ladder.

relatedness of these O25-ESBL-producing Indian isolates to the worldwide recognized clonal groups and to characterize the remaining multiresistant isolates observed. ESBL isolates were frequently (65.6%) associated with a hemolytic phenotype, with a higher rate than the non-ESBL-producing UPEC strains (58.5%). Hence, although it is a commonly accepted fact that bacterial pathogens acquire resistance determinants and express a multiresistant phenotype at the cost of their virulence properties, the frequent observation of hemolytic UPEC among our strain collection underlines the possible emergence of highly virulent multiresistant strains [36] in this area.

It is particularly worrisome that more than half of the ESBL producers (53.1%) in our collection were resistant to ciprofloxacin suggesting that they may be resistant to all available fluoroquinolones - the drug of choice for treatment of infections caused by ESBL-producing strains. Overall, nitrofurantoin and ciprofloxacin were found superior to amoxicillin and co-trimoxazole. None of the uropathogens from this study area were 100% susceptible to any of the antimicrobial substances used. Prior studies have shown a sensitivity rate of 95–100% to nitrofurantoin [37]. But in our study, nitrofurantoin showed only 57.3% sensitivity; the reason for this low sensitivity and high resistance to almost all antimicrobials in the study area may indicate difference in antimicrobial usage, infection control practices and other unrecognized factors including genetic propensity of these strains to accumulate mutations conferring MDR phenotypes. Periodic review and formulation of antibiotic policy are needed to control acquisition of drug resistance. Further studies for better understanding of the interaction of different virulence factors at molecular level are necessary as most urovirulent strains express multiple virulence factors simultaneously. We believe that the methods of detection of the above mentioned virulence markers are reasonably easy and screening them in a clinical microbiology laboratory is a worthwhile exercise.

Table 2. Distribution of various O-antigens in clinical isolates of *E. coli.*

O-Antigen	Pyelonephritis	Prostatitis	Cystitis	Simple UTI	Septicaemia	PUO	Total
O1	-	1	-	5	2	-	8
O2	-	1	-	1	-	-	2
O9	-	-	-	-	-	-	0
O14	1	-	-	-	-	-	1
O20	1	-	-	-	1	1	3
O25	6	7	11	15	2	4	45
O44	1	-	-	2	1	-	4
O45	-	-	1	-	-	-	1
O60	1		1	4	1	-	7
O64	-	-	1	1	-	-	2
O76	-	-	1	3	-	-	4
O79	-	1	-	-	-	-	1
O84	-	-	-	1	-	-	1
O102	3	1	-	8	-	1	13
O116	-	-	-	1	-	-	0
O120	2	2	3	6	-	1	14
O130	-	1	-	1	-	-	2
Rough	1		1	2	2	-	6
O 95	1	-	-	-	-	-	1
O100	-	-	-	1	-	-	1
Non- viable	-		1		-	-	1
Non *E. coli*	-	1	1	2	-	1	5
Untypeable	5	-	3	13	3	4	28
Total	22	15	24	65	12	12	150

Serotyping and genotyping

In our study, as many as 19 different serotypes (O1, O2, O9, O14, O20, O25, O44, O45, O60, O64, O76, O79, O84, O102, O116, O120, O130, O95, O100) were observed among the cultured UPEC. Out of these, 27 *E. coli* were untypeable; six expressed a rough O antigen and five were *Escherichia* species (non-*E. coli*; NEC). A majority of *E. coli* isolates expressed O antigens - O25 (31.9%), O102 (9.7%), O120 (8.3%), and O1 (5.6%). Serotype O25 was predominantly found to be isolated from patients with pyelonephritis, prostatitis, cystitis and simple UTI. Renal failure associated isolates mainly belonged to O25 and O102 serotypes (Table 2).

To determine the relatedness of the strains, a dendrogram based on rep-PCR based fingerprint data was constructed in Bionumerics®. For this study, the clinical strains from India and 50 German isolates were used while the fecal isolates were excluded as the aim of this experiment was not to prove pathogenicity of the ExPEC but to see how diverse and clonal they are and to analyze Indian isolates in juxtaposition with German strains. Apart from the occurrence of singleton strains, the dendrogram obtained could be broadly classified into 5 major clusters: Indian-German cluster I (n = 15 strains), Indian cluster I (n = 63), mixed cluster I (n = 17) and mixed clusters IIa/IIb (n = 30), which include strains from all the three locales, as depicted in Figure 3. All the strains that clustered under Indian branch (exceptionally harboring one isolate from Germany) revealed very diverse pattern, except for a few ones - it appears that the bacteria we cultured were very diverse and the ones which were close in the cluster have no phenotypic resemblances with each other in terms of antimicrobial resistance profile or serotype or other virulence markers. This may be due to the reason that the UPEC in this study area could be highly diverse at sub-species and serotype levels.

The mixed cluster I contained a group of 17 bacterial isolates from India, Germany and from global sources. This cluster predominantly comprises of APEC from cases of septicemia in chicken or goose, while the remaining seven strains were human UPEC, including strain CFT073, or they were septicemia-associated strains (SEPEC). The mixed cluster II was subdivided into two subclusters- subcluster IIa (n = 10) and subcluster IIb (n = 20). The subcluster IIa largely encompasses APEC. Eight out of ten members of this cluster were APEC and the rest were UTI pathogens from humans. In the subcluster IIb, human isolates as well as isolates from animals were grouped together. There was no discrete band pattern between strains isolated from different sources; out of twenty strains in subcluster IIb nine were APEC, seven were UPEC of humans and two from dog, one was a human SEPEC and finally the archetypical NMEC strain RS218 grouping within this subcluster. From this analysis, we may conclude that the technique of rep-PCR is not resolving enough to distinguishing strains that portray similar phenotypic markers; nevertheless the Indian ExPEC population was clearly distinguishable from German ExPEC. We also found that the isolates from different animal sources were more or less grouping into distinct clusters, indicating that this technique can also be used to find the sources of infection in a reservoir such as a water body.

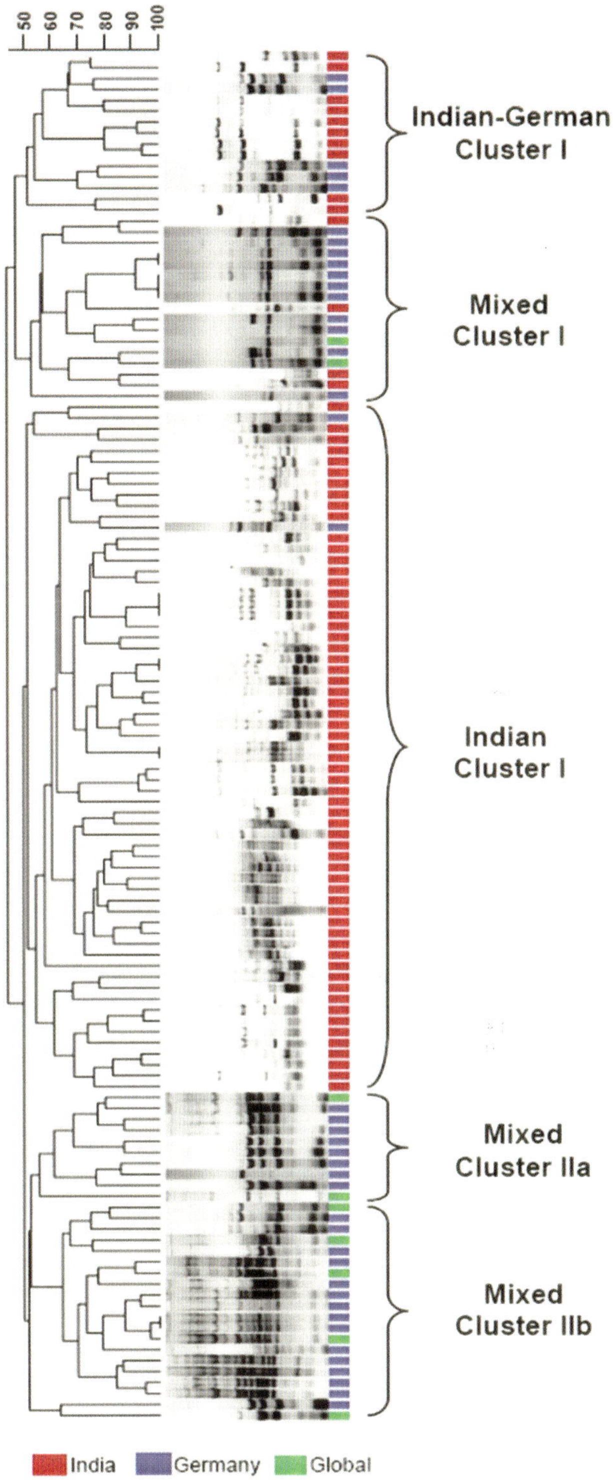

Figure 3. Dendrogram based on rep-PCR, developed in Bionumerics® revealed genetic relationships of *E. coli* representing Indian clinical isolates and ExPECs from global sources. Different geographic clusters are labeled. Upper scale denotes genetic distance.

In conclusion, our observations form an important baseline data-set towards understanding the virulence properties, antibiotic resistance profiles and genetic diversity of UPEC from India. We hope that such observations will be more meaningful towards systematically unraveling the population genetic structure of UPEC and their propensity to spread, or emerge with multi drug resistance phenotypes in new epidemiological territories. In the backdrop of this work, future studies involving decipherment of MDR mechanisms, lineage tracking based on MLST [16] and whole genome sequencing of representative isolates from different MLST clades [2] shall be imminent. Further, the 'omics' inspired studies will ultimately help understanding of the functional molecular epidemiology and infection biology of Indian UPEC at greater details. On the clinical side, it will be possible to ascertain reservoirs of infection which could be important in understanding the mechanisms of chronic and recurrent UTI [38] in a community setting and how they are maintained within or in the vicinity of different human populations of a multicultural and densely populated country such as India.

Acknowledgments

We would like to extend our thanks to Professors Jörg Hacker and Seyed E. Hasnain for their guidance and timely suggestions. We are also thankful to members of the pathogen evolution laboratory in University of Hyderabad for their help and support. We acknowledge assistance provided by Mrs. G. Navamallika at different stages of this study.

Author Contributions

Conceived and designed the experiments: NA. Performed the experiments: SJ AH SD SP. Analyzed the data: AK CE NA. Contributed reagents/materials/analysis tools: NG LHW. Wrote the manuscript: CE NA.

References

1. Fowler JE, Stamey TA (1977) Studies of introital colonization in women with recurrent urinary infections. The role of bacterial adherence. J Urol 117: 472–476.
2. Dobrindt U (2005) (Patho-)Genomics of Escherichia coli. Int J Med Microbiol 295: 357–371.
3. Johnson JR, Russo TA (2005) Molecular epidemiology of extraintestinal pathogenic (uropathogenic) Escherichia coli. Int J Med Microbiol 295: 383–404.
4. Leffler H, Svanborg-Eden C (1981) Glycolipid receptors for uropathogenic Escherichia coli on human erythrocytes and uroepithelial cells. Infect Immun 34: 920–929.
5. Hughes C, Hacker J, Roberts A, Goebel W (1983) Hemolysin production as a virulence marker in symptomatic and asymptomatic urinary tract infections caused by Escherichia coli. Infect Immun 39: 546–551.
6. Hagan EC, Mobley HL (2007) Uropathogenic Escherichia coli outer membrane antigens expressed during urinary tract infection. Infect Immun 75: 3941–3949.
7. Blanco J, Alonso MP, Blanco M, Blanco JE, Gonzalez EA, et al. (1992) Establishment of three categories of P-fimbriated Escherichia coli strains that show different toxic phenotypes and belong to particular O serogroups. FEMS Microbiol Lett 78: 131–136.
8. Blanco M, Blanco J, Blanco JE, Alonso MP, Abalia I, et al. (1995) [Virulence factors and O serogroups of Escherichia coli as a cause of community-acquired urinary infections]. Enferm Infecc Microbiol Clin 13: 236–241.
9. Mathai D, Jones RN, Pfaller MA (2001) Epidemiology and frequency of resistance among pathogens causing urinary tract infections in 1,510 hospitalized patients: a report from the SENTRY Antimicrobial Surveillance Program (North America). Diagn Microbiol Infect Dis 40: 129–136.
10. Karlowsky JA, Jones ME, Thornsberry C, Critchley I, Kelly LJ, et al. (2001) Prevalence of antimicrobial resistance among urinary tract pathogens isolated from female outpatients across the US in 1999. Int J Antimicrob Agents 18: 121–127.
11. Sahm DF, Thornsberry C, Mayfield DC, Jones ME, Karlowsky JA (2001) Multidrug-resistant urinary tract isolates of Escherichia coli: prevalence and patient demographics in the United States in 2000. Antimicrob Agents Chemother 45: 1402–1406.
12. Dombek PE, Johnson LK, Zimmerley ST, Sadowsky MJ (2000) Use of repetitive DNA sequences and the PCR To differentiate Escherichia coli isolates from human and animal sources. Appl Environ Microbiol 66: 2572–2577.
13. Quackenbush RL, Falkow S (1979) Relationship between colicin V activity and virulence in Escherichia coli. Infect Immun 24: 562–564.
14. Collee JG, Duguid JP, Fraser AG, Marmion BP, Simmons A (1996) Laboratory strategy in the diagnosis of infective syndromes. In: Collee JG, Fraser AG, Marmion BP, Simmons A, eds. Mackie and McCartney practical medical microbiology. 14th ed, Churchill Livingstone Inc: London. pp 53–94.
15. Barron EJ, Fingold MS (1990) Diagnostic Microbiology. In: Baily, Scott, eds. 8th ed. Mosby Public Philadelphia Toronto, Baltimore. pp 259–260.
16. Ewers C, Li G, Wilking H, Kiessling S, Alt K, et al. (2007) Avian pathogenic, uropathogenic, and newborn meningitis-causing Escherichia coli: how closely related are they? Int J Med Microbiol 297: 163–176.
17. Clinical and Laboratory Standards Institute (2006) 'Performing standards for antimicrobial susceptibility testing', Fifteenth information supplement, Approved standard MS45-A. Wayne, PA.
18. Babypadmini S, Appalaraju B (2004) Extended spectrum -lactamases in urinary isolates of Escherichia coli and Klebsiella pneumoniae - prevalence and susceptibility pattern in a tertiary care hospital. Indian J Med Microbiol 22: 172–174.
19. Tankhiwale SS, Jalgaonkar SV, Ahamad S, Hassani U (2004) Evaluation of extended spectrum beta lactamase in urinary isolates. Indian J Med Res 120: 553–556.
20. Sakoulas G, Eliopoulos GM, Moellering RC, Jr., Wennersten C, Venkataraman L, et al. (2002) Accessory gene regulator (agr) locus in geographically diverse Staphylococcus aureus isolates with reduced susceptibility to vancomycin. Antimicrob Agents Chemother 46: 1492–1502.
21. Siegfried L, Kmetova M, Puzova H, Molokacova M, Filka J (1994) Virulence-associated factors in Escherichia coli strains isolated from children with urinary tract infections. J Med Microbiol 41: 127–132.
22. Pezzlo M, York MK (2004) Urine Cultures. In: Isenberg HD, ed. Clinical Microbiology Procedures Handbook 2nd ed. Washington D. C.: American Society of Microbiology. pp 31211–131231.
23. Clermont O, Dhanji H, Upton M, Gibreel T, Fox A, et al. (2009) Rapid detection of the O25b-ST131 clone of Escherichia coli encompassing the CTX-M-15-producing strains. J Antimicrob Chemother 64: 274–277.
24. Versalovic J, Koeuth T, Lupski JR (1991) Distribution of repetitive DNA sequences in eubacteria and application to fingerprinting of bacterial genomes. Nucleic Acids Res 19: 6823–6831.
25. Rademaker JLW, de Bruijn FJ (1997) Characterization and classification of microbes by rep-PCR genomic fingerprinting and computer-assisted pattern analysis, 151–17. *In* Caetano-Anollés G, Gresshoff PM, eds. DNA markers: protocols, applications, and overviews, J. Wiley and Sons, New York, N.Y.
26. Gales AC, Sader HS, Jones RN (2002) Urinary tract infection trends in Latin American hospitals: report from the SENTRY antimicrobial surveillance program (1997–2000). Diagn Microbiol Infect Dis 44: 289–299.
27. Ulleryd P (2003) Febrile urinary tract infection in men. Int J Antimicrob Agents 22 Suppl 2: 89–93.
28. Johnson JR (1991) Virulence factors in Escherichia coli urinary tract infection. Clin Microbiol Rev 4: 80–128.
29. Najar GA, Nejad MM, Mansouri S (2007) The comparison between virulence factors of *Escherichia coli* isolated from urinary tract infections and fecal flora. Res Pharm Sci 2: 99 103.
30. Jacobsen SM, Stickler DJ, Mobley HL, Shirtliff ME (2008) Complicated catheter-associated urinary tract infections due to Escherichia coli and Proteus mirabilis. Clin Microbiol Rev 21: 26–59.
31. Minshew BH, Jorgensen J, Swanstrum M, Grootes-Reuvecamp GA, Falkow S (1978) Some characteristics of Escherichia coli strains isolated from extraintestinal infections of humans. J Infect Dis 137: 648–654.
32. Puzova H, Siegfried L, Kmetova M, Filka J, Takacova V, et al. (1994) Fimbriation, surface hydrophobicity and serum resistance in uropathogenic strains of Escherichia coli. FEMS Immunol Med Microbiol 9: 223–229.
33. Johnson JR (2003) Microbial virulence determinants and the pathogenesis of urinary tract infection. Infect Dis clin North Am 17(2): 261–71.
34. Ewers C, Grobbel M, Stamm I, Kopp PA, Diehl I, et al. (2010) Emergence of human pandemic O25:H4-ST131 CTX-M-15 extended-spectrum-beta-lactamase-producing Escherichia coli among companion animals. J Antimicrob Chemother 65: 651–660.
35. Nicolas-Chanoine MH, Blanco J, Leflon-Guibout V, Demarty R, Alonso MP, et al. (2008) Intercontinental emergence of Escherichia coli clone O25:H4-ST131 producing CTX-M-15. J Antimicrob Chemother 61: 273–281.
36. Wiles TJ, Kulesus RR, Mulvey MA (2008) Origins and virulence mechanisms of uropathogenic Escherichia coli. Exp Mol Pathol 85: 11–19.
37. Tambekar DH, Dhanorkar DV, Gulhane SR, Khandelwal VK, Dudhane MN (2006) Antibacterial susceptibility of some urinary tract pathogens to commonly used antibiotics. Afr J Biotechnol 5: 1562–1565.
38. Hannan TJ, Mysorekar IU, Hung CS, Isaacson-Schmid ML, Hultgren SJ (2010) Early severe inflammatory responses to uropathogenic E. coli predispose to chronic and recurrent urinary tract infection. PLoS Pathog 6: e1001042.

Trends in Antibiotic Prescribing in Adults in Dutch General Practice

Michiel B. Haeseker[1,4]*, Nicole H. T. M. Dukers-Muijrers[1,2,4], Christian J. P. A. Hoebe[1,2,4], Cathrien A. Bruggeman[1,4], Jochen W. L. Cals[3,4], Annelies Verbon[1,5]

1 Department of Medical Microbiology, Maastricht University Medical Centre, Maastricht, The Netherlands, **2** Department of Sexual Health, Infectious Diseases, and Environmental Health, Public Health Service South Limburg, Geleen, The Netherlands, **3** Department of General Practice, Maastricht University, Maastricht, The Netherlands, **4** School for Public Health and Primary Care (CAPHRI), Maastricht, The Netherlands, **5** Department of Internal Medicine Section, Infectious Disease, Erasmus Medical Centre, Rotterdam, The Netherlands

Abstract

Background: Antibiotic consumption is associated with adverse drug events (ADE) and increasing antibiotic resistance. Detailed information of antibiotic prescribing in different age categories is scarce, but necessary to develop strategies for prudent antibiotic use. The aim of this study was to determine the antibiotic prescriptions of different antibiotic classes in general practice in relation to age.

Methodology: Retrospective study of 22 rural and urban general practices from the Dutch Registration Network Family Practices (RNH). Antibiotic prescribing data were extracted from the RNH database from 2000–2009. Trends over time in antibiotic prescriptions were assessed with multivariate logistic regression including interaction terms with age. Registered ADEs as a result of antibiotic prescriptions were also analyzed.

Principal Findings: In total 658,940 patients years were analyzed. In 11.5% (n = 75,796) of the patient years at least one antibiotic was prescribed. Antibiotic prescriptions increased for all age categories during 2000–2009, but the increase in elderly patients (>80 years) was most prominent. In 2000 9% of the patients >80 years was prescribed at least one antibiotic to 22% in 2009 ($P<0.001$). Elderly patients had more ADEs with antibiotics and co-medication was identified as the only independent determinant for ADEs.

Conclusion/Discussion: The rate of antibiotic prescribing for patients who made a visit to the GP is increasing in the Netherlands with the most evident increase in the elderly patients. This may lead to more ADEs, which might lead to higher consumption of health care and more antibiotic resistance.

Editor: D. William Cameron, University of Ottawa, Canada

Funding: The authors have no support or funding to report.

Competing Interests: The authors have declared that no competing interests exist.

* E-mail: m.haeseker@mumc.nl

Introduction

The majority of antibiotics (80%) in the Netherlands are prescribed in primary care [1]. Outpatient antibiotic consumption is higher in elderly patients than in the general population [2–4] and most antibiotics are prescribed in elderly patients for respiratory tract infections (RTI) [5], skin and soft tissue infections [6] and urinary tract infections (UTI) [7]. However, detailed information of antibiotic prescribing in elderly is scarce. The majority of studies have been done in children, who also have a high antibiotic consumption [2,8,9]. The paucity of data on antibiotic use in elderly is surprising since elderly patients are more susceptible to toxic effects of antibiotics. For instance, adverse drug events (ADEs) have been described more frequently in frail elderly with co-morbidity and co-medication [10]. Additionally, elderly patients have altered pharmacokinetics, such as decreased absorption and elimination, which alters antibiotic blood levels, thereby influencing the risk of ADEs [11].

Antibiotic use is slowly, but steadily increasing in the Netherlands since 2005 [12]. It is unknown whether the increase in antibiotic use is equal in all age categories. Trends over time in antibiotic use per age category have not been studied and more information on the highest age categories is crucial as a quarter of the Dutch population will be above 65 years in the near future, similar to other European countries [13].

To determine trends in antibiotic prescribing in elderly, we have assessed antibiotic prescription rates by age categories in general practices over a ten year period in a large general practice database. Additionally, we have analyzed the incidence of registered ADEs due to antibiotics.

Methods

The data for this study are obtained retrospectively from the Dutch Registratie Netwerk Huisartsen (RNH, Registration Network Family Practices). The study group is described and regrouped into four different age categories: 18–44 years, 45–64 years, 65–79 years and ≥80 years. In these age categories, we have compared rates and trends over time in antibiotic prescriptions. Individual prescriptions per patient in a year were used as measure of prescriptions. For each prescription (at the moment of the specific consultation) information on ADE (until 4 weeks after prescription) and co-medication (at and during the prescription) were used. Data were then aggregated over a specific patient and calendar year to obtain a meaningful measure (% per patient-year).

Data Source

The RNH is a continuous, computerized and anonymous database from 22 rural and urban general practices in the south of the Netherlands, Limburg, [14]. During the study period the average number of patients >18 years in the RNH was 65,894 patients. The population was stable with respect to general sociodemographic characteristics.

The GP is responsible for the inclusion of patients. When a patient is included a unique RNH number is attributed to the patient. The GP records patient characteristics, i.e. birthdates, sex, educational level, insurance, type of household, marital status, place of residence, date of entry, last update and end of registration. The GP records all relevant health problems, only permanent, chronic and recurrent (>3 recurrences within a period of 6 months) are recorded, or when they had lasting consequences for the functional status or prognosis of the patient. Medication prescriptions (coded according to the Anatomical Therapeutic Chemical Index 2012 by the WHO Collaborating Centre for Drug Statistics Methodology) are included in the RNH database Registration. This includes type of medication, start and end date, and dose. Diagnoses are coded in a standardized fashion, according to the International Classification of Primary Care, using the criteria of the International Classification of Health in Primary Care and the current guidelines of the Dutch College of GPs [15]. Monitoring by the RNH registry ends at migration or death. All practices use MicroHIS (Torex-Hiscom), a commercially developed general practice health information software program containing a basic module, a medical module and a pharmacy module, which enable the GP to keep up an automated registration of his patients. Quarterly the RNH data collection module enables the GP to exchange all registered data to the central database. The RNH assistant checks the data and the RNH test module provides the distribution of the practice population, e.g. tables with the age distribution and the twenty most registered ICPC codes. The RNH exports the database in an SPSS data format.

A number of instruments are available in order to improve the quality and to reduce the inter-doctor variation: all GPs participating in the RNH are instructed and trained, RNH help program exists with all guidelines and criteria described, regional consensus group meeting take place at least 4 times a year to discus their registration difficulties, special software for data control in the health information system used by the GP and, special software for data control in the central database, several quality control experiments have been performed to gain insight into the quality of the database and several measures of agreement were done [14,16].

Data Analysis

Chronic diseases are selected from the classification from chronic diseases of Knottnerus [17]. We have included all chronic

Table 1. Population characteristics of the RNH in patient years.

	Antibiotic prescription		Total
	No	Yes	
Age categories			
• 18–44 yr	252,120 (43%)	28,297 (37%)	280,417 (43%)
• 45–64 yr	210,943 (36%)	26,581 (35%)	237,524 (36%)
• 65–79 yr	92,691 (16%)	15,440 (20%)	108,131 (16%)
• >80 yr	27,390 (5%)	5,478 (7%)	32,868 (5%)
Gender			
• Male	289,966 (50%)	28,655 (38%)	318,621 (48%)
• Female	293,178 (50%)	47,141 (62%)	340,319 (52%)
Education			
• Secondary school or lower secondary vocational education	188,361 (32%)	30,161 (40%)	218,522 (33%)
• Senior secondary vocational education	81,523 (14%)	11,905 (16%)	93,428 (14%)
• Higher education and University	26,248 (5%)	3,352 (4%)	29,600 (5%)
• Unknown	287,012 (49%)	30,378 (40%)	317,390 (48%)
Chronic disease			
• No	369,062 (63%)	39,161 (52%)	408,233 (62%)
• Yes	214,082 (37%)	36,635 (48%)	250,717 (38%)
General Practice			
• Rural	386,365 (66%)	45,900 (61%)	432,265 (66%)
• Urban	196,779 (34%)	29,896 (39%)	226,675 (34%)
Total	583,144 (85%)	75,796 (15%)	658,940 (100%)

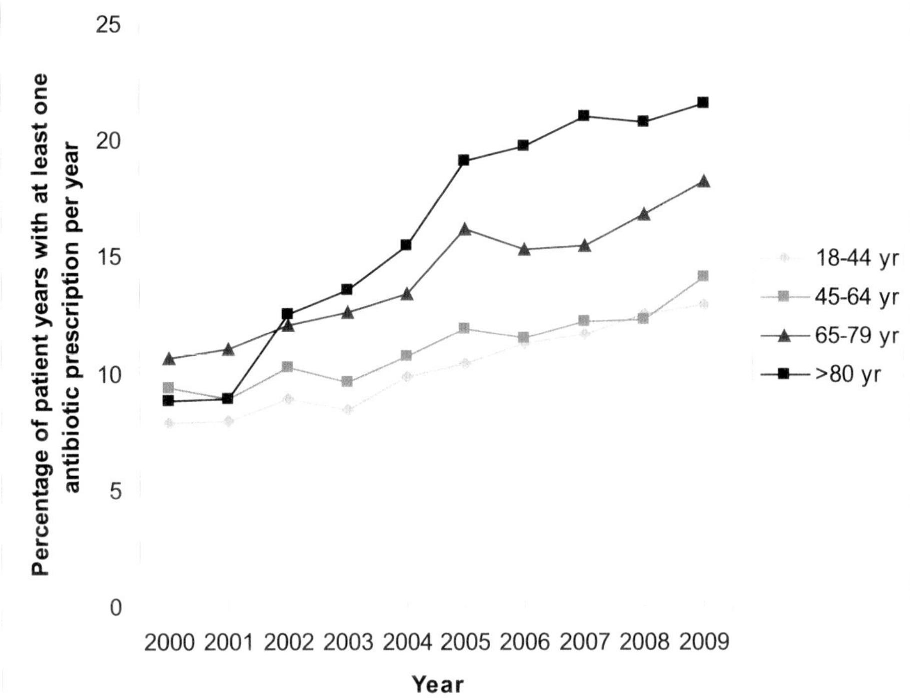

Figure 1. Percentage of patients years with at least one antibiotic prescription that year in different age categories during 2000–2009 (p<0.001).

diseases, only congenital diseases have been excluded. Using ATC code J01 for all antibacterial medication for systemic use, further discrimination is made for antibiotic classes used in general practice, i.e. tetracycline (ATC J01A), penicillins (ATC J01C), sulphonamides and trimetroprim (ATC J01E), macrolides (ATC J01F), fluoroquinolones (ATC J01MA) and nitrofuran derivates (ATC J01XE). Antifungals (J02) and anti-tuberculosis drug (J03) excluded All other medication present at the moment when antibiotics have been prescribed are considered co-medication. Co-medication is registered in the following groups of medication: drugs for peptic ulcer and gastro-esophageal reflux (ATC A02B), antithrombotic agents (ATC B01A), cardiovascular medication (ATC C), corticosteroids for systemic use (ATC H02), anti-inflammatory and anti-rheumatic products, non-steroids anti-inflammatory drugs (ATC M01A), other analgesics and anti-pyretics (ATC N02B), anxiolytics (ATC N05B), hypnotics and sedatives (ATC N05C), antidepressants (ATC N06A), and antihistamines for systemic use (ATC R06). Since 1996 the RNH is recording all ADEs as ICPC code A85. All kinds of ADEs could be recorded at the discretion of the attending GP. ADEs are considered associated with antibiotic prescription if occurring within four weeks after start of antibiotics. The ADEs are self-reported by patients and were recorded as an ADE at the discretion of the attending GP.

Statistical Analysis and Ethics

Unit of analyses are patient years, where a patient contributed one patient-year when he or she had attended a GP in that calendar year. Outcome measures included in the analyses are: antibiotic prescriptions (yes/no in a year), the number of antibiotic prescriptions (cumulated within a patient over a year) and ADEs (yes/no in a year). For antibiotic prescriptions, a multivariate model was build including age, time, gender, education level and rural versus and urban general practice, and chronic disease. In analyses with ADE as outcome restricted the study population to patient-years with antibiotic prescription and the multivariate model included age, time, gender, education level and rural versus and urban general practice, chronic disease and co-medication. The variables on age and time were presented, as these were our main focus, while controlling for the other variables. Interaction terms between age and time were explored. Statistical analysis is done with SPSS 16.0. A p-value <0.05 is considered statistically significant.

All patients included in the RNH database have been informed about the potential anonymous use of their health information. If a patient does not agree, the inclusion of this patient in the RNH database is stopped. All data in this study were analyzed anonymously, only medications and clinical data were used. The Medical Ethics Committee of the Maastricht University Medical Center approved this study (METC 12-4-053).

Results

A total of 658,940 patient years were analyzed from 2000–2009: 43% (n = 280,417) of the patients years were aged between 18–44 years, 36% (n = 237,524) between 45–64 years, 16% (n = 108,131) between 65–79 years and 5.0% (n = 32,868) ≥80 years. Forty eight percent (n = 318,621) of the patient years were comprised by male and 52% (n = 340,319) were comprised by female, see Table 1 for population characteristics of the RNH. Socio-demographical characteristics of samples in other studies, which made use of the RNH database, have shown to be comparable to the Dutch population [16]. The elderly (>65 years) are slightly

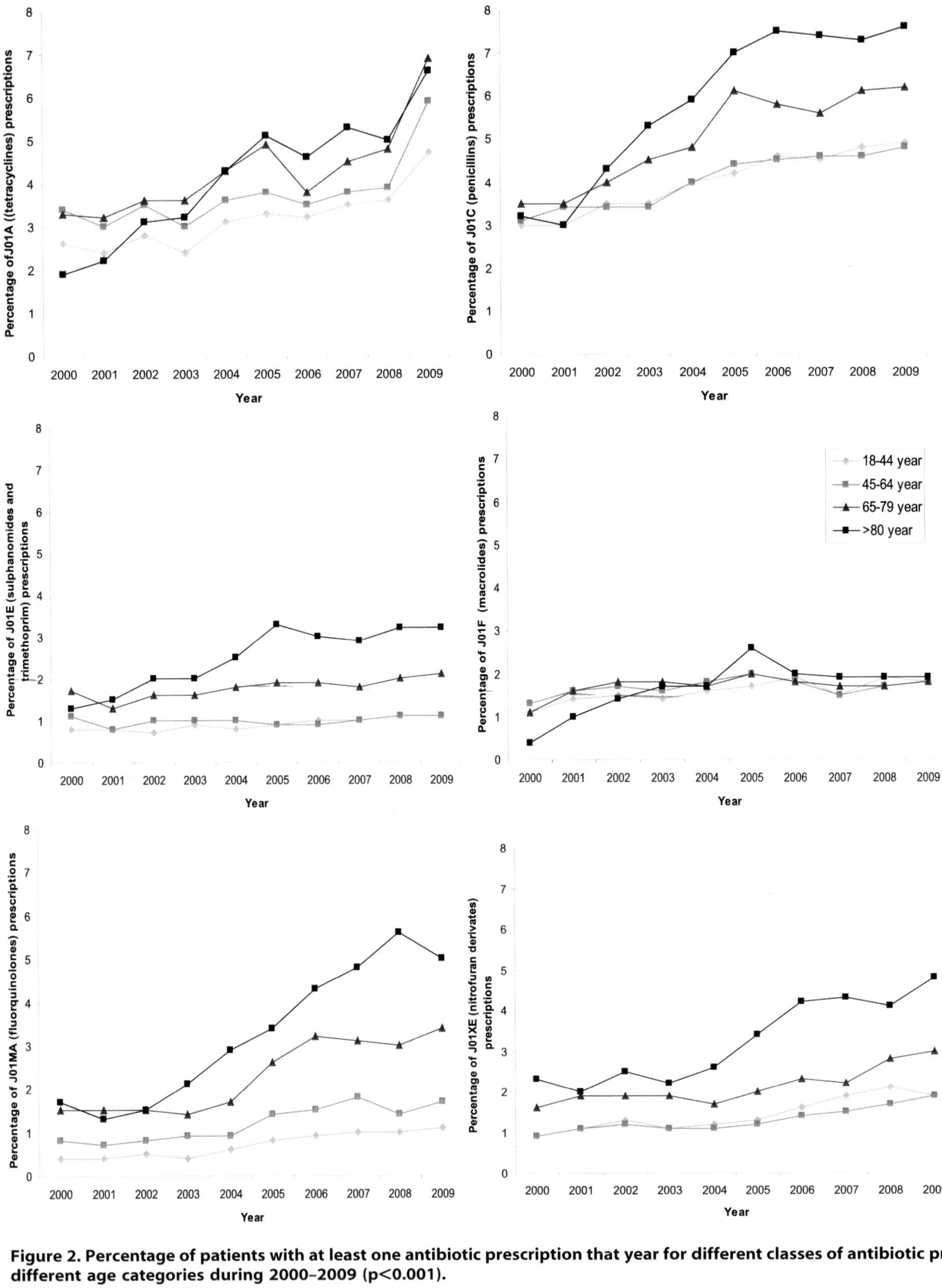

Figure 2. Percentage of patients with at least one antibiotic prescription that year for different classes of antibiotic prescriptions in different age categories during 2000–2009 (p<0.001).

overrepresented in the RNH, 22% compared to 14% in the Dutch population in 2007. Hence, we do consider our results to be accurate and representative for the Dutch population, with a high internal and external generalizability.

In total 11.5% (n = 75,796) of the patient years at least one antibiotic per year was prescribed. Antibiotics were more often prescribed in elderly patients ($p<0.001$), as shown in **Figure 1**. The association with higher age was present in all years studied. Prescription rates of all antibiotics increased in all age-categories over time (all $p<0.001$). Although an increase was observed in all age categories, the increase was strongest in patients >80 years (interaction between age and time: $p<0.001$). This increase is seen

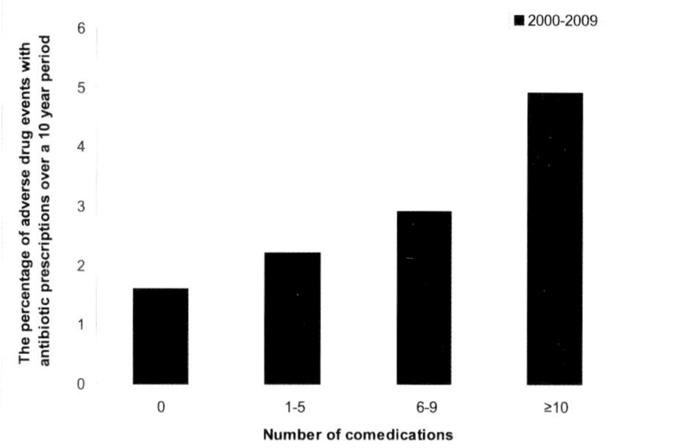

Figure 3. Percentage of adverse drug events with number of co-medication per age category during 2000–2009.

for all antibiotic classes, with the exception of the macrolides (**Figure 2**). The number of antibiotic prescriptions per patient per year increased with age ($p<0.001$): two or more antibiotic courses were prescribed for 18% (n = 1,571) of the patients years in 18–44 years, 19% (n = 5,042) in 45–64 years, 23% (n = 3,581) in 65–79 years and 29% (n = 1571) in ≥80 years. The number of prescriptions independently increased with age and independently increased over time ($p<0.001$).

ADEs, Underlying Diseases and co-medication

Of all patients who received an antibiotic prescription, the minority (2%; n = 1,526/75,796) reported an ADE in the four weeks time window. In a random sample of 4 week periods from the same patients, compared to any 4 week period, excluding antibiotic prescriptions during this period, rates found were 0.06% (n = 425/658,346) without antibiotics. No time trend in ADE reporting was observed. ADEs were not reported more frequently in the later years (2008/2009) compared to the earlier years (2000/2001). ADEs increased per age category per calendar year from 1.8% in 18–44 years, 1.9% in 45–64 years and 2.3% in 65–79 years to 2.8% in ≥80 years. However, co-medication also increased per age category from 23% (n = 6,529) in 18–44 years, 49% (n = 13,078) in 45–64 years and 70% (n = 10,978) in 65–79 years to 78% (n = 4,275) in ≥80 years. As expected, underlying chronic diseases increased by age. Of all patient years analyzed 18% (n = 50,924) were diagnosed with at least one chronic disease, 40% (n = 94,376) in the 45–64, 72% (n = 77,530) in 65–79 and 85% (n = 27,887) in >80 years age category. In the univariate analysis older age, having one or more chronic disease and co-medication were associated with occurrence of ADE. In the multivariate analysis use of co-medication remained associated with ADE ($p<0.001$) (**Figure 3**), while age and chronic disease were not.

Discussion

This large primary cohort shows that the rate of antibiotic prescribing for patients who made a visit to the GP has increased in Dutch general practice from 2000 to 2009 in all adult age categories. We have observed the highest increase in the rate of antibiotic prescriptions in elderly patients; from 9% of patients receiving at least one antibiotic in 2000 to 22% in 2009. Additionally, elderly patients more often receive two or more antibiotic prescriptions per patient than younger patients. We have shown increasing trends for all antibiotic subgroups. This is particularly striking for the fluoroquinolones, as these are not indicated as first choice in any Dutch general practice guideline. In the United States nonapproved fluoroquinolone prescribing has already been described in 2005 [18]. Only the macrolides have shown a stable prescription pattern over time and across groups. Elderly patients have more ADEs associated with antibiotics. Co-medication has been identified as the only independent determinant for ADEs. Age was not in the multivariate analysis.

Our finding that the antibiotic prescription is increasing since 2005 in the Netherlands is comparable with the increase in Europe as shown in the European Surveillance of Antimicrobial Consumption data [19]. Although, the prescription rate in the Netherlands is increasing, it is still low compared to other European countries [19]. The Dutch guidelines for GPs of common infections have not been changed significantly during these ten-years. However, the increase of the number of fluoroquinolone prescriptions suggests that guidelines are not always followed. The increase in antibiotic prescriptions might be explained by an increased consultation frequency for acute infections, such as RTIs and UTIs. Although, the consultation frequency historically has tended to decrease over the years [20], it was recently shown that consultation rates for lower RTIs are increasing in the Netherlands while RTI related consultations are stable in the UK [21]. In this study however, we did not have access to the ICPC coding for acute conditions such as acute respiratory tract infections.

To our knowledge only three previous studies, one in England/Wales, one in New Zealand and one in Italy, have shown higher antibiotic consumption in elderly patients (>75 years) [2,3]. We showed that elderly patients consistently have high antibiotic prescription rates compared to the younger patients and there is an increasing trend over time as well in these in elderly patients.

The highest risk group to develop ADEs is aged over 80 years with multiple co-morbidity and co-medication [22,23]. Inappropriate prescriptions are a leading cause for the development of ADEs [24,25]. Although, the observed rate of ADEs in our study is lower than the 5–35% found in other studies [26–28] our study is in line with studies that show that co-medication and the number of co-medication is an independent association with ADEs due to antibiotic use [23,29]. To prevent ADEs in elderly patients due to antibiotic use, the necessity of antibiotic treatment needs to be carefully determined, especially when co-medication is used. Minimizing unnecessary antibiotic treatment by even a small percentage could significantly reduce immediate and direct risks of ADE in individual patients [30].

The main strengths of this study are the long study period and the large representative study group. Since 1996 this RNH database is keeping records of all medications (including antibiotics) via a computerized medical registration program. Data accuracy can be guaranteed as data extraction takes place from electronic medical records of practices and regular training of the GPs and quality controls of the data take place [14,16]. All patients with multiple antibiotic prescriptions per year have been included only once per year. Therefore, this study group is not biased by a few fragile elderly patients with multiple antibiotic prescriptions.

However, this study has several limitations. Firstly, antibiotic prescriptions could not be given in daily defined dosages (DDDs) like some international data [31,32], limiting comparability with other studies. Secondly, we have no diagnostic information on acute infections. Thirdly, ADEs were self-reported by the patients, most probably underestimating the incidence of ADE associated with antibiotics.

Based on our findings, future strategies to decrease the antibiotic consumption and antibiotic resistance in the Netherlands should be addressed to all adult age categories. The elderly could be a specific target group and more in-depth study into the reasons for increasing antibiotic prescribing is necessary.

Acknowledgments

The authors thank Alfons Schroten, Job Metsemakers and Marjan van den Akker for the database support. The authors are also grateful to the GPs of the RNH.

Author Contributions

Conceived and designed the experiments: AV CAB NDM CJH. Performed the experiments: MBH NDM. Analyzed the data: MBH NDM CJH AV JWC. Wrote the paper: MBH NDM CJH CAB JWC AV.

References

1. Kuyvenhoven MM, van Balen FA, Verheij TJ (2003) Outpatient antibiotic prescriptions from 1992 to 2001 in the Netherlands. J Antimicrob Chemother 52: 675–678.
2. Majeed A, Moser K (1999) Age- and sex-specific antibiotic prescribing patterns in general practice in England and Wales in 1996. Br J Gen Pract 49: 735–736.
3. Norris P, Horsburgh S, Keown S, Arroll B, Lovelock K, et al. (2011) Too much and too little? Prevalence and extent of antibiotic use in a New Zealand region. J Antimicrob Chemother 66: 1921–1926.
4. Pan A, Buttazzi R, Marchi M, Gagliotti C, Resi D, et al. (2011) Secular trends in antibiotic consumption in the adult population in Emilia-Romagna, Italy, 2003–2009. Clin Microbiol Infect 17: 1698–1703.
5. Feldman C (2001) Pneumonia in the elderly. Med Clin North Am 85: 1441–1459.
6. Laube S (2004) Skin infections and ageing. Ageing Res Rev 3: 69–89.
7. Richards CL (2004) Urinary tract infections in the frail elderly: issues for diagnosis, treatment and prevention. Int Urol Nephrol 36: 457–463.
8. Finkelstein JA, Metlay JP, Davis RL, Rifas-Shiman SL, Dowell SF, et al. (2000) Antimicrobial use in defined populations of infants and young children. Arch Pediatr Adolesc Med 154: 395–400.
9. Otters HB, van der Wouden JC, Schellevis FG, van Suijlekom-Smit LW, Koes BW (2004) Trends in prescribing antibiotics for children in Dutch general practice. J Antimicrob Chemother 53: 361–366.
10. Faulkner CM, Cox HL, Williamson JC (2005) Unique aspects of antimicrobial use in older adults. Clin Infect Dis 40: 997–1004.
11. Herring AR, Williamson JC (2007) Principles of antimicrobial use in older adults. Clin Geriatr Med 23: 481–497, v.
12. SFK (2010) Antibioticagebruik groeit gestaag (Antibiotic use is growing). Available: http://www.sfk.nl/nieuws-publicaties/PW/2010/2010-07.html. Accessed 2012 Nov 14.
13. Eurostat (2010) Population projections 2010–2060 http://epp.eurostat.ec.europa.eu/cache/ITY_PUBLIC/3-08062011-BP/EN/3-08062011-BP-EN.PDF.Accessed 2012 Nov 14.
14. Akker van den M MJ, Limonard C, Knotnerus J (2004) General Practice: a gold mine for research. Data and scientific use of the Registration Network Family Practices.
15. Hofmans-Okkes IM, Lamberts H (1996) The International Classification of Primary Care (ICPC): new applications in research and computer-based patient records in family practice. Fam Pract 13: 294–302.
16. Metsemakers JF, Knottnerus JA, van Schendel GJ, Kocken RJ, Limonard CB (1996) Unlocking patients' records in general practice for research, medical education and quality assurance: the Registration Network Family Practices. Int J Biomed Comput 42: 43–50.
17. Knottnerus JA, Metsemakers J, Hoppener P, Limonard C (1992) Chronic illness in the community and the concept of 'social prevalence'. Fam Pract 9: 15–21.
18. Linder JA, Huang ES, Steinman MA, Gonzales -R, Stafford RS (2005) Fluoroquinolone prescribing in the United States: 1995 to 2002. Am J Med 118: 259–268.
19. Adriaenssens N, Coenen S, Versporten A, Muller A, Minalu G, et al. (2011) European Surveillance of Antimicrobial Consumption (ESAC): outpatient antibiotic use in Europe (1997–2009). J Antimicrob Chemother 66 Suppl 6: vi3–12.
20. Cosby JL, Francis N, Butler CC (2007) The role of evidence in the decline of antibiotic use for common respiratory infections in primary care. Lancet Infect Dis 7: 749–756.
21. Gulliford M, Latinovic R, Charlton J, Little P, van Staa T, et al. (2009) Selective decrease in consultations and antibiotic prescribing for acute respiratory tract infections in UK primary care up to 2006. J Public Health (Oxf) 31: 512–520.
22. Beard K (1992) Adverse reactions as a cause of hospital admission in the aged. Drugs Aging 2: 356–367.
23. Lazarou J, Pomeranz BH, Corey PN (1998) Incidence of adverse drug reactions in hospitalized patients: a meta-analysis of prospective studies. JAMA 279: 1200–1205.
24. Beers MH (1997) Explicit criteria for determining potentially inappropriate medication use by the elderly. An update. Arch Intern Med 157: 1531–1536.
25. O'Mahony D, Gallagher PF (2008) Inappropriate prescribing in the older population: need for new criteria. Age Ageing 37: 138–141.
26. Gandhi TK, Weingart SN, Borus J, Seger AC, Peterson J, et al. (2003) Adverse drug events in ambulatory care. N Engl J Med 348: 1556–1564.
27. Hanlon JT, Schmader KE, Koronkowski MJ, Weinberger M, Landsman PB, et al. (1997) Adverse drug events in high risk older outpatients. J Am Geriatr Soc 45: 945–948.
28. Hutchinson TA, Flegel KM, Kramer MS, Leduc DG, Kong HH (1986) Frequency, severity and risk factors for adverse drug reactions in adult outpatients: a prospective study. J Chronic Dis 39: 533–542.
29. Laroche ML, Charmes JP, Nouaille Y, Picard N, Merle L (2007) Is inappropriate medication use a major cause of adverse drug reactions in the elderly? Br J Clin Pharmacol 63: 177–186.
30. Shehab N, Patel PR, Srinivasan A, Budnitz DS (2008) Emergency department visits for antibiotic-associated adverse events. Clin Infect Dis 47: 735–743.
31. Ferech M, Coenen S, Malhotra-Kumar S, Dvorakova K, Hendrickx E, et al. (2006) European Surveillance of Antimicrobial Consumption (ESAC): outpatient antibiotic use in Europe. J Antimicrob Chemother 58: 401–407.
32. Goossens H, Ferech M, Coenen S, Stephens P (2007) Comparison of outpatient systemic antibacterial use in 2004 in the United States and 27 European countries. Clin Infect Dis 44: 1091–1095.

12

Genetic Control of the Variable Innate Immune Response to Asymptomatic Bacteriuria

Jenny Grönberg Hernández[1], Fredrik Sundén[2], John Connolly[3], Catharina Svanborg[1]*, Björn Wullt[1]

1 Department of Microbiology, Immunology and Glycobiology, Institute of Laboratory Medicine, Lund University, Lund, Sweden, 2 Department of Urology, Skåne University Hospital, Malmö, Sweden, 3 Singapore Immunology Network (SIgN), Biomedical Sciences Institutes, Agency for Science, Technology, and Research (A*STAR), Singapore, Singapore

Abstract

The severity of urinary tract infection (UTI) reflects the quality and magnitude of the host response. While strong local and systemic innate immune activation occurs in patients with acute pyelonephritis, the response to asymptomatic bacteriuria (ABU) is low. The immune response repertoire in ABU has not been characterized, due to the inherent problem to distinguish bacterial differences from host-determined variation. In this study, we investigated the host response to ABU and genetic variants affecting innate immune signaling and UTI susceptibility. Patients were subjected to therapeutic urinary tract inoculation with *E. coli* 83972 to ensure that they were exposed to the same *E. coli* strain. The innate immune response repertoire was characterized in urine samples, collected from each patient before and after inoculation with bacteria or PBS, if during the placebo arm of the study. Long-term *E. coli* 83972 ABU was established in 23 participants, who were followed for up to twelve months and the innate immune response was quantified in 233 urine samples. Neutrophil numbers increased in all but two patients and in an extended urine cytokine/chemokine analysis (31 proteins), the chemoattractants IL-8 and GRO-α, RANTES, Eotaxin-1 and MCP-1, the T cell chemoattractant and antibacterial peptide IP-10, inflammatory regulators IL-1-α and sIL-1RA and the T lymphocyte/dendritic cell product sIL-2Rα were detected and variably increased, compared to sterile samples. IL-6, which is associated with symptomatic UTI, remained low and numerous specific immune mediators were not detected. The patients were also genotyped for UTI-associated *IRF3* and *TLR4* promoter polymorphisms. Patients with ABU associated *TLR4* polymorphisms had low neutrophil numbers, IL-6, IP-10, MCP-1 and sIL-2Rα concentrations. Patients with the ABU-associated *IRF3* genotype had lower neutrophils, IL-6 and MCP-1 responses than the remaining group. The results suggest that the host-specific, low immune response to ABU mainly includes innate immune mediators and that host genetics directly influence the magnitude of this response.

Editor: Adam J. Ratner, Columbia University, United States of America

Funding: The studies were supported by grants from the Swedish Medical Research Council (2010 3070), the Crafoord, Wallenberg and Lundberg Foundations, the Österlund Foundation and the Royal Physiographic Society. Furthermore, the inoculation study was supported by the Foundations of Gösta Jönsson, Hillevi Fries, Per-Olof Ström and Greta Ekholm, Lund, Sweden; Coloplast, Copenhagen, Denmark; Riksförbundet för Trafik och Polioskadade; the Swedish Strategic Programme Against Antibiotic Resistance (STRAMA) and by Region Skåne's FoU grants. The funders had no role in study design, data collection and analysis, decision to publish, or preparation of the manuscript.

Competing Interests: The authors have declared that no competing interests exist.

* E-mail: catharina.svanborg@med.lu.se

Introduction

The symptoms and severity of urinary tract infection (UTI) reflect the host response to the infecting strain. In patients with acute pyelonephritis, bacteria trigger a local inflammatory response in the urinary tract, detected as an increase in urine neutrophils and cytokine levels [1,2,3]. In addition, the systemic involvement in acute pyelonephritis causes fever and elevated acute phase reactants like C-reactive protein (CRP) [4,5,6] and in about 30% of adults, pyelonephritis is accompanied by bacteremia. Patients with asymptomatic bacteriuria (ABU), in contrast, are protected from the development of acute pathology due to a weak host response to infection [7]. They may also be protected from re-infection, if the strain that they carry outcompetes more pathogenic strains [8]. However, variation in the host response has also been noted in patients with ABU, leading to uncertainty about the extent of innate immune reactivity in ABU. Neutrophil numbers in urine vary greatly among patients with ABU and the diagnostic value of pyuria has been debated in this patient group [6]. To use host response parameters as a basis for diagnostic and therapeutic decisions in clinical practice, such variability needs to be assessed [6,9]. More recent and extensive information on the variable immune repertoire in patients with ABU is lacking, however.

Innate immunity controls the antibacterial defense in the urinary tract and effector molecules include mucosal cytokines, chemokines and antibacterial peptides as well as recruited inflammatory cells [1,10,11,12,13]. Uroepithelial recognition of *E. coli* triggers the innate immune response and specifically, the Toll-like receptor (TLR) 4 signaling pathway is critically involved [10,14]. Downstream activation of transcription factors IRF3 or NF-κB stimulates the transcription of chemokine genes and increases e.g. IL-8 and IL-6 expression in the urinary tract [15]. Mice lacking *Tlr4* develop an ABU like state without acute tissue inflammation [10] and in patients with ABU, reduced TLR4 expression has been detected [7]. Mice lacking *Irf3*, in contrast, develop severe acute pyelonephritis with urosepsis and renal damage [15]. Polymorphisms in the *TLR4* and *IRF3* promoters have been detected [16,17] and associated to ABU [15], suggesting that the genetic repertoire of the host contributes to the reduced innate immune response in this patient group. Recent genetic screens in women with and without ABU detected an association between polymorphisms in *TLR2* and *CXCR1*, but their effect on the cellular immune response repertoire in ABU and the effects of bacterial strain diversity have not been considered [18].

Further complicating the understanding of the host response to ABU is the origin of the infecting strain and resulting variability in virulence factor expression [19,20,21,22]. To specifically evaluate the host response to ABU, we have examined samples from patients subjected to therapeutic inoculation with the ABU prototype strain *Escherichia coli* 83972 [8]. Through this unique approach, we have excluded the bacterial strain variation accompanying natural infection. The host response was characterized by broad urine proteomic profiling, and the host *TLR4* and *IRF3* genotypes were determined. The results show that ABU elicits a low, host specific innate immune response and that the patient genotype influences the propensity to mount a host response to ABU.

Results

Patients and samples

To characterize the host response to ABU, we included 23 patients participating in a placebo-controlled study of therapeutic *E. coli* 83972-inoculation (Table 1) [8]. In patients who developed *E. coli* 83972 ABU, 233 *E. coli* 83972-positive urine samples representing 260 months of observation were collected (mean 11.4, range 3.8–19.1 months). Sterile samples collected from the same patient group (20/23 patients) after saline inoculations in the placebo arm of the study, were used to distinguish the host response to *E. coli* 83972 from protein secretion into sterile urine (Figure 1).

Table 1. Patient Characteristics.

			E.coli 83972 ABU			Sterile	
Patient ID[1]	Age	CIC[2]	Inoculation attempts	Months	Urine samples	Urine samples	Diagnosis
lower motor neuron lesions, residual urine							
M1	77	+	2	9.4	11	6	Idiopathic detrusor insufficiency
F1	59	+	2	11.8	12	1	Idiopathic detrusor insufficiency
F2	66	+	1	12.2	11	3	Residual urine after urethropexia
F3	46	0	1	12.1	13	3	Detrusor insufficiency; after borreliainfection
F4	84	0	1	10.5	10	0	Idiopathic detrusor insufficiency
F5	82	+	1	12.0	10	2	Idiopathic detrusor insufficiency
F6	77	0	1	8.3	9	5	Idiopathic detrusor insufficiency; coronary by pass surgery
F7	45	0	3	5.2	4	3	Detrusor insufficiency; diabetes mellitus type 1
F8	76	0	2	3.8	4	2	Idiopathic detrusor insufficiency
F9	64	0	1	12.0	12	4	Residual urine after urethropexia; cystocele
M2	72	+	1	11.6	16	5	Detrusor insufficiency; after encephalitis
F10	32	0	1	10.7	9	5	Idiopathic detrusor insufficiency
spinal lesions							
M3	76	+	2	19.1	10	1	Tetraplegia
M4	39	0	1	11.1	10	6	Tetraplegia; spinal cord injury
M5	47	+	3	17.3	10	0	Tetraplegia; spinal cord injury, diabetes mellitus type 2, sphincterotomy.
F11	60	+	3	10.4	9	4	Tetraplegia; epidural hematoma
M6	52	+	1	16.8	14	5	Tetraplegia
F12	61	+	1	10.8	11	0	Paraplegia; slipped disc, epidural hematoma
M7	51	+	1	4.0	3	2	Tetraplegia; spinal cord injury
M8	68	+	2	16.6	11	1	Tetraplegia
M9	38	+	1	12.2	13	4	Tetraplegia; spinal cord injury
M10	55	+	1	12.2	12	3	Tetraplegia; epidural hematoma
M11	45	+	1	11.0	9	3	Paraplegia; spinal cord injury

The table displays data from trials performed between 1993 and June, 2005. All patients had incomplete bladder emptying (residual urine ≥100 ml) and UTI susceptibility with a history ≥3 UTI/ year with urinary cultures showing uropathogenic growth, two years prior to the study.

1) M = Male, F = Female.

2) Clean Intermittent Catheterization. All patients had been instructed to use CIC regularly. Of the 8 patients who did not use CIC during the study 2 patients refused because of practical reasons and the remaining 6 patients had residual urine <300 ml, and had not experienced any improvement from previously performed regular CIC.

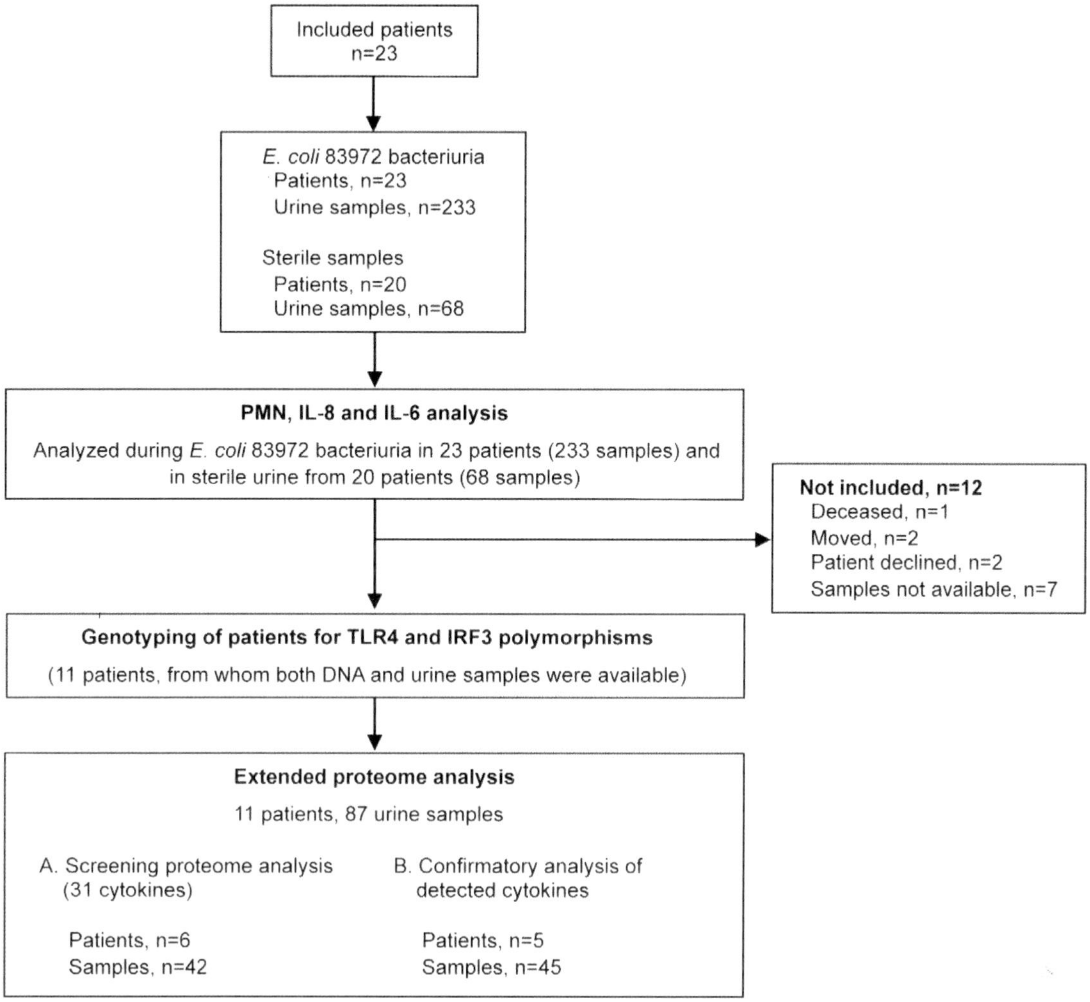

Figure 1. Patients and samples. Samples from patients participating in a clinical trial of induced *E. coli* 83972 ABU were analyzed. All collected urine samples were subjected to PMN, IL-6 and IL-8 quantification, and blood samples from eleven patients were collected for genotyping of promoter polymorphisms in TLR4 and IRF3. Blood and urine samples from these eleven patients were also selected for an extended urine protein analysis.

Basic host response parameters; PMN, IL-8 and IL-6 responses to E. coli 83972 ABU

All urine samples were initially screened for neutrophil numbers and IL-6/IL-8 concentrations. Significant PMN and IL-8 responses to ABU (both $p<0.0001$) were detected compared to sterile samples ($p<0.0001$, Figure 2A) with elevated levels in 21/23 patients (Figure 2B). Intra-individual variability during long-term *E. coli* 83972 ABU was also evaluated in repeat samples from each patient (Figure 2C). The host response variation was more limited for neutrophil numbers than for IL-8 concentrations. Variability in neutrophil counts was lower in high responders (median >100 x neutrophils/ml, $n=4$), but the opposite was observed for the IL-8 concentrations, which were more stable in the low responders (median <500 ng/l, $n=14$) (Figure 2C). No IL-6 response was detected (Figures 2A–C).

To further address if the magnitude of the host response to *E. coli* 83972 ABU was stable in each individual, PMN, IL-8 and IL-6 responses after the first and second inoculations were compared in the six patients who were colonized with *E. coli* 83972 twice and developed bacteriuria periods lasting at least three months (total $n=75$ urine samples). Neutrophil and IL-8 responses to repeat inoculations were highly reproducible (Figure 3A). The kinetics of PMN, IL-8 and IL-6 responses during the first 150 days after inoculation are shown in Figure 3B for one high and one low responder. The results suggest that ABU elicits a variable innate host response, the level of which is host specific.

Urine cytokine/chemokine proteome during E. coli 83972 ABU

Human uroepithelial cells respond to infection by secreting cytokines and chemokines. The response is further modified by the activation of other resident and recruited cells, including neutrophils that predominate in the acute cellular infiltrate during UTI [11]. To further characterize the mucosal host response repertoire in patients with *E. coli* 83972 ABU, 87 urine samples from eleven patients were subjected to extended urine cytokine/chemokine proteome analysis (Table 2 and Figure 4). Six patients (42 urine samples) were selected for an extensive urine cytokine/chemokine screening of 31 immune-related protein proteins. The IL-8 and IL-6 concentrations obtained in the screen corresponded to the results previously obtained by the Immulite method. In addition, the screen revealed the presence in urine of seven

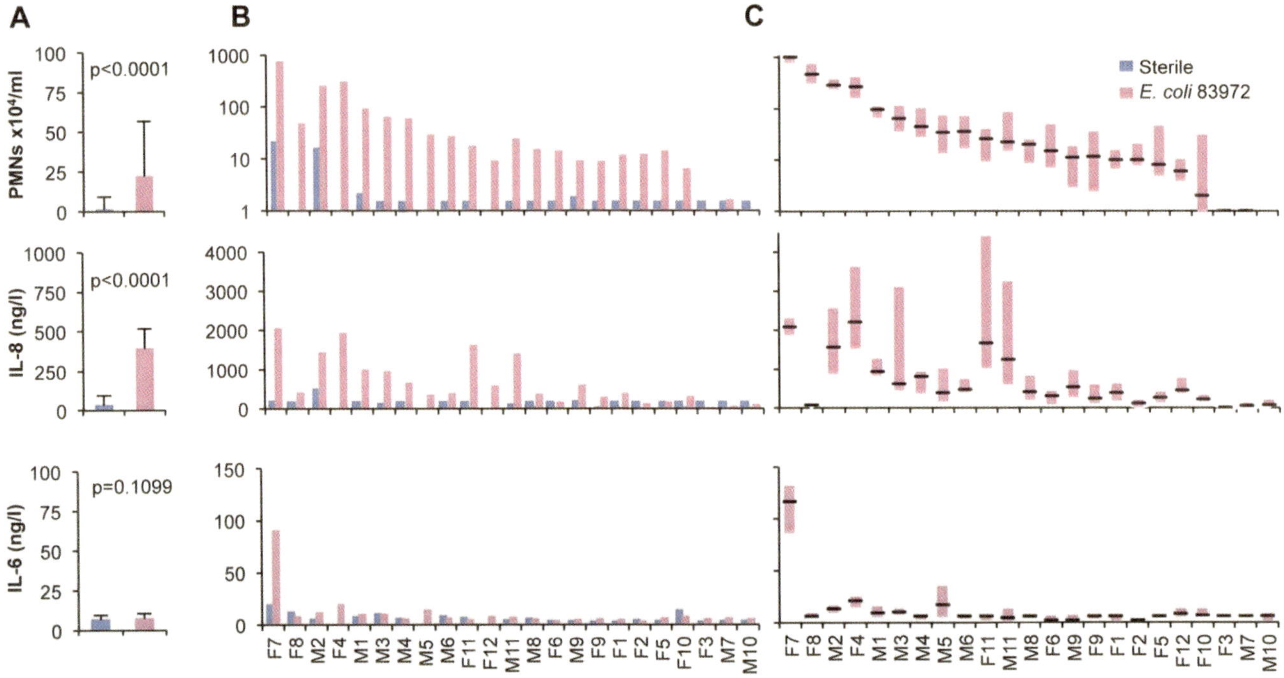

Figure 2. Host response to *E. coli* 83972 bacteriuria. *E. coli* 83972 ABU triggered an increase in PMN numbers and IL-8 concentrations ($p<0.0001$) but IL-6 levels were unchanged (n.s., Mann-Whitney test). Group-wise comparison of monthly urine samples collected during *E. coli* 83927 ABU or after PBS inoculations. Coded patient IDs are noted on the x-axis. A. Means + SEs of neutrophil numbers, IL-8 and IL-6 concentrations during *E. coli* 83972 bacteriuria (pink) or sterile conditions (blue). B. Intra-individual comparison of samples obtained during *E. coli* 83972 bacteriuria (pink) and sterile intervals (blue). C. Box-plot of intra-individual host response variation during *E. coli* 83972 ABU.

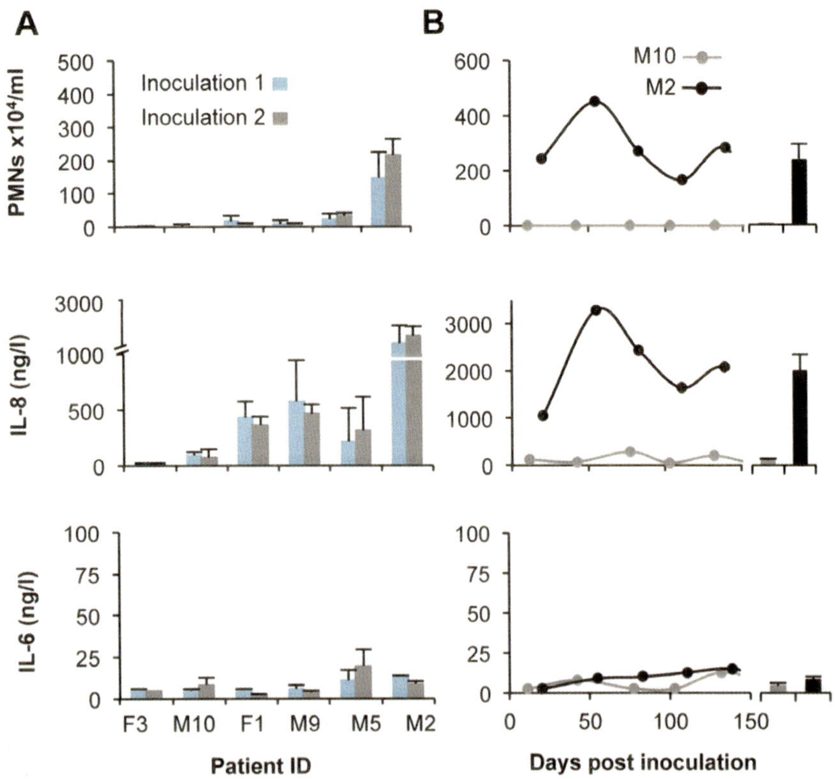

Figure 3. Consistency of the individual host response to *E. coli* 83972 inoculation. A. The host response in urine samples from the first (blue) and second inoculations (grey) were compared (Geometric means + SEs) in six patients that had received repeated inoculations. B. Kinetics of the host response during the first and second ABU episode in one high and one low responder.

Table 2. Groupwise analysis of the urine cytokine/chemokine proteome response to *E. coli* 83972 ABU.

Host response Parameter[a]	*E. coli* 83972 ABU Mean[b]		SEM	Sterile[c] Mean		SEM	p-value[d]
PMNs	46.0	±	26.8	2.1	±	1.2	0.0038
IL-8	654.8	±	209.3	50.2	±	35.9	0.0004
IL-6	5.5	±	1.0	3.2	±	0.5	0.2984
GRO-α	379.2	±	152.1	32.3	±	9.1	0.0062
IP-10	72.6	±	15.4	0.1	±	11.2	0.0138
MCP-1	265.5	±	56.8	121.6	±	22.0	0.0583
IL-1α	4.2	±	0.6	0.5	±	0.3	0.0024
IL-1RA	21.6	±	10.8	7.3	±	3.9	0.4466
sIL-2Rα	161.5	±	45.8	0.1	±	34.0	0.2537
RANTES	5.82	±	0.97	4.51	±	6.9	0.1733
Eotaxin-1	4.8	±	1.8	5.1	±	1.7	
IL-12p40	15.7	±	3.0	-			
IFN-α_2	20.5	±	-	-			

[a]Parameters were analyzed in 87 samples from 11 patients, except for RANTES which was analyzed in 64 samples from ten patients, and Eotaxin-1, IL-12p40 and IFN- α2 in 42 samples from six patients. Not detected: CCL22, MIP-1α, GM-SCF, G-CSF, MCP-3, sFasL, sICAM-1, IL-1β, IL-2, IL-3, IL-4, IL-5, IL-7, IL-10, IL-12p70, IL-13, IL-15, TNF-α, IFN-γ.
[b]Mean of individual median values for each protein from eleven patients.
[c]Mean of individual median values for each protein from nine patients, except for Eotaxin-1 (mean from 6 patients).
[d]Mann-Whitney test.

immune mediators, GRO-α, IP-10, MCP-1, sIL-2Rα, IL-1α, sIL-1RA and RANTES. Nineteen proteins were not detected and three were detected in four (Eotaxin-1, 32 samples), three (IL-12p40, 14 samples) and one patient (IFNα$_2$, one sample, see Table 2). The detected proteins were subsequently quantified in the remaining urine samples, using a custom made assay (five patients, 45 samples).

In addition to IL-8 (Table 2, $p<0.0004$), the cytokine array detected significantly increased levels of the neutrophil chemoattractant GRO-α during ABU in the entire patient group compared to all sterile controls (Table 2, $p<0.0062$) and by intra-individual analysis significantly increased levels were detected in four individuals. A significant correlation between IL-8, GRO-α concentrations and neutrophil numbers was detected in individual patients ($p=0.001$ and, $p<0.0001$ respectively, Figure 4E). By group-wise analysis, no significant MCP-1 response was detected but median levels in 9/11 patients were higher than in sterile urine and in two patients, a significant increase was observed compared to the sterile samples (Figure 4A). A correlation of the monocyte chemoattractant MCP-1 with neutrophils was also detected ($p=0.0045$, Figure 4E) but was limited to high neutrophil numbers, when the more complex inflammatory infiltrate might include monocytes.

Uroepithelial cells express IL-1 in two forms; IL-1α, which is mainly membrane-bound and IL-1β, which is a secreted cytokine [23,24]. A significant IL-1α response to ABU was detected in the entire patient group ($p=0.002$, Figure 4B), with elevated median concentrations in all patients and in four patients a significant increase was observed compared to the individual sterile samples. Increased median concentrations of the IL-1 receptor inhibitor soluble IL-1RA were present in 5/11 patients (n.s.), but the levels did not correlate with IL-1α concentrations (data not shown). The IL-2 decoy receptor, soluble IL-2Rα was detected in all patients and increased significantly after *E. coli* 83972 inoculation in three patients. Interestingly, the highest sIL-1RA and sIL-2Rα responses occurred in the same two patients.

The monocyte/T lymphocyte chemoattractant IP-10, which also has antibacterial activity [25], was significantly increased by ABU in the entire patient group ($p<0.02$, Table 2). Median levels of IP-10 during ABU were elevated in all patients compared to sterile urine, and significantly elevated in five patients compared to the sterile samples (Figure 4C). Low levels of the eosinophil and T cell chemoattractant RANTES were detected in all patients, as compared with sterile samples (Figure 4D). No significant RANTES response to *E. coli* 83972 ABU was observed, however (n.s., Table 2 and Figure 4D). Eotaxin-1, IFNα$_2$ and IL-12p40 were detected in a limited numbers of samples (Figure 4D and Table 2).

Genetic polymorphism influence the host response

To investigate if genetics influence the host response to ABU, *TLR4* and *IRF3* promoter polymorphisms were defined in the eleven subjects, whose urine was subjected to cytokine/chemokine proteome analysis. Seven of the 29 *TLR4* genotypes that occur in the Swedish population [16] were identified. The five subjects who carried *TLR4* genotypes associated with primary ABU (V, VI or VII) [16], had significantly lower IL-6, MCP-1, IP-10, sIL-2Rα and PMN responses to ABU than patients with other *TLR4* genotypes (XIX, IV, XX, IX, Figure 5A). In addition, four patients carried the heterozygous *IRF3* promoter variant (A/G – C/T) that is more common in ABU than in APN patients [15]. These patients had significantly lower urine concentrations of IL-6, MCP-1 and lower PMN numbers than homozygous patients (Figure 5B). The results suggest that genetic variation influences the innate immune response to ABU.

Discussion

ABU represents one extreme of the UTI spectrum and may even be regarded as a form of commensalism [12]. Epidemiologic studies have convincingly shown that in most cases, ABU is harmless and the demonstration that bacteriuria protects against super-infection with more virulent strains has provided the rationale for therapeutic establishment of ABU [5,11,18]. While it is now widely accepted that ABU is beneficial and should be left untreated, there have long been concerns that some patients with the appearance of ABU may have chronic renal infections, which should be treated to avoid tissue damage [26]. Distinguishing ABU from other, therapy-requiring forms of UTI therefore remains a diagnostic challenge. Refined molecular mapping of the host response repertoire is now possible, offering a promising tool to help resolve diagnostic enigmas in the future, to reduce the risk for tissue damage and the need for antibiotic treatment [27].

The mucosal cytokine response to infection was discovered in UTI and epithelial cells were identified as the first line of cytokine responder cells [28,29]. Since then, numerous studies have examined the cytokine response magnitude and repertoire in patients with different forms of UTI [30]. Early work showed that acute pyelonephritis is accompanied by an increase in urine IL-6 compared to ABU [3,31] and IL-8 levels showed a similar pattern [1,32,33], defining ABU as a condition with low mucosal host response induction. Increased serum levels of IL-6 and IL-8 were detected in bacteremic patients [31,34,35] and further work investigating the cytokine repertoire showed that febrile UTI causes an increase in GRO-α and ENA-78 in urine, and ENA-78

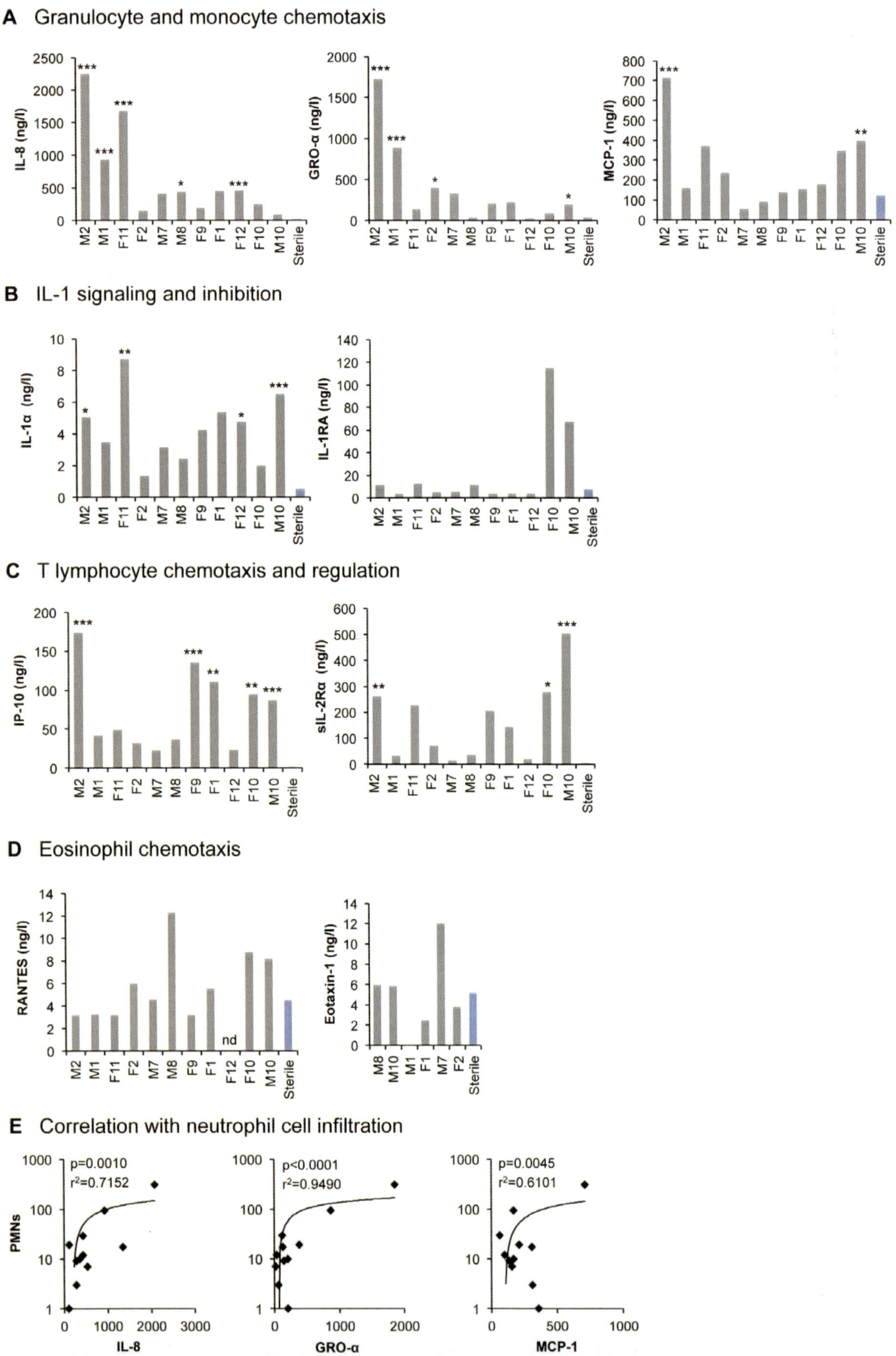
A Granulocyte and monocyte chemotaxis
IL-8 (ng/l)
GRO-α (ng/l)
MCP-1 (ng/l)
M2 M1 F11 F2 M7 M8 F9 F1 F12 F10 M10 Sterile
B IL-1 signaling and inhibition
IL-1α (ng/l)
IL-1RA (ng/l)
C T lymphocyte chemotaxis and regulation
IP-10 (ng/l)
sIL-2Rα (ng/l)
D Eosinophil chemotaxis
RANTES (ng/l)
nd
Eotaxin-1 (ng/l)
M8 M10 M1 F1 M7 F2 Sterile
E Correlation with neutrophil cell infiltration
PMNs
p=0.0010
r²=0.7152
IL-8
p<0.0001
r²=0.9490
GRO-α
p=0.0045
r²=0.6101
MCP-1

Figure 4. Urine cytokine/chemokine proteome response to *E. coli* 83972 ABU. Cytokine/chemokine levels in individual patients during ABU (grey, medians of all samples in each individual). A pool of 20 sterile urine samples from 9 patients (blue, median of all samples) is used for comparison. Coded patient IDs are noted on the x-axis, in the same order as in Figure 1. Significant differences between sterile and ABU samples from individual patients (Kruskal-Wallis, Dunn's post test) are shown (*p<0.05, **<0.01, ***<0.001). A. Granulocyte (IL-8, GRO-α) or monocyte (MCP-1) chemotaxis. B. Cytokines involved in IL-1 signaling and inhibition. C. Cytokines involved in T lymphocyte chemotaxis and regulation. D. Cytokines involved in eosinophil chemotaxis. E. Scatter diagrams illustrate significant correlations between neutrophil counts and neutrophil chemoattractants IL-8 and GRO-α, and the monocyte chemoattractant MCP-1. For the remaining proteins, no correlation with neutrophil numbers was found. For sample numbers, group means and statistical analysis see Table 2.

in serum [35]. Acute cystitis has been associated with an increase in urine IL-1α, GRO-α, IL-1β, IL-6, IL-8 and TNF-α compared to sterile samples [36,37,38]. Urine cytokine levels in ABU have been examined in transplant patients [39] and diabetic children with ABU [40]. A broader urine cytokine repertoire was examined in elderly subjects, where a group wise comparison of samples from ABU patients and sterile controls, detected a significant increase in TNF-α, IL-12, IL-18, GRO-α, IL-8, IL-6 and IL-10 in the ABU group, while MCP-1 and IL-1β were detected but not increased [38]. A comparison with acute cystitis samples showed that the levels of IL-6 and IL-8 were lower in ABU. All ABU patients in the study carried *E. coli* but the properties of the infecting strains were not recorded and host genetics were not considered.

In the present study, the host response was characterized in patients, who developed bacteriuria with the prototype ABU strain *E. coli* 83972 after therapeutic inoculation. By selecting this patient group, the study focused on host-driven differences in the innate immune response to a single ABU strain and bacterial differences accompanying natural infection were minimized. By extending the cytokine proteomic analysis to include 31 immune response related proteins, several interesting host response features were observed. *E. coli* 83972 bacteriuria stimulated a neutrophil response and the concentrations of IL-8 and GRO-α correlated well with the level of pyuria in individual samples. These neutrophil chemoattractants [1,41] are important for the recruitment neutrophils and activate their antibacterial effector functions, which are crucial to eradicate bacteria during acute UTI [42]. The monocyte chemoattractant MCP-1 showed variable levels, which are difficult to interpret, as there is little information on monocyte infiltration in response to UTI. IL-1α was increased in all patients with *E. coli* 83972 ABU. In previous studies, an IL-1α response was detected in patients with acute cystitis and acute pyelonephritis [36,37,43]. A decrease of sIL-1RA during symptomatic UTI has been recorded, suggesting that local inflammation might consume sIL-1RA [43]. As previously noted [43], IL-1α levels did not correlate with those of the inhibitor sIL-1RA. While all patients showed detectable levels of RANTES in the urine samples, there was no increase after bacterial inoculation, suggesting a basic level of activation and cytokine secretion by the mast cells in the bladder mucosa. In a parallel study, we observed a RANTES response in patients who develop acute symptoms, however, reflecting eosinophil activation and a potential role for eosinophil mediators in the development of cystitis (data not shown).

Interestingly, the response to ABU included the T cell chemoattractant IP-10, which has been found to have antibacterial activity against *E. coli* [25]. The secretion of the IL-2 decoy receptor sIL-2Rα in certain patients during both ABU and infection-free intervals may also reflect T cell- or dendritic cell activation in the urinary tract mucosa [44]. The presence of such cells has not been extensively characterized, however it is known that Peyer's patch-like cellular aggregates are formed in the bladder wall of patients with long-term ABU [45]. It may be speculated that such aggregates may include lymphocytes and dendritic cells and constitute a possible source of sIL-2Rα in patients with long-term bacteriuria, as those in the present study as well as during infection-free intervals until involution of these cellular aggregates has occurred. Most of the mediators of T cell proliferation and differentiation were not detected in patient urine, however, including IL-2, IL-3, IL-4, IL-7, IL-12p70. We did not detect T cell chemoattractants (MCP-3), B cell inhibitory cytokines (IL-14), agonists (IL-10) or regulators (IL-13), or agonists of NK cell proliferation (IL-15). Macrophage secreted proteins like the granulocyte activator MIP-1α and CCL22 were also not detected. Their absence supports the established view that adaptive immunity plays a less prominent role in UTI than innate immunity [12].

The TLR4 and IRF3 polymorphisms examined in this study were originally linked to ABU when they were shown to differ between populations who developed symptomatic infections and ABU [15,16]. The highly selected, UTI prone study populations were genotyped when their infection pattern had been established after many years of follow up. Patients with no evidence of symptomatic UTI during several years of follow up were assigned to a "primary ABU group". Children who developed ABU after a prior symptomatic infection but with no further symptomatic episodes were assigned to a "secondary ABU" group and the APN group had a history of APN, but had not developed ABU at any time during follow-up [16]. In a subsequent study, adults with a history of childhood APN were reexamined after 30 year follow up and assigned to APN or secondary ABU groups, depending on their disease patterns. Pediatric age-matched controls were enrolled at the pediatric outpatient clinic or when admitted for elective surgery for diagnoses unrelated to infection [46]. The ABU associated TLR4 genotypes used in this study were derived from the "primary ABU" group.

TLR4 promoter polymorphisms that lowered TLR4 promoter activity were associated with ABU, suggesting that genetic variation affecting TLR4 expression influences UTI susceptibility [16]. We now add data on patients with compromised urinary tracts, showing that individual patients with the ABU associated *TLR4* genotypes have reduced cytokine/chemokine responses to *E. coli* 83972, compared to patients with other *TLR4* genotypes. The transcription factor IRF3, downstream of TLR4 has also been shown to control UTI susceptibility, by affecting the efficiency of the TLR4 pathway further downstream [15]. Gene deletions result in an exaggerated, dysfunctional inflammatory response and in aggravated acute pyelonephritis in *Irf3*$^{-/-}$ mice. In patients with UTI, polymorphisms affecting the *IRF3* promoter have been detected, and the genotype associated with low promoter function is associated with acute pyelonephritis [15]. In this study, we detected an association between the *IRF3* promoter genotype and high or low responses to *E. coli* 83972, further emphasizing the importance of host genetics for the immune response in the urinary tract. In view of the fact that all patients carried the same *E. coli* strain these findings make an even stronger argument for genetic control of the host response to UTI.

The severity of UTI is explained by the virulence of the infecting strain and by the resistance to infection of individual hosts [12]. Despite the advanced understanding of molecular

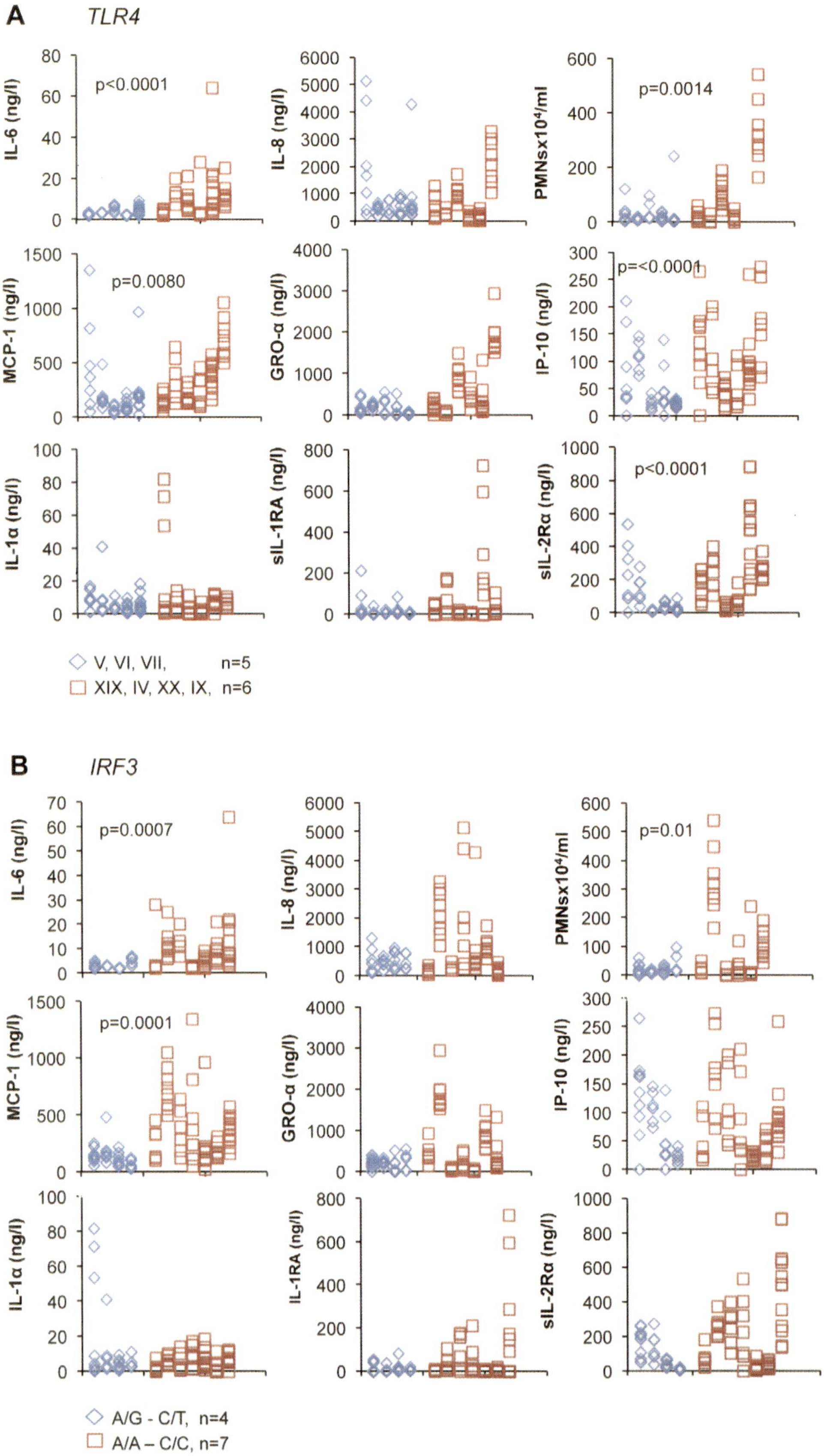
A
TLR4
IL-6 (ng/l)
p<0.0001
IL-8 (ng/l)
PMNsx10⁴/ml
p=0.0014
MCP-1 (ng/l)
p=0.0080
GRO-α (ng/l)
IP-10 (ng/l)
p=<0.0001
IL-1α (ng/l)
sIL-1RA (ng/l)
sIL-2Rα (ng/l)
p<0.0001
V, VI, VII, n=5
XIX, IV, XX, IX, n=6
B
IRF3
IL-6 (ng/l)
p=0.0007
IL-8 (ng/l)
PMNsx10⁴/ml
p=0.01
MCP-1 (ng/l)
p=0.0001
GRO-α (ng/l)
IP-10 (ng/l)
IL-1α (ng/l)
IL-1RA (ng/l)
sIL-2Rα (ng/l)
A/G - C/T, n=4
A/A – C/C, n=7

Figure 5. Promoter polymorphisms and the host response to ABU. A. Three of five *TLR4* genotypes associated with primary ABU were detected (blue hexagons) in five of the eleven patients. These patients had significantly lower neutrophil numbers ($p<0.002$) and IL-6 ($p<0.0001$), MCP-1 ($p<0.01$), IP-10 ($p<0.0001$), and sIL-2Rα ($p<0.0001$) concentrations than the patients with non-ABU associated *TLR4* genotypes XIX, IV, XX and IX (red squares). Each column represents one patient and each hexagon or square one monthly urine sample. B. The heterozygous *IRF3* promoter genotype associated with ABU (A/G-C/T, blue hexagon) was detected in four of the eleven patients, who had significantly lower neutrophil numbers ($p=0.01$) and IL-6 ($p<0.001$) and MCP-1 ($p=0.0001$) concentrations than patients with the homozygous, pyelonephritis-associated genotype (A/A-C/C, red square). Each column represents one patient and each hexagon or square one monthly urine sample.

disease mechanisms, common diagnostic procedures do not routinely include the assessment of these parameters. The traditional clinical assessment of disease severity is usually made without the support of quantitative molecular data and current diagnostic practices create a grey-zone, recognized as a cause of antibiotic over-use, and the need for improved diagnostic markers is obvious [27]. This study illustrates how an assessment of the immune response provides a powerful new tool to quantify and analyze the host response to UTI. In this case, we evaluated if patients with ABU show a local immune response to infection of characterized the repertoire of cytokines/proteins in urine. The results suggest that immune response measurements would add both qualitative and quantitative information. Supporting a positive urine culture with a urine cytokine analysis would be of special value in children, who cannot express their symptoms, in elderly, sometimes cognitively impaired patients with multiple diseases, in patients with neurogenic bladders and detrusor over-activity, in patients treated in the emergency department, and in other patients where UTI/ABU cannot be distinguished by subjective symptoms only. Distinguishing the basic immune response in the urinary tract from responses to pathogenic bacteria during symptomatic infection may also help to distinguish ABU from acute cystitis and to avoid excessive use of antibiotics in patients with compromised urinary tracts.

Materials and Methods

Ethics statement

The study was approved by the human ethics committee at Lund University and patients gave their informed consent (Clinical Trial Registration RTP-A2003 (International Committee of Medical Journal Editors, www.clinicaltrials.gov)).

Study design

Patients with incomplete bladder emptying and recurrent UTI (3-4 UTI/year for 2 years) resistant to conventional therapy participated in a placebo-controlled study of therapeutic *E. coli* 83972 inoculation [8]. The aim of the study was to establish if the deliberate establishment of asymptomatic bacteriuria with *Escherichia coli* 83972 in patients with incomplete bladder emptying and recurrent urinary tract infection protects against recurrent UTI. Exclusion criteria were upper tract UTI, renal deterioration, hydronephrosis, untreated bladder outflow obstruction, urinary calculi, immunosuppression (including corticosteroid medication) or urological malignancies. Before inclusion patients underwent renal function tests, upper urinary tract imaging, urodynamic assessment and cystoscopy. A flow-chart of patients and samples is given in Figure 1.

During phase 1 of the study the patients were randomized to blinded inoculations with *E. coli* 83972 or saline, and crossover occurred after monitoring for 12 months or after a UTI episode. During phase 2 patients were subjected to additional blinded inoculations to extend periods with and without *E. coli* 83972 bacteriuria. Outcomes were 1) the time to the first urinary tract infection in patients with and without *E. coli* 83972 bacteriuria and 2) the number of UTI episodes during 12 months with and 12 months without *E. coli* 83972 bacteriuria. There was no febrile urinary tract infection episode in either of the study arms and no significant side effects of intravesical bacterial inoculation were reported. The study concluded that deliberately induced *E. coli* 83972 bacteriuria protects patients with incomplete bladder emptying, who are prone to urinary tract infection, from recurrent urinary tract infection. The present study identified all urine samples from the patients during asymptomatic periods in the active (n = 233) and in the placebo-arm (n = 68) (Fig. 1, Table1).

Inoculation protocol

Briefly, patients were catheterized and inoculated with *E. coli* 83972 (10^5 cfu/ml in PBS, 30 ml) or placebo (sterile PBS) once daily on three consecutive days. Each patient was followed for twelve months after *E. coli* 83972 inoculation, and twelve months after PBS inoculation. In case bacteriuria was not established, the patient received a new inoculation of *E. coli* 83972. The clinical trial was double-blinded and randomized, [8] with monthly urine sampling after both *E. coli* 83972 and PBS inoculation to determine the establishment of long-term *E. coli* 83972 bacteriuria and the host response.

Urine sampling and culture

Urine samples were obtained before inoculation and during *E. coli* 83972 ABU (233 samples). 68 samples were obtained during sterile intervals after PBS inoculation. All samples were semi-quantitatively cultured. *E. coli* 83972 was identified by antibiotic resistance and a 1.565 bp plasmid was amplified by PCR. Urine samples were stored at −80°C.

Host response to E. coli 83972

In all samples, urine polymorphonuclear cell (neutrophil) numbers were quantified by hemocytometry, and Interleukin (IL) 6 and IL-8 concentrations were quantified by Immulite (Siemens, Deerfield, USA). From these samples, urine samples from eleven patients (five males and six females) were selected for further analysis of proteomic content. Sterile samples (total n = 20, from 9 patients) and samples from periods of *E. coli* 83972 ABU (n = 67) from each of the patients were chosen as controls. Samples from six patients were selected for extended proteomic analysis of infected (*E. coli* 83972 ABU) and sterile urine (total samples, n = 42). MILLIPLEX MAP Human Cytokine/Chemokine Panel (Millipore, Billarica, USA) was used to screen for protein content, and a custom-made panel detecting GRO-α, IP-10, MCP-1, sIL-2Rα, IL-1α, sIL-1RA and RANTES was used to confirm the analysis in the remaining five 45 samples (five patients).

TLR4/IRF3 genotyping

DNA was extracted from heparinized peripheral blood using QIAmp DNA Blood Midi Kit from 11 patients (see Figure 1 for details). Patients were genotyped using a Pyrosequencer (PSQ 96, Biotage, Uppsala, Sweden) after PCR amplification of patient DNA and a second biotinylated PCR for each SNP (for primers see [15,16]).

Statistics

Cytokine concentrations were evaluated using the Mann-Whitney test or Paired t-test, except for the SNP-analyses where Pearson's chi-square χ^2 test was used and for individual comparisons, Kruskal-Wallis with Dunn's post test was used. Correlations were by Spearmans rank test. The GraphPad Prism software for Mac, version 5.0, GraphPad Software was used for all calculations.

Acknowledgments

We thank those involved in the human inoculation study at the Urology and Microbiology, Immunology and Glycobiology Departments, Lund University and Orup Rehabilitation Outpatient Centre, as well as H. Jacobsson, Region Skånes Kunskaps Centrum and L. Wahlgren, Department of Statistics, Lund University. The Luminex 200 system was provided by K. Andersson and J. Vikman, Dept. of Clinical Sciences, Lund University.

Author Contributions

Conceived and designed the experiments: JGH FS BW CS. Performed the experiments: JGH FS JC. Analyzed the data: JGH. Contributed reagents/materials/analysis tools: BW CS JC. Wrote the paper: JGH BW CS.

References

1. Agace WW, Hedges SR, Ceska M, Svanborg C (1993) Interleukin-8 and the neutrophil response to mucosal gram-negative infection. J Clin Invest 92: 780–785.
2. Otto G, Burdick M, Strieter R, Godaly G (2005) Chemokine response to febrile urinary tract infection. Kidney Int 68: 62–70.
3. Benson M, Jodal U, Andreasson A, Karlsson A, Rydberg J, et al. (1994) Interleukin 6 response to urinary tract infection in childhood. Pediatr Infect Dis J 13: 612–616.
4. Hansson S, Martinell J, Stokland E, Jodal U (1997) The natural history of bacteriuria in childhood. Infectious disease clinics of North America 11: 499–512.
5. Lindberg U, Claesson I, Hanson LA, Jodal U (1975) Asymptomatic bacteriuria in schoolgirls. I. Clinical and laboratory findings. Acta paediatrica Scandinavica 64: 425–431.
6. Kunin CM (1997) Urinary Tract Infections. Detection, ed. Prevention and Management. Baltimore: Williams and Wilkins.
7. Ragnarsdottir B, Samuelsson M, Gustafsson MC, Leijonhufvud I, Karpman D, et al. (2007) Reduced toll-like receptor 4 expression in children with asymptomatic bacteriuria. J Infect Dis 196: 475–484.
8. Sunden F, Hakansson L, Ljunggren E, Wullt B (2010) Escherichia coli 83972 bacteriuria protects against recurrent lower urinary tract infections in patients with incomplete bladder emptying. The Journal of urology 184: 179–185.
9. Nanda N, Juthani-Mehta M (2009) Novel biomarkers for the diagnosis of urinary tract infection-a systematic review. Biomarker insights 4: 111–121.
10. Hagberg L, Hull R, Hull S, McGhee JR, Michalek SM, et al. (1984) Difference in susceptibility to gram-negative urinary tract infection between C3H/HeJ and C3H/HeN mice. Infect Immun 46: 839–844.
11. Ragnarsdottir B, Fischer H, Godaly G, Gronberg-Hernandez J, Gustafsson M, et al. (2008) TLR- and CXCR1-dependent innate immunity: insights into the genetics of urinary tract infections. European journal of clinical investigation 38(Suppl 2): 12–20.
12. Ragnarsdottir B, Lutay N, Gronberg-Hernandez J, Koves B, Svanborg C (2011) Genetics of innate immunity and UTI susceptibility. Nature reviews Urology 8: 449–468.
13. Chromek M, Slamova Z, Bergman P, Kovacs L, Podracka L, et al. (2006) The antimicrobial peptide cathelicidin protects the urinary tract against invasive bacterial infection. Nature medicine 12: 636–641.
14. Fischer H, Yamamoto M, Akira S, Beutler B, Svanborg C (2006) Mechanism of pathogen-specific TLR4 activation in the mucosa: fimbriae, recognition receptors and adaptor protein selection. European journal of immunology 36: 267–277.
15. Fischer H, Lutay N, Ragnarsdottir B, Yadav M, Jonsson K, et al. (2010) Pathogen specific, IRF3-dependent signaling and innate resistance to human kidney infection. PLoS pathogens 6: e1001109.
16. Ragnarsdottir B, Jonsson K, Urbano A, Gronberg-Hernandez J, Lutay N, et al. (2010) Toll-like receptor 4 promoter polymorphisms: common TLR4 variants may protect against severe urinary tract infection. PLoS One 5: e10734.
17. Akahoshi M, Nakashima H, Sadanaga A, Miyake K, Obara K, et al. (2008) Promoter polymorphisms in the IRF3 gene confer protection against systemic lupus erythematosus. Lupus 17: 568–574.
18. Hawn TR, Scholes D, Wang H, Li SS, Stapleton AE, et al. (2009) Genetic variation of the human urinary tract innate immune response and asymptomatic bacteriuria in women. PLoS One 4: e8300.
19. Eden CS, Hanson LA, Jodal U, Lindberg U, Akerlund AS (1976) Variable Adherence to Normal Human Urinary-Tract Epithelial-Cells of Escherichia-Coli Strains Associated with Various Forms of Urinary-Tract Infection. Lancet 2: 490–492.
20. Plos K, Connell H, Jodal U, Marklund BI, Marild S, et al. (1995) Intestinal carriage of P fimbriated Escherichia coli and the susceptibility to urinary tract infection in young children. The Journal of infectious diseases 171: 625–631.
21. Klemm P, Roos V, Ulett GC, Svanborg C, Schembri MA (2006) Molecular characterization of the Escherichia coli asymptomatic bacteriuria strain 83972: the taming of a pathogen. Infect Immun 74: 781–785.
22. Zdziarski J, Svanborg C, Wullt B, Hacker J, Dobrindt U (2008) Molecular basis of commensalism in the urinary tract: low virulence or virulence attenuation? Infect Immun 76: 695–703.
23. Hopp TP, Dower SK, March CJ (1986) The molecular forms of interleukin-1. Immunologic research 5: 271–280.
24. Dinarello CA (1994) The biological properties of interleukin-1. European cytokine network 5: 517–531.
25. Cole AM, Ganz T, Liese AM, Burdick MD, Liu L, et al. (2001) Cutting edge: IFN-inducible ELR- CXC chemokines display defensin-like antimicrobial activity. J Immunol 167: 623–627.
26. Jennette JC, Heptinstall RH (2007) Heptinstall's pathology of the kidney. Philadelphia, PA: Lippincott Williams & Wilkins.
27. Silver SA, Baillie L, Simor AE (2009) Positive urine cultures: A major cause of inappropriate antimicrobial use in hospitals? The Canadian journal of infectious diseases & medical microbiology = Journal canadien des maladies infectieuses et de la microbiologie medicale / AMMI Canada 20: 107–111.
28. de Man P, Jodal U, Svanborg C (1991) Dependence among host response parameters used to diagnose urinary tract infection. The Journal of infectious diseases 163: 331–335.
29. Hedges S, Anderson P, Lidin-Janson G, de Man P, Svanborg C (1991) Interleukin-6 response to deliberate colonization of the human urinary tract with gram-negative bacteria. Infection and immunity 59: 421–427.
30. Svanborg C, Godaly G, Hedlund M (1999) Cytokine responses during mucosal infections: role in disease pathogenesis and host defence. Current opinion in microbiology 2: 99–105.
31. Hedges S, Stenqvist K, Lidin-Janson G, Martinell J, Sandberg T, et al. (1992) Comparison of urine and serum concentrations of interleukin-6 in women with acute pyelonephritis or asymptomatic bacteriuria. The Journal of infectious diseases 166: 653–656.
32. Ko YC, Mukaida N, Ishiyama S, Tokue A, Kawai T, et al. (1993) Elevated interleukin-8 levels in the urine of patients with urinary tract infections. Infection and immunity 61: 1307–1314.
33. Benson M, Jodal U, Agace W, Hellstrom M, Marild S, et al. (1996) Interleukin (IL)-6 and IL-8 in children with febrile urinary tract infection and asymptomatic bacteriuria. The Journal of infectious diseases 174: 1080–1084.
34. Otto G, Braconier J, Andreasson A, Svanborg C (1999) Interleukin-6 and disease severity in patients with bacteremic and nonbacteremic febrile urinary tract infection. The Journal of infectious diseases 179: 172–179.
35. Olszyna DP, Opal SM, Prins JM, Horn DL, Speelman P, et al. (2000) Chemotactic activity of CXC chemokines interleukin-8, growth-related oncogene-alpha, and epithelial cell-derived neutrophil-activating protein-78 in urine of patients with urosepsis. The Journal of infectious diseases 182: 1731–1737.
36. Candela JV, Park E, Gerspach JM, Davidoff R, Stout L, et al. (1998) Evaluation of urinary IL-1alpha and IL-1beta in gravid females and patients with bacterial cystitis and microscopic hematuria. Urological research 26: 175–180.
37. Davidoff R, Yamaguchi R, Leach GE, Park E, Lad PM (1997) Multiple urinary cytokine levels of bacterial cystitis. The Journal of urology 157: 1980–1985.
38. Rodhe N, Lofgren S, Strindhall J, Matussek A, Molstad S (2009) Cytokines in urine in elderly subjects with acute cystitis and asymptomatic bacteriuria. Scand J Prim Health Care 27: 74–79.
39. Ciszek M, Paczek L, Bartlomiejczyk I, Mucha K (2006) Urine cytokines profile in renal transplant patients with asymptomatic bacteriuria. Transplantation 81: 1653–1657.
40. Rozsai B, Lanyi E, Berki T, Soltesz G (2006) Urinary cytokine response to asymptomatic bacteriuria in type 1 diabetic children and young adults. Pediatric diabetes 7: 153–158.
41. Godaly G, Hang L, Frendeus B, Svanborg C (2000) Transepithelial neutrophil migration is CXCR1 dependent in vitro and is defective in IL-8 receptor knockout mice. J Immunol 165: 5287–5294.
42. Shahin RD, Engberg I, Hagberg L, Svanborg Eden C (1987) Neutrophil recruitment and bacterial clearance correlated with LPS responsiveness in local gram-negative infection. Journal of immunology 138: 3475–3480.

43. Tullus K, Escobar-Billing R, Fituri O, Burman LG, Karlsson A, et al. (1996) Interleukin-1 alpha and interleukin-1 receptor antagonist in the urine of children with acute pyelonephritis and relation to renal scarring. Acta Paediatr 85: 158–162.
44. Rubin LA, Kurman CC, Fritz ME, Biddison WE, Boutin B, et al. (1985) Soluble interleukin 2 receptors are released from activated human lymphoid cells in vitro. Journal of immunology 135: 3172–3177.
45. Hansson S, Hanson E, Hjalmas K, Hultengren M, Jodal U, et al. (1990) Follicular cystitis in girls with untreated asymptomatic or covert bacteriuria. The Journal of urology 143: 330–332.
46. Lundstedt AC, McCarthy S, Gustafsson MC, Godaly G, Jodal U, et al. (2007) A genetic basis of susceptibility to acute pyelonephritis. PLoS One 2: e825.

Comparison of Adhesin Genes and Antimicrobial Susceptibilities between Uropathogenic and Intestinal Commensal *Escherichia coli* Strains

Xiaohua Qin[1], Fupin Hu[1], Shi Wu[1], Xinyu Ye[1], Demei Zhu[1], Ying Zhang[1,2], Minggui Wang[1]*

1 Huashan Hospital and Key Laboratory of Medical Molecular Virology of the Ministries of Education and Health, Shanghai Medical College, Fudan University, Shanghai, China, 2 Department of Molecular Microbiology and Immunology, Bloomberg School of Public Health, Johns Hopkins University, Baltimore, Maryland, United States of America

Abstract

The presence of adhesins is arguably an important determinant of pathogenicity for Uropathogenic *Escherichia coli* (UPEC). Antimicrobial susceptibilities were tested by agar dilution method, fifteen adhesin genes were detected by polymerase chain reaction, and multilocus sequence typing (MLST) was analyzed in 70 UPEC isolates and 41 commensal *E. coli* strains. Extended-spectrum β-lactamase (ESBL) was determined with confirmatory test. The prevalence of ESBL-producers in UPEC (53%, 37/70) was higher than the commensal intestinal isolates (7%, 3/41), and 97% (36/37) of the ESBL-producing UPEC harbored $bla_{CTX\text{-}M}$ genes. *afa* was present in 36% (10/28) UPEC isolates from recurrent lower urinary tract infection (UTI), and none in the acute pyelonephritis, acute uncomplicated cystitis or commensal strains ($P<0.0001$). *papG* was detected in 28% (20/70) of UPEC isolates, while 5% (2/41) of the commensal strains were *papG* positive ($P=0.0025$), and the prevalence of *papG* was significantly higher in acute pyelonephritis group (71%) than the other two UTI groups ($P<0.0001$). The prevalence of *flu, yqi, yadN* and *ygiL* was significantly higher in UPEC isolates than in the commensal strains. ESBL-producing UPEC showed a lower prevalence of adhesin genes compared with non-ESBL-producing strains. The MLST profiles were different between UPEC and commensal strains, with ST131 (19%, 13/70) and ST10 (20%, 8/41) being the most common MLSTs, respectively. This study demonstrated that several adhesin genes were more prevalent in UPEC isolates than in commensal *E. coli*, and *afa* may be associated with recurrent lower UTI whereas *papG* is more frequently associated with acute pyelonephritis.

Editor: Jamunarani Vadivelu, University of Malaya, Malaysia

Funding: This work was supported by a grant from the National Natural Science foundation of China (number 81102509). The funders had no role in study design, data collection and analysis, decision to publish, or preparation of the manuscript.

Competing Interests: The authors have declared that no competing interests exist.

* E-mail: mgwang@fudan.edu.cn

Introduction

Urinary tract infection (UTI) is one of the most common bacterial infections, and it is estimated that the overall lifetime prevalence of UTI in women is greater than 50% [1]. Further recurrent UTIs are reported in about 25% of women within 6 months of an acute UTI episode and pose a major health problem [2]. Uropathogenic *Escherichia coli* (UPEC) is the causative pathogen in 70–95% community-acquired UTI and over 50% nosocomial UTI [3]. Many virulence factors contribute to the pathogenesis of UPEC. The presence of adhesins is arguably the most important determinant of the pathogenicity for UPEC [4]. Adhesive organelles, including type 1, P, S/F1C, M, G and curli fimbriae, along with Afa/Dr adhesins, as well as temperature sensitive haemagglutinin (TSH), promote both bacterial attachment to and invasion of host tissues within the urinary tract [4–6].

E. coli expressing Dr/Afa adhesins may predispose the establishment of chronic or recurrent infections [7]. In previous studies, it was shown that UPEC entered the urinary epithelial cells through adhesins AfaD and AfaE, and therefore avoided the clearance of host immunosurveillance and antibiotic treatment. When the host cells shed, releasing a large amount of intracellular UPEC, a new round of infection could begin causing recurrence or relapse of UTI [8]. P fimbriae is encoded by the *pap* gene cluster, including *papG* encoding the tip adhesin PapG [9]. The three most studied PapG molecular variants, which are shown to bind distinct isoreceptors are PapG I, II and III [10]. Clinically the class II *papG* allele is primarily associated with human pyelonephritis, and class III *papG* allele with genitourinary infections in dogs and cats yet some cases of human cystitis [11]. In addition to P fimbriae, type 1 and S/F1C fimbriae, curli and M and G fimbriae which are encoded by the *fim and sfa/foc, csg, bma* and *gaf* gene clusters, respectively, may also be related to the adherence of UPEC [4,6,12]. More recently, it is discovered that adhesin Ag43, encoded by *flu* and abundant on the outer membrane of *E. coli*, enables bacterial cells to adhere to each other and form biofilm over the host urothelial cells, leading to poor clearance of the pathogens [13]. Other novel genes like *yqi, yadN and ygiL* were also found to be prevalent among UPEC strains and played an important role in colonization and pathogenesis [6,14].

Previous studies have shown that the prevalence of adhesin genes is different between UPEC and fecal commensal strains of *E. coli* [15]. However, few epidemiologic data about adhesin genes of

UPEC are available in China. The aim of the present study was to compare the prevalence of the adhesin genes and antimicrobial susceptibilities between UPEC and intestinal colonizing strains of *E. coli*, and adhesin genes between strains isolated from different types of UTIs and their association with a particular type of UTIs.

Materials and Methods

E. coli isolates

A total of 70 clinical isolates of UPEC were collected from clean midstream urine specimens of inpatients (63 female and 7 male) with urinary tract infections at Huashan Hospital, Shanghai from January 2008 to December 2010. The exclusion criteria were: 1) patients with indwelling catheter; 2) patients with urinary calculus or structural abnormalities. Isolation was performed according to standard laboratory protocols and UPEC were isolated from urine with $>10^5$ colony-forming units/ml.

Among the 70 UPEC isolates, 28 were from patients with recurrent lower UTIs. The recurrent lower UTIs were defined as at least two episodes of UTI within 6 month. Each time the patients had: a) typical clinical symptoms as urinary urgency, pain, and frequent voiding, b) pyuria, c) without fever, chill or other systematic symptoms. All of the 28 patients in recurrent lower UTI group had recurrences caused by UPEC. MLST typing of the UPEC strains from 11 randomly selected patients showed that the strains isolated from different episodes of each patient had the same MLST type.

Seventeen strains were isolated from acute pyelonephritis patients by the following criteria: a) the temperature $>38.5^\circ$C, b) positive percussion pain on kidney area, c) an elevated leukocyte count ($>11\times10^9$/L) and elevated percentage of neutrophils ($>70\%$) in the blood routine test. The remaining 25 strains were from patients with acute uncomplicated cystitis.

The intestinal commensal *E. coli* isolates (n = 41) were collected from anal swab specimens of healthy volunteers. The inclusion criteria emphasized: 1) without diarrhea or abdominal pain, 2) without antibiotic administration within the three months before taking the specimen. After isolation, all isolates were kept frozen at -70°C in 20% glycerol.

Antimicrobial susceptibility testing

The minimum inhibitory concentrations (MICs) of imipenem, cefepime, ceftazidime, cefotaxime, cefuroxime, cefazolin, piperacillin/tazobactam, piperacillin, gentamicin, amikacin, ciprofloxacin, and nitrofurantoin for both UPEC and commensal isolates were determined by agar dilution according to CLSI standards [16]. The antimicrobial concentrations were from 0.06 to 128 μg/ml. *E. coli* ATCC 25922 was used as a quality control strain.

Detection of ESBL-producing bacterial strains and ESBL genes

Extended-spectrum β-lactamase (ESBL) was determined with the previously recommended CLSI disk diffusion ESBL screening and confirmatory test [17]. CTX-M- specific genes in ESBL-producing strains were identified by polymerase chain reaction (PCR) with the primers reported previously [18].

Adhesin gene detection

The presence of genes *afa, draE, daaE, papG I, papG II, papG III, flu, fimH, sfaD, focG, bmaE, gafD, csgA, tsh, yqi, yadN* and *ygiL* was investigated by PCR amplification using primers (Sangon, Shanghai, China) as described previously [12,14,19–22]. The sequence amplified by *afa* primers, located between *afaB* and *afaC*, was conservatively shared by many subtypes of Dr/Afa adhesins [19]. All the *sfa* and *foc* PCR fragments were confirmed by sequencing as *sfa* and *foc* are highly homologous. The positive isolates identified by sequencing of PCR products in the pre-test were used as positive control in the following screening.

Analysis of UPEC by multilocus sequence typing (MLST)

All of the 70 clinical UPEC and 41 intestinal commensal isolates were analyzed by MLST. The seven housekeeping genes (*adk, fumC, icd, purA, gyrB, recA* and *mdh*) for typing [23], as well as the primer sets and PCR conditions were according to the MLST website for *E. coli* (mlst.ucc.ie/mlst/dbs/Ecoli/documents/primersColi_html). The based upon related sequence types (BURST) clustering algorithm (eburst.mlst.net) was used to analyze the allelic profiles and define clonal complexes (CCs). CCs were identified according to the number of single-locus variants (SLVs) and double-locus variants (DLVs) shared between isolates, where only STs that shared six or more loci were assigned to a defined CCs.

Statistical analysis

The comparison of prevalence rates was performed using Pearson Chi-square test or Fisher's exact test (two-tailed) with the software SPSS 16.0, and the level of significance was set at $P<0.05$.

Results

Antimicrobial susceptibility and ESBL differences of the two groups of *E. coli* strains

UPEC isolates demonstrated remarkably lower susceptibility rates to piperacillin (14%), cefazolin (21%), cefuroxime (39%), cefotaxime (43%), ceftazidime (71%), cefepime (79%), gentamicin (43%), amikacin (90%) and ciprofloxacin (23%) than intestinal commensal isolates ($P<0.05$). However, 91%–100% of *E. coli* isolates in the two groups were susceptible to piperacillin/tazobactam, imipenem and nitrofurantoin and there was no significant difference between the two groups ($P>0.05$, Table 1).

Thirty-seven (53%) of 70 UPEC isolates, while 3 (7%) out of 41 intestinal commensal isolates were ESBL-producing ($P<0.001$). bla_{CTX-M} genes were present in 97% (36/37) ESBL-producing isolates, and of these, 58% (21/36) carried $bla_{CTX-M-1}$-group ESBL genes while 42% (15/36) belonged to $bla_{CTX-M-9}$-group. ESBL genotype could not be determined in one strain. The CTX-M-2, CTX-M-8 and CTX-M-25/26 groups were not found.

Prevalence of adhesin genes

(1) Afa/Dr adhesin family member genes. *afa* was present only in 10 UPEC isolates that belonged to the recurrent lower UTIs group (10/28, 36%). None of the isolates from the acute pyelonephritis group or the acute uncomplicated cystitis group carried *afa*. No *afa* was found in 41 intestinal commensal *E. coli* isolates. Neither *draE* nor *daaE* was detected among all the strains we screened.

(2) Type P fimbriae related gene *papG*. *papG* was positive in 28% (20/70) of the UPEC isolates including 16 *papG II* and 4 *papG III*, and 5% (2/41) of the intestinal commensal isolates carried *papG II* ($P=0.0025$). The prevalence of *papG* in acute pyelonephritis (71.4%, 5/7) was significantly higher than that of recurrent lower UTI group (14.3%, 3/21, $P=0.0004$) and that of acute uncomplicated cystitis group (15.8%, 3/19, $P=0.0001$). No *papG I* was detected in any of all the tested strains.

(3) Biofilm related adhesin gene *flu* and novel genes *yqi*, *yadN* and *ygiL*. A majority (77%, 54/70) of the UPEC isolates and 41% (17/41) of the intestinal commensal isolates were found

Table 1. Comparison of the antimicrobials susceptibility between UPEC and commensal *E. coli* strains.

Antimicrobial agents	UPEC isolates (n = 70)				Commensal *E. coli* strains (n = 41)				*P* value
	MIC range (μg/ml)	MIC_{50}	MIC_{90}	S%	MIC range (μg/ml)	MIC_{50}	MIC_{90}	S%	
Piperacillin	1–256	128	256	14	0.5–256	2	64	73	<0.0001
Piperacillin/tazobactam	0.25–256	2	4	91	0.5–16	1	2	100	0.0539
Cefazolin	0.06–256	128	256	21	0.5–256	1	64	83	<0.0001
Cefuroxime	2–256	256	256	39	2–256	2	256	85	<0.0001
Cefotaxime	0.06–256	8	256	43	0.06–128	0.06	8	85	<0.0001
Ceftazidime	0.06–256	0.5	32	71	0.06–32	0.125	0.25	98	0.0007
Cefepime	0.06–256	1	16	79	0.06–8	0.06	1	100	0.0014
Imipenem	0.06–0.25	0.06	0.125	100	0.06–125	0.06	0.06	100	-
Gentamicin	0.25–256	64	128	43	0.5–256	1	64	85	<0.0001
Amikacin	1–256	2	8	90	1–4	2	2	100	0.0364
Ciprofloxacin	0.06–256	32	128	31	0.06–16	0.06	1	90	<0.0001
Nitrofurantoin	4–128	8	16	99	4–32	8	16	100	0.4420

to be *flu* positive ($P = 0.0002$). The prevalence of novel genes *yqi*, *yadN* and *ygiL* was higher in UPEC isolates than that of the commensal strains (27% *vs* 7%, 54% *vs* 32%, and 44% *vs* 17%, respectively, $P<0.05$). The prevalence differences of these four genes of *flu*, *yqi*, *yadN* and *ygiL* between the three UTI groups were not significant.

(4) Type 1 fimbrial gene *fimH* and curli fiber gene *csgA*. *fimH* was found positive in 86% (60/70) UPEC isolates and 73% (30/41) commensal isolates ($P = 0.1034$). The positive rates of *fimH* in the three UTI groups were 86%, 82% and 88%, respectively. 30% (21/70) UPEC isolates and 34% (14/41) commensal ones carried *csgA* ($P = 0.6500$).

(5) Other adhesin genes. *sfaD* was present in 5 isolates and *focG* in 2 isolates among the UPEC group. One of the *sfaD* carrying isolates was also detected *focG* positive. None of the isolates in the intestinal commensal group were *sfaD*/*focG* positive. No more than 5 isolates in UPEC or commensal groups produced amplicons with the *bmaE*, *gafD* or *tsh* primers. (Table 2)

Comparison of the prevalence of fimbrial genes between ESBL-producing and non-ESBL-producing UPEC

The prevalence of *fimH* (97%, 32/33) in the non-ESBL-producing UPEC was significantly higher than that in the ESBL-producing UPEC (76%, 28/37, $P = 0.0110$). All the six strains carrying *sfaD*/*focG* were from the non-ESBL-producing UPEC group. The prevalence of the other fimbrial genes in the non-ESBL-producing UPEC group seemed a little higher than the ESBL-producing UPEC strains, however, there were no statistically significant differences ($P>0.05$, Table 3)

MLST analysis of UPEC and commensal isolates

The 70 UPEC isolates analyzed were assigned to 26 distinct STs. The most common STs were ST131 (n = 13, 19%), followed by ST69 (9, 13%), ST405 (8, 11%), ST10 (7, 10%), ST393 (4, 6%), ST95 (4, 6%) and ST38 (3, 4%). The seven most common STs accounted for 69% (48/70) of the isolates, demonstrating the diversity of lineages. eBURST analysis revealed that 4 CCs (CC10, CC405, CC14 and CC38) encompassing 10 STs represented 25 (36%) UPEC isolates and the remaining 45 isolates included in the other 16 STs appearing as singletons (Figure 1A).

The 41 intestinal commensal isolates analyzed by MLST were grouped into 32 different STs. 28 were already included in the *E. coli* website database and 4 were new STs. ST10 (n = 8, 20%) was the most common group. A new ST had 2 strains, while the other 29 STs contained a single strain each. As analyzed by eBURST, ST10, ST34, ST167, ST48, ST559 and ST832 belonged to CC10 (Figure 1B).

Discussion

Most of the intestinal commensal isolates tested in this study were susceptible to all the tested antimicrobial agents, while the UPEC isolates were characterized by a varying degree of susceptibilities to different antimicrobials. Of 70 UPEC strains, 37 (53%) produced extended-spectrum β-lactamase (ESBL). In a previous study, 2.9% of *E. coli* isolates recovered by outpatient urine cultures in 2008 harbored ESBL in USA [24], which is much higher than previously reported but far lower than the rate in our study. The annual percentage of ESBL-producing UPEC with bla_{CTX-M} genes changed from 35% in 2003 to 64% in 2008 with the average rate of 56% in that study [24]. However, in this study, bla_{CTX-M} ESBL genes were detected in 36 (97%) of 37 ESBL positive strains, which is much higher than in the USA.

All 10 UPEC isolates harboring the *afa* belonged to recurrent lower UTI group, none was *afa* positive in isolates from other UTIs or intestinal carriage, indicating that UPEC carrying *afa* might correlate with the recurrence of UTI episodes. Blanco and colleagues screened UPEC for *afa* and found no *afa* positive strain in acute pyelonephritis isolates, however, *afa* was detected in 5 of the 116 isolates (4.3%) from cystitis patients and 1 of the 42 (2.4%) isolates from asymptomatic bacteriuria [19]. Previous studies showed that Afa/Dr fimbrial adhesins contributed to the ability of UPEC isolates to colonize and persist long term within the urinary tract and therefore more likely to cause the recurrence of UTI episodes [7–8].

The isoreceptors of adhesin PapG primarily are scattered within the kidney, including glomerulus, proximal tubulus, distal tubulus, and collecting duct. Therefore sitting on the top of type P fimbriae, adhesin PapG is thought to be associated with bacterial adhesion to the kidney [9]. The prevalence of *papG* in acute pyelonephritis

Table 2. Comparison of the prevalence of adhesin genes among different groups of *E. coli* strains.

Adhesin genes[a]	Recurrent lower UTI, n = 28 (%)	Acute pyelonephritis, n = 17 (%)	Acute uncomplicated cystitis, n = 25 (%)	Total UPEC, n = 70 (%)	Commensal isolates, n = 41(%)	*P* value (Total UPEC *vs* Commensal)
afa	36[b]	0	0	14	0	<0.0001[c]
papG	18	71[d]	12	28	5	0.0025
flu	89	65	72	77	41	0.0002
fimH	86	82	88	86	73	0.1034
sfaD	4	12	8	7	0	0.0799
focG	0	12	0	3	0	0.2747
bmaE	4	6	4	4	5	0.8845
gafD	4	0	0	1	5	0.2794
csgA	21	24	44	30	34	0.6500
tsh	0	18	8	7	5	0.6357
yqi	21	35	28	27	7	0.0114
yadN	50	76	44	54	32	0.0212
ygiL	46	43	40	44	17	0.0035

[a], *draE* and *daaE* genes were not detected in any of the isolates.
[b], Compared to the other two UTI groups, $P<0.0001$;
[c]. Recurrent lower UTI group compared to commensal isolates;
[d], Compared to the other two UTI groups, $P<0.0001$.

isolates was significantly higher (71%) than that in recurrent lower UTIs (18%) and acute uncomplicated cystitis (12%) in the present study, illustrating high correlation between the *papG* and pyelonephritis. Our findings are consistent with some previous studies. Johnson et al found 69% (118/170) acute pyonephritis strains and 25% (21/83) of cystitis strains were *papG* positive [15].

Encoded by *flu*, Ag43 is a self-recognizing adhesin that is associated with cell aggregation and biofilm formation of UPEC [13]. We found a high prevalence (77%) of *flu* in UPEC isolates, while *flu* was detected in 41% of the intestinal commensal isolates. The finding is consistent with the results of Ulett and colleagues. They reported 83% (30/36) of the UPEC isolates and 56% (35/62) of the commensal strains carried *flu* [22]. However, there was no statistically significant difference in *flu* gene prevalence between recurrent lower UTI and non-recurrent lower UTI in the present study.

It was reported that the adhesin encoding gene *yqi* was prevalent among UPEC by more than 50% while absent in all the intestinal pathogenic *E. coli* [6]. In this study, *yqi* was detected in 7% of commensal isolates, but the prevalence was significantly lower than that in UPEC strains (27%, $P=0.0114$).

yadN and *ygiL* were found to be more prevalent in UPEC (54% and 44%, respectively) than the intestinal commensal strains (32% and 17%) in the present study ($P<0.05$), which coincides with Mobley's work. It was reported that fimbriae related structure Yad and Ygi could enhance the virulence-related phenotypes, including biofilm formation and adherence to immortalized human epithelial cells [14]. In addition, we did not detect any significant prevalence difference of *yadN* or *ygiL* between UPEC strains causing recurrent lower UTI, acute pyelonephritis and uncomplicated cystitis.

Table 3. Comparison of the prevalence of fimbrial genes between ESBL-producing and non-ESBL-producing UPEC strains.

Fimbrial genes	ESBL-producing UPEC n = 37 (%)	Non-ESBL-producing UPEC n = 33 (%)	*P* value
afa	14	15	0.8450
papG	22	36	0.1729
flu	73	82	0.3790
fimH	76	97	0.0110
sfaD/focG	0	18	0.008
bmaE	3	6	0.5990
gefD	0	3	0.4710
csgA	22	39	0.1053
tsh	5	9	0.6610
yqi	22	33	0.2714
yadN	49	61	0.3161
yqiL	43	45	0.8525

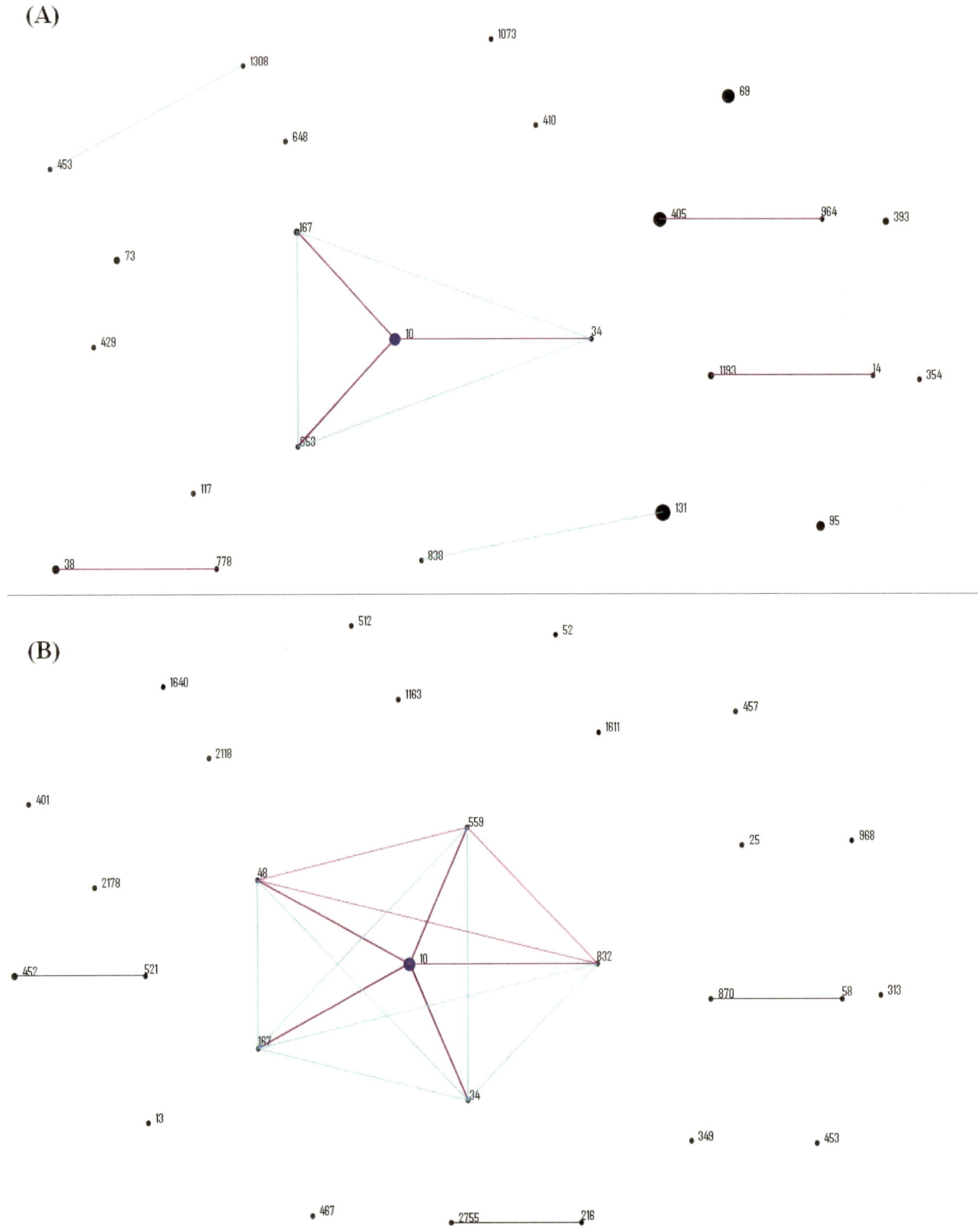

Figure 1. eBURST diagrams of UPECand intestinal commensal isolates showing related STs and individual STs. (A) referred to UPEC isolates and (B) referred to intestinal commensal isolates. Each ST is represented by a circle, the size of which correlates to the frequency of the ST. Predicted founders are positioned centrally and shown in blue, and single-locus variants and double-locus variants are shown in pink and blue, respectively.

The results showed that 86% of UPEC isolates and 73% of commensal isolates carried *fimH*, encoding the adhesin FimH as the tip fimbria for type 1 fimbriae. Wang et al detected 91% (72/79) *fimH* positive in UPEC isolates [25]. On the other hand, Schlager found that 81% (74/91) strains isolated from fecal specimen of healthy girls carried *fimH* [26]. A high prevalence of *fimH* was found in both UPEC and commensal isolates. However, the transcription and expression level of *fimH* might be different between UPEC and commensal strains, which made type 1 fimbriae an important virulence factor for UPEC [27].

In the present study, we found that ESBL-producing UPEC isolates showed a lower prevalence of fimbrial genes, *fimH* and *sfaD/focG*, compared with non-ESBL-producing ones. The results coincided with the previous findings that fimbrial genes were of reduced prevalence among UPEC resistant to extended-spectrum cephalosporins. A possible explanation is that: virulence traits like the fimbrial genes, as well as resistance genes, can be carried on conjugative plasmids; therefore, the incompatible resistance-encoding plasmids are outcompeting fimbrial factor encoding plasmids [28]. It is reported that the acquisition of antibiotic resistance may cause alterations in phenotypic and physiological characteristics, which are referred to as "biological fitness cost". The biological fitness cost on antibiotics resistance generally results in reduced growth rates. More dramatic phenotypic changes, including poor fimbrial expression, were reported in an ampicillin-resistant mutant *Acinetobacter* sp. strain DR1A comparing with the wild type strain DR1 [29]. Therefore, the decreased fimbrial genes and adherence capability in ESBL-producing UPEC might also be a fitness trade-off for the ESBL to survive antibiotics exposure. The exact explanation for the lower incidence of fimbrial genes among resistant UPEC isolates needs additional study.

In this study, 69% of the UPEC isolates were included in the seven STs (ST131, ST69, ST405, ST10, ST393, ST95 and ST38) and ST131 was the most predominant (19%). Gibreel revealed a consistent profile of STs over a 3-year period with UPEC isolates (n = 300) in the Northwest region of England primarily from 8 lineages: ST73 (16.6%), ST131 (12.3%), ST69 (9%), ST95 (6.3%), ST10 (4.3%), ST127 (3.6%), ST14 (2.7%) and ST405 (1.7%) [30]. Most of these STs (ST131, ST69, ST95, ST10 and ST405) were also prevalent in our study. The 41 commensal isolates had a richer ST diversity (32 STs) than the 70 UPEC counterparts (26 STs). A ST10 *E. coli* strain was common in UPEC (10%) as well as in intestinal commensal isolates (20%). One isolate from each group was ST453. The remaining 24 STs of the UPEC isolates were different from the other 30 STs of the commensal strains.

This study indicated that *afa* of Afa/Dr adhesin family might be associated with lower UTI recurrence, while *papG* might be correlated with acute pyelonephritis. However, we only focused on detecting the prevalence of adhesin genes by PCR, instead of the mechanism of the related adhesins of UPEC. Therefore, we could not prove the correlation between the adhesins and the pathogenesis of the UPEC. Moreover, because of the "cross-talk" among the regulators of different adhesin systems of UPEC and their functional redundancy, when a certain type of adhesin is lost, it may be quite difficult to study the relationship between the UTI recurrence and a specific kind of adhesin. Studies on other factors and mechanisms involved in pathogenesis and persistence of UPEC are required.

Author Contributions

Conceived and designed the experiments: MW. Performed the experiments: XQ FH SW. Analyzed the data: XQ. Contributed reagents/materials/analysis tools: DZ FH XY. Wrote the paper: XQ MW YZ.

References

1. Griebling TL (2005) Urologic diseases in America project trends in resource use for urinary tract infections in women. J Urol 173: 1281–1287.
2. Foxman B (1990) Recurring urinary tract infection-incidence and risk factors. Am J Public Health 80: 331–333.
3. Foxman B (2003) Epidemiology of urinary tract infections: Incidence, morbidity, and economic costs. Dis Mon 49: 53–70.
4. Mulvey MA (2002) Adhesion and entry of uropathogenic *Escherichia coli*. Cell Microbiol 4: 257–271.
5. Rosen DA, Hooton TM, Stamm WE, Humphrey PA, Hultgren SJ (2007) Detection of intracellular bacterial communities in human urinary tract infection. Plos Medicine 4: 1949–1958.
6. Antao EM, Wieler LH, Ewers C (2009) Adhesive threads of extraintestinal pathogenic *Escherichia coli*. Gut Pathog 1: 22.
7. Korotkova N, Yarova-Yarovaya Y, Tchesnokova V, Yazvenko N, Carl MA, et al. (2008) *Escherichia coli* DraE adhesin associated bacterial internalization by epithelial cells is promoted independently by decay accelerating factor and carcinoembryonic antigen related cell adhesion molecule binding and does not require the DraD invasin. Infect Immun 76: 3869–3880.
8. Dhakal BK, Kulesus RR, Mulvey MA (2008) Mechanisms and consequences of bladder cell invasion by uropathogenic *Escherichia coli*. Eur J Clin Invest 38: 2–11.
9. Lane MC, Mobley HLT (2007) Role of P-fimbrial-mediated adherence in pyelonephritis and persistence of uropathogenic *Escherichia coli* (UPEC) in the mammalian kidney. Kidney Int 72: 19–25.
10. Stromberg N, Marklund BI, Lund B, Ilver D, Hamers A, et al. (1990) Host specificity of uropathogenic *Escherichia coli* depends on differences in binding specificity to gal-alpha1-4gal containing isoreceptors. Embo Journal 9: 2001–2010.
11. Johnson JR, O'Bryan TT, Low DA, Ling G, Delavari P, et al. (2000) Evidence of commonality between canine and human extraintestinal pathogenic *Escherichia coli* strains that express *papG* allele III. Infect Immun 68: 3327–3336.
12. Johnson JR, Stell AL (2000) Extended virulence genotypes of *Escherichia coli* strains from patients with urosepsis in relation to phylogeny and host compromise. J Infect Dis 181: 261–272.
13. van der Woude MW, Henderson IR (2008) Regulation and function of Ag43 (Flu). Annu Rev Microbiol 62: 153–169.
14. Spurbeck RR, Stapleton AE, Johnson JR, Walk ST, Hooton TM, et al. (2011) Fimbrial profiles predict virulence of uropathogenic *Escherichia coli* strains: contribution of Ygi and Yad fimbriae. Infect Immun 79: 4753–4763.
15. Johnson JR, Owens K, Gajewski A, Kuskowski MA (2005) Bacterial characteristics in relation to clinical source of *Escherichia coli* isolates from women with acute cystitis or pyelonephritis and uninfected women. J Clin Microbiol 43: 6064–6072.
16. CLSI (2010) Performance strandards, for antimicrobial susceptibility testing; Twentieth informational supplement M100-S20.Standard; Twentieth informational supplement M100-S20. Wayne, PA.
17. CLSI (2009) Methods for dilution antimicrobial susceptibility tests for bacteria that grow aerobically.Standard; approved standard, 8th ed M07-A8. Wayne, PA.
18. Wang P, Hu F, Xiong Z, Ye X, Zhu D, et al. (2011) Susceptibility of extended-spectrum-beta-lactamase-producing *Enterobacteriaceae* according to the new CLSI breakpoints. J Clin Microbiol 49: 3127–3131.
19. Blanco M, Blanco JE, Alonso MP, Mora A, Balsalobre C, et al. (1997) Detection of *pap*, *sfa* and *afa* adhesin-encoding operons in uropathogenic *Escherichia coli* strains: relationship with expression of adhesins and production of toxins. Res Microbiol 148: 745–755.
20. Johnson JR, Russo TA, Brown JJ, Stapleton A (1998) *papG* alleles of *Escherichia coli* strains causing first episode or recurrent acute cystitis in adult women. J Infect Dis 177: 97–101.
21. Sokurenko EV, Feldgarden M, Trintchina E, Weissman SJ, Avagyan S, et al. (2004) Selection footprint in the FimH adhesin shows pathoadaptive niche differentiation in *Escherichia coli*. Mol Biol Evol 21: 1373–1383.
22. Ulett GC, Valle J, Beloin C, Sherlock O, Ghigo JM, et al. (2007) Functional analysis of antigen 43 in uropathogenic *Escherichia coli* reveals a role in long-term persistence in the urinary tract. Infect Immun 75: 3233–3244.
23. Tartof SY, Solberg OD, Manges AR, Riley LW (2005) Analysis of a uropathogenic *Escherichia coli* clonal group by multilocus sequence typing. J Clin Microbiol 43: 5860–5864.
24. Qi C, Pilla V, Yu JH, Reed K (2010) Changing prevalence of *Escherichia coli* with CTX-M-type extended-spectrum beta-lactamases in outpatient urinary *E. coli* between 2003 and 2008. Diagn Microbiol Infect Dis 67: 87–91.

25. Wang MC, Tseng CC, Wu AB, Huang JJ, Sheu BS, et al. (2009) Different roles of host and bacterial factors in *Escherichia coli* extra-intestinal infections. Clin Microbiol Infect 15: 372–379.
26. Schlager TA, Whittam TS, Hendley JO, Bhang JL, Wobbe CL, et al. (2003) Variation in frequency of the virulence factor gene in *Escherichia coli* clones colonizing the stools and urinary tracts of healthy prepubertal girls. J Infect Dis 188: 1059–1064.
27. Sokurenko EV, Chesnokova V, Doyle RJ, Hasty DL (1997) Diversity of the *Escherichia coli* type 1 fimbrial lectin - Differential binding to mannosides and uroepithelial cells. J Biol Chem 272: 17880–17886.
28. Zhao L, Chen X, Zhu X, Yang W, Dong L, et al. (2009) Prevalence of virulence factors and antimicrobial resistance of uropathogenic *Escherichia coli* in Jiangsu province (China). Urology 74: 702–707.
29. Kang YS, Park W (2010) Trade-off between antibiotic resistance and biological fitness in *Acinetobacter* sp. strain DR1. Environ Microbiol 12: 1304–1318.
30. Gibreel TM, Dodgson AR, Cheesbrough J, Fox AJ, Bolton FJ, et al. (2012) Population structure, virulence potential and antibiotic susceptibility of uropathogenic *Escherichia coli* from Northwest England. J Antimicrob Chemother 67: 346–356.

14

Phenotypic and Molecular Characterization of Extended-Spectrum Beta-Lactamase-Producing *Escherichia coli* in Bangladesh

Taslima T. Lina[1], Bijay K. Khajanchi[1], Ishrat J. Azmi[1], Mohammad Aminul Islam[1], Belal Mahmood[1], Mahmuda Akter[1], Atanu Banik[1], Rumana Alim[1], Armando Navarro[2], Gabriel Perez[2], Alejandro Cravioto[1], Kaisar A. Talukder[1]*

1 Centre for Food and Water Borne Diseases, International Centre for Diarrhoeal Disease Research, Bangladesh, Dhaka, Bangladesh, **2** Department of Public Health, Faculty of Medicine, Universidad Nacional Autonoma de Mexico, Mexico City, Mexico

Abstract

Background: Resistance to cephalosporins in Enterobacteriaceae is mainly due to the production of extended-spectrum beta-lactamase (ESBL). Little is known about ESBL-producing bacteria in Bangladesh. Therefore, the study presents results of phenotypic and molecular characterization of ESBL-producing *Escherichia coli* from hospitals in Bangladesh.

Methods: A total of 339 *E. coli* isolated from patients with urinary tract and wound infections attending three different medical hospitals in urban and rural areas of Bangladesh between 2003–2007 were screened for ESBL-production by the double disk diffusion test. Isolates with ESBL-phenotype were further characterized by antibiotic susceptibility testing, PCR and sequencing of different β-lactamase and virulence genes, serotyping, and *XbaI*-macrorestriction followed by pulsed-field gel electrophoresis (PFGE).

Results: We identified 40 *E. coli* with ESBL phenotype. These isolates were resistant to ceftriaxone, ceftazidime, cefotaxime, aztreonam, cefepime, and nalidixic acid but remained susceptible to imipenem. All but one isolate were additionally resistant to ciprofloxacin, and 3 isolates were resistant to cefoxitin. ESBL genes of blaCTX-M-1-group were detected in all isolates; blaTEM-type and blaOXA-1-type genes were detected in 33 (82.5%) and 19 (47.5%) isolates, respectively. Virulence genes that are present in diarrhoeagenic *E. coli* were not found. Class-1 integron was present in 20 (50%) isolates. All the ESBL-producing *E. coli* isolates harbored plasmids ranging between 1.1 and 120 MDa. PFGE-typing revealed 26 different pulsotypes, but identical pulsotype showed 6 isolates of serotype O25:H4.

Conclusion: The prevalence of multidrug-resistant ESBL-producing *E. coli* isolates appears to be high and the majority of the isolates were positive for bla_{CTX-M}. Although there was genetic heterogeneity among isolates, presence of a cluster of isolates belonging to serotype O25:H4 indicates dissemination of the pandemic uropathogenic *E. coli* clone in Bangladesh.

Editor: Ulrich Dobrindt, University of Münster, Germany

Funding: This research study was funded by icddr,b and its donors which provide unrestricted support to icddr,b for its operations and research. Current donors providing unrestricted support include: Australian Agency for International Development (AusAID), Government of the People's Republic of Bangladesh, Canadian International Development Agency (CIDA), Swedish International Development Cooperation Agency (Sida), and the Department for International Development, UK (DFID). We gratefully acknowledge these donors for their support and commitment to icddr,b's research efforts. The funders had no role in study design, data collection and analysis, decision to publish, or preparation of the manuscript.

Competing Interests: The authors have declared that no competing interests exist.

* Email: kaisar@icddrb.org

Introduction

In Gram-negative bacteria, production of beta-lactamases is one of the most common mechanisms resulting in resistance to beta-lactam antibiotics. Recently, extended-spectrum beta-lactamases (ESBLs) have contributed to the dramatic increase in resistance to new generation beta-lactam agents throughout the world [1–4]. These enzymes are usually plasmid-encoded and have the capacity to hydrolyze many antibiotics including penicillins, cephalosporins, and aztreonam and are inhibited by clavulanic acid (CA) [2,3]. These phenotypic characteristics facilitate the identification of ESBLs-producing organisms using routine laboratory tests such as double disk diffusion test or E-test. However, screening of ESBL-producing bacteria by antibiotic susceptibility testing is challenging [5]. Thus detection of specific genes by PCR and sequencing are commonly used for final confirmation of ESBL producers. The association of ESBLs and the presence of TEM, SHV, OXA and CTX-M-type enzymes have been investigated in many studies [6,7]. Previous studies have shown that CTX-M-type enzymes were the most prevalent ESBLs [7,8]. According to Lahey database in Burlington (http://www.lahey.org/Studies/) that controls numbering of new beta-lactamases, more than 130 CTX-M-type enzymes are registered, which are classified into at least five different subgroups [9]. Since ESBLs are frequently encoded by genes located on different transferable genetic elements, a variety of epidemiological situations have been documented, ranging from sporadic cases to large outbreaks [10]. Moreover, ESBL-producing strains are often resistant to antibiotics of other classes (sulfonamides, aminoglycosides, quinolones) which complicates the treatment strategies in many hospitalized patients [11].

Although ESBLs have been detected in a many different of Gram-negative bacteria, *Klebsiella pneumoniae* and *Escherichia coli* remain the major ESBL-producing organisms worldwide [6,12]. In addition, ESBL-producing organisms are frequently the cause of urinary tract infections (UTI) and also in surgical wound infections [13,14]. There is one report from Bangladesh where they found 43.2% of *E. coli* and 39.5% of *K. pneumoniae* isolated from a hospital were ESBL producers [15]. However, there is a lack of information on molecular characterization of ESBL-producing organisms isolated in Bangladesh. Therefore, the objectives of the present study were the examination of presence of beta-lactamase genes in *E. coli* from different hospitals in Bangladesh.

Materials and Methods

Bacterial isolates

Between June 2003 and December 2007 we collected 339 of *E. coli* isolates from in-patient and out-patient departments of three hospitals in Bangladesh: The Bangabandhu Sheikh Mujib Medical University (BSMMU) in Dhaka; The Sylhet Medical College Hospital (SMCH) in Sylhet and The International Centre for Diarrhoeal Disease Research, Bangladesh (icddr,b) in Dhaka. These *E. coli* were isolated from either urine samples or surgical wound swabs from 339 patients with symptoms of UTI (n = 274) and wound infection (n = 64). All urine samples were obtained from outpatient departments and all surgical wound swab samples were from inpatient department of respected hospitals. *E. coli* were isolated and identified by using standard microbiological and biochemical methods [16]. These isolates were grown in trypticase soy broth containing 0.3% yeast extract (TSBY) and stored at − 70°C after addition of 15% glycerol.

Since all isolates were collected anonymously no ethical approval was necessary for this study.

Antimicrobial susceptibility testing

Bacterial susceptibility to antimicrobial agents was determined by the disk diffusion method following the guidelines of Clinical and Laboratory Standards Institute (CLSI) using commercially available antibiotic disc (Oxoid, Basingstoke, United Kingdom). The antibiotic discs used in this study were ceftriaxone (30 µg), ceftazidime (30 µg), cefotaxime (30 µg), cefepime (30 µg), cefoxitin (30 µg), aztreonam (30 µg), imipenem (10 µg), ciprofloxacin (5 µg) and nalidixic acid (30 µg). *E. coli* (ATCC 25922) and *Staphylococcus aureus* (ATCC 25923) were used as control strains for susceptibility test [17].

All 339 *E. coli* isolates were screened for the production of ESBLs by using the double disk diffusion test as described previously [18], with some modifications [4]. After overnight incubation at 37°C, any enhancement of the zone of inhibition between a beta-lactam disk and that containing the beta-lactamase inhibitor was indicative of the presence of an ESBL.

Detection of beta-lactamase and virulence genes

PCR screening for presence of different beta-lactamase genes (*bla*TEM-type, *bla*SHV-type, *bla*OXA-1-type, *bla*CTX-M-1-group, *bla*CTX-M-2-group, *bla*CTX-M-8-group, *bla*CTX-M-9-group, *bla*CTX-M-15) and class 1 and class 2 integrons were performed as described previously [12,19–22]. The primer sequences used for the detection of virulence genes, such as, invasive plasmid antigen (*ipa*H), heat labile toxin (*lt*), heat stable toxin (*st*), attaching and effacing phenotype (*eae*), invasion associated locus (*ial*), shiga toxin 1 (stx_1), shiga toxin 2 (stx_2) and aggregative property (e_{Agg}) have been described in previous studies [19,23,24].

Amplification of qnrA, qnrB, and qnrS

Multiplex PCR of 40 ESBL isolates were performed to detect the *qnr*A, *qnr*B, and *qnr*S according to the procedure described earlier [25]. The primer sequences are 5′-AGAGGATTTCT-CACGCCAGGA-3′ and 5′-GGCTGGCCGATTAT-GATTGGT- 3′for *qnr*A, 5′-GGCTGGCCGATTAT-GATTGGT-3′ and 5′-CGCGTGCGATGAGATAACC-3′ for *qnr*B, 5′-TGCCACTTTGATGTCGCAGAT-3′ and 5′-CGCACGGAACTCTATACCGTAG-3′ for *qnr*S.

DNA sequence analysis

Chromosomal DNA from representative strains was prepared and purified by procedures described previously. Sequencing was performed to identify specific TEM and OXA type ESBL genes. Sequencing of *gyr*A and *par*C genes were performed in the *qnr* positive ESBL isolates according the procedure described elsewhere [25–28]. After PCR, the amplicons were purified with the GFX PCR DNA and gel band purification kit (Amersham Pharmacia, USA), and sequenced using the dideoxy-nucleotide chain termination method with an ABI PRISM BigDye Terminator Cycle Sequencing Reaction kit (Perkin-Elmer Applied Biosystems, Foster City, California) on an automated sequencer (ABI PRISM 310). The chromatogram sequencing files were inspected using Chromas 2.23 (Technelysium, Queensland, Australia), and contigs were prepared using SeqMan II (DNASTAR, Madison, WI). Nucleotide and protein sequence similarity searches were performed using the National Center for Biotechnology Information (NCBI, National Institutes of Health, Bethesda, MD) BLAST (Basic Local Alignment Search Tool) server on GenBank database, release 138.0 [29]. Multiple sequence alignments were developed using CLUSTALX 1.81 [30]. Sequences were manually edited in the GeneDoc version 2.6.002 alignment editor. Sequences of OXA and TEM genes reported in this paper were submitted to the Genbank using the National Center for Biotechnology Information (NCBI, Bethesda, MD) Sequin, version 7.77 under the accession number EU752482-86 and EU752487-91, respectively.

Bacterial strain typing

Serotyping. All *E. coli* with ESBL phenotype were serotyped by agglutination assays using 96-well microtitre plates with rabbit serum (SERUNAM) obtained against 187 somatic antigens and 53 flagellar antigens for *E. coli*, and against 45 somatic antigens for *Shigella* species described earlier [31].

Isolation of plasmid DNA. Plasmid DNA was prepared according to the alkaline lysis method of Kado and Liu [32] with some modifications as described previously [33]. The molecular mass of the unknown plasmid DNA was assessed by comparing with the mobility of the known molecular weight plasmids. Plasmids present in strains *E. coli* PDK-9, R1, RP_4 and V517 described previously were used as molecular mass standards [33].

Pulsed-field gel electrophoresis (PFGE). Intact agarose-embedded chromosomal DNA from clinical isolates of *E. coli* was prepared and PFGE was performed using the contour-clamped homogeneous electric field (CHEF-Mapper) apparatus from Bio-

Table 1. Characterization of ESBL-producing *E. coli*.

Strain ID	Year of Isolation	Clinical Diagnosis	Hospital	In/Out patient	Sample	TEM type[a]	OXA type[a]	CTX-M-group 1	CTX-M-15	*qnr*S	*int*-1	Plasmid pattern	Serotype	PFGE pattern
KE1	2003	UTI	BSMMU	Out	U	+	+	+	+	-	+	P1	Atypical	N
KE2	2004	WI	BSMMU	In	SWS	+	+	+	+	-	+	P13	O64:H28	J
KE3	2004	WI	BSMMU	In	SWS	+	+	+	+	-	+	P5	Atypical	B
KE4	2003	UTI	BSMMU	Out	U	+	+	+	+	-	+	P3	O1:H30	G
KE5	2004	UTI	BSMMU	Out	U	+	+	+	+	-	+	P10	O1:H6	I
KE6	2004	UTI	BSMMU	Out	U	+	+	+	+	-	+	P3	O8:H9	M
KE7	2004	UTI	BSMMU	Out	U	+	+	+	+	-	+	P3	O101:H[-]	F
KE8	2005	UTI	SMCH	Out	U	+	+	+	+	-	-	P21	O20:H[-]	C
KE9	2005	WI	BSMMU	In	SWS	+	+	+	+	-	-	P11	Atypical	E
KE10	2005	WI	BSMMU	In	SWS	+	+	+	+	-	-	P14	Atypical	T
KE11	2005	WI	BSMMU	In	SWS	+	+	+	+	-	-	P12	O8:H49	Y
KE12	2005	WI	BSMMU	In	SWS	+	+	+	+	-	-	P7	O102:H4	P
KE13	2005	WI	BSMMU	In	SWS	-	+	+	+	-	-	P15	O102:H6	U
KE14	2006	WI	BSMMU	In	SWS	-	+	+	+	-	+	P1	Atypical	L
KE15	2006	WI	BSMMU	In	SWS	-	+	+	+	-	+	P1	O25:H4	A
KE16	2006	WI	BSMMU	In	SWS	-	+	+	+	+	+	P24	O102:H6	B
KE17	2006	WI	BSMMU	In	SWS	-	+	+	+	+	+	P5	O25:H4	A
KE18	2005	UTI	BSMMU	Out	U	-	+	+	+	-	+	P17	O25:H4	Z
KE19	2005	UTI	BSMMU	Out	U	-	+	+	+	-	+	P19	O153:H6	A
KE20	2005	UTI	SMCH	Out	U	-	+	+	+	+	-	P8	O8:H9	H
KE21	2005	UTI	SMCH	Out	U	-	+	+	+	-	-	P2	O25:H9	A
KE22	2006	UTI	SMCH	Out	U	-	+	+	+	-	-	P2	O25:H4	A
KE23	2006	UTI	SMCH	Out	U	-	+	+	+	-	-	P2	O25:H4	A
KE24	2006	UTI	SMCH	Out	U	-	+	+	+	-	-	P2	O25:H4	A
KE25	2006	WI	BSMMU	In	SWS	-	+	+	+	-	-	P8	O25:H4	S
KE26	2006	WI	BSMMU	In	SWS	-	+	+	+	-	-	P1	Atypical	V
KE27	2006	WI	BSMMU	In	SWS	-	+	+	+	-	-	P6	O132:H25	C
KE28	2007	WI	BSMMU	In	SWS	-	+	+	+	-	-	P4	Atypical	A
KE29	2006	UTI	SMCH	Out	U	+	-	+	+	-	-	P7	O20:H[-]	C
KE30	2006	UTI	BSMMU	Out	U	+	-	+	+	-	-	P6	Atypical	Q
KE31	2007	UTI	BSMMU	Out	U	+	-	+	+	-	-	P18	Atypical	B
KE32	2007	WI	BSMMU	In	SWS	-	-	+	+	-	-	P25	O102:H6	X
KE33	2007	WI	BSMMU	In	SWS	+	-	+	+	-	+	P4	O146:H31	B
KE34	2007	UTI	icddr,b	Out	U	+	-	+	+	+	+	P22	Atypical	R
KE35	2007	UTI	icddr,b	Out	U	+	+	+	+	-	+	P16	Atypical	W

Table 1. Cont.

Strain ID	Year of Isolation	Clinical Diagnosis	Hospital	In/Out patient	Sample	TEM type[a]	OXA type[a]	CTX-M-group 1	CTX-M-15	*qnrS*	*int-1*	Plasmid pattern	Serotype	PFGE pattern
KE36	2007	UTI	icddr,b	Out	U	-	+	+	+	+	+	P23	Atypical	O
KE37	2007	UTI	icddr,b	Out	U	+	+	+	+	-	+	P20	O25:H4	A
KE38	2007	UTI	icddr,b	Out	U	-	+	+	+	-	+	P9	O1:H6	D
KE39	2007	UTI	icddr,b	Out	U	-	+	+	+	-	+	P9	O153:H6	D
KE40	2007	UTI	icddr,b	Out	U	-	-	+	+	-	-	P10	Atypical	K

Abbreviations: UTI: Urinary Tract Infection, WI: Wound Infection. U: Urine, SWS: Surgical Wound Swab, [a] Sequencing performed on representative strains, (+) indicates presence and (-) indicates absence.

Rad Laboratories (Richmond, CA, USA) according to the procedures described elsewhere [33]. Genomic DNA was digested with *Xba*I restriction enzyme (Gibco-BRL). The restriction fragments were separated by using CHEF-mapper system apparatus in 1% pulsed-field certified agarose in 0.5× TBE buffer. The DNA size standards used was the *Salmonella enterica* serovar Braenderup (H9812) ranging from 20.5 to 1,135 kb [34]. Banding patterns were analyzed according to the established criteria reported elsewhere [35].

Results

Of the 339 *E. coli* isolates, 11.8% (n = 40) were suspected to be ESBL producers using double disk diffusion test, of which 8.4% (23/274) were isolated from urine and 26.5% (17/64) from surgical wound samples. All *E. coli* with ESBL phenotype (n = 40) isolates were resistant to 3rd generation cephalosporins. These isolates were also resistant to monobactams, such as, aztreonam and cefepime (4th generation cephalosporin). Only 3 (7.5%) isolates were resistant to cefoxitin (2nd generation cephalosporins). In addition, all isolates except for one were resistant to ciprofloxacin and all were resistant to nalidixic acid, whereas none of the isolates were resistant to imipenem.

PCR for beta lactamase specific genes showed that all the 40 isolates contained the $bla_{CTX\text{-}M\text{-}1}$ group and $bla_{CTX\text{-}M\text{-}15}$ genes. In addition, $bla_{OXA\text{-}1}$ type and bla_{TEM}-type, genes were present in 33 (82.5%) and 19 (47.5%) isolates, respectively (Table 1). Class 1 integron gene was detected in 20 (50%) isolates. Furthermore, we also examined for the presence of different virulence genes that are usually present in diarrhoeagenic *E. coli* isolates. None of these isolates were positive for any virulence genes such as, *lt*, *st*, *eae*, *ial*, stx_1, stx_2 and e_{Agg}.

Of 40 ESBL isolates, 5 were found to carry the *qnr*S gene. In order to understand the fluoroquinolone resistance mechanism of 5 *qnr*S positive ESBL isolates, we sequenced the *gyr*A (gyrase A, a subunit of topoisomerase II) and *par*C (subunit of topoisomerase IV) genes and identified double mutations in *gyr*A (Ser^{83} → Leu, Asp^{87} → Asn) and a single mutation in *par*C (Ser^{80} → Ile) genes. Sequencing of bla_{OXA}-$_1$ type and bla_{TEM}-type genes from 5 representative isolates identified these genes as beta-lactamase genes $bla_{OXA\text{-}1}$ and $bla_{TEM\text{-}1}$ respectively.

All 40 isolates yielded heterogeneous plasmid pattern ranging in size from 1.1 to 120 MDa. Middle ranged plasmid (plasmids with a size between 30 MDa and 90 MDa) was found to be present in 65% (n = 26) isolates, while 45% (n = 18) isolates harbored 120 MDa plasmid. Plasmids ranged in size from 53 to 120 MDa were detected in all the ESBL-producing *E. coli* (Table S1).

PFGE analysis revealed 26 pulsotypes, of which 9 isolates were grouped in type A, 4 in type B, 3 in type C and 2 in type D (Figure 1) and the remaining 22 isolates yielded an individual pulsotype (Table 1). Of these 40 isolates, the predominant serotype was O25:H4 (n = 8, 20%), followed by O102:H6 (n = 3, 7.5%), O1:H6 (n = 2, 5%), O8:H9 (n = 2, 5%), O20: H- (n = 2, 5%), and O153:H6 (n = 2, 5%). Of the remaining 21 isolates, 8 (20%) belonged to a single serotype and 13 (32.5%) were atypical (Table 1). The predominant PFGE type A was mostly found in serotype O25:H4 isolates (6/8) and PFGE type B was in atypical (2/13) whereas PFGE type C is present in serotypes O20:H- (2/2) and O132:H25 (1/1). PFGE type A was identified in different hospitals and locations but PFGE type B and C were only found in BSMMU in Dhaka (Table 1).

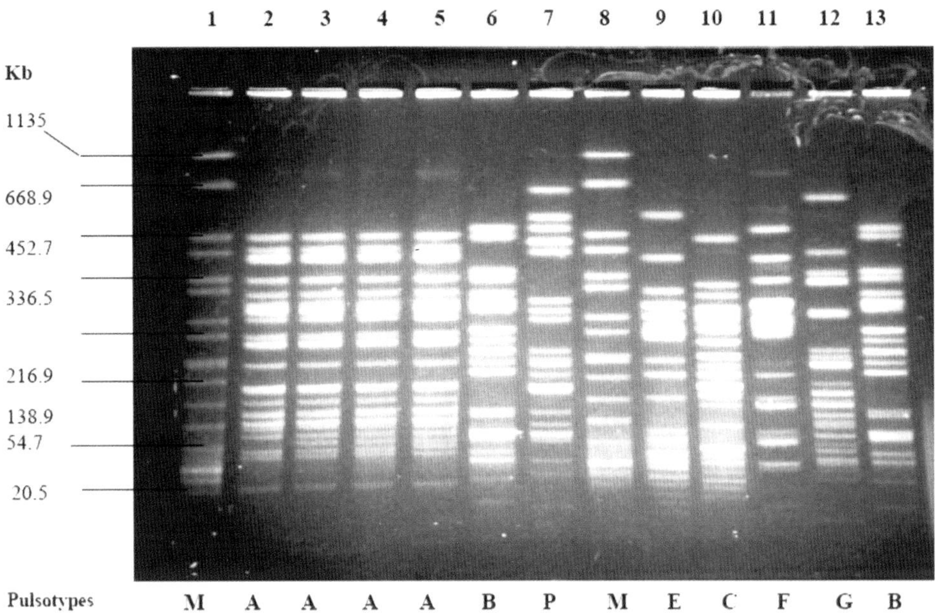

Figure 1. PFGE banding patterns of *XbaI*-digested chromosomal DNA of representative ESBL-producing *E. coli* isolates. Lane 1, *Salmonella enterica* serovar Braenderup (H9812) (marker); Lanes 2-5, PFGE type A; Lane 6, PFGE type B; Lane 7, PFGE type P; Lane 8, *Salmonella enterica* serovar Braenderup (H9812) (marker); Lane 9, PFGE type E; Lane 10, PFGE type C; Lane 11, PFGE type F; Lane 12, PFGE type G; Lane 13, PFGE type B. Four isolates belonged to PFGE pattern A were isolated from UTI patients attending SMCH hospital.

Discussion

The emergence of ESBL-producing organisms has been reported in many parts of the world [1–4]. In 2004, a study in Bangladesh showed that high prevalence (43.2%) of ESBL-producing *E. coli* was found in an urban Hospital in Dhaka [15]. The present study showed that around 12% of *E. coli* isolates obtained from patients with UTI and wound infections were ESBL-producers. The difference in prevalence between these two studies would be due to the sampling from different hospitals and from different geographic locations, which is the case for this study (Table 1) whereas in the previous study, samples were collected only from single hospital setting. However, occurrence of ESBL-producing bacteria in clinical specimens at present might be different than the rate that we found in this study as we analyzed the isolates collected during the period 2003–2007.

In present study, among 40 ESBL-producing *E. coli* strains, O25:H4 was identified as the predominant serotype (n = 8, 20%). Importantly, a particular clone detected by multilocus sequence typing (MLST) in this serogroup (O25:H4-ST131) of ESBL-producing *E. coli* has disseminated in many countries in Europe and in Asia [36,37]. O25:H4 is mainly associated with production of CTX-M-15. Ceftazidime resistance indicated presence of CTX-M-15 in our O25:H4 isolates and we confirmed the presence of CTX-M-1group and CTX-M-15 in all isolates. Based on our results it is highly probable that the ESBL-producing clone *E. coli* O25:H4-ST131 is present in our study collection from different hospitals. Thus, further analyses especially MLST are needed to investigate the dissemination of this clone in future.

The antibiotic susceptibility data indicated that ESBL-producing *E. coli* isolates acquired resistance mechanisms against different classes of antibiotics that are frequently used for empirical treatment of UTIs and other extra intestinal infections. Interestingly, all 40 ESBL-producing isolates except for one were resistant to ciprofloxacin (n = 39, 97.5%), of which 5 isolates were positive for plasmid mediated quinolone resistance gene *qnr*S along with mutations in gyrA/parC genes demonstrating underlying causes of resistance to fluoroquinolones. In our previous study, we found ciprofloxacin resistance ESBL-producing *E. coli* were positive for *qnr*S gene [38] and similar findings were found in a study from Spain in 2008 [27]. This may reflect the indiscriminate and inappropriate use of antibiotics in Bangladesh where these drugs are often sold over the counter without a physician's prescription [15]. All ESBL-producing *E. coli* isolates were susceptible to carbapenems, the current drug of choice for the treatment of patients infected with multidrug-resistant ESBL-producing bacteria.

Similar to other studies within or outside of Bangladesh, we found that all clinical isolates were positive for CTX-M-1 group and CTX-M-15 specific genes [7,39]. Moreover, previous reports from Bangladesh showed a high prevalence of CTX-M-15 group in ESBL producing *E. coli* isolated from household tap water and pigeons [37,38,40]. The CTX-M type beta-lactamases represent a rapidly emerging group worldwide, which have been found predominantly in *Enterobacteriaceae*, particularly in *E. coli*, *Klebsiella. pneumoniae*, *Proteus mirabilis* and *Salmonella Typhimurium* [2,8,41–43].

Sequence analysis of PCR product of TEM-1 and OXA-1 genes from selected isolates showed that all strains were identical to TEM-1 and OXA-1 which correlates with other studies [44,45]. ESBL genes located on integrons-like structures are being increasingly reported worldwide [10,41]. Hence, we examined the presence of class 1 and class 2 integrons. In our study, 50% (n = 20) of *E. coli* isolates harbored class 1 integron while none of the isolates contained class 2 integron as found in previous studies [46,47]. However, further study is needed to investigate the association between class 1 integron production and dissemination of ESBL type genes in *E. coli* from Bangladesh.

Interestingly, we identified no virulence genes (*ipa*H, *ial*, *lt*, *st*, *eae*, stx_1, stx_2, and e_{Agg} genes). These virulence genes are normally present in diarrhoeagenic *E. coli* which cause gastrointestinal infections [48]. Therefore, it can be explained that *E. coli* causing extra-intestinal infections such as UTI and surgical wound infection might have a different set of virulence factors than that of *E. coli* causing intestinal infection.

Apart from serotyping, plasmid profiles of all 40 isolates were compared between each other to demonstrate variation and epidemiological linkage among ESBL producing isolates. All isolates contained multiple plasmids ranging in size from 1.1 to 120 MDa and plasmid patterns of these isolates were heterogeneous (Table S1), which correlates with previous findings [38]. Plasmids ranged in size either 53 or>120 MDa or both were detected in all the ESBL-producing *E. coli* strains supporting previous findings that plasmids carrying beta-lactamase genes are ranged in size from 53 to 200 MDa [49]. Due to possible occurrence of intrinsic $bla_{CTX\text{-}M}$ genes further analyses are needed to determine the exact location of the $bla_{CTX\text{-}M}$ genes.

PFGE profile analysis showed heterogeneity among majority of isolates except for a few that could be clustered into a single PFGE type (9 isolates in type A, 4 isolates in type B, 3 isolates in type C and 2 isolates type D) (Table 1). It is interesting to note that isolates grouped into PFGE pattern A were mostly belonged to serotype O25:H4 (6/8) of which 4 were from patients with UTI at outpatient department and the remaining 2 were from patients with wound infections attending hospitals. These isolates were isolated in 2006 from three different hospitals which are geographically distant from each other. However, PFGE analysis of the majority of isolates demonstrated a low clonal relationship (26 clones/40 isolates), similar findings reported in previous studies [6,50]. These findings can be explained by the fact that ESBL production might be a consequence of horizontal gene transfer between bacteria rather than the spread of specific bacterial clones.

In conclusion, high prevalence (11.8%) and presence of variety of beta-lactamase genes in ESBL-producing *E. coli* possibly reflects the overuse and misuse of antibiotics in Bangladesh and severely limits the therapeutic options in Bangladesh. Surveillance of multidrug-resistant Gram negative bacteria causing intestinal and extra-intestinal infections is essential to guide the empirical treatment strategies for these infections in Bangladesh. Nevertheless, this is the first effort to characterize the ESBL-producing clinical isolates in Bangladesh using molecular techniques.

Ethical statement

The Enteric and Food Microbiology laboratory of icddr,b is a research laboratory where all anonymous samples were tested for respective pathogens, and for this present analysis anonymous samples were collected from different hospitals. So no ethical approval was needed.

Author Contributions

Conceived and designed the experiments: TTL BKK IJA BM MA AB KAT. Performed the experiments: TTL BKK IJA BM. Analyzed the data: TTL BKK IJA BM MA AB KAT. Contributed reagents/materials/analysis tools: KAT RA AN GP. Wrote the paper: TTL BKK IJA BM AB AN GP AC KAT MAI. Critical review: RA AN GP AC KAT MAI.

References

1. Knothe H, Shah P, Krcmery V, Antal M, Mitsuhashi S (1983) Transferable resistance to cefotaxime, cefoxitin, cefamandole and cefuroxime in clinical isolates of *Klebsiella pneumoniae* and *Serratia marcescens*. Infection 11: 315–317.
2. Bradford PA (2001) Extended-spectrum beta-lactamases in the 21st century: characterization, epidemiology, and detection of this important resistance threat. Clin Microbiol Rev 14: 933–951, table of contents.
3. Bush K (2001) New beta-lactamases in gram-negative bacteria: diversity and impact on the selection of antimicrobial therapy. Clin Infect Dis 32: 1085–1089.
4. Coudron PE, Moland ES, Sanders CC (1997) Occurrence and detection of extended-spectrum beta-lactamases in members of the family *Enterobacteriaceae* at a veterans medical center: seek and you may find. J Clin Microbiol 35: 2593–2597.
5. Dashti AA, West P, Paton R, Amyes SG (2006) Characterization of extended-spectrum beta-lactamase (ESBL)-producing Kuwait and UK strains identified by the Vitek system, and subsequent comparison of the Vitek system with other commercial ESBL-testing systems using these strains. J Med Microbiol 55: 417–421.
6. Hernandez JR, Martinez-Martinez L, Canton R, Coque TM, Pascual A (2005) Nationwide study of *Escherichia coli* and *Klebsiella pneumoniae* producing extended-spectrum beta-lactamases in Spain. Antimicrob Agents Chemother 49: 2122–2125.
7. Mugnaioli C, Luzzaro F, De Luca F, Brigante G, Perilli M, et al. (2006) CTX-M-type extended-spectrum beta-lactamases in Italy: molecular epidemiology of an emerging countrywide problem. Antimicrob Agents Chemother 50: 2700–2706.
8. Radice M, Power P, Di Conza J, Gutkind G (2002) Early dissemination of CTX-M-derived enzymes in South America. Antimicrob Agents Chemother 46: 602–604.
9. Suzuki S, Shibata N, Yamane K, Wachino J, Ito K, et al. (2009) Change in the prevalence of extended-spectrum-beta-lactamase-producing *Escherichia coli* in Japan by clonal spread. J Antimicrob Chemother 63: 72–79.
10. Canton R, Coque TM, Baquero F (2003) Multi-resistant Gram-negative bacilli: from epidemics to endemics. Curr Opin Infect Dis 16: 315–325.
11. Fang H, Ataker F, Hedin G, Dornbusch K (2008) Molecular epidemiology of extended-spectrum beta-lactamases among *Escherichia coli* isolates collected in a Swedish hospital and its associated health care facilities from 2001 to 2006. J Clin Microbiol 46: 707–712.
12. Ryoo NH, Kim EC, Hong SG, Park YJ, Lee K, et al. (2005) Dissemination of SHV-12 and CTX-M-type extended-spectrum beta-lactamases among clinical isolates of *Escherichia coli* and *Klebsiella pneumoniae* and emergence of GES-3 in Korea. J Antimicrob Chemother 56: 698–702.
13. Dromigny JA, Nabeth P, Juergens-Behr A, Perrier-Gros-Claude JD (2005) Risk factors for antibiotic-resistant *Escherichia coli* isolated from community-acquired urinary tract infections in Dakar, Senegal. J Antimicrob Chemother 56: 236–239.
14. Mehrgan H, Rahbar M (2008) Prevalence of extended-spectrum beta-lactamase-producing *Escherichia coli* in a tertiary care hospital in Tehran, Iran. Int J Antimicrob Agents 31: 147–151.
15. Rahman MM, Haq JA, Hossain MA, Sultana R, Islam F, et al. (2004) Prevalence of extended-spectrum beta-lactamase-producing *Escherichia coli* and *Klebsiella pneumoniae* in an urban hospital in Dhaka, Bangladesh. Int J Antimicrob Agents 24: 508–510.
16. Forbes BA SD, Weissfeld AS (2001) Overview of conventional methods for bacterial identification. In: Edmiston CE, editor. Bailey and Scott's Diagnostic Microbiology. St Loius, MO:Elsevier Health Sciences.
17. CLSI (2010) Performance Standards for Antimicrobial Susceptibility Testing. Approved Standard M100–S20-U, 20th Informational Supplement (June 2010, Update). Wayne, PA: Clinical and Laboratory Standards Institute.
18. Jarlier V, Nicolas MH, Fournier G, Philippon A (1988) Extended broad-spectrum beta-lactamases conferring transferable resistance to newer beta-lactam agents in *Enterobacteriaceae*: hospital prevalence and susceptibility patterns. Rev Infect Dis 10: 867–878.
19. Heuvelink AE DBE, Wernars K (1994) Detection of *Escherichia coli* 0157:H7 in raw beef by polymerase chain reaction. De ware Chemicus 24: 25–43.
20. Pitout JD, Thomson KS, Hanson ND, Ehrhardt AF, Moland ES, et al. (1998) beta-Lactamases responsible for resistance to expanded-spectrum cephalosporins in *Klebsiella pneumoniae*, *Escherichia coli*, and *Proteus mirabilis* isolates recovered in South Africa. Antimicrob Agents Chemother 42: 1350–1354.
21. Guerra B, Soto SM, Argüelles JM (2001) Multidrug resistance is mediated by large plasmids carrying a class 1 integron in the emergent *Salmonella* enterica serotype [4,5,12:i:-]. Antimicrob Agents Chemother 45: 1305–8.
22. Muzaheed, Doi Y, Adams-Haduch JM, Endimiani A, Sidjabat HE, et al. (2008) High prevalence of CTX-M-15-producing Klebsiella pneumoniae among inpatients and outpatients with urinary tract infection in Southern India. J Antimicrob Chemother 61: 1393–1394.
23. Vargas M, Gascon J, Jimenez De Anta MT, Vila J (1999) Prevalence of *Shigella* enterotoxins 1 and 2 among *Shigella* strains isolated from patients with traveler's diarrhea. J Clin Microbiol 37: 3608–3611.
24. Chakraborty S, Deokule JS, Garg P, Bhattacharya SK, Nandy RK, et al. (2001) Concomitant infection of enterotoxigenic *Escherichia coli* in an outbreak of

cholera caused by *Vibrio cholerae* O1 and O139 in Ahmedabad, India. J Clin Microbiol 39: 3241–6.
25. Islam MA, Talukdar PK, Hoque A, Huq M, Nabi A, et al. (2012) Emergence of multidrug-resistant NDM-1-producing Gram-negative bacteria in Bangladesh. Eur J Clin Microbiol Infect Dis.31(10): 2593–600.
26. Talukder KA, Khajanchi BK, Islam MA, Islam Z, Dutta DK, et al. (2006) Fluoroquinolone resistance linked to both *gyrA* and *parC* mutations in the quinolone resistance-determining region of *Shigella dysenteriae* type 1. Curr Microbiol 52: 108–111.
27. Lavilla S, Gonzalez-Lopez JJ, Sabate M, Garcia-Fernandez A, Larrosa MN, et al. (2008) Prevalence of *qnr* genes among extended-spectrum beta-lactamase-producing enterobacterial isolates in Barcelona, Spain. J Antimicrob Chemother 61: 291–295.
28. Morgan-Linnell SK, Zechiedrich L (2007) Contributions of the combined effects of topoisomerase mutations toward fluoroquinolone resistance in *Escherichia coli*. Antimicrob Agents Chemother 51: 4205–4208.
29. Altschul SF, Gish W, Miller W, Myers EW, Lipman DJ (1990) Basic local alignment search tool. J Mol Biol 215: 403–410.
30. Thompson JD, Gibson TJ, Plewniak F, Jeanmougin F, Higgins DG (1997) The CLUSTAL_X windows interface: flexible strategies for multiple sequence alignment aided by quality analysis tools. Nucleic Acids Res 25: 4876–4882.
31. Ørskov F, Ørskov I (1984) Serotyping of *Escherichia coli*. In T. Bergan (Ed). Methods in Microbiology. Academic Press Ltd, London 14: 43–112.
32. Kado CI, Liu ST (1981) Rapid procedure for detection and isolation of large and small plasmids. J Bacteriol 145: 1365–1373.
33. Talukder KA, Islam MA, Dutta DK, Hassan F, Safa A, et al. (2002) Phenotypic and genotypic characterization of serologically atypical strains of *Shigella flexneri* type 4 isolated in Dhaka, Bangladesh. J Clin Microbiol 40: 2490–2497.
34. Hunter SB, Vauterin P, Lambert-Fair MA, Van Duyne MS, Kubota K, et al. (2005) Establishment of a universal size standard strain for use with the PulseNet standardized pulsed-field gel electrophoresis protocols: converting the national databases to the new size standard. J Clin Microbiol 43: 1045–1050.
35. Tenover FC, Arbeit RD, Goering RV, Mickelsen PA, Murray BE, et al. (1995) Interpreting chromosomal DNA restriction patterns produced by pulsed-field gel electrophoresis: criteria for bacterial strain typing. J Clin Microbiol 33: 2233–2239.
36. Lau SH, Kaufmann ME, Livermore DM, Woodford N, Willshaw GA, et al. (2008) UK epidemic *Escherichia coli* strains A-E, with CTX-M-15 beta-lactamase, all belong to the international O25:H4-ST131 clone. J Antimicrob Chemother 62: 1241–1244.
37. Nicolas-Chanoine MH, Blanco J, Leflon-Guibout V, Demarty R, Alonso MP, et al. (2008) Intercontinental emergence of *Escherichia coli* clone O25:H4-ST131 producing CTX-M-15. J Antimicrob Chemother 61: 273–281.
38. Talukdar PK, Rahman M, Nabi A, Islam Z, Hoque MM, et al. (2013) Antimicrobial resistance, virulence factors and genetic diversity of *Escherichia coli* isolates from household water supply in Dhaka, Bangladesh. PLoS One 8(4): e61090.
39. Prelog M, Fille M, Prodinger W, Grif K, Brunner A, et al. (2008) CTX-M-1-related extended-spectrum beta-lactamases producing *Escherichia coli*: so far a sporadic event in Western Austria. Infection 36: 362–367.
40. Hasan B, Islam K, Ahsan M, Hossain Z, Rashid M, et al. (2014) Fecal carriage of multi-drug resistant and extended spectrum beta-lactamases producing *E. coli* in household pigeons, Bangladesh. Vet Microbiol 168: 221–224.
41. Bonnet R (2004) Growing group of extended-spectrum beta-lactamases: the CTX-M enzymes. Antimicrob Agents Chemother 48: 1–14.
42. Doublet B, Granier SA, Robin F, Bonnet R, Fabre L, et al. (2009) Novel plasmid-encoded ceftazidime-hydrolyzing CTX-M-53 extended-spectrum beta-lactamase from *Salmonella enterica* serotypes Westhampton and Senftenberg. Antimicrob Agents Chemother 53: 1944–1951.
43. Liu W, Chen L, Li H, Duan H, Zhang Y, et al. (2009) Novel CTX-M {beta}-lactamase genotype distribution and spread into multiple species of *Enterobacteriaceae* in Changsha, Southern China. J Antimicrob Chemother 63: 895–900.
44. Boyd DA, Mulvey MR (2006) OXA-1 is OXA-30 is OXA-1. J Antimicrob Chemother 58: 224–225.
45. Carattoli A, Garcia-Fernandez A, Varesi P, Fortini D, Gerardi S, et al. (2008) Molecular epidemiology of *Escherichia coli* producing extended-spectrum beta-lactamases isolated in Rome, Italy. J Clin Microbiol 46: 103–108.
46. Villa L, Pezzella C, Tosini F, Visca P, Petrucca A, et al. (2000) Multiple-antibiotic resistance mediated by structurally related IncL/M plasmids carrying an extended-spectrum beta-lactamase gene and a class 1 integron. Antimicrob Agents Chemother 44: 2911–2914.
47. Machado E, Canton R, Baquero F, Galan JC, Rollan A, et al. (2005) Integron content of extended-spectrum-beta-lactamase-producing *Escherichia coli* strains over 12 years in a single hospital in Madrid, Spain. Antimicrob Agents Chemother 49: 1823–1829.
48. Salyers AA WD (2005) *Escherichia coli* Gastrointestinal Infections. In: Bacterial Pathogenesis a Molecular Approach. Washington, D.C.
49. Jacoby GA, Sutton L (1991) Properties of plasmids responsible for production of extended-spectrum beta-lactamases. Antimicrob Agents Chemother 35: 164–169.
50. Valverde A, Coque TM, Sanchez-Moreno MP, Rollan A, Baquero F, et al. (2004) Dramatic increase in prevalence of fecal carriage of extended-spectrum beta-lactamase-producing *Enterobacteriaceae* during nonoutbreak situations in Spain. J Clin Microbiol 42: 4769–4775.

Role of Capsule and O Antigen in the Virulence of Uropathogenic *Escherichia coli*

Sohinee Sarkar[1], Glen C. Ulett[2], Makrina Totsika[1], Minh-Duy Phan[1], Mark A. Schembri[1]*

1 Australian Infectious Disease Research Centre, School of Chemistry and Molecular Biosciences, The University of Queensland, Brisbane, Queensland, Australia, **2** School of Medical Sciences, Griffith Health Institute, Griffith University, Gold Coast, Queensland, Australia

Abstract

Urinary tract infection (UTI) is one of the most common bacterial infections in humans, with uropathogenic *Escherichia coli* (UPEC) the leading causative organism. UPEC has a number of virulence factors that enable it to overcome host defenses within the urinary tract and establish infection. The O antigen and the capsular polysaccharide are two such factors that provide a survival advantage to UPEC. Here we describe the application of the *rpsL* counter selection system to construct capsule (*kpsD*) and O antigen (*waaL*) mutants and complemented derivatives of three reference UPEC strains: CFT073 (O6:K2:H1), RS218 (O18:K1:H7) and 1177 (O1:K1:H7). We observed that while the O1, O6 and O18 antigens were required for survival in human serum, the role of the capsule was less clear and linked to O antigen type. In contrast, both the K1 and K2 capsular antigens provided a survival advantage to UPEC in whole blood. In the mouse urinary tract, mutation of the O6 antigen significantly attenuated CFT073 bladder colonization. Overall, this study contrasts the role of capsule and O antigen in three common UPEC serotypes using defined mutant and complemented strains. The combined mutagenesis-complementation strategy can be applied to study other virulence factors with complex functions both *in vitro* and *in vivo*.

Editor: Christiane Forestier, Université d'Auvergne Clermont 1, France

Funding: This work was supported by grants from the Australian National Health and Medical Research Council (APP1012076 and APP1005315). GCU and MAS are supported by Australian Research Council Future Fellowships (FT110101048 and FT100100662, respectively). MT is supported by an Australian Research Council Discovery Early Career Researcher Award (DE130101169). The funders had no role in study design, data collection and analysis, decision to publish, or preparation of the manuscript.

Competing Interests: The authors have declared that no competing interests exist.

* E-mail: m.schembri@uq.edu.au

Introduction

Urinary tract infections (UTIs) are one of the most common types of bacterial infection in humans. Approximately 150 million cases of UTI are estimated to occur across the globe annually [1]. UTI occurs frequently in women; it is estimated that 40–50% of adult healthy women experience at least one UTI episode in their lifetime [2]. Catheterized patients, the elderly and children are also at a higher risk for UTI [3–5]. If untreated, UTI may progress from the bladder to the kidneys and even cause life-threatening urosepsis. The estimated annual cost of treating UTI in the USA alone is greater than $1.6 billion, thus emphasizing the global economic burden these infections place on health care systems [2].

Uropathogenic *Escherichia coli* (UPEC) is the primary causative organism in more than 80% of all UTI cases [6]. UPEC isolates exhibit a high degree of genetic diversity, primarily due to the possession of specialized virulence genes located on mobile genetic elements called pathogenicity islands [7,8]. Although no single virulence factor is uniquely definitive of UPEC, their ability to cause symptomatic UTI is enhanced by adhesins (e.g. type 1, and P fimbriae), toxins (e.g. hemolysin), iron acquisition systems and cell surface polysaccharides [9–11]. The capsule and the O antigen represent two cell-surface associated polysaccharides that contribute to UPEC virulence [12–14]. These extracellular polysaccharides protect UPEC against phagocytosis by immune cells such as neutrophils and inhibit complement-mediated killing [15,16].

Bacterial lipopolysaccharide (LPS) plays a primary role in mediating UPEC resistance to the bactericidal activity of human serum [17]. LPS consists of the highly conserved lipid A-core and repeating O antigen subunits that differ greatly between strains based on the sugar residues and their linkage patterns within the repeating subunits [18]. More than 180 different serotypes have been reported for *E. coli* [18,19], with some O antigen types such as O1, O2, O4, O6, O7, O8, O16, O18, O25, and O75 being common among UPEC strains [20]. This variation is imparted by differences in the genes that encode for glycosyltransferase enzymes that modify O antigen structure. The lipid A-core and the O antigen subunits are assembled in separate pathways that come together for ligation at the inner membrane [21]. WaaL is a conserved O antigen ligase and the only known membrane enzyme implicated in the ligation of pre-assembled undecaprenyl-diphosphate (Und-PP)-linked O antigen to lipid A-core oligosaccharide [22]. *E. coli* K-12 *waaL* deletion mutants are unable to cap the lipid A-core and are therefore disrupted in the expression of O antigen at the cell surface [23].

Like the O antigen, there is also significant variation in the *E. coli* capsule. More than 80 distinct types of *E. coli* capsule have been identified, with four major groups defined based on genetic assembly, biochemistry and physical attributes [24]. The group 2 capsular polysaccharides have mostly been associated with UPEC strains [12,25]. The role of the capsule in protecting UPEC from phagocytosis has been defined [26,27], however, its role in resistance to serum-mediated killing is unclear, with several conflicting reports in the literature [28–31]. Understanding the role of the capsule in UPEC serum resistance is further complicated by the use of multiple strains with different O antigen and capsule types. For example, a multi-strain study by Stawski *et al.* found that the contribution of capsule to serum resistance varied between strains and ranged from being important to having no protective role [32]. The genes involved in capsule production are located in the *kpsFEDUCS* operon [24,33]. KpsD is a 60 kDa outer membrane protein involved in the export of group 2 capsular polysaccharides across the outer membrane [34]. Mutation of *kpsD* results in the loss of surface expression of the capsule and accumulation of polysaccharide within the periplasmic space [35].

Given the importance of O antigen and capsule in UPEC virulence, we studied the function of these polysaccharides in three well-characterized UPEC strains (CFT073, RS218 and 1177) bearing different O and K antigens. We employed a recently described counter-selection strategy based on streptomycin-kanamycin resistance (mediated by the *rpsL* and *neo* genes, respectively) for the mutation of single genes and the subsequent repair of these mutations to generate complemented strains [36]. This enabled us to generate a defined set of wild-type (WT), mutant and complemented strains that were used to test the contributions of O antigen and capsule to UPEC virulence. Our study is the first to demonstrate the use of the *rpsL-neo* counter-selection system in UPEC, and shows that the O antigen is the major polysaccharide responsible for UPEC serum resistance and survival in the mouse urinary tract.

Results

Construction of capsule and O antigen insertion mutants

A prerequisite for the *rpsL-neo* counter-selection system is that the bacterial strain should be streptomycin resistant (Strep^R) and that this resistance is the direct effect of a mutation within the *rpsL* gene. Streptomycin resistance is a recessive trait and in the presence of both WT and mutant alleles, the strain is sensitive to streptomycin (Strep^S) [37]. This trait can be exploited for the rapid mutation and repair of mutated genes, and a schematic outline of the strategy we employed is presented in Figure 1. Strep^R derivatives of the UPEC strains CFT073 (O6:K2), 1177 (O1:K1) and RS218 (O18:K1) were generated spontaneously by sequential plating on increasing concentrations of streptomycin. These Strep^R strains (CFT073^{Strep}, 1177^{Strep}, RS218^{Strep}) were then transformed with pRedET, a temperature sensitive expression plasmid harboring the λ-Red recombinase genes. Mutation of the *waaL* (O antigen) and *kpsD* (capsule) genes in the pRedET-containing strains was performed by insertional inactivation following homologous recombination between the bacterial chromosome and the *rpsL-neo* cassette flanked by 50 bp homology regions and subsequent growth on kanamycin LB-agar. These mutants, which became sensitive to streptomycin due to the presence of a functional *rpsL* gene, were referred to as CFT073*waaL*, CFT073*kpsD*, 1177*waaL*, 1177*kpsD*, RS218*waaL* and RS218*kpsD*, respectively.

Generation of complemented strains

To repair the mutation and generate complemented strains, pRedET was re-introduced into the mutant strains and they were transformed with a 100 bp oligonucleotide that contained the same sequence as the WT strain in the regions flanking the point of insertion of the *rpsL-neo* cassette (Figure 1). The re-constructed WT strains were selected based on resistance to streptomycin, as loss of a functional *rpsL* gene reverted them to a Strep^R phenotype. These strains were referred to as CFT073*waaL*^{C}, CFT073*kpsD*^{C}, 1177*waaL*^{C}, 1177*kpsD*^{C}, RS218*waaL*^{C} and RS218*kpsD*^{C}, respectively. In summary, we therefore generated a series of O antigen and capsule mutants, as well as repaired/complemented strains, in three UPEC strains with different O and K antigens. Hereon, all references to WT strains denote the Strep^R derivatives of CFT073, *E. coli* 1177 and RS218, respectively.

Phenotypic characterization of capsule mutants and complements

The K1 phage assay was used to detect the presence of a K1 capsule on the surface of UPEC strains 1177 and RS218 (Figure 2). In this assay, the 1177 and RS218 WT strains were killed upon encountering the phage due to its specific attachment to the K1 capsule and subsequent lytic replication life-cycle. In contrast, the *kpsD* mutants exhibited normal growth beyond the streak line, indicating a loss of K1 capsule expression and thus resistance to phage killing. A WT phenotype was fully restored in the complemented strains. In separate experiments, counter-current immunoelectrophoresis using K2 antiserum was used to detect K2 capsule on the surface of CFT073. Capsular extracts from CFT073, CFT073*kpsD* and CFT073*kpsD*^{C} were electrophoresed against K2 antisera. A precipitin band was observed for CFT073 and CFT073*kpsD*^{C}, while this was absent in CFT073*kpsD*. Taken together, these results confirm the K1 or K2 capsule phenotype of the three mutated and complemented UPEC strains.

Phenotypic characterization of O antigen mutants and complemented strains

The *waaL* gene encodes an O antigen ligase and its mutation abolishes the attachment of the O antigen to the LPS core, resulting in a rough phenotype. In order to phenotypically characterize the *waaL* mutants and their complemented strains, LPS extracts were prepared from standardized late log phase cultures, separated by TSDS-PAGE and viewed by silver staining (Figure 3). As expected, due to their different O types, the LPS banding patterns from WT CFT073, 1177 and RS218 varied. *E. coli* 1177 (O1) possessed an even distribution of short, medium and long O antigen side chains, while CFT073 (O6) and RS218 (O18) possessed predominantly short and long O antigen side chains. Disruption of the *waaL* gene resulted in complete loss of the bands corresponding to the O antigen subunits from all strains, with only the lipid A-core detected. In each of the complemented strains, the O antigen-banding profile was restored to WT.

O antigen is the major determinant of serum resistance

To compare the relative contribution of O antigen and capsule to UPEC serum resistance we tested our WT, mutant and complemented strains in a serum survival assay. In this assay, bacterial survival was measured as colony forming units (CFU) before and after incubation with pooled normal human sera. As expected, the WT strains CFT073, 1177 and RS218 were resistant to killing by human serum (Figure 4). In contrast, the CFT073*waaL*, 1177*waaL* and RS218*waaL* mutants were all highly sensitive to human serum and displayed a high serum sensitivity index (SSI; $P<0.05$, paired *t* test). This phenotype reverted back to WT (i.e. resistant) in each of the respective complemented strains. The contribution of the capsule to serum resistance was less clear. The CFT073*kpsD* mutant was most sensitive ($SSI = 2$, $P = 0.046$), while RS218*kpsD* displayed reduced sensitivity ($SSI = 1$, $P = 0.027$). Complementation of the *kpsD* mutation in CFT073*kpsD* and RS218*kpsD* resulted in reversion to a WT resistance phenotype. The 1177*kpsD* mutant, on the other hand, was completely resistant

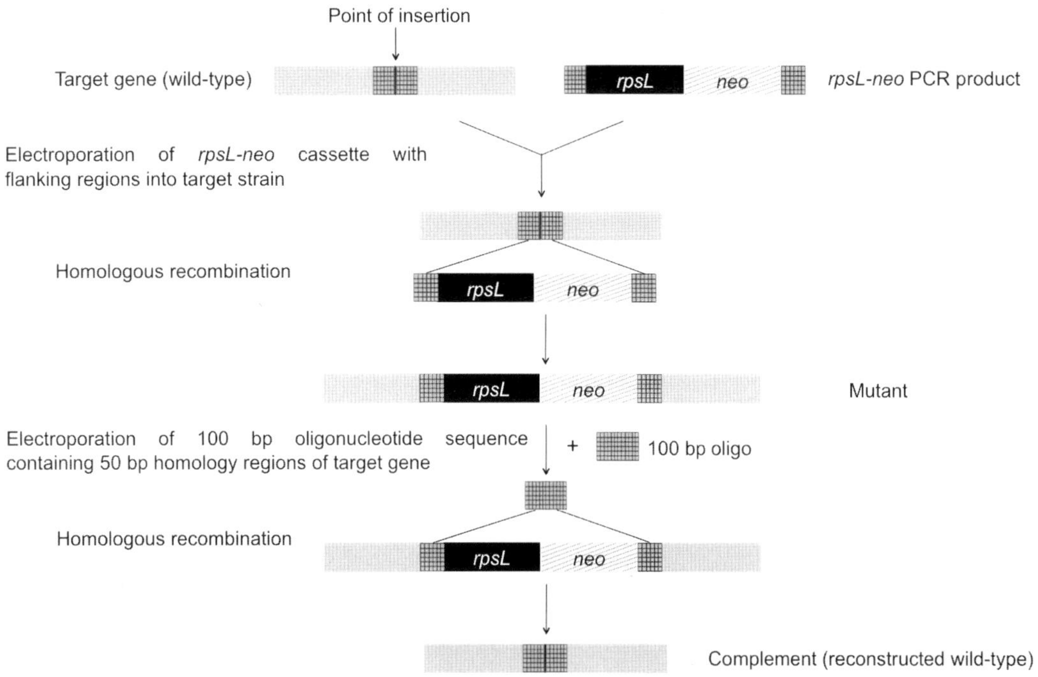

Figure 1. Schematic representation of the mutagenesis strategy utilizing *rpsL* counter selection. A 100 bp conserved region (shown as patterned region in WT sequence) was selected for the *kpsD* and *waaL*; Strep^R strains harboring the pRedET plasmid were transformed with PCR product consisting of the *rpsL-neo* cassette flanked by 50 bp regions homologous to sequences on either side of the chosen point of insertion; double cross-over events during homologous recombination make the mutant strains Strep^S Kan^R due to integration of the *rpsL-neo* cassette; for complementation, mutant strains were transformed with 100 bp oligonucleotides bearing the same sequence as the WT across the region of insertion; complemented strains were again Strep^R due to loss of the *rpsL-neo* cassette and restoration of the parental genotype; streptomycin resistant (Strep^R), streptomycin sensitive (Strep^S), kanamycin resistant (Kan^R). The methodology depicted in this figure is a modification of the *rpsL* counter-selection technique previously used for site-directed mutagenesis in bacterial artificial chromosomes [57–59].

to serum killing. The *E. coli* K12 strain MG1655 was used as a control for the integrity of serum, and was completely killed in all assays. All the strains were resistant to heat-inactivated normal human sera (data not shown). Taken together, our data show that O antigen is the major determinant of serum resistance in the UPEC strains tested. Furthermore, given that 1177 and RS218 are K1 capsule type, the observed difference in their serum sensitivities indicate that the contribution of the capsule to serum resistance is closely linked to O antigen serotype.

UPEC survival in whole blood

The most well-characterized virulence-related role of capsular expression in UPEC relates to bacterial resistance to uptake and killing by phagocytes such as neutrophils and monocytes [15]. In view of this, and the data from the above assays that showed a less clear contribution of the capsule to serum resistance compared to O antigen, we performed a series of whole blood killing assays. These assays incorporate both of the cell types relevant to UPEC phagocytosis. In these experiments, the CFT073*kpsD* and 1177*kpsD* mutants displayed significantly enhanced sensitivity to killing by whole blood compared to their respective WT counterparts (Figure 5; $P<0.05$, independent samples t test); in contrast, RS218 WT was so sensitive to killing in this assay that the data on the *kpsD* mutants could not be interpreted. Complementation of the *kpsD* mutation in CFT073*kpsD* and 1177*kpsD* restored survival to WT levels. Given that 1177 and RS218 both produce a K1 capsule, these data suggest that there may be differences in the composition of their K1 antigen, or that the role of the K1 capsule in resistance to killing by whole blood is strongly linked to O antigen type, as observed in serum killing assays.

The O6 antigen and K2 capsule are required for colonization of the mouse urinary tract

Analysis of plasmid-based complemented strains *in vivo* is challenging as it is difficult to ensure consistent expression of the cloned gene or maintenance of the plasmid in the pathogen during infection. A major advantage of the counter selection strategy described here is that complementation is performed by repair of the mutated chromosomal gene, and thus the complemented strains can be tested *in vivo*. In order to demonstrate this, we analyzed the CFT073 WT, capsule and O antigen mutant and complemented strains in a mouse UTI model. Experiments were performed as mixed competition assays, whereby mice were inoculated with a 1:1 mix of CFT073:CFT073*kpsD*, CFT073*kpsD*:CFT073*kpsD*^{C}, CFT073:CFT073*waaL* or CFT073*waaL*:CFT073-*waaL*^{C} and the number of colonizing bacteria was calculated at 18 h post infection. In these assays, both the capsule and O antigen mutants were significantly outcompeted by the WT and complemented strains in colonization of the bladder (Figure 6; $P<0.05$). No significant colonization of the kidneys was observed (data not shown); this is consistent with previous data from our laboratory using C57BL/6 mice [38–41]. Taken together, these data demonstrate that the O6 antigen has a major impact on the colonization of the urinary tract by CFT073, and that the K2 capsular antigen, while less important, also contributes to this phenotype.

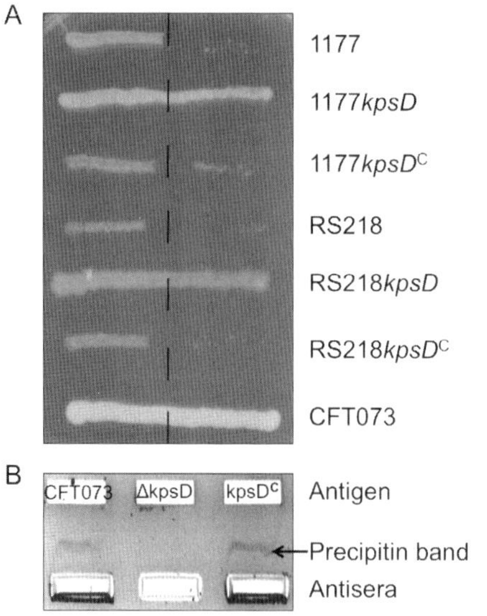

Figure 2. Phenotypic characterization of capsule mutants (*kpsD*) and complemented (*kpsD*^{C}) UPEC strains. A) Agar slab showing K1 phage reactions of 1177 and RS218 strains with CFT073 (expressing K2 antigen) as negative control; dashed lined through the center denotes line of phage suspension. Wild-type and complemented strains expressing K1 antigen are lysed by the phage and exhibit inhibited growth upon crossing the line of phage suspension. Growth of capsule mutants and the negative control strain is unaffected. B) Agarose gel showing precipitin bands arising from cross-linking of K2 antigen and antisera post electrophoresis. CFT073 WT and capsule complement show a positive reaction; no band is observed for the *kpsD* mutant due to loss of surface expression of the K2 antigen.

Discussion

The polysaccharide capsule and O antigen are well-described UPEC virulence determinants that contribute to resistance against host defenses. Specific O and K types are associated with UPEC infection, often to different degrees depending on the serotype of the strain. In this study, we investigated the role of different O and K antigens in mediating resistance to serum and whole blood, and colonization of the urinary tract, using a novel set of WT, mutant and complemented strains.

Gene disruption in bacteria using λ-Red mediated homologous recombination is a widely used and highly efficient technique [42]. In this method, the mutation of a gene or set of genes is attained by insertional inactivation using an antibiotic cassette that can subsequently be removed by FLP-mediated recombination to leave a characteristic scar sequence at the target site. Several modifications have been made to λ-Red recombineering to improve recombination frequency that can otherwise be a major limitation in certain applications. These include using transformation amplimers with large flanking regions [43], the removal of endogenous nucleases from the host strain [44], and the use of three-way overlapping PCR methods that negate the need for multiple intermediary cloning steps [45,46]. Complementation of a specific mutation, a common procedure used to prove the function of a gene and fulfill Koch's postulates, is normally achieved *in trans* by introduction of the relevant gene into the cell on a plasmid. This approach, while effective, can be complicated by the need for antibiotic selection to maintain the plasmid [47,48], differences in copy number of the complemented gene due to its location on a plasmid [49] and differences in expression of the complemented gene [50]. These issues are often compounded when complementation is attempted in an animal infection model. Another approach for complementation involves the use of a transducing phage to repair the mutation on the chromosome [51]. This involves the replacement of up to 40 kb of the chromosomal region surrounding the target gene, and also requires the use of a strain-specific phage. A different allelic exchange strategy using suicide vectors can be employed when several rounds of modification are required, however problems such as the need for large flanking regions to facilitate recombination, loss of temperature sensitivity of the vector or drastically reduced recombination efficiency due to mismatched bases with target DNA sequences make this method less than ideal when dealing with non genome-sequenced clinical isolates [52]. Transposable elements also provide an alternative to λ-Red

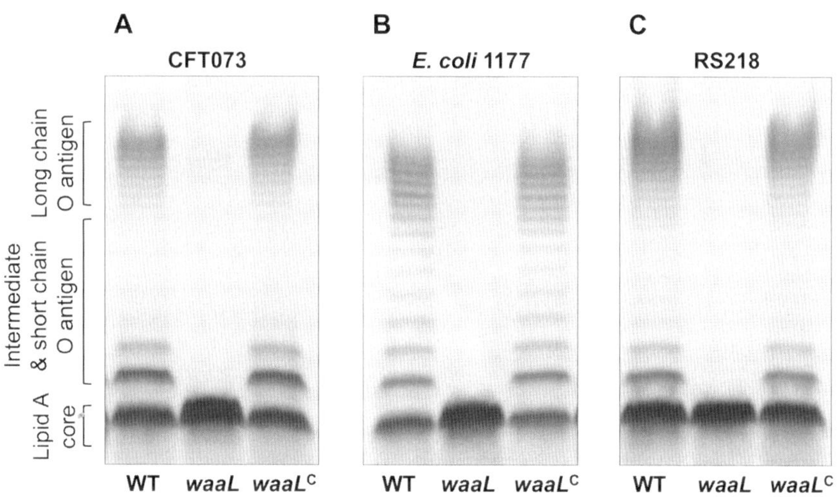

Figure 3. Analysis of lipopolysaccharide profiles by silver staining. Silver stained LPS profiles from strains listed below the gels. LPS banding patterns vary according to serotype; CFT073:O6 (A), *E. coli* 1177:O1 (B), RS218:O18 (C). Wild-type, O antigen mutant (*waaL*) and its complemented strain (*waaL*^{C}) are ordered from left to right. The thick band at the bottom represents the lipid A core and is intact in all the strains. The bands stacked on top of the core represent different O antigen side chains of different lengths that disappear in the *waaL* mutant strains. Banding patterns are restored in the complemented strains and appear to be the same as the WT.

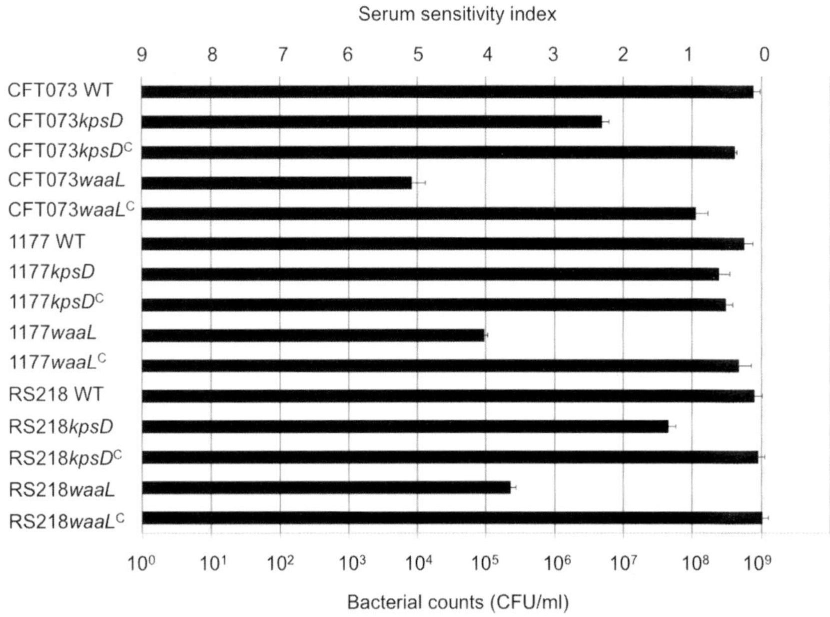

Figure 4. UPEC survival in human serum. Bacteria (approximately 4×10^8 CFU/ml) were incubated in fresh human serum for 90 min and colony counts were used to determine serum sensitivity index (SSI) for each strain, shown at the top of the graph. SSI of 0 represents a resistant strain; 1,2,3,4,5 represent equivalent reduction in log values of colony forming units (CFU/ml) post incubation with serum. The WT strains CFT073, 1177 and RS218 were resistant; CFT073*waaL*, 1177*waaL* and RS218*waaL* mutants were all highly sensitive to human serum (SSI; $P<0.05$, paired t test) and the complemented strains (*waaL*^{C}) were resistant. CFT073*kpsD* and RS218*kpsD* mutants displayed reduced sensitivity (SSI = 2 and 1, respectively); complemented strains (*kpsD*^{C}) were resistant. The 1177*kpsD* mutant was completely resistant to serum killing.

mediated homologous recombination. Transposition based strategies involving transposons such as Tn-5 and Tn-7, as well as their derivatives, have been used successfully to generate transposon mutant libraries [53,54] for site specific tagging [55] and for the generation of transcriptional/translational target gene fusions [56].

The *rpsL* counter selection system has been used previously for the modification of bacterial artificial chromosomes in viral and eukaryotic systems [57-59]. In *E. coli*, this system has been used in conjunction with *loxP* to generate markerless chromosomal deletions [60] and to introduce point mutations at specific sites on the chromosome [36]. Here, we have demonstrated its application in the construction of mutant and complemented UPEC strains. The method for complementation was highly efficient, and only required the use of a 100 base oligonucleotide that matched the target region. Since the complementation method stably generates the parental genotype without the need for a selectable marker, complemented strains can be used in animal infection experiments without antibiotic selection. This method is analogous to that previously described for *sacB*, another widely used counter selectable marker [61]. However, an advantage of *rpsL* counter selection is that unlike the *sacB* system, it can still be used in strains containing a native ColE1 replicon

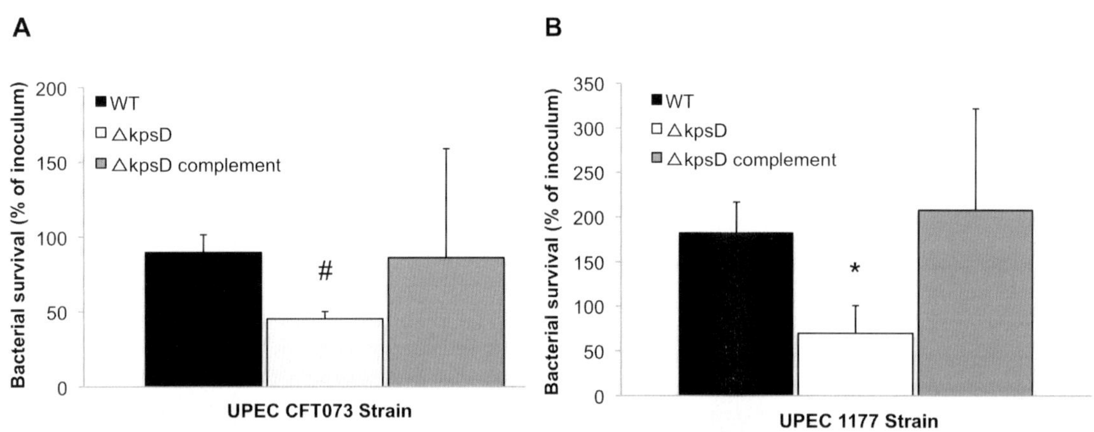

Figure 5. Survival of UPEC CFT073 (A) and 1177 (B) WT, mutant and complemented strains in whole blood killing assays. Bacteria were incubated in fresh whole blood for 3–5 h and colony counts were used to compare survival phenotypes of mutants and complemented strains to the WT parents. Fitness of the CFT073 and 1177 capsule (*kpsD*) mutants was significantly impaired compared to the WT, and was restored completely in the respective capsule complemented (*kpsD*^{C}) strains. The survival data for the RS218 WT derivatives could not be analyzed due to the high sensitivity of WT strain to killing by whole blood. *P* values, as determined by the independent samples, t test were as follows: # 0.038, * 0.042.

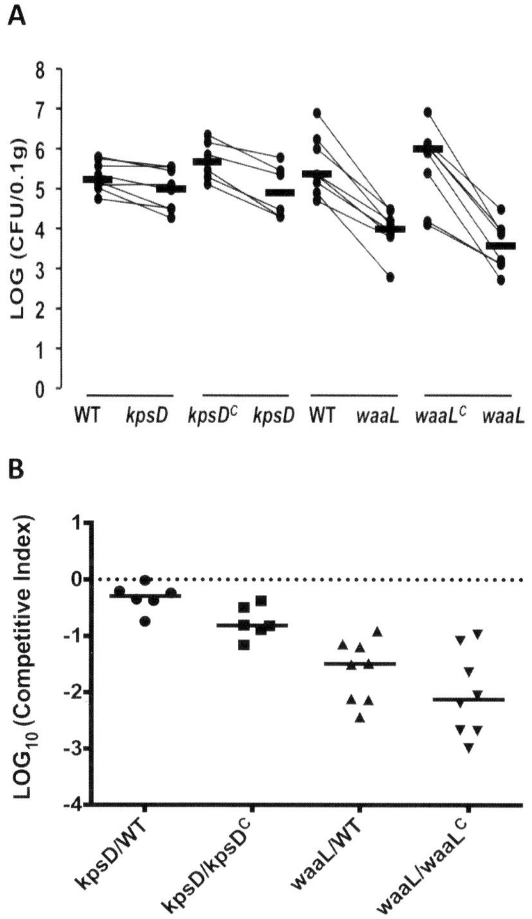

Figure 6. Fitness of CFT073 capsule (*kpsD*) and O antigen (*waaL*) mutants during *in vivo* competition with CFT073 WT and corresponding complemented (*kpsD*^C^, *waaL*^C^) strains. C57B/L6 mice were infected transurethally with a 1:1 mixture of CFT073*kpsD* and CFT073 WT or CFT073*kpsD*^{C}; CFT073*waaL* and CFT073 WT or CFT073*waaL*^{C}. (A) Each marker represents LOG_{10} total CFU recovered from each mouse per 0.1 g of bladder tissue. Lines connect data points for the same mouse, and horizontal bars represent median values. (B) Each marker represents the LOG_{10} competitive index calculated for each individual mouse; competitive indices are the ratio of the mutant 0.1 g of bladder tissue to that of WT or complemented strain. Dashed lines represent hypothetical competitive index of 1 ($LOG_{10}1 = 0$), which indicates no difference in fitness between the two strains. Horizontal bars represent group medians, and each competition group had 6 to 8 mice. All mutants were significantly outcompeted by CFT073 WT or their respective complemented strains for bladder colonization ($P<0.05$). The O6 antigen was significantly more important than the K2 capsular antigen for bladder colonization ($P<0.05$).

[62,63]. A disadvantage of the *rpsL* counter selection system is that it requires the generation of a spontaneous streptomycin resistant derivative of the strain to be studied, and it cannot be applied directly to strains with an existing streptomycin resistance cassette [64,65]. Mutations in the native *rpsL* gene have also been shown to result in a fitness cost on *E. coli* growth, with the decline in bacterial fitness dependent on the type of *rpsL* mutation and the carbon source available in the medium [66,67]. Thus, this issue needs to be considered when comparing the virulence of knockout and complemented strains where one is Strep^{R} and the other is Strep^{S}. In this study, we used spontaneously generated Strep^{R} derivatives of each parent strain (referred to as WT for simplicity), as well as mutants and repaired/complemented strains generated from these Strep^{R} derivatives. Although we did observe a slight decrease in exponential growth rate for the Strep^{R} strains, several of our mutants (which were Strep^{S}) still exhibited clear phenotypes with respect to serum resistance, whole blood killing and bladder colonization. Furthermore, our spontaneous CFT073 Strep^{R} derivate (CFT0073^{Strep}) colonized the C57BL/6 mouse bladder at a similar level to that we have reported previously for CFT073 [38,68].

Three UPEC strains with different O and K antigens were used to demonstrate the application of the *rpsL* counter selection system. For UPEC, the potential influence of *waaL* deletion and disruption of expression of O antigen on virulence is undefined except for a recent study that showed *waaL* was required for efficient colonization of mouse bladder [14]. Disruption of the *waaL* gene has been shown to result in uncapped lipid A-core due to the absence of a functional O antigen ligase [23,69]. Our *waaL* mutants had a similar lipid A-core region, while the characteristic O antigen was absent (and restored in complemented strains). The role of O antigen in mediating serum resistance in multiple bacterial pathogens has been extensively reported in the literature [32,43,70,71]. Our results demonstrate that the O1, O6 and O18 antigens are important for survival in serum. This is consistent with previous studies on the O18 antigen, which has been extensively studied in the context of neonatal meningitis strains [72–74]. Our results for the O1 and O6 antigens, while expected, represent to the best of our knowledge the first demonstration of this phenotype in well-defined mutant and complemented strains.

Mutation of the *kpsD* gene resulted in mutants lacking any surface exposed K antigen, and this was restored by complementation. In our experiments, the K2 capsule contributed to the resistance of CFT073 against the bactericidal activity of human serum. A study by Buckles *et al.* has shown the importance of the K2 capsule in UTI pathogenesis and its role in preventing complement mediated killing [31]. Notably, the serum sensitivity index for the K2 mutant in our study was significantly lower than its corresponding O antigen mutant ($P<0.01$). However, both of the strains were resistant to heat-inactivated normal human sera indicating a role for complement attack that depends at least in part, on the presence of O antigen. There are conflicting reports in the literature about the importance of K1 capsule in effecting bacterial survival in serum. A study by Leying *et al.* has suggested that K1 expression is a prerequisite for serum resistance [28]. However, the mutants used were not defined and complementation was not described. Likewise, Kim *et al.* reported that the K1 capsule plays a more important role than the O18 antigen in establishing bacteremia in a neonatal rat meningitis model [29]. In contrast, an earlier report concluded that in a similar animal model, the K1 capsule, while important for establishing meningitis, had no effect on bacterial survival in serum [75]. Several other reports have corroborated these findings [30,76,77]. Both the RS218 and 1177 strains used in our study produce a K1 capsule. We observed that while the absence of the capsule renders RS218 slightly susceptible to the bactericidal activity of serum, it had no significant effect on 1177. We also analyzed UPEC survival in whole blood to elucidate the role of capsule in protecting against whole blood killing. Survival of the CFT073 and 1177 capsule mutants was significantly impaired, which is similar to the role of K5 capsule antigen that mediates resistance to phagocytosis in UPEC [15]. The RS218 WT strain exhibited a poor survival rate and its corresponding mutants could not be analyzed by this assay. Thus, the importance of the K1 capsule in mediating serum resistance and survival in whole blood is variable, and possibly linked to the O antigen type and other factors such as hemolysin

Table 1. Bacterial strains used in this study

Strain	Relevant Characteristics	Reference
***E. coli* K12 strains**		
MG1655	OR:K-	[94]
MC1061*hsdR*	*hsdR, mcrB, araD,* 139_(araABCleu) 7679 ΔlacX74 galU galK rpsL thi	[47,95]
UPEC WT strains		
CFT073	O6:K2	[96]
E. coli 1177	O1:K1	[97]
RS218	O18:K1	[98]
Streptomycin resistant strains		
CFT073 $Strep^R$	CFT073*rpsL*, $Strep^R$	This study
E. coli 1177 $Strep^R$	*E.coli* 1177*rpsL*, $Strep^R$	This study
RS218 $Strep^R$	RS218*rpsL*, $Strep^R$	This study
CFT073 strains		
CFT073(pRedET)	CFT073*rpsL* (pRedET), $Strep^R$, Tet^R	This study
CFT073*kpsD*	CFT073*kpsD::rpsl-neo*, Kan^R	This study
CFT073*kpsD*(pRedET)	CFT073*kpsD::rpsl-neo*(pRedET), Kan^R, Tet^R	This study
CFT073*kpsD*^{C}	Re-constructed CFT073 from CFT073*kpsD*, $Strep^R$	This study
CFT073*waaL*	CFT073*waaL::rpsl-neo*, Kan^R	This study
CFT073*waaL*(pRedET)	CFT073*waaL::rpsl-neo*(pRedET), Kan^R, Tet^R	This study
CFT073*waaL*^{C}	Re-constructed CFT073 from CFT073*waaL*, $Strep^R$	This study
E. coli 1177 strains		
1177(pRedET)	1177*rpsL* (pRedET), $Strep^R$, Tet^R	This study
1177*kpsD*	1177*kpsD::rpsl-neo*, Kan^R	This study
1177*kpsD*(pRedET)	1177*kpsD::rpsl-neo*(pRedET), Kan^R, Tet^R	This study
1177*kpsD*^{C}	Re-constructed 1177 from 1177*kpsD*, $Strep^R$	This study
1177*waaL*	1177*waaL::rpsl-neo*, Kan^R	This study
1177*waaL*(pRedET)	1177*waaL::rpsl-neo*(pRedET), Kan^R, Tet^R	This study
1177*waaL*^{C}	Re-constructed 1177 from 1177*waaL*, $Strep^R$	This study
RS218 strains		
RS218(pRedET)	RS218*rpsL* (pRedET), $Strep^R$, Tet^R	This study
RS218*kpsD*	RS218*kpsD::rpsl-neo*, Kan^R	This study
RS218*kpsD*(pRedET)	RS218*kpsD::rpsl-neo*(pRedET), Kan^R, Tet^R	This study
RS218*kpsD*^{C}	Re-constructed RS218 from RS218*kpsD*, $Strep^R$	This study
RS218*waaL*	RS218*waaL::rpsl-neo*, Kan^R	This study
RS218*waaL*(pRedET)	RS218*waaL::rpsl-neo*(pRedET), Kan^R, Tet^R	This study
RS218*waaL*^{C}	Re-constructed RS218 from RS218*waaL*, $Strep^R$	This study

[78], outer membrane proteins (OmpA, OmpC) [79,80] and plasmid-encoded virulence factors (TraT, Iss) [81,82].

A key advantage of the *rpsL* counter selection strategy is that mutants can be complemented and studied *in vivo*. To demonstrate this, the ability of the CFT073 capsule and O antigen mutant strains to cause disease in a mouse UTI model was analyzed. We observed that both the K2 and O6 mutants were outcompeted by the WT and the complemented strains in bladder colonization during mixed infection challenges. However, based on competitive index the O6 antigen was significantly more important for disease pathogenesis than the K2 capsule. These results confirm the importance of the O6 antigen and, to some extent, the K2 capsular antigen, as colonization factors of the mouse urinary tract. The results are also consistent with a recent report demonstrating that restoration of the O-antigen producing capacity of the *E. coli* K12 strain MG1655 was sufficient for it to kill *Caenorhabditis elegans* at rates comparable to other pathogenic bacteria [83]. The expression of O antigen and capsule on the bacterial surface can also affect the function of other virulence factors [84,85]. Differences in the role of other UPEC K capsular antigens during infection have also been described previously. For example, the K15 antigen is important for virulence but not for serum resistance in a neonatal mouse UTI model [86], while a protective role for O4 but not for the K54 antigen has been described during colonization of the mouse urinary tract [87].

The O antigen and capsule are well known virulence factors of UPEC, however the interplay between common O and K antigens remains to be assessed using defined mutant and complemented strains. Here we have described a strategy to make single gene mutants and their complements that can be analyzed *in vitro* and *in vivo*. With the aid of mutant and complemented strain sets we have shown that the surface expression of the O1, O6 and O18 antigens and to a lesser extent, the K2 antigen, are important for bacterial survival in human serum. O1, O6, K1 and K2 antigens were all found to provide a survival advantage in the presence of whole blood. The O6 antigen was shown to be more important than the K2 antigen for colonization of the mouse bladder. The strategy described herein can be applied to study other virulence factors with complex functions and thus avoid the use of plasmid-based systems for complementation.

Materials and Methods

Ethical approval

This study was carried out in strict accordance with the recommendations in the Animal Care and Protection Act (Queensland, 2002) and the Australian Code of Practice for the Care and Use of Animals for Scientific Purposes (7th edition, 2004). Approval for mouse infection studies was obtained from the University of Queensland Animal Ethics Committee (SCMB/471/09/NHMRC (NF)). Approvals for the collection of human blood for serum sensitivity and whole blood killing assays were obtained from the University of Queensland Medical Research Ethics Committee (2008001123) and the Griffith University Human Research Ethics Committee (MSC/18/10/HREC), respectively.

Bacterial strains and growth conditions

The UPEC strains used in this study are listed in Table 1. Wild-type clinical isolates and their derivatives were routinely cultured at 28°C or 37°C on solid or in liquid Luria-Bertani (LB) medium [88] supplemented with the appropriate antibiotics: streptomycin (Strep, 100 µg/ml), kanamycin (Kan, 50 µg/ml), tetracycline (Tet, 5 µg/ml). Streptomycin-resistant derivatives of UPEC strains CFT073, 1177 and RS218 were generated by sequential growth on increasing concentrations of streptomycin (10 µg/ml, 25 µg/ml, 50 µg/ml and 100 µg/ml).

DNA manipulations and genetic techniques

Oligonucleotides used in this study were sourced from Sigma-Aldrich (Australia). Plasmid pRedET and the *rpsL-neo* template were obtained from the Counter selection BAC modification kit (GeneBridges). Isolation of plasmid DNA was carried out using the QIAprep Spin Miniprep Kit (Qiagen). All polymerase chain reactions were performed using *Taq* DNA polymerase (New England Biolabs) under standard conditions except for reactions requiring high fidelity, in which case Phusion DNA polymerase (Thermo Scientific) was used. DNA sequencing for mutant and complement validation was performed using the Big Dye v3.1 kit (Applied Biosystems) at the Australian Equine Genetics Research Centre, University of Queensland.

Construction of capsule and O antigen insertion mutants

Primers were designed using Vector NTI Advance 10 software (Invitrogen). Due to the unavailability of the RS218 and *E. coli* 1177 genome sequence, sequences of *kpsD* and *waaL* genes from UPEC strains CFT073, APEC01, 536 and UTI89 were aligned to identify 100 bp regions of complete sequence conservation. These sequences were incorporated as the 50 bp homology regions at the 5′ end of the forward and reverse knockout primers. The 3′ end of the primers contained the 24 base sequences specified in the Counter selection BAC modification kit (GeneBridges), which were used to amplify the *rpsL-neo* cassette. The primer sequences used are as follows: *kpsD* forward (F): TCCAACGTCAACGTC-TACGCCTCCTTATTACAGGCGCAGCCAGTAAAAGTGG-CCTGGTGATGATGGCGGGATCG; *kpsD* reverse (R): ACGT-CACACCGCCATACAGACCAGGATTACGCACAAATCCG-GTCACGTACTCAGAAGAACTCGTCAAGAAGGCG; *waaL* F: CGCGTGCAGCCATATTAGTGTTTCCATTCTTTGCG-TTACTATTAATCGTAGGCCTGGTGATGATGGCGGGA-TCG; *waaL* R: ATAAAACAATATAACTTATAATTAATTCG-CTTATTAATATAACTATCCATTCAGAAGAACTCGTCAA-GAAGGCG. Screening primers were designed at least 70 bp upstream and downstream of the homology regions, respectively. Their sequences are as follows: *kpsD* screen F: GATGGTGCGT-TACAGGTTGATC; *kpsD* screen R: CCGCGCTTGACCA-CAATATC; *waaL* screen F: CAACAGCAGGCTACATCATCC; *waaL* screen R: CTTCATACATTGCCAGACGG. Streptomycin resistant UPEC strains CFT073, 1177 and RS218 were transformed with pRedET by electroporation and selected in the presence of tetracycline. These strains were then grown at 28°C to an optical density at 600nm ($OD_{600\ nm}$) of 0.3, induced with L-arabinose (0.3% w/v) for approximately 1 h to allow expression of the recombinase genes, and then electroporated with the *rpsL-neo* cassette bearing the 50 bp homology regions. Mutants that were streptomycin sensitive ($Strep^S$) and kanamycin resistant (Kan^R) were identified and insertion of the *rpsL-neo* cassette within the *kpsD* and *waaL* genes, respectively, was confirmed by PCR and sequencing.

Complementation of capsule and O antigen insertion mutants

Plasmid pRedET was re-introduced into the CFT073, 1177, and RS218 *waaL* and *kpsD* mutants, respectively. To repair the *waaL* and *kpsD* mutations, these strains were prepared as described above and transformed with 2 µM single-stranded 100 base oligonucleotides comprising a sequence identical to the WT strain in the mutated region (*kpsD*:TCCAACGTCAACGTCTACG-CCTCCTTATTACAGGCGCAGCCAGTAAAAGTGTACG-TGACCGGATTTGTGCGTAATCCTGGTCTGTATGGC-GGTGTGACGT; *waaL*:CGCGTGCAGCCATATTAGTGTT-TCCATTCTTTGCGTTACTATTAATCGTAATGGATAGT-TATATTAATAAGCGAATTAATTATAAGTTATATTGTTT-TAT). Repair of the specific *waaL* or *kpsD* mutation in $Strep^R$ colonies was confirmed by PCR screening and sequencing.

K1 phage assay

K1 phage solution was sourced from the Statens Serum Institut (Denmark). The cross-brush method recommended by the manufacturer was used to determine the presence of K1 antigen [89]. Briefly, a vertical line of phage suspension was streaked across an agar plate and allowed to dry. Horizontal lines of overnight *E. coli* broth cultures were then streaked from left to right across the phage suspension and plates were incubated at 37°C for 12 h. Inhibited growth or complete killing of bacteria after crossing the phage suspension was deemed a positive reaction. A negative reaction, in the absence of K1, was characterized by normal bacterial growth across the entire bacterial streak. CFT073 WT strain with K2 capsule was used as a negative control for the assay.

Counter current immunoelectrophoresis

E. coli diagnostic K2 antisera (Statens Serum Institut, Denmark) was used to detect the presence of the K2 antigen. Capsule extracts were made according to manufacturer guidelines. Briefly, the bacterial cells from an agar plate were suspended in 1 ml phosphate buffered saline (PBS) (pH 7.4) and incubated at 60°C for 20 min. The cell suspension was then centrifuged for 30 min at 14,000 rpm and the supernatant transferred to a fresh tube and heated for 1 h at 95°C. Extracts were then diluted in PBS (1:50) for electrophoresis. A 1.5% agarose gel was applied to a glass plate with 2 rows of wells and a distance of 5 mm between each row. 15 µl of K2 antisera and diluted capsule extracts were loaded at the anode and cathode ends, respectively. Counter-current immunoelectrophoresis was performed for 70 min at 80 V in 1X TAE buffer. A precipitin band between the wells demonstrated the presence of a K2 capsule.

LPS isolation and silver staining

LPS was extracted as described previously by West *et al.* [90]. Tricine-SDS PAGE (TSDS PAGE) was used to obtain a high resolution of LPS. Gels were cast with a 16.5% resolving phase containing 4 M urea, overlaid with a 4% stacking phase. A two-buffer system was used for electrophoresis as previously described [91]. Electrophoresis was performed in the Mini-PROTEAN gel apparatus (BioRad) at 50 V for 30 min and then at 150 V for 70 min. A modified silver staining method originally described by Tsai and Frasch [92] was used to view LPS bands. Gels were transferred to a glass tray and fixed overnight (40% ethanol, 5% glacial acetic acid) at room temperature. The fixing solution was replaced with an oxidizing solution (40% ethanol, 5% glacial acetic acid, 0.7% periodic acid) and incubated for 7 min. Gels were washed repeatedly in copious amounts of milliQ water and then stained (20 mM sodium hydroxide, 0.4% ammonium hydroxide, 0.7% silver nitrate) for 10 min. The staining solution was removed and gels were incubated in the dark in a developing solution (0.02% formaldehyde, 0.26 mM citric acid) until distinct bands were visible. Gels were then washed in water to stop the reaction.

Serum killing assay

Overnight bacterial cultures were washed in PBS and then standardized to a final $OD_{600} = 0.8$ (approximately 4×10^8 CFU/ml). A volume of 50 µl of each standardized culture was mixed with an equal volume of PBS and serially diluted for colony counts on agar to enumerate CFU prior to serum treatment (t = 0 min). Fresh blood was collected in EDTA-free vacutainer tubes on the day of the assay from two healthy human donors who gave informed consent. The same donors were used for all assays in order to reduce serum variability. Blood was allowed to clot for 15 min and the tubes were centrifuged at 1500 *g* for 10 min. A volume of 50 µl of each standardized culture (approximately 3×10^7 CFU) was mixed with an equal volume of pooled human sera, mixed and incubated for 90 min at 37°C. All experiments were performed in triplicate. Colony counts were used to enumerate bacterial cells post treatment (t = 90 min). *E. coli* MG1655 was used as a serum sensitive control strain. All the strains were tested similarly in a parallel assay using heat-inactivated normal human sera (Millipore). Strains showing at least a $\log_{10}$ difference (i.e. 10-fold) in CFU/ml were deemed to have altered sensitivity to serum as compared to WT. Serum sensitivity indices (SSI) were calculated according to these differences. Paired samples t tests were performed on CFU/ml values at the two time points (0 min and 90 min) to determine statistical significance.

Whole blood killing assay

Approximately 10^4 colony forming units (CFU) of UPEC prepared from a late exponential phase culture in LB were added to 1.5 ml of whole blood collected from a healthy human volunteer using plasma preparation tubes (PPT) containing 9.0 mg K2EDTA (BD Vacutainer, NJ, USA). The infected cultures were incubated rolling at 37°C and after 3–5 h diluted blood samples were plated in triplicate onto agar to enumerate the surviving bacteria. The survival rate was calculated as a percentage of the starting inoculum ([CFU (at a given time point)/CFU (at the start)] ×100) and *P* values were determined using the independent samples t test.

Mouse model of UTI

The mouse model of UTI described by Roos *et al.* (2006) was used in this study [93]. Female C57BL/6 mice (8–10 weeks) were purchased from the University of Queensland Animal Facility and housed in sterile cages with *ad libitum* access to sterile water. All strains used in this experiment were enriched for type 1 fimbriae expression after 3 passages under static conditions. Bacterial cultures were prepared by overnight static growth in LB broth; all strains were strongly positive for type 1 fimbriae expression as determined by yeast cell agglutination. For competitive (mixed infection) assays, inocula contained 1:1 strain mixtures of CFT073*kpsD* and CFT073 WT (group 1) or CFT073*kpsD*^{C} (complement; group 2); CFT073*waaL* and CFT073 WT (group 3) or CFT073*waaL*^{C} (group 4). An inoculum of 20–40 µl, containing 5×10^8 CFU of bacteria in PBS was injected directly into the bladder of each mouse. Urine was collected from mice 18 h after challenge following which they were euthanized by cervical dislocation. Bladders were then excised aseptically, weighed, and homogenized in PBS. Urine and bladder homogenates were serially diluted in PBS and plated onto streptomycin and kanamycin-containing LB agar for colony counts. The two strains in each group were differentiated by their resistance to streptomycin (WT and complements) or kanamycin (*kpsD* and *waaL* mutants). Significance was determined using the two-tailed Wilcoxon matched pairs test on CFU/ml urine, or CFU/0.1 g bladder tissue using Prism6 (GraphPad). *P* values <0.05 were considered significant.

Acknowledgments

We thank Barbara Arnts and Kendall Hepple for expert technical assistance with the mouse UTI model.

Author Contributions

Conceived and designed the experiments: SS GCU MT MDP MAS. Performed the experiments: SS GCU. Analyzed the data: SS GCU. Contributed reagents/materials/analysis tools: GCU MAS. Wrote the paper: SS GCU MT MDP MAS.

References

1. Stamm WE, Norrby SR (2001) Urinary tract infections: disease panorama and challenges. J Infect Dis 183 Suppl 1: S1–4.
2. Foxman B (2002) Epidemiology of urinary tract infections: Incidence, morbidity, and economic costs. American Journal of Medicine 113: 5S–13S.
3. Chenoweth CE, Saint S (2011) Urinary tract infections. Infect Dis Clin North Am 25: 103–115.
4. Buonsenso D, Cataldi L (2012) Urinary tract infections in children: a review. Minerva Pediatr 64: 145–157.
5. Nicolle LE (2001) Urinary tract infections in long-term-care facilities. Infect Control Hosp Epidemiol 22: 167–175.
6. Stamm WE, Hooton TM (1993) Management of Urinary-Tract Infections in Adults. New England Journal of Medicine 329: 1328–1334.
7. Hacker J, Bender L, Ott M, Wingender J, Lund B, et al. (1990) Deletions of chromosomal regions coding for fimbriae and hemolysins occur in vitro and in vivo in various extraintestinal Escherichia coli isolates. Microb Pathog 8: 213–225.

8. Oelschlaeger TA, Dobrindt U, Hacker J (2002) Pathogenicity islands of uropathogenic E. coli and the evolution of virulence. Int J Antimicrob Agents 19: 517–521.
9. Klemm P, Schembri MA (2000) Bacterial adhesins: function and structure. International Journal of Medical Microbiology 290: 27–35.
10. Oelschlaeger TA, Dobrindt U, Hacker J (2002) Virulence factors of uropathogens. Curr Opin Urol 12: 33–38.
11. Garcia EC, Brumbaugh AR, Mobley HL (2011) Redundancy and specificity of Escherichia coli iron acquisition systems during urinary tract infection. Infect Immun 79: 1225–1235.
12. Johnson JR (1991) Virulence Factors in *Escherichia coli* Urinary Tract Infection. Clin Microbiol Rev 4: 80–128.
13. Bahrani-Mougeot FK, Buckles EL, Lockatell CV, Hebel JR, Johnson DE, et al. (2002) Type 1 fimbriae and extracellular polysaccharides are preeminent uropathogenic Escherichia coli virulence determinants in the murine urinary tract. Mol Microbiol 45: 1079–1093.
14. Billips BK, Yaggie RE, Cashy JP, Schaeffer AJ, Klumpp DJ (2009) A Live-Attenuated Vaccine for the Treatment of Urinary Tract Infection by Uropathogenic Escherichia coli. Journal of Infectious Diseases 200: 263–272.
15. Burns SM, Hull SI (1999) Loss of resistance to ingestion and phagocytic killing by O(-) and K(-) mutants of a uropathogenic Escherichia coli O75:K5 strain. Infect Immun 67: 3757–3762.
16. Burns SM, Hull SI (1998) Comparison of loss of serum resistance by defined lipopolysaccharide mutants and an acapsular mutant of uropathogenic Escherichia coli O75:K5. Infect Immun 66: 4244–4253.
17. Tomas JM, Ciurana B, Benedi VJ, Juarez A (1988) Role of Lipopolysaccharide and Complement in Susceptibility of Escherichia-Coli and Salmonella-Typhimurium to Non-Immune Serum. Journal of General Microbiology 134: 1009–1016.
18. Stenutz R, Weintraub A, Widmalm G (2006) The structures of Escherichia coli O-polysaccharide antigens. Fems Microbiology Reviews 30: 382–403.
19. Orskov I, Orskov F, Jann B, Jann K (1977) Serology, Chemistry, and Genetics of O and K Antigens of Escherichia-Coli. Bacteriological Reviews 41: 667–710.
20. Totsika M, Moriel DG, Idris A, Rogers BA, Wurpel DJ, et al. (2012) Uropathogenic Escherichia coli mediated urinary tract infection. Curr Drug Targets 13: 1386–1399.
21. Raetz CR, Whitfield C (2002) Lipopolysaccharide endotoxins. Annu Rev Biochem 71: 635–700.
22. Perez JM, McGarry MA, Marolda CL, Valvano MA (2008) Functional analysis of the large periplasmic loop of the Escherichia coli K-12 WaaL O-antigen ligase. Mol Microbiol 70: 1424–1440.
23. Heinrichs DE, Monteiro MA, Perry MB, Whitfield C (1998) The assembly system for the lipopolysaccharide R2 core-type of Escherichia coli is a hybrid of those found in Escherichia coli K-12 and Salmonella enterica - Structure and function of the R2 WaaK and WaaL homologs. Journal of Biological Chemistry 273: 8849–8859.
24. Whitfield C, Roberts IS (1999) Structure, assembly and regulation of expression of capsules in Escherichia coli. Mol Microbiol 31: 1307–1319.
25. Roberts IS (1996) The biochemistry and genetics of capsular polysaccharide production in bacteria. Annual Review of Microbiology 50: 285–315.
26. Weiss J, Victor M, Cross AS, Elsbach P (1982) Sensitivity of K1-Encapsulated Escherichia-Coli to Killing by the Bactericidal Permeability-Increasing Protein of Rabbit and Human-Neutrophils. Infect Immun 38: 1149–1153.
27. Howard CJ, Glynn AA (1971) Virulence for mice of strains of *Escherichia coli* related to effects of K antigens on their resistance to phagocytosis and killing by complement. Immunology 20: 767–&.
28. Leying H, Suerbaum S, Kroll HP, Stahl D, Opferkuch W (1990) The capsular polysaccharide is a major determinant of serum resistance in K-1-positive blood culture isolates of Escherichia coli. Infect Immun 58: 222–227.
29. Kim KS, Itabashi H, Gemski P, Sadoff J, Warren RL, et al. (1992) The K1-Capsule Is the Critical Determinant in the Development of Escherichia-Coli Meningitis in the Rat. Journal of Clinical Investigation 90: 897–905.
30. Bjorksten B, Bortolussi R, Gothefors L, Quie PG (1976) Interaction of E. coli strains with human serum: lack of relationship to K1 antigen. J Pediatr 89: 892–897.
31. Buckles EL, Wang XL, Lane MC, Lockatell CV, Johnson DE, et al. (2009) Role of the K2 Capsule in Escherichia coli Urinary Tract Infection and Serum Resistance. Journal of Infectious Diseases 199: 1689–1697.
32. Stawski G, Nielsen L, Orskov F, Orskov I (1990) Serum sensitivity of a diversity of Escherichia coli antigenic reference strains. Correlation with an LPS variation phenomenon. Apmis 98: 828–838.
33. Silver RP, Vann WF, Aaronson W (1984) Genetic and molecular analyses of Escherichia coli K1 antigen genes. J Bacteriol 157: 568–575.
34. Silver RP, Aaronson W, Vann WF (1987) Translocation of capsular polysaccharides in pathogenic strains of Escherichia coli requires a 60-kilodalton periplasmic protein. J Bacteriol 169: 5489–5495.
35. Wunder DE, Aaronson W, Hayes SF, Bliss JM, Silver RP (1994) Nucleotide sequence and mutational analysis of the gene encoding kpsD, a periplasmic protein involved in transport of polysialic acid in Escherichia coli K1. J Bacteriol 176: 4025–4033.
36. Heermann R, Zeppenfeld T, Jung K (2008) Simple generation of site-directed point mutations in the Escherichia coli chromosome using Red(R)/ET(R) Recombination. Microb Cell Fact 7: 14.
37. Lederberg J (1951) Streptomycin resistance; a genetically recessive mutation. J Bacteriol 61: 549–550.
38. Ulett GC, Valle J, Beloin C, Sherlock O, Ghigo JM, et al. (2007) Functional analysis of antigen 43 in uropathogenic Escherichia coli reveals a role in long-term persistence in the urinary tract. Infect Immun 75: 3233–3244.
39. Allsopp LP, Totsika M, Tree JJ, Ulett GC, Mabbett AN, et al. (2010) UpaH is a newly identified autotransporter protein that contributes to biofilm formation and bladder colonization by uropathogenic Escherichia coli CFT073. Infect Immun 78: 1659–1669.
40. Duell BL, Carey AJ, Tan CK, Cui X, Webb RI, et al. (2012) Innate transcriptional networks activated in bladder in response to uropathogenic Escherichia coli drive diverse biological pathways and rapid synthesis of IL-10 for defense against bacterial urinary tract infection. J Immunol 188: 781–792.
41. Tan CK, Carey AJ, Cui X, Webb RI, Ipe D, et al. (2012) Genome-wide mapping of cystitis due to Streptococcus agalactiae and Escherichia coli in mice identifies a unique bladder transcriptome that signifies pathogen-specific antimicrobial defense against urinary tract infection. Infect Immun 80: 3145–3160.
42. Datsenko KA, Wanner BL (2000) One-step inactivation of chromosomal genes in Escherichia coli K-12 using PCR products. Proc Natl Acad Sci U S A 97: 6640–6645.
43. Phan MD, Peters KM, Sarkar S, Lukowski SW, Allsopp LP, et al. (2013) The Serum Resistome of a Globally Disseminated Multidrug Resistant Uropathogenic Clone. PLoS Genet 9: e1003834.
44. Mosberg JA, Gregg CJ, Lajoie MJ, Wang HH, Church GM (2012) Improving lambda red genome engineering in Escherichia coli via rational removal of endogenous nucleases. PLoS One 7: e44638.
45. Webb JS, Nikolakakis KC, Willett JL, Aoki SK, Hayes CS, et al. (2013) Delivery of CdiA nuclease toxins into target cells during contact-dependent growth inhibition. PLoS One 8: e57609.
46. Derbise A, Lesic B, Dacheux D, Ghigo JM, Carniel E (2003) A rapid and simple method for inactivating chromosomal genes in Yersinia. FEMS Immunol Med Microbiol 38: 113–116.
47. Meissner PS, Sisk WP, Berman ML (1987) Bacteriophage lambda cloning system for the construction of directional cDNA libraries. Proc Natl Acad Sci U S A 84: 4171–4175.
48. Soussy CJ, Wolfson JS, Ng EY, Hooper DC (1993) Limitations of plasmid complementation test for determination of quinolone resistance due to changes in the gyrase A protein and identification of conditional quinolone resistance locus. Antimicrob Agents Chemother 37: 2588–2592.
49. Watve MM, Dahanukar N, Watve MG (2010) Sociobiological control of plasmid copy number in bacteria. PLoS One 5: e9328.
50. Siegele DA, Hu JC (1997) Gene expression from plasmids containing the araBAD promoter at subsaturating inducer concentrations represents mixed populations. Proc Natl Acad Sci U S A 94: 8168–8172.
51. Battaglioli EJ, Baisa GA, Weeks AE, Schroll RA, Hryckowian AJ, et al. (2011) Isolation of generalized transducing bacteriophages for uropathogenic strains of Escherichia coli. Appl Environ Microbiol 77: 6630–6635.
52. Emmerson JR, Gally DL, Roe AJ (2006) Generation of gene deletions and gene replacements in Escherichia coli O157: H7 using a temperature sensitive allelic exchange system. Biological Procedures Online 8: 153–162.
53. Goryshin IY, Naumann TA, Apodaca J, Reznikoff WS (2003) Chromosomal deletion formation system based on Tn5 double transposition: use for making minimal genomes and essential gene analysis. Genome Res 13: 644–653.
54. Winterberg KM, Luecke J, Bruegl AS, Reznikoff WS (2005) Phenotypic screening of Escherichia coli K-12 Tn5 insertion libraries, using whole-genome oligonucleotide microarrays. Appl Environ Microbiol 71: 451–459.
55. Lambertsen L, Sternberg C, Molin S (2004) Mini-Tn7 transposons for site-specific tagging of bacteria with fluorescent proteins. Environ Microbiol 6: 726–732.
56. Biery MC, Stewart FJ, Stellwagen AE, Raleigh EA, Craig NL (2000) A simple in vitro Tn7-based transposition system with low target site selectivity for genome and gene analysis. Nucleic Acids Res 28: 1067–1077.
57. Bird AW, Erler A, Fu J, Heriche JK, Maresca M, et al. (2012) High-efficiency counterselection recombineering for site-directed mutagenesis in bacterial artificial chromosomes. Nat Methods 9: 103–109.
58. Schwartz JA, Brittle EE, Reynolds AE, Enquist LW, Silverstein SJ (2006) UL54-null pseudorabies virus is attenuated in mice but productively infects cells in culture. J Virol 80: 769–784.
59. White EA, Spector DH (2005) Exon 3 of the human cytomegalovirus major immediate-early region is required for efficient viral gene expression and for cellular cyclin modulation. J Virol 79: 7438–7452.
60. Tuntufye HN, Goddeeris BM (2011) Use of lambda Red-mediated recombineering and Cre/lox for generation of markerless chromosomal deletions in avian pathogenic Escherichia coli. FEMS Microbiol Lett 325: 140–147.
61. Blomfield IC, Vaughn V, Rest RF, Eisenstein BI (1991) Allelic Exchange in Escherichia-Coli Using the Bacillus-Subtilis Sacb Gene and a Temperature-Sensitive Psc101 Replicon. Molecular Microbiology 5: 1447–1457.
62. Marx CJ (2008) Development of a broad-host-range sacB-based vector for unmarked allelic exchange. BMC Res Notes 1: 1.
63. Hamilton CM, Aldea M, Washburn BK, Babitzke P, Kushner SR (1989) New method for generating deletions and gene replacements in Escherichia coli. J Bacteriol 171: 4617–4622.

64. Sandvang D (1999) Novel streptomycin and spectinomycin resistance gene as a gene cassette within a class 1 integron isolated from Escherichia coli. Antimicrob Agents Chemother 43: 3036–3038.
65. Hollingshead S, Vapnek D (1985) Nucleotide sequence analysis of a gene encoding a streptomycin/spectinomycin adenylyltransferase. Plasmid 13: 17–30.
66. Paulander W, Maisnier-Patin S, Andersson DI (2009) The fitness cost of streptomycin resistance depends on rpsL mutation, carbon source and RpoS (sigmaS). Genetics 183: 539–546, 531SI–532SI.
67. Enne VI, Delsol AA, Davis GR, Hayward SL, Roe JM, et al. (2005) Assessment of the fitness impacts on Escherichia coli of acquisition of antibiotic resistance genes encoded by different types of genetic element. J Antimicrob Chemother 56: 544–551.
68. Tree JJ, Ulett GC, Ong CL, Trott DJ, McEwan AG, et al. (2008) Trade-off between iron uptake and protection against oxidative stress: deletion of cueO promotes uropathogenic Escherichia coli virulence in a mouse model of urinary tract infection. J Bacteriol 190: 6909–6912.
69. Abeyrathne PD, Daniels C, Poon KKH, Matewish MJ, Lam JS (2005) Functional characterization of WaaL, a ligase associated with linking O-antigen polysaccharide to the core of Pseudomonas aeruginosa lipopolysaccharide. J Bacteriol 187: 3002–3012.
70. DeShazer D, Brett PJ, Woods DE (1998) The type II O-antigenic polysaccharide moiety of Burkholderia pseudomallei lipopolysaccharide is required for serum resistance and virulence. Mol Microbiol 30: 1081–1100.
71. Bravo D, Silva C, Carter JA, Hoare A, Alvarez SA, et al. (2008) Growth-phase regulation of lipopolysaccharide O-antigen chain length influences serum resistance in serovars of Salmonella. J Med Microbiol 57: 938–946.
72. Pluschke G, Mayden J, Achtman M, Levine RP (1983) Role of the capsule and the O antigen in resistance of O18:K1 Escherichia coli to complement-mediated killing. Infect Immun 42: 907–913.
73. Hughes C, Phillips R, Roberts AP (1982) Serum resistance among Escherichia coli strains causing urinary tract infection in relation to O type and the carriage of hemolysin, colicin, and antibiotic resistance determinants. Infect Immun 35: 270–275.
74. Cryz SJ, Jr., Cross AS, Sadoff JC, Furer E (1990) Synthesis and characterization of Escherichia coli O18 O-polysaccharide conjugate vaccines. Infect Immun 58: 373–377.
75. Bortolussi R, Ferrieri P, Bjorksten B, Quie PG (1979) Capsular K1-Polysaccharide of Escherichia-Coli - Relationship to Virulence in Newborn Rats and Resistance to Phagocytosis. Infect Immun 25: 293–298.
76. McCabe WR, Kaijser B, Olling S, Uwaydah M, Hanson LA (1978) Escherichia coli in bacteremia: K and O antigens and serum sensitivity of strains from adults and neonates. J Infect Dis 138: 33–41.
77. Taylor PW (1976) Immunochemical investigations on lipopolysaccharides and acidic polysaccharides from serum-sensitive and serum-resistant strains of Escherichia coli isolated from urinary-tract infections. J Med Microbiol 9: 405–421.
78. Gadeberg OV, Mansa B (1990) In vitro cytotoxic effect of alpha-hemolytic Escherichia coli on human blood granulocytes. Inhibition by alpha-hemolysin antibody. Zentralbl Bakteriol 273: 492–500.
79. Prasadarao NV, Blom AM, Villoutreix BO, Linsangan LC (2002) A novel interaction of outer membrane protein A with C4b binding protein mediates serum resistance of Escherichia coli K1. J Immunol 169: 6352–6360.
80. Liu YF, Yan JJ, Lei HY, Teng CH, Wang MC, et al. (2012) Loss of outer membrane protein C in Escherichia coli contributes to both antibiotic resistance and escaping antibody-dependent bactericidal activity. Infect Immun 80: 1815–1822.
81. Montenegro MA, Bitter-Suermann D, Timmis JK, Aguero ME, Cabello FC, et al. (1985) traT gene sequences, serum resistance and pathogenicity-related factors in clinical isolates of Escherichia coli and other gram-negative bacteria. J Gen Microbiol 131: 1511–1521.
82. Binns MM, Mayden J, Levine RP (1982) Further characterization of complement resistance conferred on Escherichia coli by the plasmid genes traT of R100 and iss of ColV,I-K94. Infect Immun 35: 654–659.
83. Browning DF, Wells TJ, Franca FL, Morris FC, Sevastsyanovich YR, et al. (2013) Laboratory adapted Escherichia coli K-12 becomes a pathogen of Caenorhabditis elegans upon restoration of O antigen biosynthesis. Mol Microbiol 87: 939–950.
84. Schembri MA, Dalsgaard D, Klemm P (2004) Capsule shields the function of short bacterial adhesins. J Bacteriol 186: 1249–1257.
85. Schembri MA, Blom J, Krogfelt KA, Klemm P (2005) Capsule and fimbria interaction in Klebsiella pneumoniae. Infect Immun 73: 4626–4633.
86. Schneider G, Dobrindt U, Bruggemann H, Nagy G, Janke B, et al. (2004) The pathogenicity island-associated K15 capsule determinant exhibits a novel genetic structure and correlates with virulence in uropathogenic Escherichia coli strain 536. Infect Immun 72: 5993–6001.
87. Russo TA, Brown JJ, Jodush ST, Johnson JR (1996) The O4 specific antigen moiety of lipopolysaccharide but not the K54 group 2 capsule is important for urovirulence of an extraintestinal isolate of Escherichia coli. Infect Immun 64: 2343–2348.
88. Bertani G (1951) Studies on lysogenesis. I. The mode of phage liberation by lysogenic Escherichia coli. J Bacteriol 62: 293–300.
89. Orskov F, Orskov I (1984) Serotyping of Escherichia coli. In: Bergan T, editor. Methods in Microbiology: Academic Press. pp. 43–112.
90. West NP, Jungnitz H, Fitter JT, McArthur JD, Guzman CA, et al. (2000) Role of phosphoglucomutase of Bordetella bronchiseptica in lipopolysaccharide biosynthesis and virulence. Infect Immun 68: 4673–4680.
91. Lesse AJ, Campagnari AA, Bittner WE, Apicella MA (1990) Increased Resolution of Lipopolysaccharides and Lipooligosaccharides Utilizing Tricine-Sodium Dodecyl Sulfate-Polyacrylamide Gel-Electrophoresis. Journal of Immunological Methods 126: 109–117.
92. Tsai CM, Frasch CE (1982) A sensitive silver stain for detecting lipopolysaccharides in polyacrylamide gels. Anal Biochem 119: 115–119.
93. Roos V, Schembri MA, Ulett GC, Klemm P (2006) Asymptomatic bacteriuria Escherichia coli strain 83972 carries mutations in the foc locus and is unable to express F1C fimbriae. Microbiology 152: 1799–1806.
94. Bachmann BJ (1972) Pedigrees of some mutant strains of Escherichia coli K-12. Bacteriol Rev 36: 525–557.
95. Casadaban MJ, Cohen SN (1980) Analysis of gene control signals by DNA fusion and cloning in Escherichia coli. J Mol Biol 138: 179–207.
96. Mobley HL, Green DM, Trifillis AL, Johnson DE, Chippendale GR, et al. (1990) Pyelonephritogenic Escherichia coli and killing of cultured human renal proximal tubular epithelial cells: role of hemolysin in some strains. Infect Immun 58: 1281–1289.
97. Svanborg Eden C, Gotschlich EC, Korhonen TK, Leffler H, Schoolnik G (1983) Aspects on structure and function of pili on uropathogenic Escherichia coli. Prog Allergy 33: 189–202.
98. Silver RP, Aaronson W, Sutton A, Schneerson R (1980) Comparative analysis of plasmids and some metabolic characteristics of Escherichia coli K1 from diseased and healthy individuals. Infect Immun 29: 200–206.

Increased Risk of Urinary Tract Cancer in ESRD Patients Associated with Usage of Chinese Herbal Products Suspected of Containing Aristolochic Acid

Shuo-Meng Wang[1,4], Ming-Nan Lai[2], Alan Wei[3], Ya-Yin Chen[1,2], Yeong-Shiau Pu[1], Pau-Chung Chen[4], Jung-Der Wang[5,6]*

1 Department of Urology, National Taiwan University Hospital, Taipei, Taiwan, **2** Department of Statistics, Feng Chia University, Taichung, Taiwan, **3** School of Medicine, Stony Brook University, Stony Brook, New York, United States of America, **4** Institute of Occupational Medicine and Industrial Hygiene, College of Public Health, National Taiwan University, Taipei, Taiwan, **5** Department of Public Health, National Cheng Kung University Medical College, Tainan City, Taiwan, **6** Departments of Internal Medicine and Occupational and Environmental Medicine, National Cheng Kung University Hospital, Tainan City, Taiwan

Abstract

Introduction: Both end-stage renal disease (ESRD) and urothelial cancer (UC) are associated with the consumption of Chinese herbal products containing aristolochic acid (AA) by the general population. The objective of this study was to determine the risk of UC associated with AA-related Chinese herbal products among ESRD patients.

Methods: We conducted a cohort study using the National Health Insurance reimbursement database to enroll all ESRD patients in Taiwan from 1998–2002. Cox regression models were constructed and hazard ratios and confidence intervals were estimated after controlling for potential confounders, including age, sex, residence in region with endemic black foot disease, urinary tract infection, and use of non-steroidal anti-inflammatory drugs and acetaminophen.

Results: A total of 38,995 ESRD patients were included in the final analysis, and 320 patients developed UC after ESRD. Having been prescribed Mu Tong that was adulterated with Guan Mu Tong (*Aristolochia manshuriensis*) before 2004, or an estimated consumption of more than 1–100 mg of aristolochic acid, were both associated with an increased risk of UC in the multivariable analyses. Analgesic consumption of more than 150 pills was also associated with an increased risk of UC, although there was little correlation between the two risk factors.

Conclusion: Consumption of aristolochic acid-related Chinese herbal products was associated with an increased risk of developing UC in ESRD patients. Regular follow-up screening for UC in ESRD patients who have consumed Chinese herbal products is thus necessary.

Editor: Francisco X. Real, Centro Nacional de Investigaciones Oncológicas (CNIO), Spain

Funding: This study was supported by the National Health Research Institutes of Taiwan (intramural project EO-100-EO-PP04), and a grant from the Headquarters of University Advancement at the National Cheng Kung University. The funders had no role in study design, data collection and analysis, decision to publish, or preparation of the manuscript.

Competing Interests: The authors have declared that no competing interests exist.

* Email: jdwang121@gmail.com

Introduction

Aristolochic acid nephropathy—a progressive form of renal interstitial fibrosis—was first reported in a group of young Belgian patients with end-stage renal disease in 1993, and was thought to be caused by the use of Chinese herbal medicines that contained aristolochic acid [1–3]. Aristolochic acid has been shown to be associated with urothelial cancer (UC) in many studies of clinical cases around the world, in animal models, and by the detection of aristolochic acid–DNA adducts in the kidney and ureteral tissues [4][5,6]. Prior studies observed increased risks of developing UC and ESRD in the general population in association with the consumption of Chinese herbal products [7][8], and patients with ESRD have a higher incidence of malignancies than the general population [9–12]. We have noticed an extraordinarily high incidence of UC in uremic or ESRD patients in the past decade in Taiwan [13–16], but the reason for this remains unknown. Some researchers suggest that chronic bladder irritation, a decreased urinary washout effect, atrophic involution of the bladder, compound analgesic abuse [17–19], use of Chinese herbs [4,5,20], groundwater intake (arsenic exposure) [21,22], and uremia per se [15,16] may play roles in the development of UC. A report published by the International Agency in Research on Cancer (IARC) [23] stated that the risk factors associated with UC include analgesics (phenacetin), herbal usage (aristolochic acid), heavy metals (arsenic) and tobacco smoking.

Although the IARC classifies aristolochic acid as a group 1 carcinogen, to the best of our knowledge there have been no cohort studies that examine the association between urinary tract cancer and the use of herbs or herbal products containing aristolochic acid in ESRD patients. In March of 1995, Taiwan established the National Health Insurance (NHI) program, which covers more than 99% of the population [24]. The NHI routinely reimburses enrollees for the cost of prescribed medicines, including Chinese herbal products containing aristolochic acid, which were widely prescribed before being banned in December 2003. We thus used the NHI reimbursement database to conduct an ESRD population-based cohort study to examine the association between having been prescribed Chinese herbal products that contain substantial amounts of aristolochic acid, including Guan Mu Tong and Guang Fangchi, and the risk of urinary tract cancer, as well as the possibility of a dose–response relationship between the two.

Materials and Methods

Study Population

Established in Taiwan in March 1995, the National Health Insurance program (NHI) covers over 99% of the population residents [24]. Standard mixtures of Chinese herbal products (CHP) are included in the regular schedule of reimbursement. The National Health Research Institutes (NHRI) transformed the NHI reimbursement data into files suitable for use by researchers, and which contain detailed information about the usage of conventional drugs and CHP [25]. This study was conducted using ESRD patient data obtained from the database of approximately more than 22 million people enrolled in the NHI. The data collection period began in 1996, but became more comprehensive after January 1997. As noted above, the NHRI anonymized and converted the reimbursement data into research-ready files, called the National Health Insurance Research Database (NHIRD) [25]. The identification numbers of all the individuals in the database were doubly encrypted to ensure their privacy.

The dataset to which we had access provided detailed demographic data (including birth date and sex) and information regarding the health-care services provided for each patient, including all payments for outpatient visits, hospitalizations, and prescriptions, as well as where each patient lived. The data for each hospitalization contained up to five diagnoses that were coded according to the International Classification of Diseases, Ninth Revision (ICD-9) [26], all drugs prescribed and the doses (i.e., conventional medicines, including generic and commercial brands of acetaminophen and non-steroidal anti-inflammatory drugs, as well as Chinese herbal products), and the date of each prescription. During the study period (i.e., from January 1, 1998, to December 31, 2002), all prescribed medications were covered under the NHI of Taiwan, and no drug could be dispensed at a pharmacy without a doctor's prescription.

To select potential case subjects for this study, we first obtained the NHI catastrophic illness registry files for all patients who were diagnosed with end-stage renal disease from January 1, 1998, to December 31, 2002. Because all patients who are registered as having a catastrophic illness are exempt from all copayments, their data is very comprehensive and has been carefully validated. A diagnosis of urinary tract cancer or end-stage renal disease made by doctors and officials of the NHI is usually accurate: urinary tract cancer must be proven by tissue pathology, and is classified as cancer of the upper urinary tract, which includes the renal pelvis and ureter (ICD-9 codes 189.1 and 189.2, respectively) or bladder cancer (ICD-9 code 188). The database contains 38,675 Non-UTC and 839 UTC prevalent cases of end-stage renal disease that were diagnosed from January 1, 1998, to December 31, 2002.Within this population, we identified 320 patients who were newly diagnosed with urinary tract cancer from January 1, 2001, to December 31, 2002, to allow at least four years between January 1, 1997, and the date of diagnosis to give sufficient time for the case subjects to accumulate sufficient doses of herbal products to induce UTC.

Exposure Assessment

The reimbursement database contained all the details of the prescribed conventional medicines, which included acetaminophen and the commercial names of 45 kinds of non-steroidal anti-inflammatory drugs (NSAIDs), shown in the File S1.

As phenacetin has been totally banned by the Department of Health since 1986, it was not included. Doses of each drug were determined according to the number of pills prescribed and cumulative doses were calculated before ESRD. The use of 600–1000 pills of acetaminophen, NSAIDs, or mixed analgesics has been associated with an increased risk of renal damage or renal cancer in previous studies [27,28]. We thus accumulated the total number of analgesics pills for each subject before dialysis during 1998–2002.

According to the standard prescription recommended by the Committee on Chinese Medicine and Pharmacy (CCMP) in Taiwan, the following Chinese herbal products may contain AA: Xi-Xin (Asarum heterotoppoides), Guan-Mu-Tong (Aristolochia manshuriensis), and Guang-Fangchi (A. fangchi). However, Guan-Mu-Tong and Guang-Fangchi were once offered under the names Mu-Tong (Akebia sp.) and Fangchi (Stephania sp.), respectively, in Taiwan before 2003, because of similarities of gross morphology and common practices [29]. In addition, according to an investigation by the Bureau of Food and Drug Analysis in Taiwan, as well as some studies, approximately 89.2–100% of Fangchi preparations were actually Guang-Fangchi [30–32] and 84% of Mu-Tong were actually Guan-Mu-Tong [33]. These three herbs were prescribed as single products or included as components of some mixed CHP. Each pharmaceutical company has published and submitted the detailed composition of every product it produces, and data on this can be retrieved from the website of the Committee on Chinese Medicine and Pharmacy of the Department of Health [29]. With this information, the original amounts of herbs, in grams, could be determined for each mixture of CHP, and the cumulative dose for each herb prescribed to an individual before developing ESRD could thus be calculated. We also calculated the estimated cumulative dose of aristolochic acid for each subject by using the following estimates obtained in previous studies: the estimated average doses of aristolochic acid per 1 g of Guan Mu Tong, Guang Fangchi, and Xi Xin are 2.59 mg, 2.04 mg, and 0.042 mg, respectively [30,32–35].

The reimbursement database also has data on where all the subjects lived. We identified subjects who lived in the four townships in Taiwan that have been reported to be areas endemic for black foot disease—Pu-Tai and Yi-Chu in Chiayi County, and Hsueh-Chia and Pei-Men in Tainan County [36,37]. Black foot disease is a peripheral vascular disease that has been endemic to the coastal region of Taiwan for the past 60 years, and is associated with drinking water from artesian wells containing arsenic, and has been documented to be associated with an increased incidence of bladder cancer [36,37]. We controlled for this factor (townships) as a surrogate for arsenic exposure.

According to the Committee on Chinese Medicine and Pharmacy [29], Mu Tong is usually prescribed for the treatment of hepatitis, urinary tract infection, rhinitis, dysmenorrhea, and eczema. Recurrent or chronic urinary tract infection, associated with Schistosomiasis or prolonged indwelling catheters in patients with spinal cord injury, is associated with an increase risk of bladder cancer [38,39], whereas urinary tract infection from other causes does not show any consistent association with bladder cancer risk [38,40]. We thus defined patients with chronic urinary tract infection (UTI) as those who had such a diagnosis at least 12 times up to one year before the diagnosis of UC, and we controlled for the above potential confounders during the risk-estimate analysis. The patients with diabetes or hypertension were also ascertained based on the related diagnosis numbers in ICD-9 before ESRD diagnosis.

Statistical Analyses

To assess the independent association of various risk factors with new occurrences of UC, univariate and multivariable Cox regression models were used to analyze the population of ESRD patients and those cases that developed UC subsequent to ESRD diagnosis. Potential risk factors, including age, sex, hypertension, diabetes mellitus, chronic UTI, and prescriptions of NSAIDs, acetaminophen or any of the aforementioned Chinese herbs suspected to contain AA, were assessed for independent association with new occurrences of UC. We constructed models for two different types of exposure assessment: prescribed dosages of Chinese herbs (model 1) and different estimated dosages of AA as risk factors (model 2). The dose–response association between cumulative dose of Chinese herbs, analgesics and occurrence of UC was tested by the Mantel–Haenszel extension for the trend. For each potential risk factor, multivariate Cox proportional hazards models were constructed to estimate the relative risk and its 95% confidence interval (CI) for UC incidence. An estimate with the 95% CI that did not contain the number 1 was considered statistically significant. We also ran a correlation analysis between the total numbers of analgesics pills and cumulative doses (in mg) of AA. All the above analyses were conducted using the SAS ver. 9.2 software package (SAS Institute, Cary, NC, USA).

Results

After excluding people with incomplete data or aged over 100 years, a total of 39,514 prevalent cases of end-stage renal disease were included in the data, with 839 of these developing UTC between January 1, 1998 and December 31, 2002. Among these patients, there were 38,675 cases without UTC and 320 UTC cases who were newly diagnosed with urinary tract cancer between January 1, 2001 and December 31, 2002. A total of 38,995 ESRD patients were thus included in the final analysis, with 18,522 (47.5%) men and 20,473 (52.5%) women. There were high prevalence rates of hypertension (88.5%) and diabetes mellitus (55.7%). The average crude incidence rate of UTC for these ESRD patients was 1,368 per million person-years.

Table 1 summarizes the frequency data of the ESRD patient population with respect to different potential risk factors, including sex, age, follow-up time after ESRD diagnosis, residence in township with endemic black foot disease, hypertension, diabetes, chronic UTI, and analgesics (NSAID and acetaminophen) consumption. The patient population was also characterized in terms of Chinese herb consumption for individual herbs (Mu-Tong, Fangchi, and Xi-Xin), as well as total estimated consumption of AA calculated based on total consumption of Chinese herbs containing this substance. The incidence rate of UTC appears to increase with the time after diagnosis of ESRD (Table 1).

Because only one UTC patient and 254 non-UTC controls had lived in area with endemic black foot disease (Table 1), we decided to exclude subjects with this characteristic in the final analysis for both cases and controls.

The number of new UTC cases and adjusted hazard ratios (aHR) calculated from the Cox regression models for multiple risk factors (sex, age, diabetes, hypertension, chronic UTI, analgesics and cumulative doses for different herbs) are summarized in Table 2. The crude and adjusted HR (aHR) for development of UTC increased significantly for older patients, whereas the crude and adjusted HR for development of UTC was not significantly related to either hypertension or diabetes. Crude HR's also increased for prescribed cumulative doses of Mu-Tong greater than 1 g, Fangchi 1–30 g, >100 g, as well as for prescribed Xi-Xin and for estimated AA consumptions of 1–100 mg, 101–200 g, and >300 mg. Prescription of analgesics also increased the crude HR. After control of potential confounding by other risk factors, we found that the aHR for development of UTC increased for ESRD patients prescribed Mu Tong, and that the various estimated consumptions of AA were each associated with an increased risk of UTC in the multivariable analyses (Mu Tong: at 1–30 g, aHR = 1.8, 95% CI = 1.3 to 2.6, and each 30 g increase, aHR = 1.3, 95% CI = 1.2 to 1.5; AA: at 1–100 mg, aHR = 2.1, 95% CI = 1.6 to 2.6, and each 100 mg increase, aHR = 1.6, 95% CI = 1.4 to 1.8). Prescription of analgesics is associated with a greater risk of urothelial cancer, with an increased aHR of 1.3 (95% CI = 1.2 to 1.4) for each increment of 150 pills, as summarized in models 1 and 2 of Table 2. However, there is little association between the prescribed numbers of analgesic pills and cumulative doses of AA, as shown in Figure 1.

Discussion

To the best of our knowledge, this is the first population-based study to document a linear dose–response relationship between prescription of Chinese herbal products containing AA and the risk of UTC in ESRD patients after controlling for confounding by age, sex, living in a township endemic for black foot disease (a surrogate of arsenic contamination in the water supply), analgesic consumption, and history of chronic urinary tract infection. In fact, because the NHI reimbursement database collects all prescription information prospectively, we can rule out the possibility of recall bias for the intake doses of various Chinese herbal products. Since we included all ESRD patients newly diagnosed in Taiwan from 1998 to 2002, and the diagnosis of urinary tract cancer or end-stage renal disease made by doctors and officials of the NHI is usually accurate, we can also rule out the possibility of selection bias. Moreover, we excluded all subjects who had lived in townships endemic for black foot disease (a surrogate of high arsenic exposure) to prevent confounding the results due to the carcinogenic effects of arsenic exposure. Although increased prescription of analgesics was also associated with UTC (Table 2), the effect has been controlled in the multivariable regression model, and Figure 1 also shows no association between the number of analgesics pills and cumulative dose of AA. Finally, this study has documented a dose-dependent association between the cumulative estimated prescribed dose of AA and urinary tract cancer, as well as a dose-dependent association between the cumulative prescribed dose of Mu-Tong and UTC. We thus tentatively conclude that the urothelial cancers developed by ESRD patients are associated with prescription of AA-associated Chinese herbal products.

This study found a consistent dose-response relationship between the estimated intake of AA (or prescribed dose of AA-containing CHP) and urinary tract cancer in ESRD patients, suggesting that AA may be responsible for increased cancer risk of these patients. Fangchi and Xi-Xin both showed increased hazard ratios at higher doses, but these results did not reach statistical significance after adjustment for risk factors, likely due to the small number of case subjects. However, the increased hazard ratios for the occurrence of UC were found to be significantly higher in

Table 1. Frequency distributions of various risk factors for the occurrence of urinary tract cancers (UTC) stratified by different inclusion criteria in 38,995 patients with end-stage renal disease (ESRD).

	All ESRD Patients	
Risk Factors	**UTC Cases (n = 320)**	**Non-UTC Cases (n = 38675)**
Sex		
Men	131 (40.94%)	18391 (47.55%)
Women	189 (59.06%)	20284 (52.45%)
Age (year)		
<50	67 (20.94%)	9804 (25.35%)
50–59	80 (25.00%)	7790 (20.14%)
60–69	99 (30.94%)	10572 (27.34%)
70–99	74 (23.13%)	10509 (27.17%)
Residence in township where black foot disease was endemic		
No	319 (99.69%)	38421 (99.34%)
Yes	1 (0.31%)	254 (0.66%)
Hypertension		
No	68 (21.25%)	4297 (11.11%)
Yes	252 (78.75%)	34378 (88.89%)
Diabetes		
No	219 (68.44%)	17045 (44.07%)
Yes	101 (31.56%)	21630 (55.93%)
Chronic UTI		
No	312 (97.50%)	38511 (99.58%)
Yes	8 (2.50%)	164 (0.42%)
Analgesics *(pills) NSAID & acetaminophen		
0–150	123 (38.44%)	16116 (41.65%)
151–300	74 (23.13%)	8187 (21.16%)
351–450	32 (10.00%)	4405 (11.40%)
451–600	25 (7.81%)	2665 (6.90%)
>600	66 (20.63%)	7306 (18.88%)
Mu-Tong (g) total amount prescribed		
0	286 (89.38%)	35968 (93.00%)
1–30	20 (6.25%)	1845 (4.77%)
30–60	3 (0.94%)	348 (0.90%)
61–100	3 (0.94%)	179 (0.46%)
101–200	4 (1.25%)	164 (0.42%)
>200	4 (1.25%)	171 (0.44%)
Fangchi (g) total amount prescribed		
0	295 (92.19%)	35731 (92.39%)
1–30	19 (5.94%)	2417 (6.25%)
31–60 (31–100)	4 (1.25%)	271 (0.70%)
61–100	0 (0%)	121 (0.31%)
101–200 (>100)	2 (0.63%)	86 (0.22%)
>200	0 (0%)	49 (0.13%)
Xi-Xin (g) total amount prescribed		
0	283 (88.44%)	34679 (89.67%)
1–30	22 (6.88%)	2995 (7.74%)
31–60	5 (1.56%)	465 (1.20%)
61–100	5 (1.56%)	231 (0.60%)
101–200	3 (0.94%)	185 (0.48%)
>200	2 (0.63%)	120 (0.32%)
Aristolochic acid (mg) estimated total consumption		

Table 1. Cont.

	All ESRD Patients	
Risk Factors	**UTC Cases (n = 320)**	**Non-UTC Cases (n = 38675)**
0	270 (84.38%)	32550 (84.16%)
1–100	33 (10.31%)	5363 (13.09%)
101–200	4 (1.25%)	464 (1.20%)
201–300	4 (1.25%)	197 (0.51%)
>300	9 (2.81%)	.04%)

Analgesics *, sum of acetaminophen and non-steroidal anti-inflammatory drugs (NSAIDs).

ESRD patients when over 1–30 g of Mu-Tong or over 1–100 mg cumulative AA were prescribed. Because these doses are much smaller than those reported by Belgian scholars [4] and our previous report [7], it suggests that patients with ESRD might be more vulnerable to the carcinogenic effects of AA. Although these subgroups do not correlate with a cumulative dose of higher than 147-mg AA, as reported in the Belgian report [4], the observation of increased hazard ratios at lower cumulative levels of AA-containing Chinese herbal products in ESRD patients who consume these products suggests potential pathogenic effects at lower doses, and this is an issue that deserves further investigation, with more long-term follow-up of these patients.

Forty-five percent of the UTC cases in this study were upper urinary tract cancer, which is similar to the rates seen in the general population, as reported by the National Cancer Registry and in a previous clinical report examining pathology-confirmed urinary tract cancer cases in Taiwan [41]. However, these rates are much higher than those in other countries, in which less than 10% of all UTC cases are upper urinary tract cancer. In this study, prescription of Chinese herbal products was associated with urothelial cancers that occurred in all parts of the urinary tract, similar to what was reported in a recent case study of Belgian women who received kidney transplants for end-stage AA nephropathy, in which 44.7% had upper urinary tract cancer and 39.5% had bladder cancer [42]. We thus hypothesize that AA induces urothelial cancers in the upper urinary tract and bladder with approximately equal tendency.

We also found a dose-dependent association between analgesics and occurrence of UTC among patients with ESRD, corroborating previous reports [17–19]. Unfortunately, we did not have a sufficiently large sample size to further explore this issue. Future studies are thus recommended to collect more UTC cases among patients with ESRD, and determine if the effect is associated with acetaminophen, aspirin, or any other NSAID.

There are some limitations to this study, as follows. First, because patient identities were not obtainable from the NHI reimbursement database, histopathology reports were unavailable to confirm the diagnoses. However, accurate diagnosis of UTC in the NHI database is based on pathology and/or cytology evidence and made after serious consideration with histopathologic proof in 95% of bladder cancers and 91%–92% of upper urinary tract cancers [43]. Second, we were unable to contact patients directly about their use of herbs due to anonymization of the database; therefore, we were unable to rule out the possibility that subjects may have taken additional nephrotoxic herbs or agents that were not prescribed. However, the comprehensive coverage and copayment for prescriptions is universally 50 NT$ (approximately equal to US $1.5), which is generally less than the cost of herbs

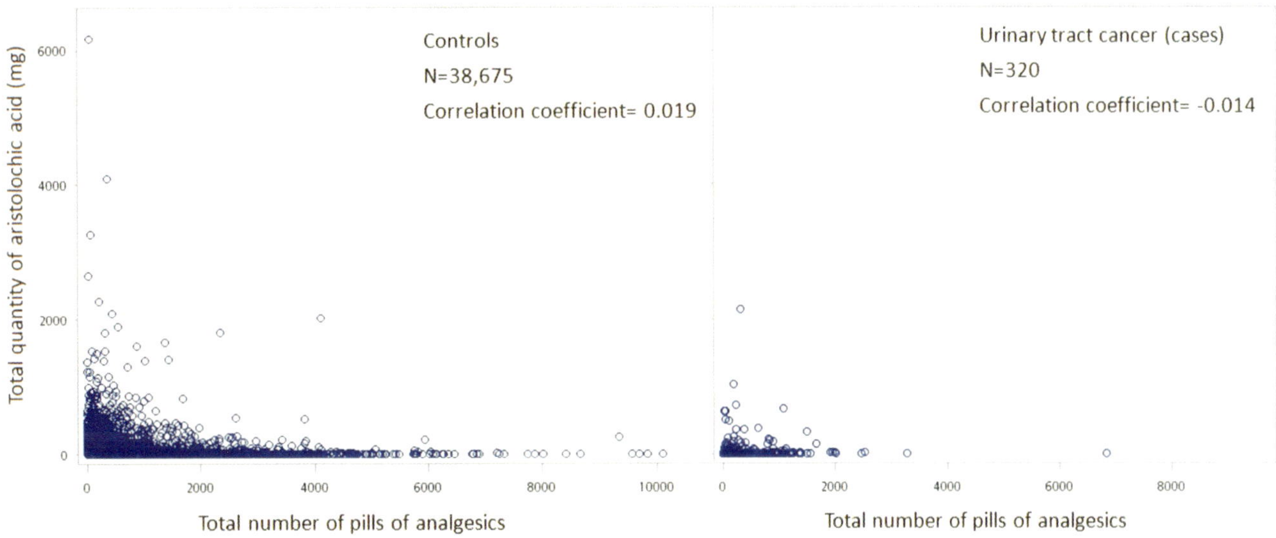

Figure 1. Correlation analysis between prescription of analgesics (number of pills) and cumulative dose of aristolochic acid for both cases and controls.

Table 2. Crude and adjusted hazards ratios (HR), and 95% confidence intervals (CI) estimated from multivariate Cox regression models for urinary tract cancer developed in patients with ESRD.

		Model 1	Model 2
Risk Factors	**Crude HR (95% CI)**	**Adjusted HR (95% CI)†**	**Adjusted HR (95% CI)†**
Sex			
Men	1	1	1
Women	1.02 (0.82 to 1.27)	0.89 (0.71 to 1.12)	0.91 (0.73 to 1.14)
Age (years)			
<50	1	1	1
50–59	1.38 (1.04 to 1.85)*	1.43 (1.06 to 1.93)*	1.44 (1.07 to 1.92)*
60–69	1.77 (1.34 to 2.35)**	1.75 (1.30 to 2.36)**	1.73 (1.29 to 2.32)**
70–99	1.93 (1.39 to 2.66)**	1.90 (1.35 to 2.67)**	1.83 (1.31 to 2.56)**
Diabetes			
No	1	1	1
Yes	1.12 (0.90 to 1.40)	0.95 (0.76 to 1.20)	0.94 (0.75 to 1.19)
Hypertension			
No	1	1	1
Yes	1.00 (0.78 to 1.29)	0.74 (0.57 to 0.97)*	0.78 (0.60 to 1.01)
Chronic UTI			
No	1	1	1
Yes	4.77 (2.46 to 9.26)**	6.85 (3.52 to 13.34)**	6.68 (3.43 to 12.99)**
Analgesics (pills)			
0–150	1	1	1
151–300	2.03 (1.54 to 2.67)**	1.91 (1.44 to 2.53)**	1.93 (1.46 to 2.55)**
301–450	2.26 (1.55 to 3.28)**	1.97 (1.35 to 2.89)**	2.02 (1.39 to 2.95)**
451–600	2.92 (1.93 to 4.43)**	2.70 (1.75 to 4.15)**	2.72 (1.78 to 4.16)**
>600	3.36 (2.51 to 4.49)**	2.98 (2.19 to 4.06)**	2.83 (2.09 to 3.83)**
Each 150 pills increase	1.35 (1.26 to 1.44)**	1.32 (1.23 to 1.41)**	1.31 (1.22 to 1.40)**
Mu-Tong (g) total amount prescribed			
0	1	1	-
1–30	2.38 (1.79 to 3.16)**	1.83 (1.30 to 2.57)**	-
31–60	2.21 (1.29 to 3.82)‡	1.98 (1.07 to 3.69)*	-
61–100	3.08 (1.58 to 6.02)**	2.51 (1.19 to 5.28)*	-
101–200	2.73 (1.61 to 4.63)**	3.16 (1.63 to 6.14)**	-
>200	3.45 (1.88 to 6.36)**	3.46 (1.70 to 7.03)**	-
Each 30 g increase	1.33 (1.23 to 1.44)**	1.31 (1.17 to 1.48)**	-
Fangchi (g) total amount prescribed			
0	1	1	-
1–30	2.24 (1.73 to 2.92)**	1.23 (0.91 to 1.67)	-
31–100	1.41 (0.75 to 2.66)	0.84 (0.43 to 1.62)	-
>100	3.18 (1.31 to 7.70)*	1.89 (0.76 to 4.68)	-
Each 30 g increase	1.56 (1.33 to 1.84)**	1.22 (1.00 to 1.48)	
Xi-Xin (g) total amount prescribed			
0	1	1	-
1–30	2.02 (1.55 to 2.63)**	1.27 (0.91 to 1.78)	-
31–60	2.40 (1.44 to 3.99)**	1.50 (0.84 to 2.70)	-
61–100	2.90 (1.62 to 5.20)**	1.34 (0.69 to 2.60)	-
101–200	2.47 (1.26 to 4.83)‡	1.17 (0.53 to 2.59)	-
>200	2.25 (1.15 to 4.21)*	0.78 (0.34 to 1.81)	-
Each 30 g increase	1.28 (1.18 to 1.39)**	1.02 (0.89 to 1.16)	
Aristolochic acid (mg) estimated total consumption			
0	1	-	1

Table 2. Cont.

		Model 1	Model 2
Risk Factors	**Crude HR (95% CI)**	**Adjusted HR (95% CI)†**	**Adjusted HR (95% CI)†**
1–100	1.21 (0.83 to 1.78)	-	2.05 (1.61 to 2.60)**
101–200	2.16 (0.80 to 5.80)	-	2.84 (1.66 to 4.86)**
201–300	4.80 (1.79 to 12.91)‡	-	2.42 (0.89 to 6.55)
>300	6.29 (3.23 to 12.26)**	-	5.18 (2.86 to 9.40)**
Each 100 mg increase	1.56 (1.40 to 1.74)**	-	1.57 (1.40 to 1.75)**

†Logistic regression models for different dosages of Chinese herbs (model 1) and different estimated dosages of aristolochic acid as risk factors (model 2) were adjusted for age, sex, residence in township with endemic black foot disease, and history of chronic UTI.
*$P<0.05$.
‡$P<0.01$.
**$P<0.001$.

sold in Taiwan's markets. It is thus unlikely that the subjects purchased AA-containing herbs or nephrotoxic drugs without a prescription. Third, we also could not validate the actual intake of prescribed herbal product by the patients. Because 95% of the dosing frequenciesfor Chinese herbal products last for only one week [44], a large cumulative dose indicates that patients on long-term prescriptions actually consumed the prescribed medication. However, if the patients did not take all of the prescribed medication, our findings would underestimate the effects of AA-related Chinese herbal consumption. Fourth, because the NHI data did not include smoking history, we could not control for this variable in our models. However, because smoking rates in Taiwan in the last two decades have ranged from 47% to 62% and from 2.3% to 5.3%, for males and females, respectively, male patients with ESRD would be expected to have a higher risk of developing UTC if smoking were a major contributing risk factor [45]. As we did not find any increased risk of UTC in males compared to females, our results do not seem to be confounded by smoking.

Conclusions

This study finds that AA from Chinese herbal products and analgesics is associated with increased risk of developing UTC in ESRD patients, due to these having been prescribed low doses of Mu-Tong. The linear dose-response relationships found in this work may be useful in consideration of a total ban or establishment of limits on the consumption of such herbal products among patients with ESRD and/or chronic kidney disease. More studies are needed to examine the potential carcinogenic effects of analgesics on patients with ESRD and/or chronic renal failure. In addition, regular follow-up screening for UC in ESRD patients who have consumed AA-related Chinese herbal products is also necessary.

Author Contributions

Conceived and designed the experiments: SMW JD. Performed the experiments: JDW PC. Analyzed the data: SMW. Contributed reagents/materials/analysis tools: PCC. Wrote the paper: SMW. Contributed to the idea and design in this work: MNL AW YYC YSP.

References

1. Vanherweghem JL, Depierreux M, Tielemans C, Abramowicz D, Dratwa M, et al. (1993) Rapidly progressive interstitial renal fibrosis in young women: association with slimming regimen including Chinese herbs. Lancet 341: 387–391.
2. Vanhaelen M, Vanhaelen-Fastre R, But P, Vanherweghem JL (1994) Identification of aristolochic acid in Chinese herbs. Lancet 343: 174.
3. Cosyns JP (2003) Aristolochic acid and 'Chinese herbs nephropathy': a review of the evidence to date. Drug safety : an international journal of medical toxicology and drug experience 26: 33–48.
4. Nortier JL, Martinez MC, Schmeiser HH, Arlt VM, Bieler CA, et al. (2000) Urothelial carcinoma associated with the use of a Chinese herb (Aristolochia fangchi). N Engl J Med 342: 1686–1692.
5. Cosyns JP, Jadoul M, Squifflet JP, Wese FX, van Ypersele de Strihou C (1999) Urothelial lesions in Chinese-herb nephropathy. American journal of kidney diseases : the official journal of the National Kidney Foundation 33: 1011–1017.
6. Arlt VM, Stiborova M, Schmeiser HH (2002) Aristolochic acid as a probable human cancer hazard in herbal remedies: a review. Mutagenesis 17: 265–277.
7. Lai MN, Wang SM, Chen PC, Chen YY, Wang JD (2010) Population-based case-control study of Chinese herbal products containing aristolochic acid and urinary tract cancer risk. J Natl Cancer Inst 102: 179–186.
8. Lai MN, Wang SM, Chen PC, Chen YY, Wang JD (2009) Population-based case-control study of Chinese herbal products containing aristolochic acid and urinary tract cancer risk. J Natl Cancer Inst 102: 179–186.
9. Matas AJ, Simmons RL, Kjellstrand CM, Buselmeier TJ, Najarian JS (1975) Increased incidence of malignancy during chronic renal failure. Lancet 1: 883–886.
10. Port FK, Ragheb NE, Schwartz AG, Hawthorne VM (1989) Neoplasms in dialysis patients: a population-based study. American journal of kidney diseases : the official journal of the National Kidney Foundation 14: 119–123.
11. Kjellstrand CM (1979) Are malignancies increased in uremia? Nephron 23: 159–161.
12. Maisonneuve P, Agodoa L, Gellert R, Stewart JH, Buccianti G, et al. (1999) Cancer in patients on dialysis for end-stage renal disease: an international collaborative study. Lancet 354: 93–99.
13. Chuang CH, Lee CT, Tsai TL, Chen JB, Hsu KT, et al. (2002) Urological malignancy in chronic dialysis patients. Acta Nephrologica 16: 19–24.
14. Chang CH, Yang CM, Yang AH (2007) Renal diagnosis of chronic hemodialysis patients with urinary tract transitional cell carcinoma in Taiwan. Cancer 109: 1487–1492.
15. Ou JH, Pan CC, Lin JS, Tzai TS, Yang WH, et al. (2000) Transitional cell carcinoma in dialysis patients. European urology 37: 90–94.
16. Chen KS, Lai MK, Huang CC, Chu SH, Leu ML (1995) Urologic cancers in uremic patients. American journal of kidney diseases : the official journal of the National Kidney Foundation 25: 694–700.
17. Gonwa TA, Corbett WT, Schey HM, Buckalew VM, Jr. (1980) Analgesic-associated nephropathy and transitional cell carcinoma of the urinary tract. Annals of internal medicine 93: 249–252.

18. Swindle P, Falk M, Rigby R, Petrie J, Hawley C, et al. (1998) Transitional cell carcinoma in renal transplant recipients: the influence of compound analgesics. British journal of urology 81: 229–233.
19. Kliem V, Thon W, Krautzig S, Kolditz M, Behrend M, et al. (1996) High mortality from urothelial carcinoma despite regular tumor screening in patients with analgesic nephropathy after renal transplantation. Transplant international : official journal of the European Society for Organ Transplantation 9: 231–235.
20. Vanherweghem LJ (1998) Misuse of herbal remedies: the case of an outbreak of terminal renal failure in Belgium (Chinese herbs nephropathy). Journal of alternative and complementary medicine 4: 9–13.
21. Chiang HS, Guo HR, Hong CL, Lin SM, Lee EF (1993) The incidence of bladder cancer in the black foot disease endemic area in Taiwan. British journal of urology 71: 274–278.
22. Chiou HY, Chiou ST, Hsu YH, Chou YL, Tseng CH, et al. (2001) Incidence of transitional cell carcinoma and arsenic in drinking water: a follow-up study of 8,102 residents in an arseniasis-endemic area in northeastern Taiwan. American journal of epidemiology 153: 411–418.
23. Wiessler M (1994) DNA adducts of pyrrolizidine alkaloids, nitroimidazoles and aristolochic acid. IARC Sci Publ: 165–177.
24. TaiwanYearbook2009 Public Health: Health Insurance.
25. NHRI-Taiwan (2003) National Health Research Database.
26. Centers_for_Disease_Control_and_Prevention (2009) International Classification of Diseases, Ninth Revision (ICD-9). Atlanta, Georgia.
27. Perneger TV, Whelton PK, Klag MJ (1994) Risk of kidney failure associated with the use of acetaminophen, aspirin, and nonsteroidal antiinflammatory drugs. N Engl J Med 331: 1675–1679.
28. Gago-Dominguez M, Yuan JM, Castelao JE, Ross RK, Yu MC (1999) Regular use of analgesics is a risk factor for renal cell carcinoma. Br J Cancer 81: 542–548.
29. Committee Chinese Medicine and Pharmacy DOH-T (2002) Unified Formulas.
30. Hsu Y, Tseng H, Wen K (1997) Determination of aristolochic acid in Fangchi radix. Ann Rept NLFD Taiwan ROC: 136–142 (In Chinese).
31. Tung C, Ho Y, Tsai H, Chong Y (1999) Studies on the commonly musused and adulterated Chinese crude drug species in Taiwan. Chin Med Coll J: 35–46.
32. Deng J (2002) Quality evaluation of Fang-Ji and analysis of marker constituents [dissertation]. Taiwan: Institute of Chiense Pharmaceutical Sciences, China Medical University: 75–77.
33. Chuang M, Hsu Y, Chang H, Lin J, Liao C (2002) Studies on adulteration and misusage of marketed Akebiae caulisn. Ann Rept NLFD Taiwan ROC: 104–119 (In Chinese).
34. Jong TT, Lee MR, Hsiao SS, Hsai JL, Wu TS, et al. (2003) Analysis of aristolochic acid in nine sources of Xixin, a traditional Chinese medicine, by liquid chromatography/atmospheric pressure chemical ionization/tandem mass spectrometry. J Pharm Biomed Anal 33: 831–837.
35. Hsu Y, Lo C, Chang H, Lin J (2003) Studies on adulteration and misusage of Asari radi in the market. Ann Rept NLFD Taiwan ROC: 153–167 (In Chinese).
36. Chen CJ, Chuang YC, Lin TM, Wu HY (1985) Malignant neoplasms among residents of a blackfoot disease-endemic area in Taiwan: high-arsenic artesian well water and cancers. Cancer research 45: 5895–5899.
37. Chen CJ, Chuang YC, You SL, Lin TM, Wu HY (1986) A retrospective study on malignant neoplasms of bladder, lung and liver in blackfoot disease endemic area in Taiwan. British journal of cancer 53: 399–405.
38. Johansson SL, Cohen SM (1997) Epidemiology and etiology of bladder cancer. Seminars in surgical oncology 13: 291–298.
39. Groah SL, Weitzenkamp DA, Lammertse DP, Whiteneck GG, Lezotte DC, et al. (2002) Excess risk of bladder cancer in spinal cord injury: Evidence for an association between indwelling catheter use and bladder cancer. Archives of Physical Medicine and Rehabilitation 83: 346–351.
40. Jiang X, Castelao JE, Groshen S, Cortessis VK, Shibata D, et al. (2009) Urinary tract infections and reduced risk of bladder cancer in Los Angeles. British journal of cancer 100: 834–839.
41. (2008) Cancer Incidence Rate in Taiwan, 1998–2002 & 2003–2007 http://tcr.cph.ntu.edu.tw/main.php?Page = N2: Taiwan cancer registry.
42. Achenbach H, Fischer A (1997) 6-O-beta-D-glucoside of aristolochic acid IIIa and other components from the roots of Aristolochia baetica. Planta Med 63: 579.
43. TaiwanCancerRegistry (2009) Cancer incidence rate in Taiwan, 1998–2002.
44. Hsieh SC, Lai JN, Lee CF, Hu FC, Tseng WL, et al. (2008) The prescribing of Chinese herbal products in Taiwan: a cross-sectional analysis of the national health insurance reimbursement database. Pharmacoepidemiology and drug safety 17: 609–619.
45. (2013) Adult Smoking Behavior Surveillance System,ASBS. Taipei, Taiwan.

A Novel Role for D-Alanylation of Lipoteichoic Acid of *Enterococcus faecalis* in Urinary Tract Infection

Dominique Wobser[1], Liaqat Ali[1,2], Elisabeth Grohmann[1,2], Johannes Huebner[1,3], Türkan Sakinc[1]*

1 Division of Infectious Diseases, Department of Internal Medicine II, University Hospital Freiburg, Freiburg, Germany, 2 Faculty of Biology, Albert Ludwigs University of Freiburg, Freiburg, Germany, 3 Division of Pediatric Infectious Diseases, Dr. Von Hauner Children's Hospital, Ludwig Maximilian University Munich, Munich, Germany

Abstract

Background: Enterococci are the third most common cause of healthcare-associated infections, which include urinary tract infections, bacteremia and endocarditis. Cell-surface structures such as lipoteichoic acid (LTA) have been poorly examined in *E. faecalis*, especially with respect to urinary tract infections (UTIs). The *dlt* operon is responsible for the D-alanylation of LTA and includes the gene *dlt*A, which encodes the D-alanyl carrier protein ligase (Dcl). The involvement of LTA in UTI infection by *E. faecalis* has not been studied so far. Here, we examined the role of teichoic acid alanylation in the adhesion of enterococci to uroepithelial cells.

Results: In a mouse model of urinary tract infection, we showed that *E. faecalis* 12030Δ*dlt*A mutant colonizes uroepithelial surfaces more efficiently than wild type bacteria. We also demonstrated that this mutant adhered four fold better to human bladder carcinoma cell line T24 compared to the wild type strain. Bacterial adherence could be significantly inhibited by purified lipoteichoic acid (LTA) and inhibition was specific.

Conclusion: In contrast to bacteraemia model and adherence to colon surfaces, *E. faecalis* 12030Δ*dlt*A mutant colonized uroepithelial surfaces more efficiently than wild-type bacteria. In the case of the uroepithelial surface the adherence to specific host cells could be prevented by purified LTA. Our results therefore suggest a novel function of alanylation of LTA in *E. faecalis*.

Editor: José A Lemos, University of Rochester Medical Center, United States of America

Funding: This work was supported by grants from the German Ministry of Science and Education (BMBF:UroGenOmics0315833C). The funders had no role in study design, data collection and analysis, decision to publish, or preparation of the manuscript.

Competing Interests: The authors have declared that no competing interests exist.

* Email: tuerkan.sakinc@uniklinik-freiburg.de

Introduction

Enterococci are the third most common cause of healthcare-associated infections, which include urinary tract infections, bacteremia and endocarditis. Risk groups for invasive enterococcal infections include neonates, Intensive Care Unit (ICU) patients and immunocompromised hosts [1]. The increasing identification of enterococcal strains resistant to multiple antibiotics in recent decades represents a serious threat to therapy and emphasizes the need for a better understanding of the pathogenicity of these microbes.

Bacterial adherence is an important step in the disease process by facilitating colonization and translocation across the mucosal barrier, which eventually results in systemic dissemination within the host [2]. Like other Gram-positive bacteria (e.g., *Staphylococcus aureus*), the surface of *E. faecalis* is rich in exposed adhesins that mediate binding to human receptors or to various components of the extracellular matrix (ECM); they are thus considered a member of MSCRAMM-microbial surface component–recognizing adhesive matrix molecules [3]. Basically, MSCRAMMs are cell wall–anchored surface proteins that have characteristic immunoglobulin-like folds [4].

Attachment of microorganisms to mucosal surfaces of the urinary tract is important for the pathogenesis of UTI, because the mechanical removal of colonizing bacteria by the urine flow is an important innate defense mechanism. In the process of bacterial cell adherence, infectious agents interfere with specific molecules on epithelial cells [5–6]. Furthermore, it has been shown that the tendency of certain bacteria to infect specific tissues is often related to their ability to adhere to a specific target cell.

While UTI-specific virulence factors of *E. coli* have been studied extensively, relatively little is known about *E. faecalis* cell-surface structures with respect to UTIs [7–10 & 11]. In a model of ascending UTI, the presence of an enterococcal surface protein encoded by an acquired gene was shown to increase the persistence of bacteria in the urinary bladders of mice [7] whereas [9] demonstrated that *E. faecalis* has greater tropism for the kidneys. Using a similar model, the MSCRAMM adhesion of collagen of *E. faecalis* (Ace) was recently identified as a putative virulence factor involved in colonization of renal tissue [12–13]. In another study, Torelli *et al.* reported that a PavA-like fibronectin-binding protein in *E. faecalis* called enterococcal fibronectin-binding protein A (EfbA) contributes to the pathogenesis of enterococcal UTIs. The EfbA mutant shows attenuated colonization in a mouse model of mounting UTI [11]. Ebp, a biofilm-associated pilus, produces immunogenic and pleomorphic pili [14] and also plays a role in UTI pathogenesis [15].

Generally, the functions of most *E. faecalis* cell surface structures have been poorly investigated, especially with respect to UTIs [7–10,16]. The enterococcal cell wall contains peptidoglycan (PG) and a number of accessory cell-wall polysaccharides and glycoconjugates such as LTA wall teichoic acid (WTA), a rhamnose-containing cell-wall polysaccharide *epa* (enterococcal polysaccharide antigen) [17–20] and a diheteroglycan [21]. Lipoteichoic acid (LTA) is an amphiphilic polymer consisting of polyglycerolphosphate and a glycolipid anchor inserted into the cell membrane [22–23]. The *dlt* operon includes four genes and is responsible for the D-alanylation of LTA [24]. One of these genes, *dlt*A, encodes the D-alanyl carrier protein ligase (Dcl), which activates the D-alanine and ligates it to the D-alanyl carrier protein (Dcp). The involvement of LTA in UTI infection by *E. faecalis* has not been studied. Here we examined the role of teichoic acid alanylation in the adhesion of enterococci to uroepithelial cells.

Materials and Methods

Cell culture

T24 human bladder carcinoma cells (Cell Line Service, Eppelheim, Germany) were cultured in Dulbeccos Modified Eagles Medium (DMEM, Sigma Aldrich), nutrient mixture F-12 Ham, supplemented with 5% fetal bovine serum (FBS Superior, Biochrom AG) in a humidified 5% CO_2 atmosphere at 37°C.

Bacterial strains and chemicals

E. faecalis 12030 strain is a clinical isolate obtained in Cleveland, OH. It is a strong biofilm producer and is opsonized by antibodies against its LTA [25]. *E. faecalis* 12030Δ*dlt*A mutant and its complemented strain *E. faecalis* 12030Δ*dlt*Acompl were kindly provided by C. Theilacker and F. Fabretti. All bacterial strains were grown at 37°C without agitation in Caso Bouillon (Carl Roth), and reagents were obtained from Sigma.

LTA extraction

LTA from *E. faecalis* 12030 wild type were isolated as described [26] and with modifications by Theilacker *et al.*, 2006 [25]. Bacterial cells were grown in tryptic soy broth, harvested after 3 h and resuspended in 0.1 M citrate buffer (pH 4.7). The harvested cells were disrupted using glass beads (Beadbeater; Glenn Mills, Clifton, NJ) and stirred with an equal volume of n-butanol for 30 min at room temperature. After centrifugation, the aqueous layer was dialyzed against 0.1 M ammonium acetate (pH 4.7) and lyophilized. The material was redissolved in 15% n-propanol in 0.1 M ammonium acetate (pH 4.7) and applied to an octyl Sepharose column for hydrophobic interaction chromatography. Bound material was eluted with a gradient of 15–80% n-propanol. Fractions were assayed for total phosphorus and by immunoblot assay [26].

Invasion/Adherence assay

For the adherence assay, cells were cultivated in 24-well plates to a density of approximately 1×10^5 cells/well for 16 h. Bacteria were inoculated at ($OD_{600\ nm}$ ~ 0.1) and grown to mid-log phase ($OD_{600\ nm}$ ~ 0.4) at 37°C in Caso Bouillon. T24 cells were incubated with bacteria for 2 h at a multiplicity of infection of 100:1. After infection of the monolayer, human bladder carcinoma cells were washed five times with bovine serum albumin (PBS, Biochrom AG) and lysed with DMEM F-12 Ham + 5% FBS + 0.25% Triton-X100 buffer for 15 min. Surface adherent and intracellular bacteria were enumerated by quantitative bacterial counts. Six replicates (wells) of each stimulation were prepared and the full experiment was repeated 3 times.

Inhibition assays

For inhibition of enterococcal binding to T24 cells, purified LTA (10–500 µg/mL) from wild type *E. faecalis* 12030 was added to the cells 30 min before infection. The assay was then performed as described above.

Mouse Urinary Tract Infection model

Female BALB/C mice (6–8 weeks old, Charles River, Sulzfeld, Germany) were used for the experiments. To prepare the inoculum, bacteria were grown in 5 mL for ~ 16 h at 37°C with gentle shaking. For inoculum preparation the overnight culture was diluted 1:100 in 50 mL fresh medium and grown to an OD_{600nm} ~ 0.3 at 37°C with shaking. The cells were pelleted for 10 min (6.000×g at 10°C) and resuspended in half of the volume of 0.9% saline. Further dilutions were prepared in Caso Bouillon and then plated to determine the actual inoculum. Before starting the experiment, the bladder of the mouse was emptied by catheter (20 mm). Subsequently, isoflurane-anesthetized mice were infected via urethral catheterization with 100 µL of the bacterial suspension (3–5×10^8 CFU/mL). After 2 h the same amount of bacteria was injected again to achieve consistent infection. The urethral catheter was removed immediately after this step, and all animals had free access to food and water during the course of study. Mice were euthanized by CO_2 inhalation at 24 h and 48 h after transurethral challenge. The urinary bladder and kidney pairs were excised, weighed, and homogenized in 1 mL of 0.9% saline + 0.025% Triton X-100, and dilutions were plated onto Caso Agar without antibiotics. The CFU/100 mg of bacteria for each tissue (bladder or kidney) was calculated for each animal.

Statistical analysis

If not stated otherwise, the experiments were repeated three times. All cell culture tests were made by multigroup comparisons using ANOVA (PRISM4, GraphPad software). P value less than 0.05 was considered significant. Comparisons among groups were made using the Mann-Whitney U test. P value less than 0.05 was considered significant.

Ethics Statement

All animal experiments were performed in compliance with the German animal protection law (TierSchG). The mice were housed and handled in accordance with good animal practice as defined by FELASA and the national animal welfare body GV-SOLAS. The animal welfare committees of the University of Freiburg (Regierungspräsidium Freiburg Az 35/9185.81/G-11/118) approved all animal experiments.

Results

E. faecalis 12030Δ*dlt*A mutant shows strong adherence to uroepithelial cells

To investigate the importance of LTA D-alanylation to in vitro adherence to uroepithelia, we used T24 human bladder cell lines, *E. faecalis* 12030Δ*dlt*A mutant and the wild type *E. faecalis* 12030. As control, the *E. faecalis* 12030Δ*dlt*A complemented strain was used. As shown in Figure 1a, compared to the wild type strain (0.6×10^6 CFU/mL), the *E. faecalis* 12030Δ*dlt*A mutant showed up to four fold increased adherence (2.9×10^6 CFU/mL,

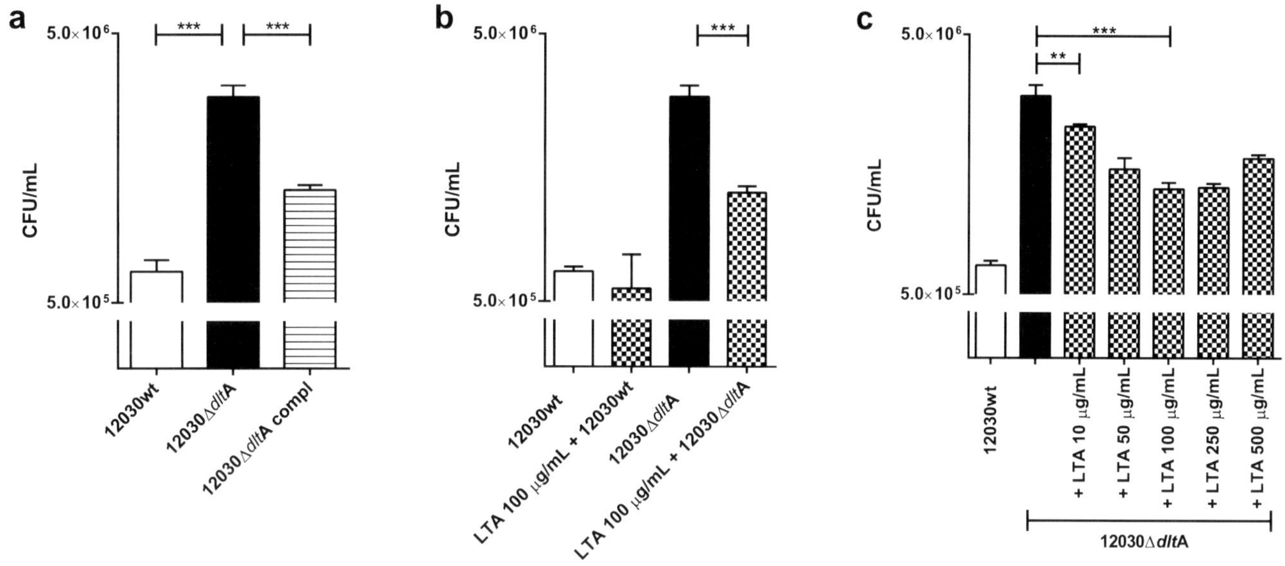

Figure 1. Attachment to T24 cells. (**A**) *E. faecalis* 12030 wild type, *E. faecalis* 12030Δ*dlt*A mutant and the *E. faecalis* 12030Δ*dlt*A complemented strain were tested for their ability to adhere to and/or invade T24 uroepithelial cells. Bacterial titers in logarithmic scale (log scale). T24 cells were cultivated in 24-well plates to a density of 1×10^5 cells/well and incubated for 2 h with bacteria grown to mid-log phase ($OD_{600nm}\sim0.4$) at a bacteria-to-cell ratio of 100:1. Total cell-associated bacteria include surface-adherent and intracellular bacteria. Bars represent average ± S.E. The *E. faecalis* 12030Δ*dlt*A mutant shows strongly increased adherence to uroepithelial cells compared to the wild type ($p<0.001$). **B**) Treatment of cells with purified LTA. *E. faecalis* 12030 wild type and the *E. faecalis* 12030Δ*dlt*A mutant were tested. Concentration of purified LTA was 100 μg/mL. The adherence to uroepithelial cells was significantly reduced by *E. faecalis* 12030Δ*dlt*A mutant ($p<0.01$) after LTA treatment and no differences were obtained by wild type strain. In each experiment 6 replicates (wells) of each stimulation were prepared. The full experiment was repeated 3 times. Multigroup comparisons were made by ANOVA (PRISM4, GraphPad software). P-values of <0.05 (*), <0.005 (**) and <0.0005 (***) were considered statistically significant. **C**) Dose-dependent reduction in adhesion using purified LTA. *E. faecalis* 12030Δ*dlt*A mutant were tested with increasing concentrations of LTA (10 – 500 μg/mL).

$p<0.001$) to uroepithelial cells. The complemented mutant strain *E. faecalis* 12030Δ*dlt*Acompl showed a partially restored effect of the mutation (1.2×10^6 CFU/mL, $p<0.001$).

Bacterial adherence could be inhibited by purified LTA

To study the specific interaction between bacteria and a still-unknown receptor, T24 cells were first incubated with 100 μg/mL purified LTA from wild type *E. faecalis* 12030 strain to saturate binding sites and subsequently they were inoculated with bacteria. As shown in Figure 1b, the *E. faecalis* 12030Δ*dltA* mutant with LTA treatment showed significantly less adherence (1.25×10^6 CFU/mL, $p<0.01$) to the bladder epithelial cell line as compared to without LTA treatment (2.9×10^6 CFU/mL). In the wild type, no significant differences in adherence properties were observed using purified LTA and a dose dependent reduction of adherence using LTA could also demonstrated in Figure 1c.

E. faecalis 12030Δ*dlt*A colonizes uroepithelial surfaces more efficiently than wild type bacteria

To study the effect of lipoteichoic acid on urinary tract infection, a modified mouse urinary infection model was used [9]. The wild type strain *E. faecalis* 12030 and the mutant *E. faecalis* 12030Δ*dlt*A were tested. The bacterial counts in the bladder and in both kidneys were determined after 24 h and 48 h of incubation as described elsewhere [9]. As shown in Figure 2 after 24 h, the mutant colonized the bladder (4×10^5 CFU/100 mg) significantly better compared to the wild type strain (9×10^3 CFU/100 mg), i.e. up to 1.5 log more bacteria ($p<0.001$). This difference in colonization behaviour between mutant and wild type strains was 2.4 logs higher in kidneys ($p<0.001$). The mutant showed 3×10^6 CFU/100 mg tissue compared to wild type 9×10^3 CFU/100 mg. We observed colonization differences between mutant and wild type strains to bladder and kidney epithelia after the prolonged incubation time of 48 h. A statistically significant difference ($p<0.05$) was observed only in kidneys. Here the mutant colonized up to 9×10^5 CFU/100 mg tissue whereas the wild type achieved only 1×10^3 CFU/100 mg. In fact, the *E. faecalis* 12030Δ*dlt*A mutant colonized the kidneys at both time points considerably better than the wild-type strain.

Discussion

Attachment of microorganisms to mucosal surfaces of the urinary tract is important for the pathogenesis of UTI because the mechanical removal of colonizing bacteria by the urine flow is an important innate defense mechanism. In the process of bacterial cell adherence, infectious agents interfere with specific molecules on epithelial cells [17,20,5–6,27,28]. While UTI-specific virulence factors of *E. coli* have been studied extensively, relatively little is known about *E. faecalis* cell-surface structures with respect to UTIs [7–10 & 11].

In a model of ascending UTI, the presence of an enterococcal surface protein was shown to increase the persistence of bacteria in the urinary bladders of mice without histological changes [7] whereas Kau *et al.* demonstrated that *E. faecalis* has greater tropism for the kidneys [9]. Using a similar model, the MSCRAMMs of *E. faecalis* such as collagen adhesion protein (Ace) [12–13], PavA-like fibronectin-binding protein (EfbA) [11], and a biofilm-associated pilus (Ebp) [14,15] contributed to the pathogenesis of enterococcal UTIs.

The D-Ala-LTA formation racks up several functions, such as cationic homeostasis maintenance, integration of metal cations

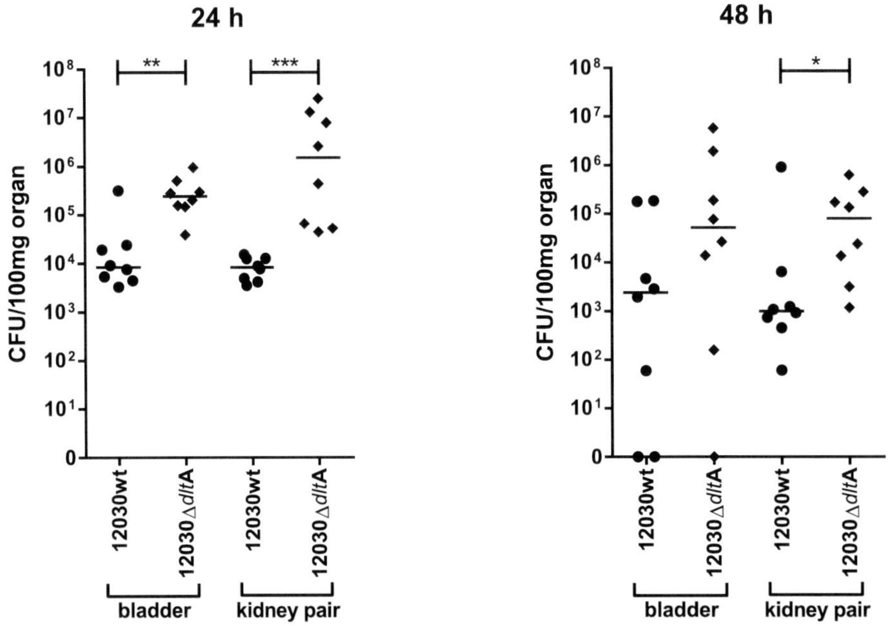

Figure 2. Monoinfection with wild-type *E. faecalis* 12030 (12030 wt) and mutant *E. faecalis* 12030Δ*dltA*. Bacterial titers in logarithmic scale (log scale). Data are from 8 mice infected with 3–5×10^8 CFU; results are expressed as CFU per 100 mg of kidney and bladder homogenates 24 h and 48 h after transurethral challenge. The CFU from both kidneys were averaged. A value of 1 CFU was assigned to kidneys without bacteria. Circles represent wild-type *E. faecalis* 12030, squares represent *E. faecalis* 12030Δ*dltA*. Horizontal bars represent the geometric mean. Values that are significantly different by the Mann-Whitney U test are indicated as follows: P-value of $<$0.05 (*), $<$0.005 (**) and $<$0.0005 (***).

and inflection of autolytic actions and several other electromechanical properties of the bacterial envelope when the surface of gram-positive bacteria is exposed to disparate microenvironments. The cell wall of gram-positive bacteria contains different types of anionic molecules. Two different teichoic acids are present on the surface of gram-positive bacteria: lipoteichoic acid (LTA), an amphiphilic polymer non-covalently inserted into the cellular membrane, and wall teichoic acid (WTA), covalently linked to the peptidoglycan of the cell wall. These two molecules are synthesized by separate biosynthetic pathways that have been well characterized in *Bacillus subtilis* and other gram-positive bacteria [29]. Nevertheless, D-alanyl-ester substituents of WTA originally derive from LTA and are later transferred to WTA by transacylation. It is a single *dlt* operon encoding the genes responsible for the D-alanine incorporation [30–32].

The *dltA* operon has been studied in several gram-positive bacteria revealing an identical organization [33]. Bacteria with mutations in the *dlt* operon showed a variety of phenotypic changes that could be attributed to the resulting charge modification of their cell surface. The lack of D-alanine esters resulted in a stronger negative net charge, because D-alanine esters introduce positively charged groups into the otherwise negatively charged teichoic acids [34]. In *B. subtilis* and *S. aureus*, the absence of D-alanine has been shown to cause alterations in the activity of autolytic enzymes [35,36]. Also possible is an altered host immune response, leading to enhanced proliferation/persistence.

In this work, the *E. faecalis* 12030Δ*dlt*A mutant has been investigated with regard to adherence to T24 bladder carcinoma cells. Surprisingly, we observed that it displayed more than four-fold increased adherence to human bladder carcinoma cells compared to the wild-type strain. We could partially restore this adherence to 1.310^6 CFU/mL using a complemented mutant strain (Figure 1a). Moreover, using purified LTA it was possible to significantly inhibit adherence to human bladder cells, demonstrating the specificity of binding (Figure 1b). A dose dependent reduction of adherence using LTA could also be demonstrated (data not shown). Interestingly, in contrast to our previous data, which showed that the same mutant exhibits less binding to Caco2 colonic epithelial cells than wild-type bacteria, here we obtained higher adherence to uroepithelial cells [3,25,37]. In addition, these data are in contrast to previous studies using *S. aureus* and *Listeria monocytogenes*, in which elimination of D-alanylation of LTA impaired adherence to mammalian cells [38–40].

To assess the relevance of these results and the differences in vivo, a modified mouse urinary infection model was used; our results confirmed that the *E. faecalis* 12030Δ*dlt*A mutant colonized the kidneys significantly better than the wild-type strain after 24 and 48 h (Figure 2). In addition, the mutant colonized the bladder significantly better after 24 and 48 h albeit the differences observed at 48 h were not statistically significant. This is assumed by the fact that *E. faecalis* usually does not persist in the bladder, resulting in decrease number of colony counts, because of clearance of bacteria from the bladder by mechanical forces of urine flow.

However, the same *E. faecalis* 12030Δ*dlt*A mutant demonstrated less colonization in a mouse sepsis model [37]. This disparate finding suggests the existence of specific receptors on bladder and/or uroepithelial cell surfaces. Our results therefore show that D-alanylation of LTA can decrease adherence to specific host cells and therefore suggest a novel function of alanylation of LTA in *E. faecalis*. Differential expression of the *dlt* locus may allow enterococci to adapt to specific ecological niches.

Acknowledgments

This work was supported by grants from the German Ministry of Science and Education (BMBF:UroGenOmics0315833C).

Author Contributions

Conceived and designed the experiments: TS JH. Performed the experiments: DW LA. Analyzed the data: TS DW LA. Contributed reagents/materials/analysis tools: JH EG. Wrote the paper: TS LA.

References

1. Hidron AI, Edwards JR, Patel J, Horan TC, Sievert DM, et al. (2009) National Healthcare Safety Network Team; Participating National Healthcare Safety Network Facilities: NHSN annual update: antimicrobial-resistant pathogens associated with healthcare-associated infections: annual summary of data reported to the National Healthcare Safety Network at the Centers for Disease Control and Prevention, 2006-2007. Infect Control Hosp Epidemiol 30: 107.
2. Koch S, Hufnagel M, Theilacker C, Huebner J (2004) Enterococcal infections: host response, therapeutic, and prophylactic possibilities. Vaccine 22: 822–30.
3. Sava IG, Heikens E, Huebner J (2010) Pathogenesis and immunity in enterococcal infections. Clin Microbiol Infect 16: 533–40.
4. Sillanpää J, Xu Y, Nallapareddy SR, Murray BE, Höök M (2004) A family of putative MSCRAMMs from *Enterococcus faecalis*. Microbiology 150: 2069–78.
5. Kunin CM (1994) Urinary tract infections in females. Clin Infect Dis 18: 1–12.
6. Svenborg Eden C, Hagberg L, Hanson LA (1993) Bacterial adherence a pathogenetic mechanism in urinary tract infections caused in *Escherichia coli*. *Prog Allergy* 33: 175–188.
7. Shankar N, Lockatell CV, Baghdayan AS, Drachenberg C, Gilmore MS, et al. (2001) Role of *Enterococcus faecalis* surface protein Esp in the pathogenesis of ascending urinary tract infection. Infect & Immun 69: 4366–72.
8. Johnson JR, Clabots C, Hirt H, Waters C, Dunny G (2004) Enterococcal aggregation substance and binding substance are not major contributors to urinary tract colonization by *Enterococcus faecalis* in a mouse model of ascending unobstructed urinary tract infection. Infect Immun 72: 2445–8.
9. Kau AL, Martin SM, Lyon W, Hayes E, Caparon MG, et al. (2005) *Enterococcus faecalis* tropism for the kidneys in the urinary tract of C57BL/6J mice. Infect Immun 73: 2461–8.
10. Guiton PS, Hung CS, Hancock LE, Caparon MG, Hultgren SJ (2010) Enterococcal biofilm formation and virulence in an optimized murine model of foreign body-associated urinary tract infections. Infect Immun 78: 4166–75.
11. Torelli R, Serror P, Bugli F, Paroni Sterbini F, Florio AR, et al. (2012) The PavA-like fibronectin-binding protein of *Enterococcus faecalis*, EfbA, is important for virulence in a mouse model of ascending urinary tract infection. J Infect Dis 15: 952–60.
12. Nallapareddy SR, Singh KV, Sillanpää J, Zhao M, Murray BE (2011) Relative contributions of Ebp Pili and the collagen adhesin *ace* to host extracellular matrix protein adherence and experimental urinary tract infection by *Enterococcus faecalis* OG1RF. Infect Immun 79: 2901–10.
13. Lebreton F, Riboulet-Bisson E, Serror P, Sanguinetti M, Posteraro B, et al. (2009) Ace, which encodes an adhesin in *Enterococcus faecalis*, is regulated by Ers and is involved in virulence. Infect Immun 77: 2832–9.
14. Nallapareddy SR, Singh KV, Sillanpää J, Garsin DA, Höök M, et al. (2006) Endocarditis and biofilm-associated pili of Enterococcus faecalis. J Clin Invest 116: 2799–807.
15. Singh KV, Nallapareddy SR, Murray BE (2007) Importance of the *ebp* (endocarditis- and biofilm-associated pilus) locus in the pathogenesis of *Enterococcus faecalis* ascending urinary tract infection. J Infect Dis 195: 1671–1677.
16. Nallapareddy SR, Singh KV, Sillanpää J, Garsin DA, Höök M, et al. (2006) Endocarditis and biofilm-associated pili of *Enterococcus faecalis*. J Clin Invest 116: 2799–2807.
17. Teng F, Jacques-Palaz KD, Weinstock GM, Murray BE (2002) Evidence that the enterococcal polysaccharide antigen gene (*epa*) cluster is widespread in *Enterococcus faecalis* and influences resistance to phagocytic killing of *E. faecalis*. Infect Immun 70: 2010–5.
18. Teng F, Singh KV, Bourgogne A, Zeng J, Murray BE (2009) Further characterization of the *epa* gene cluster and Epa polysaccharides of *Enterococcus faecalis*. Infect Immun 77: 3759–67.
19. Xu Y, Murray BE, Weinstock GM(1998) A cluster of genes involved in polysaccharide biosynthesis from *Enterococcus faecalis* OG1RF. Infect Immun 66: 4313–23.
20. Xu Y, Singh KV, Qin X, Murray BE, Weinstock GM (2000) Analysis of a gene cluster of *Enterococcus faecalis* involved in polysaccharide biosynthesis. Infect Immun 68: 815–23.
21. Theilacker C, Kaczyński Z, Kropec A, Sava I, Ye L, et al. (2011) Serodiversity of opsonic antibodies against *Enterococcus faecalis* glycans of the cell wall revisited. PLoS ONE 6: e17839.
22. Fischer W (1988) Physiology of lipoteichoic acids in bacteria. Adv Microb Physiol 29: 233–302.
23. Fischer W, Mannsfeld T, Hagen G (1990) On the basic structure of poly(glycerophosphate) lipoteichoic acids. Biochem Cell Biol 68: 33–43.
24. Neuhaus FC, Baddiley J (2003) A continuum of anionic charge: structures and functions of D-alanyl-teichoic acids in gram-positive bacteria. Microbiol Mol Biol Rev 67: 686–723.
25. Theilacker C, Kaczynski Z, Kropec A, Fabretti F, Sange T, et al. (2006) Opsonic antibodies to *Enterococcus faecalis* strain 12030 are directed against lipoteichoic acid. Infect Immun 74: 5703–12.
26. Morath SA, Geyer, Hartung T (2001) Structure-function relationship of cytokine induction by lipoteichoic acid from *Staphylococcus aureus*. J Exp Med 193: 393–397.
27. Guzman CA, Pruzzo C, Plate M, Guardati MC, Calegari L (1991) Serum dependent expression of *Enterococcus faecalis* adhesins involved in the colonization of heart cells. Microb Pathog 11: 399–409.
28. Hufnagel M, Carey VJ, Baldassarri L, Reinert RR, Huebner J (2006) Distribution of four capsular serotypes of *Enterococcus faecalis* among clinical isolates from different geographical origins and infection sites. Infection 34: 22–5.
29. Neumeister B, Mond JJ, Peschel A (2004) Role of teichoic acids in *Staphylococcus aureus* nasal colonization, a major risk factor in nosocomial infections. Nat Med 10: 243–5.
30. Kristian SA, Datta V, Weidenmaier C, Kansal R, Fedtke I, et al. (2005) D-alanylation of teichoic acids promotes group a streptococcus antimicrobial peptide resistance, neutrophil survival, and epithelial cell invasion. J Bacteriol 187: 6719–25.
31. Perego M, Glaser P, Minutello A, Strauch MA, Leopold K, et al. (1995) Incorporation of D-alanine into lipoteichoic acid and wall teichoic acid in *Bacillus subtilis*. Identification of genes and regulation. J Biol Chem 270: 15598–606.
32. Peschel A, Otto M, Jack RW, Kalbacher H, Jung G, et al. (1999) Inactivation of the dlt operon in *Staphylococcus aureus* confers sensitivity to defensins, protegrins, and other antimicrobial peptides. J Biol Chem 274: 8405–10.
33. Poyart C, Pellegrini E, Marceau M, Baptista M, Jaubert F, et al. (2003) Attenuated virulence of *Streptococcus agalactiae* deficient in D-alanyl-lipoteichoic acid is due to an increased susceptibility to defensins and phagocytic cells. Mol. Microbiol. 49:1615–1625.
34. Boyd DA, Cvitkovitch DG, Bleiweis AS, Kiriukhin MY, Debabov DV, et al. (2000) Defects in d-alanyl-lipoteichoic acid synthesis in *Streptococcus mutants* results in acid sensitivity. J Bacteriol 182: 6055–6065.
35. Peschel AC, Vuong, Otto M, Gotz F (2000) The D-alanine residues of *Staphylococcus aureus* teichoic acids alter the susceptibility to vancomycin and the activity of autolytic enzymes. Antimicrob Agents Chemother 44: 2845–2847.
36. Wecke J, Perego M, Fischer W (1996) D-Alanine deprivation of *Bacillus subtilis* teichoic acids is without effect on cell growth and morphology but affects the autolytic activity. Microb *Drug Resist* 2: 123–129.
37. Fabretti F, Theilacker C, Baldassarri L, Kaczynski Z, Kropec A, et al. (2006) Alanine esters of enterococcal lipoteichoic acid play a role in biofilm formation and resistance to antimicrobial peptides. Infect Immun 74: 4164–71.
38. Abachin E, Poyart C, Pellegrini E, Milohanic E, Fiedler F, et al. (2002) Formation of D-alanyl-lipoteichoic acid is required for adhesion and virulence of *Listeria monocytogenes*. Mol Microbiol 43: 1–14.
39. Weidenmaier C, Kokai-Kun JF, Kristian SA, Chanturiya T, Kalbacher H, et al. (2004) Role of teichoic acids in *Staphylococcus aureus* nasal colonization, a major risk factor in nosocomial infections. Nat Med 10: 243–5.
40. Weidenmaier C, Peschel A, Kempf VA, Lucindo N, Yeaman MR, et al. (2005) DltABCD- and MprF-mediated cell envelope modifications of *Staphylococcus aureus* confer resistance to platelet microbicidal proteins and contribute to virulence in a rabbit endocarditis model. Infect Immun 73: 8033–8.

Robustness and Plasticity of Metabolic Pathway Flux among Uropathogenic Isolates of *Pseudomonas aeruginosa*

Antje Berger[1], Katrin Dohnt[1], Petra Tielen[2], Dieter Jahn[2], Judith Becker[1,3], Christoph Wittmann[1,3]*

1 Institute of Biochemical Engineering, Technische Universität Braunschweig, Braunschweig, Germany, **2** Institute of Microbiology, Technische Universität Braunschweig, Braunschweig, Germany, **3** Institute of Systems Biotechnology, Saarland University, Saarbrücken, Germany

Abstract

Pseudomonas aeruginosa is a human pathogen that frequently causes urinary tract and catheter-associated urinary tract infections. Here, using ^{13}C-metabolic flux analysis, we conducted quantitative analysis of metabolic fluxes in the model strain *P. aeruginosa* PAO1 and 17 clinical isolates. All *P. aeruginosa* strains catabolized glucose through the Entner-Doudoroff pathway with fully respiratory metabolism and no overflow. Together with other NADPH supplying reactions, this high-flux pathway provided by far more NADPH than needed for anabolism: a benefit for the pathogen to counteract oxidative stress imposed by the host. *P. aeruginosa* recruited the pentose phosphate pathway exclusively for biosynthesis. In contrast to glycolytic metabolism, which was conserved among all isolates, the flux through pyruvate metabolism, the tricarboxylic acid cycle, and the glyoxylate shunt was highly variable, likely caused by adaptive processes in individual strains during infection. This aspect of metabolism was niche-specific with respect to the corresponding flux because strains isolated from the urinary tract clustered separately from those originating from catheter-associated infections. Interestingly, most glucose-grown strains exhibited significant flux through the glyoxylate shunt. Projection into the theoretical flux space, which was computed using elementary flux-mode analysis, indicated that *P. aeruginosa* metabolism is optimized for efficient growth and exhibits significant potential for increasing NADPH supply to drive oxidative stress response.

Editor: Stephen S. Fong, Virginia Commonwealth University, United States of America

Funding: This work was financially supported by the German Federal Ministry of Eduction and Research (www.bmbf.de) through grant 315833D in the initiative Medical Infection Genomics. The funders had no role in study design, data collection and analysis, decision to publish, or preparation of the manuscript.

Competing Interests: The authors have declared that no competing interests exist.

* E-mail: christoph.wittmann@uni-saarland.de

Introduction

Pseudomonas aeruginosa is a metabolically versatile bacterium that resides in a wide range of biotic and abiotic habitats and is a human pathogen that causes numerous acute and opportunistic infections [1]. The clinical spectrum of *P. aeruginosa* infections includes wound and urinary tract infections, meningitis, and necrotizing pneumonia [2]. In particular, urinary tract infections and catheter-associated urinary tract infections are the most common bacterial infections in clinical practice [3,4] and pose a severe health threat with more than one million hospitalizations annually [5].

Research on *P. aeruginosa* has focused its virulence [1], resistance [6], and adaptation [7] as well as therapeutic strategies [8]. Microevolution through resistance-mediating mutations in the bacterium's resistome involves a large subset of its genetic repertoire and a complex network of metabolic pathways that mediate adaptive resistance and adaptive metabolism [9–11]. Therefore, a systems-level understanding of the network that drives the pathogenesis of *P. aeruginosa* is important for devising specific control strategies [1]. In particular, ^{13}C-metabolic flux analysis (fluxomics) detects common and specific pathways employed by pathogens and identifies candidate pathways as targets for therapy [12,13].

This network-wide approach provides information on the activities of central enzymes and pathways most directly linked to phenotype [14]. However, to our knowledge, such analyses of *P. aeruginosa* have not been published. Here, we investigated the laboratory strain *P. aeruginosa* PAO1 at the level of carbon fluxes by using ^{13}C-metabolic flux analysis that combined isotopic tracer experiments with mass spectrometric labeling analysis and stoichiometric and isotopomer balancing for flux calculation [15]. This was extended to a collection of 17 *P. aeruginosa* clinical isolates from patients with urinary tract infections and catheter-associated urinary tract infections. These strains are genetically diverse, differ from strains that cause chronic lung infections in patients with cystic fibrosis, and exhibit heterogeneous production of virulence factors *in vitro* [16].

Materials and Methods

Bacteria

The model strain, *P. aeruginosa* PAO1 served as a reference [17]. Uropathogenic *P. aeruginosa* isolates from patients with direct urinary tract infections included the strains MH06u, MH09u, RN12u, RN13u, MH16u, MH17u, MH26u, and MH29u. Isolates from patients with catheter-associated urinary tract infections included the strains MH15c, MH25c, MH33c, MH34c, MH36c,

MH37c, MH39c, MH56c, and MH57c [16]. *Corynebacterium glutamicum* ATCC 13032 and *P. putida* KT2440 were acquired from the German Collection of Strains and Cell Cultures (DSMZ, Braunschweig, Germany). All strains were stored in 10% (w/v) glycerol at −80°C.

Culture media

Starter cultures were grown in complex LB medium containing 5 g·L^{-1} yeast extract (Becton, Dickinson and Company, Sparks, MD, USA), 10 g·L^{-1} peptone (Becton, Dickinson and Company) and 10 g·L^{-1} NaCl. For the second and main cultures, a minimal medium developed during the study ensured balanced growth of all strains, an important prerequisite for the ^{13}C-flux approach [15]. The osmolality of this medium was 500 mosmol·kg^{-1}, which reflects that of human urine [18]. The medium contained the following (per liter): 2.5 g glucose, 13.0 g $KH_2PO_4 \times 2\ H_2O$, 20.6 g K_2HPO_4, 0.49 g $MgSO_4 \times 7\ H_2O$, 2.5 g NH_4Cl, 1.41 g Na_2SO_4, 0.085 g $CaCl_2 \times 2\ H_2O$, 1.2 mg $FeSO_4 \times 7\ H_2O$, and 25 mg 3,4-dihydroxybenzoate. For ^{13}C-flux experiments, naturally labeled glucose was replaced with 99% [1-^{13}C] glucose (Cambridge Isotope Laboratories, Inc., Andover, MA, USA).

Culture conditions

Cultures were shaken at 1,050 rpm and 37°C in 10 mL deep-well plates (HJ Bioanalytik, Mönchengladbach, Germany) with a working volume of 1.4 mL (Titramax 1000, Heidolph Instruments, Schwabach, Germany). Starter cultures were prepared by inoculating LB medium with 20 µL of a glycerol stock. After 6 h of incubation, 50 µL of cell suspension was transferred to a second culture in minimal medium. Subsequently, exponentially growing cells (50 µL) were used as inoculum for main cultures, and strains were grown in 30 mL of minimal medium in 300 mL baffled shake flasks. These were incubated at 37°C with shaking at 200 rpm on an orbital shaker (Aquatron, Infors AG, Switzerland). Dissolved oxygen was monitored online using shake flasks with integrated sensor spots (PreSens SFR, PreSens Precision Sensing GmbH, Regensburg, Germany). The sensor device was installed in the orbital shaker as described previously [19]. In cultures incubated with ^{13}C-tracer, the inoculum level was always kept below 1% of the final sampled cell concentration to exclude potential interference of a differently labeled inoculum on subsequent calculation of flux [15].

Quantification of cell concentration

Cell growth was monitored spectrophotometrically at 578 nm (OD_{578}) (Libra S11, Biochrome, Cambridge, UK). Cell dry weight (CDW) was determined as follows: Dried plastic tubes were filled with 20 mL cell suspension, and cells were harvested by centrifugation (25,800× *g*, 4°C, 10 min); subsequently, pellets were washed twice with deionized water, and then dried to a constant weight.

Quantification of substrates and products

The concentration of glucose was determined from filtered supernatants (Minisart, 0.2 µm, Sartorius, Göttingen, Germany) using a YSI 2700 Select biochemical analyzer (Kreienbaum, Langenfeld, Germany). The analysis of organic acids (oxalic acid, citric acid, α-ketoglutaric acid, gluconic acid, glyoxylic acid, pyruvic acid, succinic acid, glycolic acid, lactic acid, fumaric acid, acetic acid, propanoic acid, and butyric acid) and amino acids in the culture supernatant was conducted using high-pressure liquid chromatography [20]. The limit of detection was below 10 µM for organic acids and below 1 µM for amino acids, respectively.

Enzyme assays

Cultures (10 mL) were harvested by centrifugation (25,800× *g*, 4°C, 5 min), washed with 100 mM Tris-HCl (pH 7.5) containing 10 mM $MgCl_2$ and 0.75 mM dithiothreitol, and then resuspended in the same buffer. The cells were then mechanically disrupted (100 µm silica glass beads, 2×20 s, 6.0 m·s^{-1}, FastPrep-24, MP Biomedicals, Eschwege, Germany). Total protein concentration of the obtained cell extract was determined using Roti-Quant (Carl Roth GmbH, Karlsruhe, Germany). Phosphofructokinase activity was determined spectrophotometrically at 340 nm [21]. The reaction mixture contained 100 mM Tris-HCl (pH 8.0), 0.5 U·mL^{-1} aldolase, 1 U·mL^{-1} triosephosphate isomerase, 0.5 U·ml^{-1} glycerol-phosphate dehydrogenase, 5 mM $MgCl_2$, 0.25 mM NADH, 0.1 mM ATP, and 4 mM fructose 6-phosphate. The activity of isocitrate lyase was determined as described previously [22]. Reactions were initiated by adding substrate, and reactions without substrate served as negative controls. One unit (U) of activity represents the conversion of 1 µmol substrate per minute.

Mass isotopomer labeling analysis of proteinogenic amino acids

Cells (0.5 mg CDW) were harvested in the mid-exponential growth phase by centrifugation (3 min, 16,000× *g*, 4°C, Biofuge Fresco, Heraeus, Hanau, Germany), washed twice with deionized water, and incubated with 30 µL 6 M HCl for 24 h at 100°C. The obtained hydrolysate was filtered (0.2 µm, Ultrafree MC, Millipore, Bedford, MA, USA) and then lyophilized. The proteinogenic amino acids in the lyophilisate were dissolved in 50 µL *N*, *N*-dimethylformamide containing 1% (v/v) pyridine and then derivatized at 80°C for 30 min with 50 µL N-methyl-*t*-butyldimethylsilyl-trifluoroacetamide (Macherey-Nagel, Düren, Germany). Mass isotopomer distributions of selected ion clusters of the analytes were then quantified using gas chromatography-mass spectrometry (GC-MS) (HP6890, M 5973, Agilent Technologies, Waldbronn, Germany) as described earlier [23]. All samples were first measured in scan mode to exclude isobaric overlay, and were analyzed in triplicate by selective ion monitoring to determine relative fractions of the mass isotopomers of interest [15].

Metabolic reaction network and flux calculation

A large-scale model of the central metabolism of *P. aeruginosa* was assembled according to the genome-scale model of *P. aeruginosa* PAO1 [24], KEGG database [25], and the *Pseudomonas* genome database [26]. The network compromised the Entner-Doudoroff pathway (EDP), incomplete Embden-Meyerhof-Parnas pathway lacking phosphofructokinase (EMPP), pentose phosphate pathway (PPP), gluconeogenesis, reactions of pyruvate carboxylase, PEP carboxylase, PEP carboxykinase, malic enzyme, tricarboxylic acid (TCA) cycle, glyoxylate pathway, and anabolic pathways generating biomass. The chemical composition of *P. aeruginosa* cells was adapted from that of closely related *Pseudomonas* species [27,28]. Because *P. aeruginosa* uniquely synthesizes the capsular polysaccharide alginate [29], the cellular content of this polymer was measured (Table S1, [30]), and the corresponding precursor demand was considered for all strains. The calculation of metabolic flux through the network was performed using OpenFLUX software [31]. For each strain,

Table 1. Kinetics and stoichiometry of glucose-grown *P. aeruginosa* PAO1 and uropathogenic *P. aeruginosa* isolates obtained from patients with catheter-associated urinary tract infection or urinary tract infections.

Strain	Maximum specific growth rate (h^{-1})	Biomass yield ($g_{CDW}\ g_{Glucose}^{-1}$)	Glucose uptake rate (mmol $g_{CDW}^{-1}\ h^{-1}$)
PAO1	0.91±0.02	0.53±0.01	9.52±0.21
MH15c	0.35±0.01	0.36±0.01	5.37±0.29
MH25c	0.67±0.04	0.45±0.00	8.28±0.58
MH33c	0.91±0.02	0.51±0.01	9.87±0.17
MH34c	0.88±0.03	0.53±0.01	9.30±0.16
MH36c	0.70±0.02	0.44±0.01	8.92±0.35
MH37c	0.62±0.02	0.43±0.01	8.08±0.40
MH39c	0.60±0.01	0.41±0.01	8.04±0.05
MH56c	0.93±0.01	0.51±0.01	10.16±0.07
MH57c	0.85±0.02	0.39±0.00	12.22±0.28
MH06u	0.81±0.04	0.49±0.01	9.31±0.58
MH09u	0.74±0.03	0.49±0.02	8.33±0.11
RN12u	0.67±0.02	0.47±0.00	7.94±0.25
RN13u	0.82±0.03	0.48±0.02	9.49±0.40
MH16u	0.52±0.01	0.51±0.02	5.75±0.10
MH17u	0.59±0.01	0.50±0.02	6.66±0.25
MH26u	0.65±0.02	0.44±0.02	8.24±0.17
MH29u	0.82±0.03	0.53±0.00	8.65±0.33

The corresponding cultivation profiles for all strains are provided in Supporting Information (Figure S3). Values indicate means and standard deviations of three biological replicates. By-products in the supernatants were not detected; concentrations were below the detection limit (1 μM for amino acids and 10 μM for organic acids).

the mass isotopomer distributions of the derivatized amino acid residues [M-57] of alanine (*m/z* 260), glycine (*m/z* 246), valine (*m/z* 288), serine (*m/z* 390), threonine (*m/z* 404), phenylalanine (*m/z* 336), aspartate (*m/z* 418), glutamate (*m/z* 432), tyrosine (*m/z* 466), and the [M-85] fragment of serine (*m/z* 362) were used as input after correction for natural isotopes [32]. Multiple flux estimations using statistically varied starting values for free flux parameters confirmed the identification of a global minimum. For all flux data, 95% confidence intervals were calculated using a Monte Carlo approach [33].

Elementary flux mode analysis

The metabolic network of *P. aeruginosa* was investigated using in silico pathway analysis involving the computation of elementary flux modes. The network topology agreed with that of the related species *P. putida* [34]. The energy demand for polymerization of building blocks and biomass assembly was based on the genome model of *P. aeruginosa* PAO1 [24]. Elementary flux modes were calculated as described previously [35]. Evaluation of the modes was carried out using Excel (MS Office, Windows, 2007) and provided relative pathway flux and yields for each of the modes [34,35].

Statistical analysis

Hierarchical clustering analysis (HCA) and principal component analysis (PCA) were conducted using MATLAB (Version R2011b, The MathWorks). PCA was used to convert the set of ^{13}C-labeling data to a set of linearly uncorrelated variables, i.e., the principal components [36]. HCA was carried out using the complete linkage, the Euclidean distance, as a measure of proximity of experimental data to inspect strain similarity [37].

Results

Quantitative metabolism of *P. aeruginosa* PAO1 and the clinical isolates

P. aeruginosa PAO1 consumed glucose from an early time point (Figure S1), and its growth rate was approximately 0.91/h, corresponding to a doubling time of 45 min (Table 1). Biomass and CO_2 were considered to be the only products formed, because secreted by-products were not detected. Note that the strain grew fully aerobically as verified by on-line monitoring of the dissolved oxygen level (Figure S2). Next, we analyzed *P. aeruginosa* isolates from urinary tract infections (8 strains) and catheter-associated urinary tract infections (9 strains). All individual growth profiles are presented in the Supporting Information (Figure S3). The strains showed high variability in growth (Table 1).

The efficiency for recruiting glucose for anabolism, i.e., the biomass yield, differed by more than a factor of 1.5. Strain MH15c produced the lowest biomass yield, which was approximately 65% of the value of the two most efficient strains, MH34c and MH29u, which yielded a biomass 0.53 $g \cdot g^{-1}$. This approached the theoretical optimum (0.54 $g \cdot g^{-1}$), a value derived by in silico pathway simulation. Briefly, the corresponding simulation for the carbon core network of *P. aeruginosa* provided 13,138 elementary modes, each representing a theoretical metabolic state of the cell. Together, all modes span the feasible flux space of the organism and contain the optimum growth mode with maximum possible yield [35]. Differences between growth kinetics of the strains were even larger. Whereas certain strains grew rather slowly and

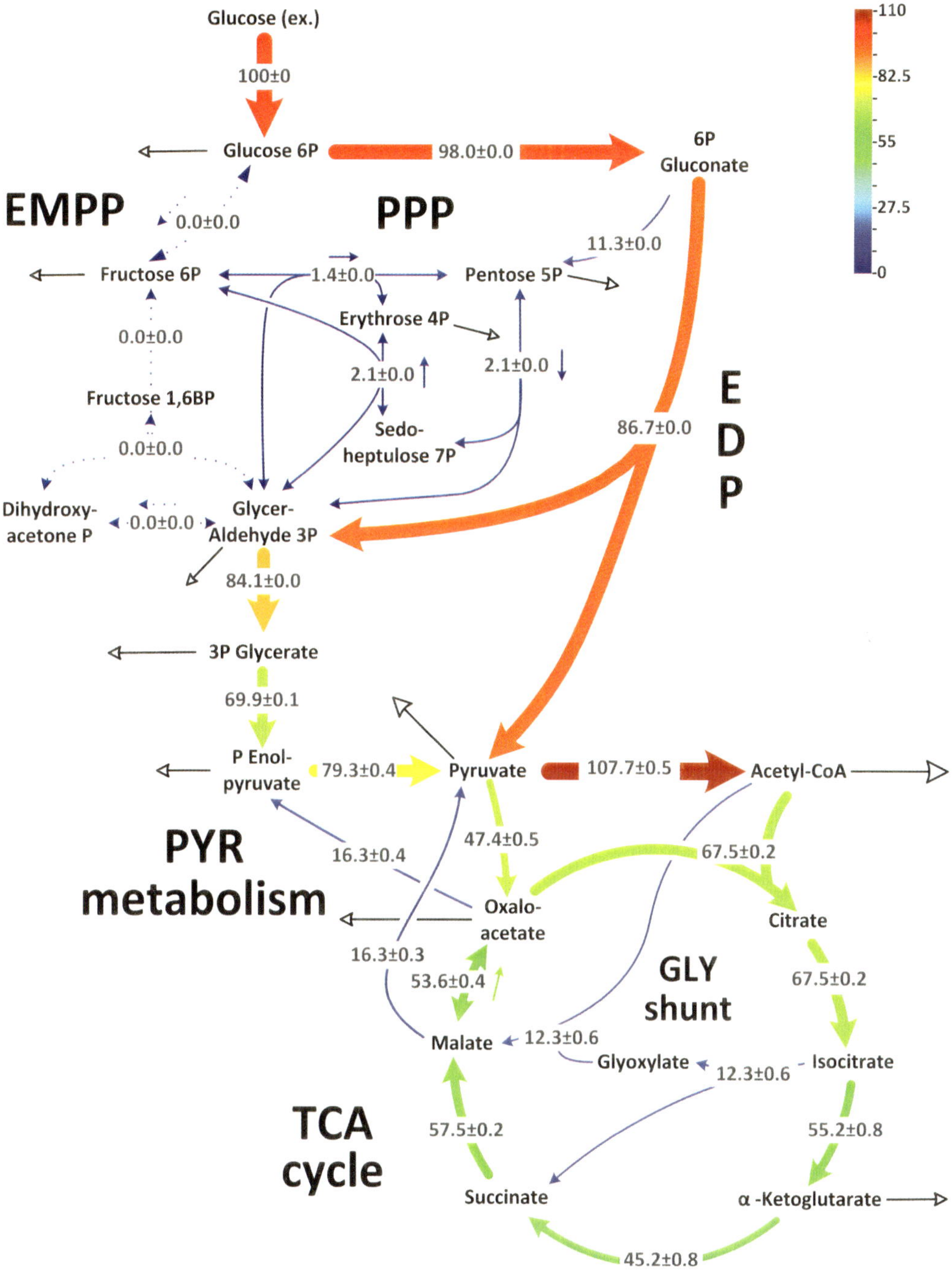

Figure 1. In vivo carbon flux distribution in the central metabolism of *P. aeruginosa* PAO1. Flux is expressed as a molar percentage of the specific glucose uptake rate of 9.5 mmol g^{-1} h^{-1}. Open arrows indicate the flux toward biomass. For reversible reactions, the direction of the net flux is indicated by a dashed arrow. The errors given for each flux reflect the corresponding 90% confidence intervals. The full flux data set is presented in Supporting Information. Metabolic and isotopic steady states were ensured by constant stoichiometry, kinetics, and the constant ^{13}C-labeling patterns of recruited metabolites during cultivation (see Figure S1, Figure S5). The abbreviations are as follows: Entner-Doudoroff pathway (EDP), Embden-Meyerhof-Parnas pathway (EMPP), pentose phosphate pathway (PPP), glyoxylate (Gly) shunt, tricarboxylic acid (TCA) cycle, and pyruvate metabolism.

exhibited doubling times of about 120 min, others duplicated within only 40 min. Similarly, specific uptake rates for glucose differed significantly.

Glucose catabolism by *P. aeruginosa* PAO1

P. aeruginosa PAO1 was grown on [1-^{13}C] glucose to estimate metabolic flux and exhibited metabolic and isotopic steady state growth (see Supporting Information). This fulfilled an important prerequisite for the ^{13}C-flux approach [15]. The simulated labeling data, corresponding to the optimal fit, agreed closely with experimental values (Table S2) and indicated high consistency of the flux values. Glucose was mainly consumed through the EDP (Figure 1). The flux through 6-phosphogluconate dehydrogenase, which catalyzes the first reaction of the oxidative

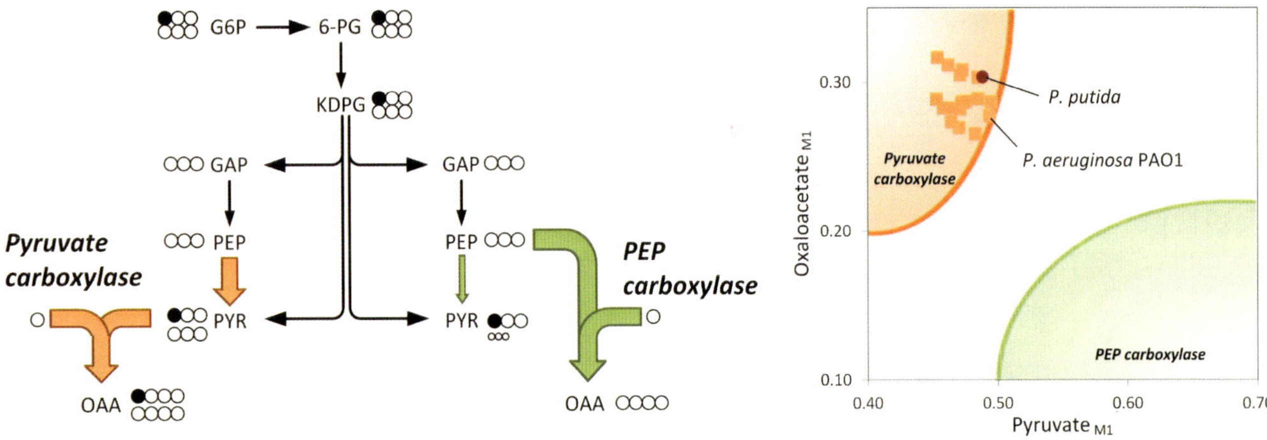

Figure 2. Resolution of anaplerotic flux in [1-^{13}C]-glucose-grown uropathogenic *P. aeruginosa*, *P. aeruginosa* PAO1, and *P. putida*. For exclusive use of the ED pathway for glucose catabolism, the contribution of PEP carboxylase resulted in low ^{13}C-enrichment of oxaloacetate (deduced from aspartate), whereas the ^{13}C accumulated in pyruvate (alanine), which creates an excess of its single-labeled (M1) mass isotopomer (green region). In contrast, the action of pyruvate carboxylase reduced and increased the levels of pyruvate and oxaloacetate (orange region), respectively. This allowed for discrimination between these enzymes according to the combined labeling of the two molecules. Prior to inspection, the ^{13}C-labelling data were corrected for the contribution of natural isotopes [32].

PPP, was low. The PPP exclusively served for anabolic purposes. Both, oxidative and non-oxidative PPP, contributed to supply of ribose 5-phosphate, erythrose 4-phosphate, and fructose 6-phosphate for anabolism. EMPP activity was undetectable, likely caused by lack of cytoplasmic phosphofructokinase activity (<0.01 mU·mg^{-1}). Accordingly, *P. aeruginosa* PAO1 catabolized glucose only through the EDP to subsequent glycolytic steps and further to pyruvate.

Pyruvate metabolism, anaplerosis, and the TCA cycle in *P. aeruginosa* PAO1

The activity of a functional PEP carboxylase (anaplerotic reaction from phosphoenolpyruvate to oxaloacetate) could not be confirmed. During growth on [1-^{13}C] glucose, the combination of ^{13}C enrichment in pyruvate and oxaloacetate can be used to discriminative between PEP and pyruvate carboxylase (Figure 2). The weak signal generated by the singly labeled pyruvate mass isotopomer (M1), i.e., the low ^{13}C-enrichment in the molecule, together with a relatively high value for the corresponding M1

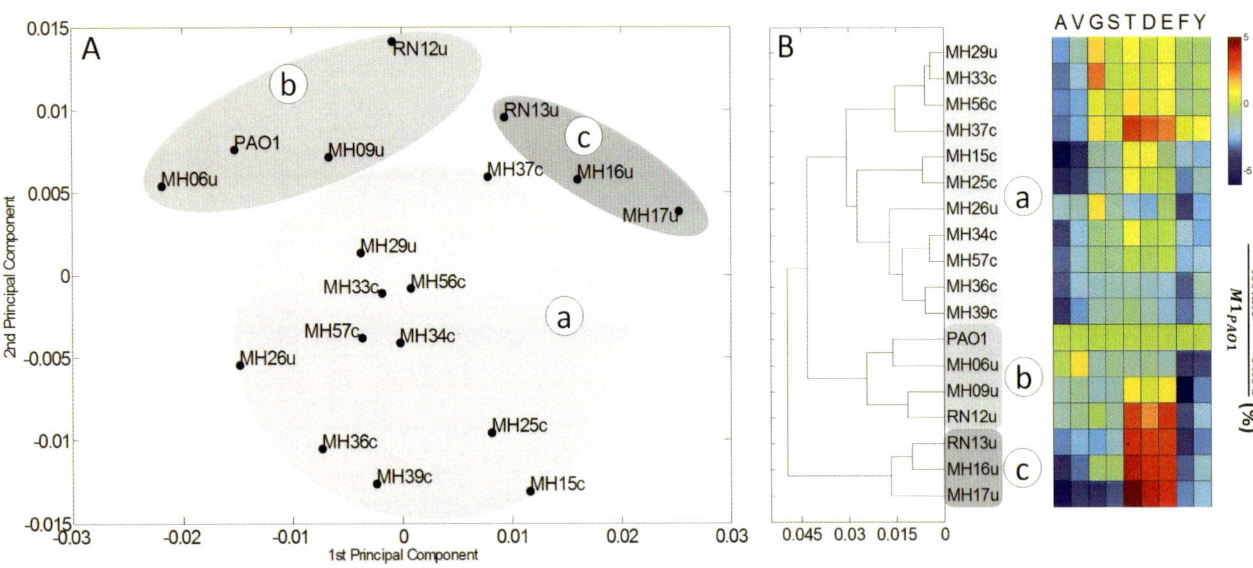

Figure 3. Statistical analysis of carbon core metabolism of uropathogenic *P. aeruginosa* isolates and *P. aeruginosa* PAO1 based on ^{13}C-labeled amino acid enrichment data from the tracer studies. Principal component analysis provided a clustering of the strains according to the two major components (A). Hierarchical cluster analysis revealed the degree of similarity, shown as a Euclidian tree (B). The relative fraction of the single labeled (M1) mass isotopomer of each amino acid was considered after normalization to the value of *P. aeruginosa* PAO1. The relative ^{13}C-enrichment is displayed in color. The amino acids are denoted by their single letter code.

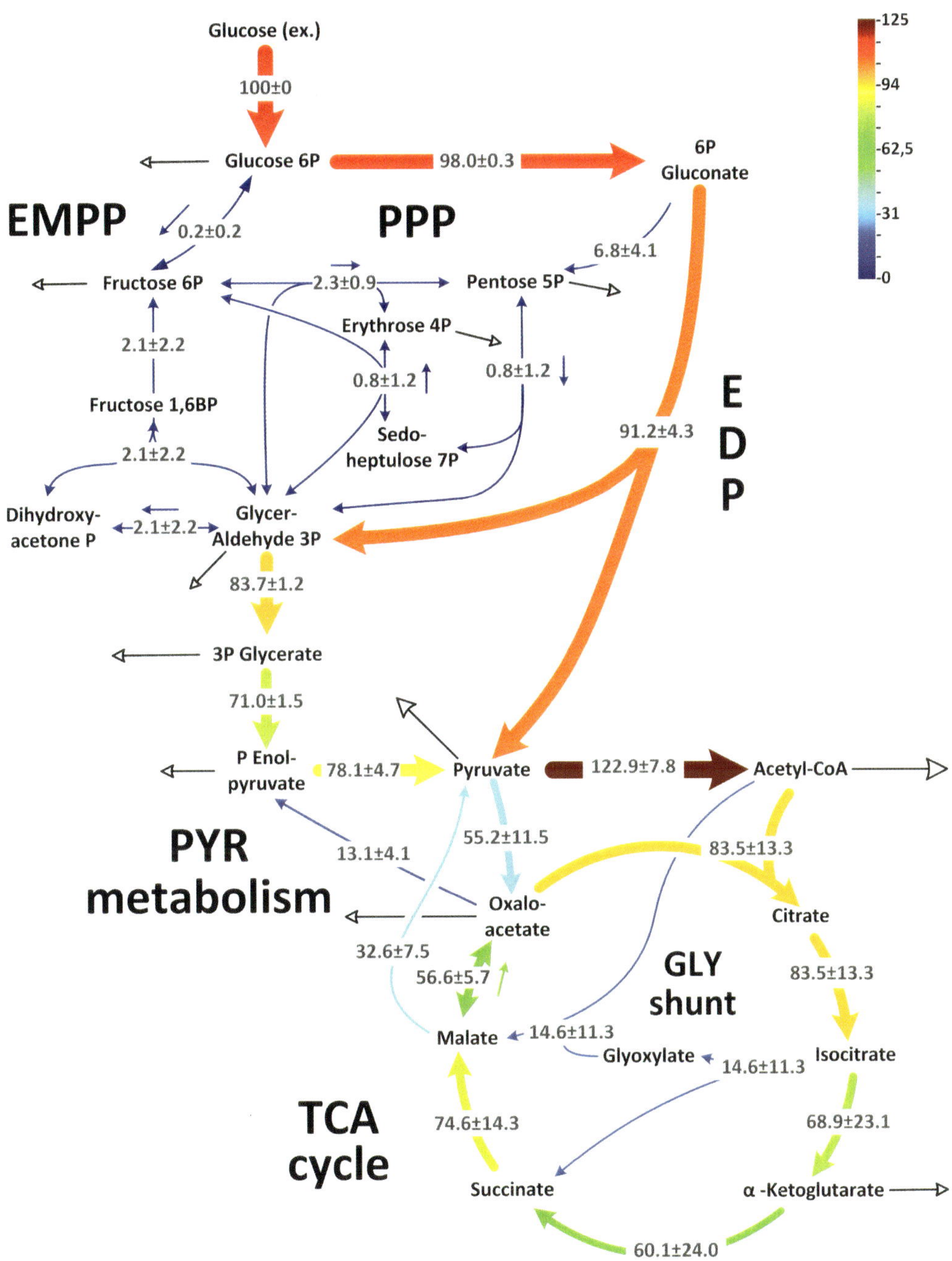

Figure 4. In vivo carbon flux distributions in central metabolism of uropathogenic *P. aeruginosa* isolates during growth on glucose. Flux is given as average flux of all strains and is expressed as a molar percentage of the average glucose uptake rate of all strains (8.6 mmol g^{-1} h^{-1}, calculated from the individual rates in Table 1). Open arrows indicate flux toward biomass. For reversible reactions, the direction of net flux is indicated by a dashed arrow. The errors given for each flux reflect the corresponding 90% confidence intervals. The full flux data sets are presented in Supporting Information. Metabolic and isotopic steady states are ensured by constant stoichiometry, kinetics, and the constant ^{13}C-labeling patterns of recruited metabolites during cultivation (see Figure S1, Figure S5). Abbreviations are as follows: Entner-Doudoroff pathway (EDP), Embden-Meyerhof-Parnas pathway (EMPP), pentose phosphate pathway (PPP), glyoxylate (Gly) shunt, and tricarboxylic acid (TCA) cycle.

isotopomer of oxaloacetate, matched the expected pattern for pyruvate carboxylase. In contrast, it differed significantly from possible combinations for pyruvate and oxaloacetate, which would result from PEP carboxylase. Thus, pyruvate was the source of anaplerotic oxaloacetate.

P. putida expresses pyruvate carboxylase [27] and shows the same pattern (Figure 2). On flux level, decarboxylating phosphoenolpyruvate carboxykinase and malic enzyme returned carbon to the glycolytic pools (Figure 1). Accordingly, malic enzyme powered the pyruvate shunt (malate conversion to pyruvate by malic enzyme and further to oxaloacetate by pyruvate carboxylase) [27]. The overall net flux toward the TCA cycle generated by the concerted action of the carboxylating and decarboxylating enzymes was rather low (14.8%). Therefore, this anaplerotic route alone was not sufficient to replenish the TCA cycle, which was continuously depleted by the anabolic requirement for its

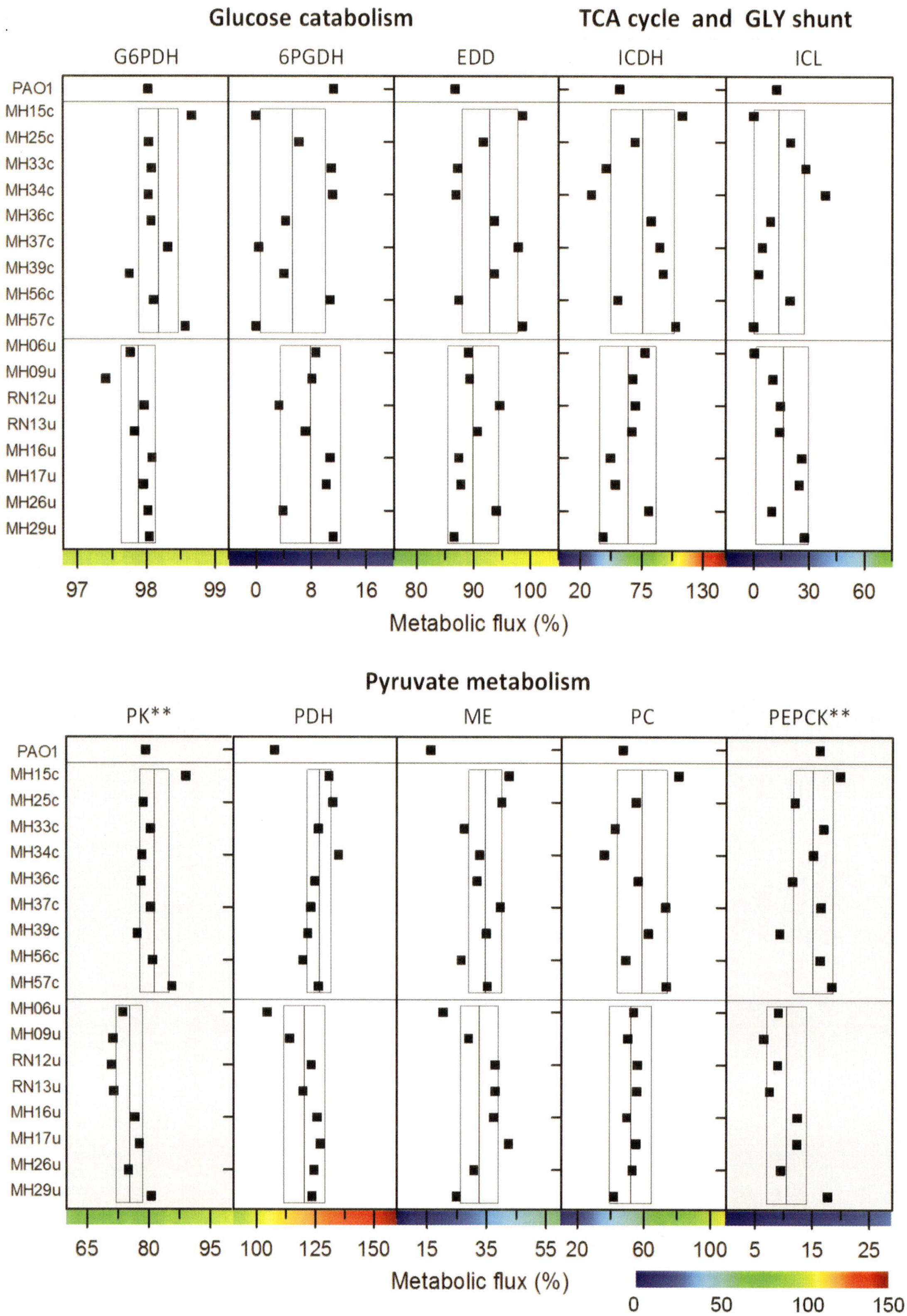

Figure 5. In vivo carbon fluxes through central metabolic pathways of uropathogenic *P. aeruginosa* during growth on glucose. The data reflect the individual flux for each isolate. All fluxes are expressed as a molar percentage of the corresponding specific glucose uptake rate (Table 1). Statistical differences of flux between strains from urinary tract infections and from catheter-associated infections were assessed using a *t* test. Significant differences (**$P<0.05$) are indicated. Abbreviations are as follows: glucose 6-phosphate dehydrogenase (G6PDH), 6-phosphogluconate dehydrogenase (6PGDH), 6-phosphogluconate dehydratase (EDD), isocitrate dehydrogenase (ICDH), isocitrate lyase (ICL), pyruvate kinase (PK), pyruvate dehydrogenase (PDH), malic enzyme (ME), pyruvate carboxylase (PC), and phosphoenolpyruvate carboxykinase (PEPCK). The full flux data sets for all strains are presented in the Supporting Information.

Table 2. Metabolic flux in *P. aeruginosa* PAO1 and select gram-negative and gram-positive bacteria.

Organism	EDP [%]	EMPP [%]	PPP [%]	Gly shunt [%]	Reference
P. aeruginosa PAO1	87	-*	11	12	this work
P. putida KT2440	89	-	11	n.d.**	[27]
P. fluorescens	91	-	9	n.d.	[65]
E. coli	3	73	25	0	[53]
C. glutamicum	-	67	33	0	[66]

Flux refers to the Entner-Doudoroff pathway (EDP), Embden-Meyerhof-Parnas pathway (EMPP), pentose phosphate pathway (PPP), and glyoxylate (Gly) shunt and reflects relative values normalized to the corresponding glucose uptake rate, defined as 100%.
* functional pathway not encoded.
** n.d. = not determined.

intermediates oxaloacetate (17%) and 2-oxoglutarate (10%). Note that the cells recruited the glyoxylate shunt as an anaplerotic pathway. At the level of isocitrate, approximately 20% of carbon was channeled into the shunt, matched by a relative flux of 12%. The activity of this pathway seemed surprising at first, because it is typically not required in glucose-grown cells. We therefore performed *in-vitro* measurements to detect isocitrate lyase, the key enzyme of this pathway. Indeed, isocitrate lyase was present in the cytoplasm (124 ± 1 mU· (mg protein)$^{-1}$). Further studies showed that acetate as sole carbon source activated isocitrate lyase by approximately a factor of four (Figure S4).

Metabolic analysis of clinical isolates using [1-^{13}C] glucose

The *P. aeruginosa* isolates grown on [1-^{13}C] glucose exhibited balanced growth and reached a metabolic steady state (Figure S5). The ^{13}C-labeling patterns of proteinogenic amino acids (Table S2) were first explored by unsupervised statistical analysis because they were informative for directly discriminating between different types of metabolism and pathway use [38] and provided an initial qualitative overview of the strains. Briefly, the ^{13}C-data were analyzed using PCA (Figure 3A) and HCA (Figure 3B). The 18 strains clustered into three subgroups, designated as clusters *a*, *b* and *c* in the Euclidian tree. This revealed site-specific metabolism. Clusters *b* and *c* comprised only isolates from urinary tract infections. In contrast, all strains from catheter-related infections grouped in cluster *a*. The only strains assigned to cluster *a* from the urinary tract infections were MH26u and MH29u. The clustering resulted from differences in distinct amino acids and were therefore of metabolic origin. A prominent example is the high enrichment of label in threonine, aspartate, and glutamate, which was specific for the strains of cluster *c* (Figure 3B). The three clusters were also identified using PCA (Figure 3A), which described 98% of the labeling information.

Metabolic flux of *P. aeruginosa* isolates

The full set of flux analysis as well as all experimental and simulated labeling patterns, which reflect optimal fit, are presented in Table S2. Figure 4 provides an integrated view of pathway use. Briefly, flux through each reaction displays the average value of all strains, whereas the deviation indicates the corresponding variability. Flux through the initial metabolic pathways, i.e., EDP, PPP and EMPP, respectively, was conserved. This was inferred from the flux data of the single isolates (Figure 5) where the corresponding pathways showed similar activity.

Only three catheter-associated strains (MH15c, MH37c, and MH57c) did not use 6-phosphogluconate dehydrogenase, whereas all other strains channeled carbon through this enzyme into the PPP. Using an *in-vitro* assay, phosphofructokinase activity was not detected in any isolate (<0.01 mU (mg protein)$^{-1}$). All isolates, as well as PAO1, recruited pyruvate carboxylase but not PEP carboxylase (Figure 2). Interestingly, flux varied downstream from the pyruvate node. This involved the TCA cycle and the reactions interconnecting the cycle with the glycolytic intermediates, i.e., the anaplerotic and gluconeogenetic reactions.

The most variable metabolic reactions were localized around the isocitrate node, where the isolates differed significantly in the flux partitioning between the glyoxylate shunt and the TCA cycle (Figure 4). This is even more apparent when inspecting individual strains (Figure 5). In certain isolates, the glyoxylate shunt was completely inactive, whereas others showed high flux (44%). As exemplified by MH34c, strains with an active shunt showed isocitrate lyase activity (see Figure S4). Similarly, the TCA cycle (17–112%) and other enzymes, positioned near the pyruvate node varied strongly in flux. Note that flux through pyruvate kinase and phosphoenolpyruvate carboxykinase was significantly different between the two clinical subgroups (Figure 5). The catheter-associated isolates carried higher flux through these reactions ($P<0.05$) compared with strains isolated from patients with urinary tract infections.

Discussion

The present study describes the analysis of metabolic fluxes in *P. aeruginosa* PAO1 as well as uropathogenic isolates and provides novel insights into function and regulation of carbon core metabolism of this important pathogen. We show here that *P. aeruginosa* isolates catabolize glucose through the EDP with fully respiratory metabolism and without overflow (Figure 2, Figure 4, Figure 5). They further recruit the oxidative and non-oxidative PPP exclusively for biosynthesis, but do not exhibit a functional EMPP. All strains utilize pyruvate carboxylase but not PEP carboxylase (Figure 2), and the glyoxylate shunt operates as anaplerotic pathway. Hierarchical clustering of the strains according to their flux reveals a site-specific metabolism among the isolates, which might indicate that *P. aeruginosa* differently adapts to its environment: the urinary tract and the surface of catheters infections, respectively. The isolates differ strongly in glucose uptake rate and growth efficiency. Faster uptake of nutrients and their more efficient conversion into biomass might provide an advantage to compete and persist during infection. However, one should be cautious with this particular interpretation due to potential metabolic differences, caused by different levels of oxygen in our aerobic experimental setup and the oxygen limited infection environments, in which *P. aeruginosa* thrives [39].

The exclusive use of the EDP as a glycolytic strategy is conserved among *P. aeruginosa* and other pseudomonads

The predominant use of the EDP is identical to that of other glucose-grown pseudomonads, including *P. putida*, *P. fluorescens*, and *P. denitrificans* previously studied at the flux level (Table 2). This finding is attributed to the lack of phosphofructokinase, an essential enzyme of the alternative glycolytic EMPP [27]. However, this glycolytic strategy is uncommon among prokaryotes, and only 12% of bacteria rely solely on the EDP [40], whereas the more energy-efficient EMPP is nearly ubiquitous [41].

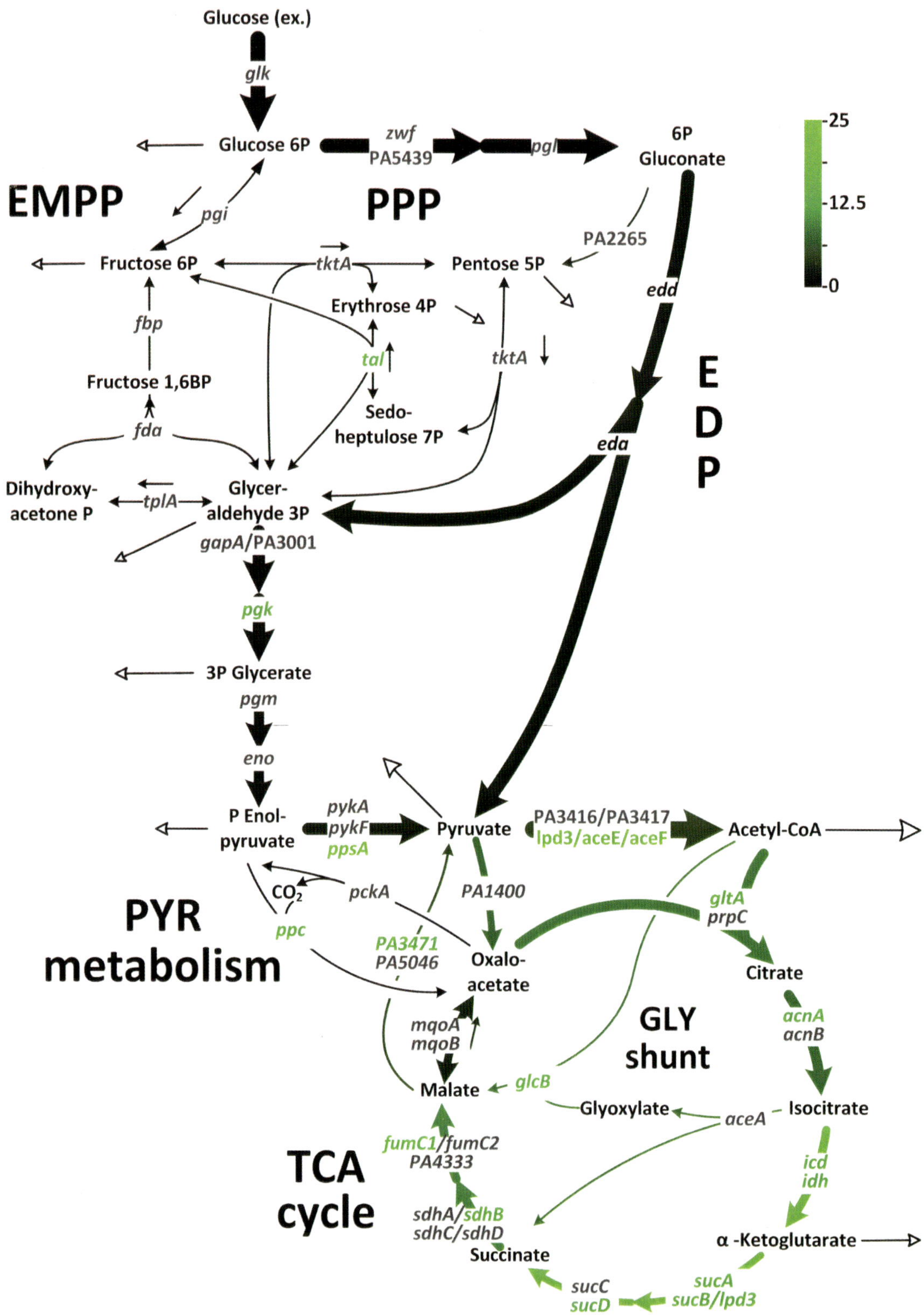

Figure 6. Metabolic adaption of pathogenic *P. aeruginosa*. The network representation integrates changes of flux determined for uropathogenic isolates and *P. aeruginosa* PAO1 (this work) and changes in transcription transcript level previously determined for successive isolates of *P. aeruginosa* from patients with chronic cystic fibrosis [11]. The variation of metabolic flux among strains is indicated by color (black = conserved, green = changed). Genes with changed or unchanged transcript levels are shown in green or black, respectively. Abbreviations are as follows: Entner-Doudoroff pathway (EDP), Embden-Meyerhof-Parnas pathway (EMPP), pentose phosphate pathway (PPP), glyoxylate (Gly) shunt, and tricarboxylic acid (TCA) cycle.

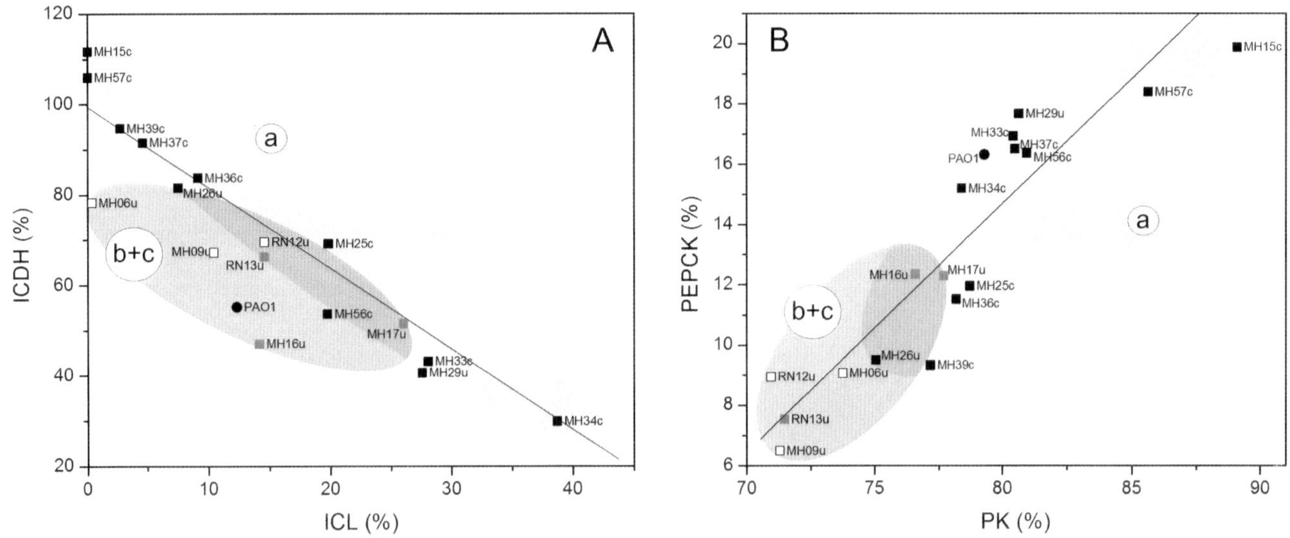

Figure 7. Niche-specific metabolic flux in uropathogenic *P. aeruginosa*, including flux through isocitrate dehydrogenase and isocitrate lyase (A) and through pyruvate kinase and phosphoenolpyruvate carboxykinase (B). Each data point refers to a distinct isolate. The clustering represents statistical analysis using principal components (see Figure 4) that discriminated between isolates from catheter-associated infections (cluster *a*) and strains from urinary tract infections (clusters *b* and *c*). The full flux data sets for all strains are presented in Supporting Information. All flux values are normalized to the average glucose uptake rate for all strains (100%).

However, the EDP mediates superior resistance to oxidative stress [42]. In this study, the expression of a functional EMPP in *P. putida*, which forced the organism to redirect flux from the natural ED route, significantly decreased its robust response to oxidative stress [42], because the EMP pathway does not yield NADPH required by various antioxidant defense mechanisms [43–46]. In contrast, the ED pathway provides NADPH [40].

Accordingly, bacteria that reside in the environment, such as *P. putida*, favor the ED pathway to better cope with naturally occurring oxidative stress [42]. We conclude, therefore, that the high ED flux of *P. aeruginosa* provides a major benefit for this pathogen, which must counteract oxidative stress imposed by the host as a response to infection. Moreover, *P. aeruginosa* senses the redox state and switches its metabolism as a reaction to the host immune defense and other oxidative stress conditions, which involves the activation of catalase, thiol reductase, and superoxide dismutase, all of which use NADPH as a cofactor [47].

Anaplerotic and TCA cycle flux of uropathogenic *P. aeruginosa* reveal high plasticity

Microevolution of *P. aeruginosa* during chronic pulmonary infection creates a metabolic shift to support adaptation to the host environment [7,48]. Transcriptome profiling has shown that this predominantly involves its carbon core machinery [11]. Briefly, adaptive evolution affected only specific pathways such as pyruvate metabolism, the TCA cycle, and the linked pathways of anaplerosis and gluconeogenesis. In contrast, the reactions that metabolize glucose to pyruvate via the EDP remained unchanged.

The integration of observations of distinct metabolic changes in *P. aeruginosa* during chronic lung infection determined at the transcript level [11] taken together with the metabolic flux changes in uropathogenic isolates presented here, reveal a striking picture (Figure 6). It seems that the pathogen undergoes a similar metabolic adaptation in two very different infection environments: the lung and the urinary tract. The conserved upstream steps of metabolism, i.e. conversion of glucose to pyruvate, are combined with variations in metabolic flux through the downstream steps of metabolic pathways among all strains. For example, the isolates varied in the flux-partitioning ratio at isocitrate, i.e., toward the glyoxylate shunt and TCA cycle (Figure 7 A). Further, flux at the PEP pool showed significant differences (Figure 7B). Similarly, these reactions were also affected during chronic lung infection [11] (Figure 6). This may reflect a more general underlying strategy that allows *P. aeruginosa* to adapt to the host environment. The validity of this conclusion is limited by our study's use of isolates from different patients, which did not allow a time-resolved reconstruction of the evolving flux changes during infection. Nevertheless, the alterations in metabolism detected among these isolates are likely involved in adaptation and supports their survival in the host. Further flux studies on strains, experimentally evolved in the laboratory [49,50], and on evolutive lineages of clinical isolates [10,11] seem straightforward to confirm this assumption.

The isocitrate node displays a flexible switch-point in the metabolism of *P. aeruginosa*

The glyoxylate shunt, comprising isocitrate lyase and malate synthase, is widespread [51]. First discovered in *P. aeruginosa* [52], it has been commonly considered as a by-pass of the TCA cycle to assimilate carbon from C2 compounds [22] and to overcome limitations in the junction between glycolysis and TCA cycle under stress [53]. The use of the shunt in non-pathogenic bacteria grown on glucose was not significant (Table 2). In contrast, most of the *P. aeruginosa* clinical isolates exhibited significant flux through this pathway (Figure 5). The presence of the glyoxylate shunt, a bit surprising at first, was confirmed by enzyme assays (Figure S4). Its use in the presence of glucose differed from other bacteria, which repress the shunt (Figure S4), as shown previously [54].

The enhancement of isocitrate lyase activity by a factor of 4 for acetate-grown *P. aeruginosa* indicates transcriptional regulation of the pathway, which is known for *C. glutamicum* [54]. At the level of isocitrate dehydrogenase, the glyoxylate shunt competes with the TCA cycle, i.e., cells can direct carbon toward either pathway. Consistent with this, flux through both pathways is coupled

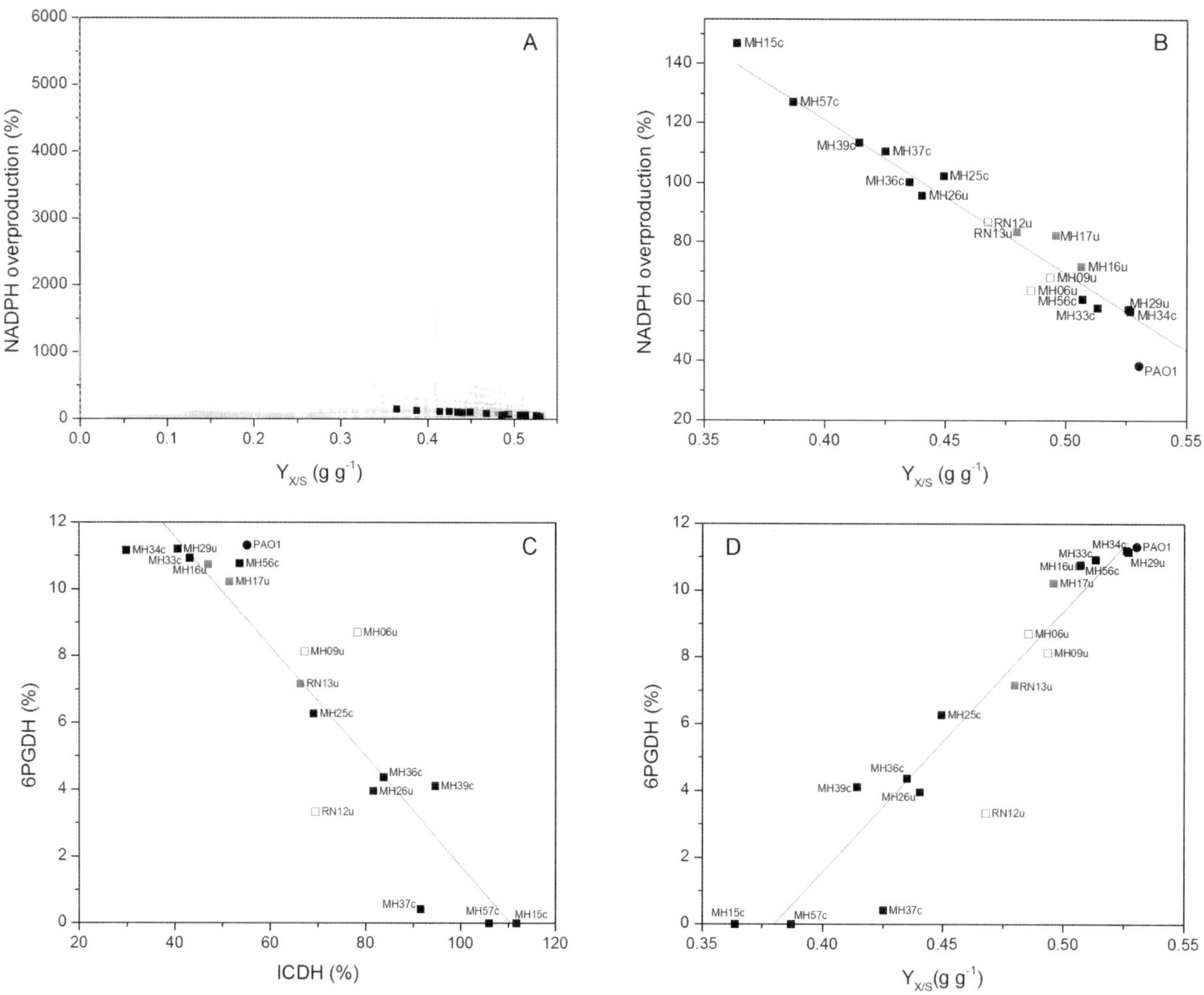

Figure 8. Metabolic properties of uropathogenic *P. aeruginosa* isolates and *P. aeruginosa* PAO1. Integration of flux phenotypes into the theoretical flux space on basis of anabolism (considering the biomass yield coefficient $Y_{X/S}$, given in Table 1) and of NADPH metabolism (considering the NADPH balance as described below). In order to evaluate individual flux phenotypes, experimental values for biomass yield and apparent NADPH excess, respectively, (black squares) are integrated into the flux space created by elementary flux mode analysis (grey squares). Most strains localize close to the growth optimum. (A), Correlation of biomass formation and NADPH metabolism (B), contribution of isocitrate dehydrogenase and 6-phosphogluconate dehydrogenase to supply of reducing power (C), correlation of biomass formation and flux through the oxidative pentose phosphate pathway (D). NADPH metabolism was inspected by balancing of the redox cofactor. For this purpose, the NADPH formation flux by concerted action of glucose 6-phosphate dehydrogenase, 6-phosphogluconate dehydrogenase, isocitrate dehydrogenase, and malic enzyme was balanced with the NADPH consumption flux for anabolism. For all strains, NADPH formation was higher than consumption. The resulting apparent excess flux of NADPH supply is presented here. The full flux data sets for all strains are presented in Supporting Information. The flux values are normalized to the corresponding glucose uptake rate for each strain (set to 100%).

(Figure 7A). Here, the isolates differed significantly in the relative activation of the glyoxylate shunt. Note that the shunt plays a major role in bacterial pathogenesis [55]. For example, isocitrate lyase is up-regulated in *P. aeruginosa* during infection [56]. Mutants lacking a functional glyoxylate pathway show reduced virulence in plants and mammals [57]. However, the shunt is essential for the survival of other pathogens inside the host, including *Mycobacterium tuberculosis* [58], *Salmonella enterica* [59], and *Rhodococcus equi* [60]. *P. aeruginosa* isolates show an enhanced turnover of fatty acids and lipids that are abundantly found in the host's environment [11]. The metabolism of such substrates ultimately requires the glyoxylate shunt to metabolize the C2 intermediate acetyl CoA formed during their degradation. Therefore, the changed flux might reflect an adaptation to nutrients available in the host.

Uropathogenic *P. aeruginosa* is optimized for growth efficiency

For the metabolic network of *P. aeruginosa*, computer-based analysis yielded 12,955 elementary flux modes, each a unique, minimal combination of reactions with fluxes that support steady state operation of cellular metabolism [34]. Together, all modes spanned the theoretical flux space [35]. Here, we focused on growth efficiency and redox metabolism of *P. aeruginosa*. The model allowed for NADPH overproduction. Particularly, we were interested in scenarios, which produce more NADPH than needed for anabolism, i.e. reveal apparent NADPH excess. We assumed that this extra amount of reducing power approximately reflects tolerance against oxidative stress, because NADPH drives many antioxidant mechanisms [43–45].Two-dimensional visualization grouped the obtained elementary modes according to their efficiency for growth and NADPH production (Figure 8 A). Therefore, we defined the yield coefficient for biomass ($Y_{X/S}$) associated with a particular mode as measure of growth efficiency. As measure of NADPH metabolism, we defined the surplus NADPH that resulted from balancing of this cofactor: For each mode, the NADPH formation flux through glucose 6-phosphate dehydrogenase, 6-phosphogluconate dehydrogenase, isocitrate dehydrogenase, and malic enzyme was balanced with the NADPH consumption flux for anabolism.

In order to evaluate the isolates, we placed their flux phenotypes, i.e. the experimental biomass yield coefficient (Figure 8 A) and the flux of apparent NADPH overproduction (Figure 8 B) into this space of feasible physiological states and looked for their distance to certain points of optimality.

The elementary modes (grey squares) span a triangle with the extremes at the corners, reflecting the corresponding theoretical maximum yield for biomass ($Y_{X/S} = 0.54\ g \cdot g^{-1}$) and the maximum flux for NADPH overproduction (6,000%), respectively. The experimentally determined yields and the NADPH overproduction flux of all isolates (black squares) clearly localize close to optimum growth (Figure 8 A). We conclude that the metabolism of these strains is optimized for growth. However, the metabolic network exhibits a significant potential for enhancing NADPH overproduction, if needed. Growth efficiency occurred at the expense of the NADPH supply, because flux closely coupled in the isolates (Figure 8 B). Therefore, the amount of extra NADPH, not needed for anabolism, was decreased in efficient growers. However, they all exhibited an apparent excess, which was not required for anabolism.

We conclude that, under the conditions studied, *P. aeruginosa* recruits a transhydrogenase to direct the extra NADPH to NADH and the respiratory chain for energy generation. Under stress, the extra amount of NADPH, which is not required for anabolism, could immediately serve for protection against oxidative stress [46].Two nucleotide transhydrogenases, the soluble Sth and the membrane-bound Pnt, respectively, are annotated in the genome of *P. aeruginosa* [24] and might be involved in this inter conversion process. It is unlikely that the transhydrogenases operate in the NADH-to-NADPH direction, although the flux data do not allow a definite conclusion.

Improved growth efficiency relates to preferential use of the PPP but reduced the production of excess NADPH

The *P. aeruginosa* isolates differed in their relative use of the oxidative PPP (Figures 8 C and D), and this is directly related to their growth efficiency. Strains with an increased biomass yield recruited the PPP to a higher extent. We conclude that the activated PPP represented by its entry enzyme, 6-phosphogluconate dehydrogenase, served for biosynthesis. First, it supplied anabolic precursors such as erythrose 4-phosphate and ribose 5-phosphate. Second, it compensated for reduced flux through isocitrate dehydrogenase that catalyzes the synthesis of NADPH in the TCA cycle, which was reduced as a function of increased biomass formation. Thus, the PPP may provide a significant source of redox potential. Similarly, these enzymes complement each other, supplying NADPH as in other bacteria [32].

P. aeruginosa shows niche-specific traits in carbon core metabolism related to the type of infection

The flux data indicate that the metabolism of strains isolated from urinary tract infections differed from those isolated from catheter-associated infections. This represents potential adaptations to the specific conditions during infection. The strains were grouped into three clusters according to flux level. In particular, the differences involved the ^{13}C-labeling of amino acids generated by the TCA cycle (Figure 3 B) and the flux at the junction between the cycles, the pyruvate node, and the glyoxylate shunt (Figures 5, 6, and 7A and B). Other studies demonstrate site-specific phenotypes of *P. aeruginosa* isolates [16,61,62]. These differences include extracellular enzymes such as phospholipase [16] or elastase [63], reflecting specific adaptation to nutrient status in the corresponding host environment. Changes in biofilm formation, cell adhesion, and polymer formation indicate adaptions to sessile life styles [16]. Note that the clustering of the *P. aeruginosa* isolates at the phenotypic flux level (Figure 3 B) was completely different from a previously reported clustering at the genetic level [16]. At seems clear that a different number of changes in the genome could have the same effect on cell activity or even no effect [64]. Consequently, characterization of function, i.e., metabolic level, promises to provide a more direct understanding of the adaption processes. In particular, central metabolic pathways, activated during the infection, appear relevant. Future metabolic flux analysis of direct evolutionary lineages of *P. aeruginosa* [10,11] and under conditions of oxygen limitation, typically present in the afflicted tissues in which these isolates thrive [39], should be straightforward and promises to shed more light on this interesting question.

Supporting Information

Figure S1 Growth characteristics and validation of the experimental approach exemplified for the reference strain *P. aeruginosa* PAO1. Cultivation profile on minimal glucose medium (A). Metabolic and isotopic steady-state are visualized by constant yield for biomass, derived as slope from the profiles of consumed glucose concentration and formed cell dry weight (B). Isotopic steady state is indicated by constant labeling patterns over time, as shown for single-labeled mass isotopomers (M1) of [M-57] amino acid fragments (C). The growth behavior in shake flasks and deep-well plates was identical regarding growth stoichiometry (B) and ^{13}C labeling data (D) justifying the joint use of data. Accordingly, cell dry weight measurements from shake flask cultures could be integrated with growth and labeling data from deep-well plates for flux calculations, when needed. Experiments were performed in three replicates.

Figure S2 Dissolved oxygen during cultivation of *P. aeruginosa* on minimal medium in shake flask culture. To ensure sufficient aeration during cultivation, the level of dissolved oxygen was monitored on-line. As exemplified for *P. aeruginosa* PAO1, the oxygen level was above 80% of saturation so that fully aerobic conditions were given (one of three replicates shown). The excellent agreement of growth kinetics and stoichiometry and of the ^{13}C labeling fingerprint (Figure S1), confirmed that this was obviously also the case for the deep-well plate cultures.

Figure S3 Growth characteristics of uropathogenic *P. aeruginosa* isolates. Cultivation profiles on minimal glucose medium (three biological replicates each). For none of the strains, extracellular by-products were detected.

Figure S4 Enzymatic analysis of isocitrate lyase as key enzyme of the glyoxylate shunt. *C. glutamicum* and *P.*

aeruginosa were cultivated in minimal medium, supplemented either with 40 mM acetate or with 14 mM glucose as sole carbon source, respectively.

Figure S5 Metabolic profiles of consumed glucose concentration and formed cell dry weight of clinical *P. aeruginosa* isolates on minimal glucose medium (three biological replicates each). Metabolic steady-state is inferred from the constant yield for biomass, derived as slope from the profiles.

Table S1 Refinement of the cellular composition of *P. aeruginosa* by quantification of the alginate capsule and the corresponding anabolic demand for F6P for its biosynthesis. For quantification, alginate was detached from the cells, and then analyzed by the sulfamate-biphenyl method [1]. Shortly, cells were harvested, washed once with deionized water. Subsequently, the alginate was detached by shaking for 5 h (300 μL 0.14 M NaCl suspension, 1400 min^{-1}, 25°C). The supernatant (200 μL), obtained by centrifugation (15 min, 16,000× *g*, 4°C), was then amended with 20 μL 4 M sulfamate and with 1.2 mL 0.075 M tetraborate, dissolved in concentrated H_2SO_4, and then incubated for 20 min at 99°C. Afterwards, the suspension was transferred to an ice bath (5 min), followed by addition of 40 μL 0.15% 3-hydroxybiphenyl, dissolved in 0.5% NaOH. The mixture was incubated for 10 min at room temperature. Alginate was quantified by photometry at 525 nm, using isolated alginate from mucoid *P. aeruginosa* FRD1 as external standard [2]. The data reflect the F6P demand for alginate biosynthesis and are given as relative flux, normalized to the specific glucose uptake rate (Table 1). These values were additionally considered in the anabolic requirement for flux analysis by correcting the demand for F6P (Table S2). Generally, the requirement was low.

Table S2 Supporting information on metabolic flux analysis. The data include the ^{13}C labelling analysis of proteinogenic amino acids by GC-MS for all strains, the entire set of estimated metabolic fluxes, and information on the goodness of fit, i.e. the comparison of experimental and simulated labelling data, corresponding to the optimized fit.

Author Contributions

Conceived and designed the experiments: CW. Performed the experiments: AB. Analyzed the data: AB JB PT CW. Contributed reagents/materials/analysis tools: KD. Wrote the paper: AB JB DJ CW. Drafted metabolic network and performed in silico pathway analysis: JB. Provided clinical isolates: PT.

References

1. Balasubramanian D, Schneper L, Kumari H, Mathee K (2012) A dynamic and intricate regulatory network determines *Pseudomonas aeruginosa* virulence. Nucleic Acids Res 41: 1–20.
2. Bereket W, Hemalatha K, Getenet B, Wondwossen T, Solomon A, et al. (2012) Update on bacterial nosocomial infections. Eur Rev Med Pharmacol Sci 16: 1039–1044.
3. Kucheria R (2005) Urinary tract infections: new insights into a common problem. Postgrad Med J 81: 83–86.
4. Chang SL, Shortliffe LD (2006) Pediatric urinary tract infections. Pediatr Clin N Am 53: 379–400.
5. Mittal R, Aggarwal S, Sharma S, Chhibber S, Harjai K (2009) Urinary tract infections caused by *Pseudomonas aeruginosa*: A minireview. Journal Infect Public Health 2: 101–111.
6. Damron FH, Goldberg JB (2012) Proteolytic regulation of alginate overproduction in *Pseudomonas aeruginosa*. Mol Microbiol 84: 595–607.
7. Hogardt M, Heesemann J (2013) Microevolution of *Pseudomonas aeruginosa* to a chronic pathogen of the cystic fibrosis lung. Curr Top Microbiol 358: 91–118.
8. Tamma PD, Cosgrove SE, Maragakis LL (2012) Combination therapy for treatment of infections with gram-negative bacteria. Clin Microbiol Rev 25: 450–470.
9. Breidenstein EB, La Fuente-Núñez C de, Hancock RE (2011) *Pseudomonas aeruginosa*: all roads lead to resistance. Trends Microbiol 19: 419–426.
10. Folkesson A, Jelsbak L, Yang L, Johansen HK, Ciofu O, et al. (2012) Adaptation of *Pseudomonas aeruginosa* to the cystic fibrosis airway: an evolutionary perspective. Nat Rev Micro 10: 841–851.
11. Hoboth C, Hoffmann R, Eichner A, Henke C, Schmoldt S, et al. (2009) Dynamics of adaptive microevolution of hypermutable *Pseudomonas aeruginosa* during chronic pulmonary infection in patients with cystic fibrosis. J Infect Dis 200: 118–130.
12. Munger J, Bennett BD, Parikh A, Feng X, McArdle J, et al. (2008) Systems-level metabolic flux profiling identifies fatty acid synthesis as a target for antiviral therapy. Nat Biotechnol 26: 1179–1186.
13. Kelleher JK (2001) Flux estimation using isotopic tracers: Common ground for metabolic physiology and metabolic engineering. Metab Eng 3: 100–110.
14. Kohlstedt M, Becker J, Wittmann C (2010) Metabolic fluxes and beyond—systems biology understanding and engineering of microbial metabolism. Appl Microbiol Biotechnol 88: 1065–1075.
15. Wittmann C (2007) Fluxome analysis using GC-MS. Microb Cell Fact 6: 6.
16. Tielen P, Narten M, Rosin N, Biegler I, Haddad I, et al. (2011) Genotypic and phenotypic characterization of *Pseudomonas aeruginosa* isolates from urinary tract infections. Int J Med Microbiol 301: 282–292.
17. Stover CK, Pham XQ, Erwin AL, Mizoguchi SD, Warrener P, et al. (2000) Complete genome sequence of *Pseudomonas aeruginosa* PAO1, an opportunistic pathogen. Nature 406: 959–964.
18. Dohnt K, Sauer M, Müller M, Atallah K, Weidemann M, et al. (2011) An in vitro urinary tract catheter system to investigate biofilm development in catheter-associated urinary tract infections. J Microbiol Meth 87: 302–308.
19. Schneider K, Schütz V, John GT, Heinzle E (2010) Optical device for parallel online measurement of dissolved oxygen and pH in shake flask cultures. Bioprocess Biosyst Eng 33: 541–547.
20. Kind S, Becker J, Wittmann C (2013) Increased lysine production by flux coupling of the tricarboxylic acid cycle and the lysine biosynthetic pathway—Metabolic engineering of the availability of succinyl-CoA in *Corynebacterium glutamicum*. Metab Eng 15: 184–195.
21. Fürch T, Preusse M, Tomasch J, Zech H, Wagner-Döbler I, et al. (2009) Metabolic fluxes in the central carbon metabolism of *Dinoroseobacter shibae* and *Phaeobacter gallaeciensis*, two members of the marine *Roseobacter* clade. BMC Microbiol 9: 209.
22. Kretzschmar U, Khodaverdi V, Jeoung J, Görisch H (2008) Function and transcriptional regulation of the isocitrate lyase in *Pseudomonas aeruginosa*. Arch Microbiol 190: 151–158.
23. Wittmann C, Hans M, Heinzle E (2002) In vivo analysis of intracellular amino acid labelings by GC/MS. Anal Biochem 307: 379–382.
24. Oberhardt MA, Puchałka J, Martins dos Santos VAP, Papin JA, Bourne PE (2011) Reconciliation of genome-scale metabolic reconstructions for comparative systems analysis. PLoS Comput Biol 7: e1001116.
25. Kanehisa M, Goto S, Sato Y, Furumichi M, Tanabe M (2011) KEGG for integration and interpretation of large-scale molecular data sets. Nucleic Acids Res 40: D109–D114.
26. Winsor GL, Lam DKW, Fleming L, Lo R, Whiteside MD, et al. (2010) *Pseudomonas* genome database: improved comparative analysis and population genomics capability for *Pseudomonas* genomes. Nucleic Acids Res 39: D596–D600.
27. Blank LM, Ionidis G, Ebert BE, Bühler B, Schmid A (2008) Metabolic response of *Pseudomonas putida* during redox biocatalysis in the presence of a second octanol phase. FEBS J 275: 5173–5190.
28. Neidhardt FC, Ingraham JL, Schächter M (1990) Physiology of the bacterial cell: a molecular approach. Sunderland, MA: Sinauer.
29. Mann EE, Wozniak DJ (2012) *Pseudomonas* biofilm matrix composition and niche biology. FEMS Microbiol Rev 36: 893–916.
30. Filisetti-Cozzi TM, Carpita NC (1991) Measurement of uronic acids without interference from neutral sugars. Anal Biochem 197: 157–162.
31. Quek L, Wittmann C, Nielsen LK, Krömer JO (2009) OpenFLUX: efficient modelling software for ^{13}C-based metabolic flux analysis. Microb Cell Fact 8: 25.
32. van Winden WA, Wittmann C, Heinzle E, Heijnen JJ (2002) Correcting mass isotopomer distributions for naturally occurring isotopes. Biotechnol Bioeng 80: 477–479.
33. Wittmann C, Heinzle E (2002) Genealogy profiling through strain improvement by using metabolic network analysis: metabolic flux genealogy of several generations of lysine-producing corynebacteria. Appl Environ Microb 68: 5843–5859.
34. Poblete-Castro I, Binger D, Rodrigues A, Becker J, Martins Dos Santos VA, et al. (2013) In-silico-driven metabolic engineering of *Pseudomonas putida* for enhanced production of poly-hydroxyalkanoates. Metab Eng 15:113–123

35. Melzer G, Esfandabadi M, Franco-Lara E, Wittmann C (2009) Flux design: In silico design of cell factories based on correlation of pathway fluxes to desired properties. BMC Syst Biol 3: 120.
36. Pearson K (1901) On lines and planes of closest fit to systems of points in space. Philos Mag 2: 559–572.
37. Dash M, Liu H, Scheuermann P, Tan KL (2003) Fast hierarchical clustering and its validation. Data Knowl Eng 44: 109–138.
38. Zamboni N, Sauer U (2004) Model-independent fluxome profiling from ^{2}H and ^{13}C experiments for metabolic variant discrimination. Genome Biol 5: R99.
39. Eschbach E, Schreiber K, Trunk K, Buer J, Jahn D, et al. (2006) Long-term anaerobic survival of the opportunistic pathogen *Pseudomonas aeruginosa* via pyruvate fermentation. J Bacteriol. 186: 4596–4604.64.
40. Flamholz A, Noor E, Bar-Even A, Liebermeister W, Milo R (2013) Glycolytic strategy as a tradeoff between energy yield and protein cost. P Natl A Sci 110: 10039–10044.
41. Romano A, Conway T (1996) Evolution of carbohydrate metabolic pathways. Res Microb 147: 448–455.
42. Chavarría M, Nikel PI, Pérez-Pantoja D, Lorenzo V de (2013) The Entner-Doudoroff pathway empowers *Pseudomonas putida* KT2440 with a high tolerance to oxidative stress. Environ Microbiol 15: 1772–1785.
43. Storz G, Tartaglia LA, Farr SB, Ames BN (1990) Bacterial defenses against oxidative stress. Trends Genet 6: 363–368.
44. Storz G, Imlay JA (1999) Oxidative stress. Curr Opin Microb 2: 188–194.
45. Singh R, Mailloux RJ, Puiseux-Dao S, Appanna VD (2007) Oxidative stress evokes a metabolic adaptation that favors increased NADPH synthesis and decreased NADH production in *Pseudomonas fluorescens*. J Bacteriol 189: 6665–6675.
46. Krömer JO, Bolten CJ, Heinzle E, Schröder H, Wittmann C (2008) Physiological response of *Corynebacterium glutamicum* to oxidative stress induced by deletion of the transcriptional repressor McbR. Microbiology 154: 3917–3930.
47. Chen PR, Brugarolas P, He C (2011) Redox signaling in human pathogens. Antioxid & Redox Sign 14: 1107–1118.
48. Hogardt M, Heesemann J (2010) Adaptation of *Pseudomonas aeruginosa* during persistence in the cystic fibrosis lung. Int J Med Microbiol 300: 557–562.
49. Le Gac M, Plucain J, Hindré T, Lenski RE, Schneider D (2012) Ecological and evolutionary dynamics of coexisting lineages during a long-term experiment with *Escherichia coli*. Proc Natl Acad Sci U S A. 109: 9487–9492.
50. Hindré T, Knibbe C, Beslon G, Schneider D (2012) New insights into bacterial adaptation through in vivo and in silico experimental evolution. Nat Rev Microbiol.10:352–365.
51. Kondrashov FA, Koonin EV, Morgunov IG, Finogenova TV, Kondrashova MN (2006) Evolution of glyoxylate cycle enzymes in *Metazoa*: Evidence of multiple horizontal transfer events and pseudogene formation. Biol Direct 1: 31.
52. Smith RA, Gunsalus IC (1957) Isocitritase; enzyme properties and reaction equilibrium. J Biol Chem 229: 305–319.
53. Wittmann C, Weber J, Betiku E, Krömer J, Böhm D, et al. (2007) Response of fluxome and metabolome to temperature-induced recombinant protein synthesis in *Escherichia coli*. J Biotechnol 132: 375–384.
54. Reinscheid DJ, Eikmanns BJ, Sahm H (1994) Characterization of the isocitrate lyase gene from *Corynebacterium glutamicum* and biochemical analysis of the enzyme. J Bacteriol 176: 3474–3483.
55. Dunn MF, Ramirez-Trujillo JA, Hernandez-Lucas I (2009) Major roles of isocitrate lyase and malate synthase in bacterial and fungal pathogenesis. Microbiology 155: 3166–3175.
56. Son MS, Matthews WJ, Kang Y, Nguyen DT, Hoang TT (2007) In vivo evidence of *Pseudomonas aeruginosa* nutrient acquisition and pathogenesis in the lungs of cystic fibrosis patients. Infection and Immunity 75: 5313–5324.
57. Lindsey TL, Hagins JM, Sokol PA, Silo-Suh LA (2008) Virulence determinants from a cystic fibrosis isolate of *Pseudomonas aeruginosa* include isocitrate lyase. Microbiology 154: 1616–1627.
58. McKinney JD, Bentrup KH zu, Muñoz-Elías EJ, Miczak A, Chen B, et al. (2000) Persistence of *Mycobacterium tuberculosis* in macrophages and mice requires the glyoxylate shunt enzyme isocitrate lyase. Nature 406: 735–738.
59. Fang FC, Libby SJ, Castor ME, Fung AM (2005) Isocitrate lyase (AceA) is required for *Salmonella* persistence but not for acute lethal infection in mice. Infect Immun 73: 2547–2549.
60. Wall DM, Duffy PS, DuPont C, Prescott JF, Meijer WG (2005) Isocitrate lyase activity is required for virulence of the intracellular pathogen *Rhodococcus equi*. Infect Immun 73: 6736–6741.
61. Hamood AN, Griswold JA, Duhan CM (1996) Production of extracellular virulence factors by *Pseudomonas aeruginosa* isolates obtained from tracheal, urinary tract, and wound infections. J Surg Res 61: 425–432.
62. Rumbaugh K, Griswold J, Hamood A (1999) *Pseudomonas aeruginosa* strains obtained from patients with tracheal, urinary tract and wound infection: variations in virulence factors and virulence genes. J Hosp Infect 43: 211–218.
63. Rosenbloom J, Koo H, Howard PS, Mecham R, Macarak EJ (1995) Elastic fibers and their role in bladder extracellular matrix. Adv Exp Med Biol 385: 161–72.
64. Hellerstein MK (2008) A critique of the molecular target-based drug discovery paradigm based on principles of metabolic control: Advantages of pathway-based discovery. Metab Eng 10: 1–9.
65. Fuhrer T, Fischer E, Sauer U (2005) Experimental identification and quantification of glucose metabolism in seven bacterial species. J Bacteriol 187: 1581–1590.
66. Marx A, Graaf AA de, Wiechert W, Eggeling L, Sahm H (1996) Determination of the fluxes in the central metabolism of *Corynebacterium glutamicum* by nuclear magnetic resonance spectroscopy combined with metabolite balancing. Biotechnol Bioeng 49: 111–129.

Asymptomatic Bacteriuria *Escherichia coli* Are Live Biotherapeutics for UTI

Charles N. Rudick[1¶], Aisha K. Taylor[1¶¤], Ryan E. Yaggie[1], Anthony J. Schaeffer[1], David J. Klumpp[1,2*]

1 Department of Urology, Feinberg School of Medicine, Northwestern University, Chicago, Illinois, United States of America, 2 Microbiology-Immunology, Feinberg School of Medicine, Northwestern University, Chicago, Illinois, United States of America

Abstract

Urinary tract infections (UTI) account for approximately 8 million clinic visits annually with symptoms that include acute pelvic pain, dysuria, and irritative voiding. Empiric UTI management with antimicrobials is complicated by increasing antimicrobial resistance among uropathogens, but live biotherapeutics products (LBPs), such as asymptomatic bacteriuria (ASB) strains of *E. coli*, offer the potential to circumvent antimicrobial resistance. Here we evaluated ASB *E. coli* as LBPs, relative to ciprofloxacin, for efficacy against infection and visceral pain in a murine UTI model. Visceral pain was quantified as tactile allodynia of the pelvic region in response to mechanical stimulation with von Frey filaments. Whereas ciprofloxacin promoted clearance of uropathogenic *E. coli* (UPEC), it did not reduce pelvic tactile allodynia, a measure of visceral pain. In contrast, ASB *E. coli* administered intravesically or intravaginally provided comparable reduction of allodynia similar to intravesical lidocaine. Moreover, ASB *E. coli* were similarly effective against UTI allodynia induced by *Proteus mirabilis, Enterococccus faecalis* and *Klebsiella pneumoniae*. Therefore, ASB *E. coli* have anti-infective activity comparable to the current standard of care yet also provide superior analgesia. These studies suggest that ASB *E. coli* represent novel LBPs for UTI symptoms.

Editor: Neil A. Bhowmick, Cedars Sinai Medical Center, United States of America

Funding: These studies were funded by the National Institute of Diabetes and Digestive and Kidney Diseases (http://www.niddk.nih.gov/Pages/default.aspx). Funding was through awards R01 DK042648 and U01 DK8234201 to D.J.K. and A.J.S. Award U01 DK8234201 is within the Multi-Disciplinary Approaches to Chronic Pelvic Pain Research Network (MAPP, www.mappnetwork.org). This work was approved for publication by the MAPP Publications Committee. The funders had no role in study design, data collection and analysis, decision to publish, or preparation of the manuscript.

Competing Interests: The authors have the following interests: Northwestern University holds a patent for skewing immune responses by strains with altered LPS structures (Billips et al., Live-attenuated compositions for bacterial infections, US 8,709,444 B2, issued 29 April, 2014) and a pending application for pain therapies based on analgesic bacteria (Rudick et al., Compositions and methods for treatment of pain, provisional 61.450,937, filed 09 March, 2011). D.J.K. and A.J.S. are incorporated in the State of Illinois as ProbioTx, Inc. and pursue commercial development of strains described here, with the support of Northwestern University and the Chicago Innovation Mentors program. D.J.K. and A.J.S. are also officers in Gold Coast Therapeutics, Inc., a company targeting mast cells in urologic disease. All proprietary bacterial strains from Northwestern University described in provisional patent 61.450,937 and this article will be shared upon request through Northwestern's INVO under a Material Transfer Agreement authorizing non-commercial use.

* Email: d-klumpp@northwestern.edu

¤ Current address: Department of Urology, Case Western Reserve, Cleveland, OH, United States of America

¶ These authors contributed equally to this work.

Introduction

Urinary tract infection (UTI) is the second-most common infectious disease, resulting in millions of cases in the U.S. annually and costing billions of dollars for associated treatment [1,2]. The standard of care for UTI is antimicrobial therapy, where such therapy effectively sterilizes the urine of susceptible bacteria [3]. Unfortunately, uropathogenic bacteria are increasingly resistant to frontline antimicrobials, and multi-drug resistant strains are emerging rapidly [4,5]. In addition to waning efficacy due to resistance, it is unclear that acute antimicrobial therapy is sufficient to prevent recurrent UTI. Data from murine models and clinical studies demonstrate that UPEC and other uropathogens establish quiescent reservoirs within bladder urothelium that can trigger subsequent acute infection [6]. These quiescent reservoirs are resistant to antimicrobial therapy, indicating a need for alternative approaches. While antimicrobial therapies are effective at sterilizing urine of susceptible bacteria, it is unclear that antimicrobial activity is the basis for symptomatic relief of UTI [4]. Indeed, recent studies in murine UTI suggest that symptom kinetics are mediated by initial receptor-mediated responses to bacterial surface molecules, not bacterial loads [7].

Given the rapid rise in antimicrobial resistance and the potential for collateral damage caused by conventional therapies [8–11], alternative approaches are needed, and live biotherapeutic products (LBPs) such as vaccines and probiotics offer the potential to treat UTIs without concerns about antimicrobial resistance. Lactobacilli are normally a major component of the vaginal microflora of fertile women that act as a natural barrier against ascending infection by uropathogens [12]. Clinical trials have demonstrated that vaginal application of *L. crispatus* reduces UTI occurrence, presumably by restoring or augmenting the natural

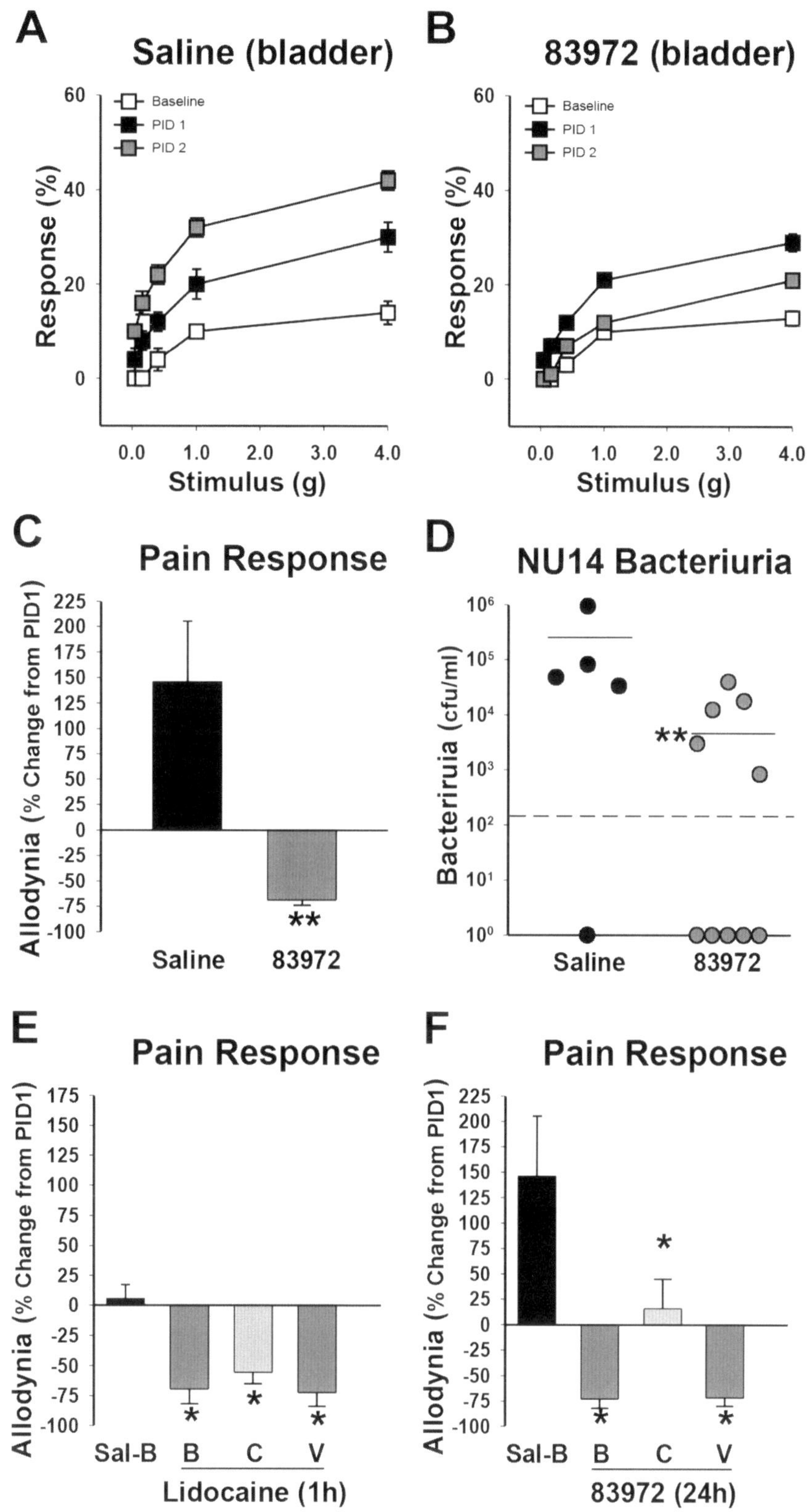

Figure 1. *E. coli* 83972 attenuates NU14-induced bacteriuria and pelvic pain. A) Referred visceral hyperalgesia was measured as responses to mechanical stimulation of the pelvic region with von Frey filaments of 5 intensities. Responses were quantified at baseline, PID1 following NU14 infection, and 24 hours following of saline (n = 5) or 83972 (n = 10) instillation (PID2). B) NU14-infected mice exhibited a significant decrease in allodynia 24 hours following 83972 instillation. C) Percent increase in allodynia from PID1 was 146.2% in saline-treated mice, but decreased by over 68.9% in 83972-treated mice ($P<0.01$). D) Mice treated with 83972 exhibited a significantly less NU14 bacteriuria compared to saline-treated mice ($P<0.01$). Dashed line represents limit of detection. E) At PID1, NU14-infected mice were instilled with saline into the bladder or 2% lidocaine in the

bladder, vaginal introitus or colon. Allodynia was significantly reduced at 1 h after lidocaine into any compartment, relative to bladder saline (*$P < 0.05$; n = 9 saline, n = 10 bladder lidocaine, n = 11 colon lidocaine, n = 12 vaginal lidocaine). F) NU14-infected mice exhibited increased allodynia 24 hours after bladder instillation of saline, relative to PID1 (n = 10). Allodynia was significantly decreased at 24 hours following 83972 instillation into the bladder, colon or vaginal introitus (*$P<0.05$, n = 10 all groups). Data are reported as the mean ± SEM (A–C, E & F).

protective barrier against ascending infection [13–15]. Alternatively, asymptomatic bacteriuria (ASB) *E. coli* have been harnessed to prevent UTI. Since the American Urologic Association Guidelines are to not treat ASB, ASB *E. coli* have been instilled into patients to occupy this biological niche and thereby prevent infection by "bacterial interference" [16]. Clinical inoculation of the prototypic ASB *E. coli* strain 83972 was shown to significantly reduce UTI among spinal cord injury patients with chronic indwelling or intermittent catheterization while protecting patients with incomplete bladder emptying from recurrent UTI [17]. Similarly, clinical trials with HU2117, a P fimbriae-deficient mutant of 83972, demonstrated significantly increased time between symptomatic UTI in neurogenic bladder patients [18]. These studies with 83972 suggest that ASB *E. coli* strains possess biologic activities that thwart uropathogens and/or alter UTI symptoms. These clinical studies were not designed to test the bacterial interference hypothesis directly so mechanism of ASB *E. coli* impact UTI pathogenesis is unknown.

We recently characterized pelvic pain responses in a murine model of UTI. Using tactile allodynia as a behavioral correlate to pelvic pain, we quantified pelvic allodynia in response to UPEC strain NU14 or ASB strain 83972. NU14 induced pelvic allodynia that was not observed in response to 83972, yet similar inflammatory responses were induced by either bacterial infection or by lipopolysaccharide (LPS) purified from either strain [7,19]. Although neither instillation of 83972 nor its purified LPS induced pelvic allodynia, we found that 83972 LPS significantly reduced allodynia associated with NU14 infection, suggesting that ASB *E. coli* possess analgesic activity [19]. Here, we evaluated ASB *E. coli* strains for efficacy treating colonization of the urinary tract by uropathogens and for efficacy treating pain associated with UTI. We found that ASB *E. coli* exhibit anti-infective and analgesic activities in murine UTI, suggesting a potential use of ASB *E. coli*-based LBPs for treating UTI and other symptom-based disorders.

Methods

Animals

Adult female mice C57BL/6J 10–14 weeks of age were purchased from Jackson Laboratory. All experiments were performed using protocols approved by Northwestern University Animal Care and Use Committee as previously described [7,19].

Bacterial strains

NU14 is a clinical isolate of *E. coli* originally obtained from the urine of a cystitis patient and is considered archetypal for UPEC [20]. ASB strain 83972 was isolated from a young Swedish girl who was infected for at least 3 years without symptoms [21,22] and is one of the most extensively characterized ABS strains [23,24]. ASB *E. coli* strains were previously collected as a panel of consecutive clinical isolates [25] or isolates from the Northwestern Urology Clinic for the purposes of this study. *Proteus mirabilis*, *Enterococcus faecalis* and *Klebsiella pneumoniae* were isolated from discarded urine of uncomplicated cystitis patients. All clinical isolates obtained for this study were identified by standard microbiologic testing, including Gram staining and Microscan (Siemens Healthcare). Bacteria were cultured by serial passage in Luria broth at 37° in static broth [26,27]. *E. coli* strains were differentiated by plating onto selective agar: NU14 is resistant to streptomycin, 2–12 is resistant to streptomycin/ampicillin, and 83972 is resistant to chloramphenicol.

Infection and behavioral testing

Female mice were anesthetized with isoflurane and instilled via transurethral catheter with a volume of 10 µl containing 1×10^8 CFU bacteria in saline [28]. Following termination of the experiment the bladders were harvested, homogenized and plated on agar with or without antibiotic selection for colonization. Mice were tested prior to bacterial infection (baseline) and up to PID 20. Referred hyperalgesia and tactile allodynia was tested, as previously described [29,30], using von Frey filaments applied to the abdomen [29,30].

Treatments

Lidocaine was administered as a 2% lidocaine solution in water that was instilled via a Hamilton syringe and polyethylene catheter as previously described [30]. Ciprofloxacin (10 mg/kg/0.15 ml) drug therapy was administered daily as a 3-day course via I.P. via injection.

Statistical analyses

Colonization, inflammation and behavioral data were analyzed with the student t-test or a Kruskal-Wallis test followed by Dunn's post test or repeated ANOVA followed by a Dunnett's post test using Prism software from GraphPad Inc. as appropriate. A value of $P<0.05$ was considered statistically significant.

Ethics statement

These studies were conducted under Northwestern University IACUC protocols 2010–1788 and 2009–1677.

Results

ASB isolate 83972 attenuates UTI allodynia and bacteriuria

Since 83972 LPS attenuated UTI-associated allodynia [19], we hypothesized that intact 83972 bacteria would exhibit similar analgesic activity. To test this, female B6 mice were instilled with the UPEC strain NU14 via transurethral catheter to initiate UTI; after 24 h, mice were instilled with saline or 83972. Allodynia was quantified at baseline and daily throughout the experiment by assessing responsiveness to stimulation of the pelvic region with a graded series of von Frey filaments [30]. Saline-treated mice exhibited significant pelvic allodynia (Figs. 1A and C) relative to 83972-treated mice that showed a significantly reduced allodynia (Figs. 1B and C, $P<0.01$). Since 83972 is thought to prevent UTI by bacterial interference, we also quantified bacteriuria. 83972 significantly reduced urinary NU14, relative to saline instillation (Fig. 1D, $P<0.01$).

ASB isolate 83972 mediates analgesia via crosstalk

We have shown previously that colonic lidocaine attenuates pelvic pain in a neurogenic cystitis model as effectively as intravesical lidocaine, demonstrating organ crosstalk in pelvic pain relief [30]. We used a similar strategy to evaluate whether

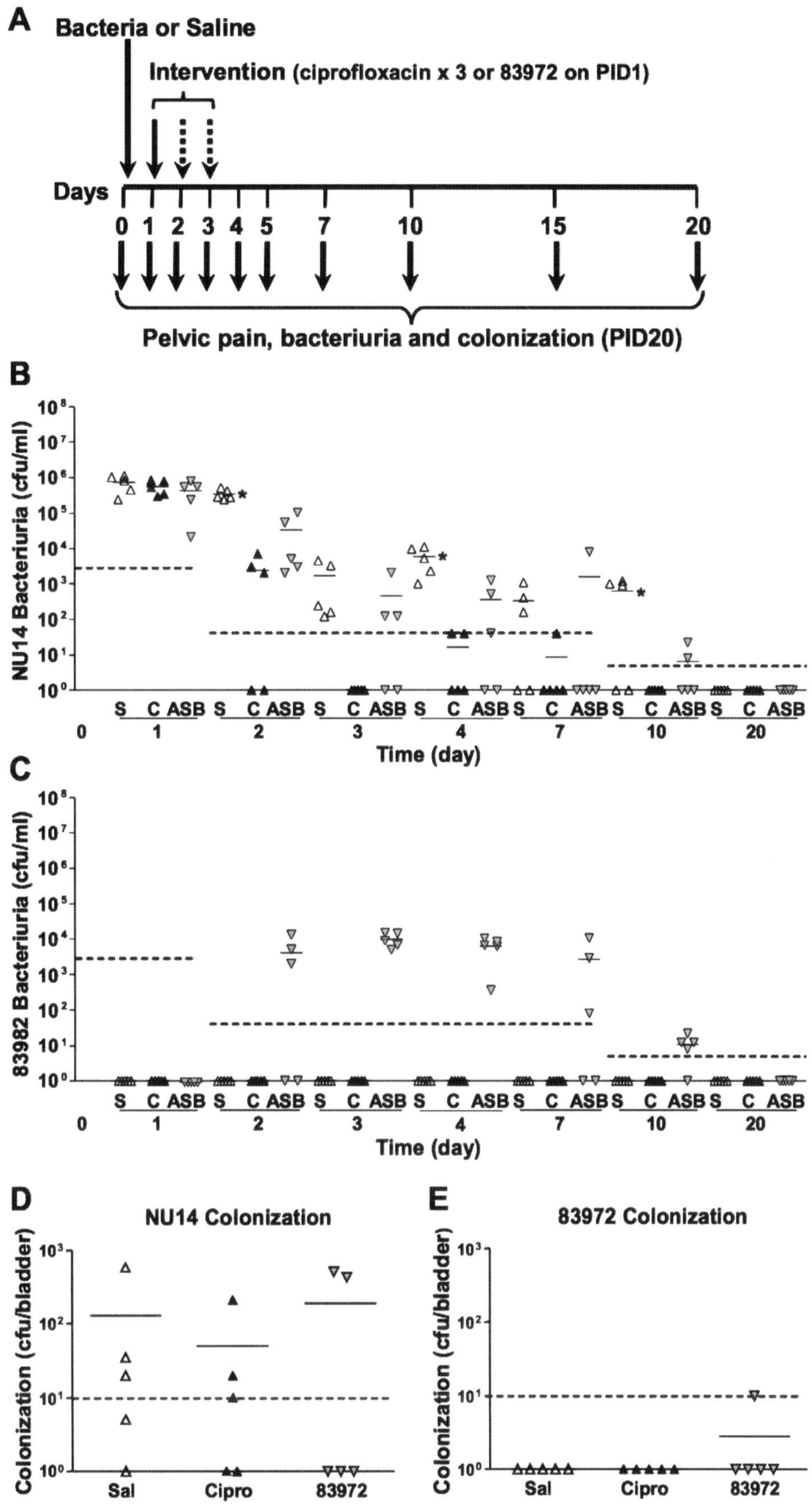

Figure 2. *E. coli* 83972 attenuates NU14 bacteriuria. A) Experimental scheme for assessing efficacy of a single administration of ASB therapy relative to 3-day course of ciprofloxacin (n = 5 for all groups). B) Mice infected with NU14 exhibited a significant decrease in NU14 bacteriuria 24 hours

after initiation of ciprofloxacin (group C, back triangles, PID2, 4, 10), relative to saline-treated mice (group S, white triangles, *P<0.05). A single instillation of 83972 (group ASB, grey inverted triangles) also resulted in a significant decrease in NU14 bacteriuria after 24 hours (PID2, 4, 10, *P< 0.05). C) Urinary 83972 for all three groups during the experiment. D and E) Bladder colonization on PID20 was not significantly different between the groups tested. Dashed lines represent limits of detection.

analgesic activity of ASB *E. coli* was capable of crosstalk during UTI. Allodynia was quantified 1 hour after lidocaine administration to mice that were infected with NU14 24 h prior (Fig. 1E); as a result, allodynia was not increased in the saline group (compare saline group in Fig. 1F). Relative to bladder instillation of saline, 2% lidocaine significantly and similarly attenuated UTI allodynia whether administered into the bladder, colon, or vagina (Fig. 1E, P<0.05). Analgesic activity of 83972 was evaluated at 24 h, and colonic 83972 significantly reduced saline-treated UTI allodynia (Fig. 1F, P<0.05), consistent with our previous findings for colonic modulation of cystitis pain [30]. 83972 significantly and similarly attenuated NU14-induced allodynia when administered intravesically or intravaginally (P<0.05). Remarkably, 83972 analgesic activity was comparable to lidocaine, whether acting directly or via crosstalk from the vagina (compare Figs. 1E and F).

ASB isolate 83972 attenuates bacteriuria comparable to ciprofloxacin

Since 83972 significantly reduced NU14 bacteriuria (Fig. 1D), we evaluated the anti-infective activity of intravesical 83972 relative to a three-day course of ciprofloxacin, a standard clinical regimen for uncomplicated UTI. All three groups exhibited similar levels of bacteriuria at post-infection day 1 (PID1) and had sterile urine by PID20 (Fig. 2B). Mice receiving ciprofloxacin or 83972 exhibited significantly reduced NU14 bacteriuria from PID2, 4 and 10, compared to the saline group (Fig. 2B, P<0.05). 83972 also became transiently established in the urinary tract, as indicated by 83972 bacteriuria from PID2 to PID10 (Fig. 2C). At PID20, most mice exhibited low levels of residual bladder colonization consistent with previous reports [31], no differences in NU14 colonization were observed between bladders of treated and untreated mice, and 83972 was largely cleared (Figs. 2D and E). While not significantly different here, we cannot exclude the possibility that ciprofloxacin therapy would exhibit increased antimicrobial activity relative to 83972 with larger samples. Nonetheless, these data suggest that the antimicrobial activity of ciprofloxacin and the anti-infective activity of 83972 are comparable and are manifested at the level of bacteriuria without fully sterilizing the bladder of bacterial reservoirs.

ASB *E. coli* differentially attenuate UTI allodynia

To determine whether analgesic activity was a unique property of 83972, we screened a panel of ASB *E. coli* strains including 3 strains collected from the Northwestern Urology Clinic for this study and 12 ASB strains from a panel of 54 consecutive clinical isolates [25]. As in Figure 1, mice were instilled with NU14 and then instilled with saline or an ASB panel strain 24 hours later and evaluated for pelvic responsiveness prior to instillation, 24 hours after NU14 instillation, and daily after saline or ASB treatment; strains were then grouped arbitrarily by relative analgesic activity (panels of Fig. 3A). All ASB isolates attenuated NU14-induced pelvic allodynia when compared to saline-instilled controls, but the magnitude of attenuation varied (Figs. 3A & B). While some mice exhibited an increase in pelvic pain 24 hours after infection with an ASB isolate (Fig. 3A, left panel), indicating only modest analgesic activity, they were significantly decreased compared to the saline-instilled control (Fig. 3B, black bars, P<0.05). Eight strains exhibited an intermediate analgesic phenotype, ranging from no increase in allodynia from PID1 to 70% reduction in allodynia (Fig. 3A, middle panel, and Fig. 3B, white bars). A third group was comprised of 6 ASB isolates that displayed a high analgesic phenotype, relative to PID1, attenuating cystitis allodynia from 75% to 85% (Fig. 3A, right panel, and Fig. 3B, grey bars). Since we recently showed that serial infections with could reveal a pain phenotype in an *E. coli* strain otherwise exhibiting no pain phenotype [7], three serial infections were performed with strains from the ASB panel (Fig. 3C). None of the ASB isolates tested induced pain following serial infections, consistent with our recent report that serial infection with 83972 did not induce pain [7]. These data demonstrate that ASB *E. coli* exhibit a range of analgesic phenotypes, and that the prototypic ASB strain, 83972, possesses a highly analgesic phenotype. However, since strain 2–12 had the greatest analgesic activity against cystitis pain, 85%, we focused on 2–12 for further study.

ASB isolate 2–12 is superior to ciprofloxacin for analgesia

We evaluated the effect of 2–12 on NU14-induced cystitis pain, relative to sham treatment or a 3-day course of ciprofloxacin using the schemed depicted in Figure 2A. Since we observed that 83972 could exert analgesic activity via crosstalk (Fig. 1F), we also evaluated 2–12 administered intravesically and intravaginally. Control groups instilled with saline then treated with 3 injections of saline or ciprofloxacin did not develop detectable allodynia (Fig. 4A). Consistent with previous observations [19], mice instilled with NU14 developed allodynia that decayed over two or three weeks, but ciprofloxacin therapy did not reduce allodynia better than saline during the course of the experiment (Fig. 4A). In contrast, mice receiving a single therapeutic dose of ASB isolate 2–12 exhibited a rapid and significant decrease in allodynia, whether that dose was administered to the bladder or vaginal introitus (Fig. 4A, P<0.05).

ASB isolate 2–12 is a superior analgesic against diverse uropathogens

Since ASB *E. coli* strains possess anti-infective and analgesic activity against UPEC, we examined effects against non-*E. coli* uropathogens. Allodynia was quantified in murine models of UTI Gram-positive bacteria, and responses to 2–12 therapy were compared with saline and ciprofloxacin. A single clinical isolate of *Proteus mirabilis* (PM1, Gram negative), *Enteroccus faecalis* (EF1, Gram positive) and *Klebsiella pneumoniae* (KP1, Gram negative) was obtained from urines of the Northwestern Urology Clinic and typed using standard microbiologic procedures. PM1-induced acute pelvic allodynia that was unaltered by a 3-day course of ciprofloxacin (Fig. 4B). However, PM1-induced allodynia was significantly attenuated in mice instilled with 2–12 on PID3 and PID4 (P<0.05). Similarly, 2–12 significantly reduced allodynia associated with EF1 or KP1 infection (Figs. 4C and D, respectively, P<0.05). Thus, 2–12 exhibits superior analgesic activity to current antimicrobial therapy in multiple urine UTI models.

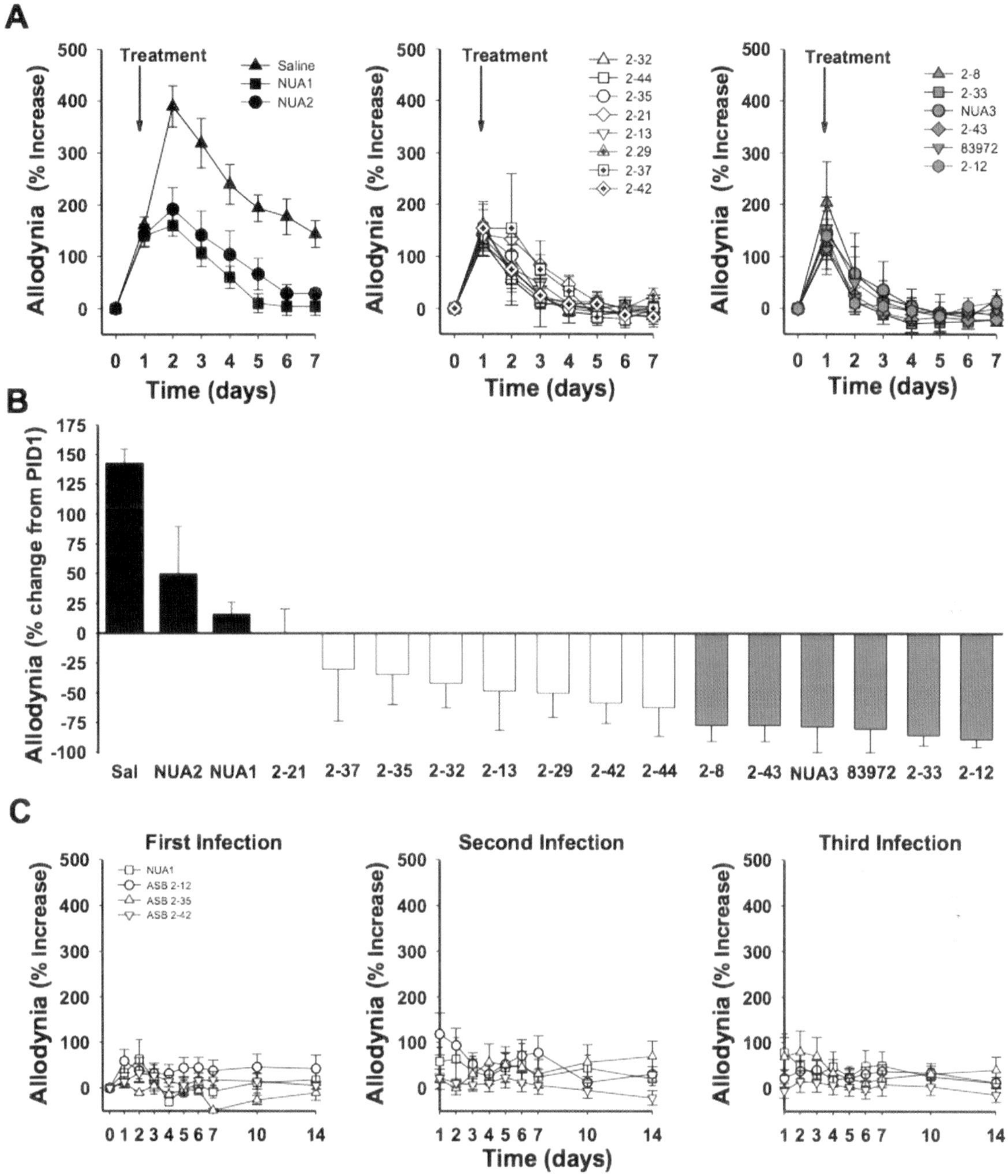

Figure 3. ASB strains differentially attenuate UTI visceral pain. Modulation of UTI visceral pain by a panel of 16 ASB *E. coli* strains. A) Mice were infected with NU14 and then instilled with saline or ASB *E. coli* at PID1, and allodynia was quantified through PID7 (n = 6 for all groups). For clarity, timecourses of allodynia for all 17 conditions were divided among 3 panels. All 16 ASB strains attenuated NU14-induced pelvic pain compared to the saline treated group. B) The relative analgesic activity of ASB strains was arbitrary grouped according to the magnitude of analgesia: strains with analgesic relative to saline but increased allodynia from PID1 (black bars), those that exhibited no increase in allodynia from PID1 to less than 75% reduction in visceral pain from PID1 (white bars), and those that exhibited greater than 75% reduction (gray bars). C) Representative ASB strains from each group in (B) were used in serial infections at two-week intervals. Serial infection did not induce allodynia. Data are reported as the mean ± SEM.

Discussion

Our findings demonstrate that ASB *E. coli* 83972 exhibit anti-infective activities comparable to ciprofloxacin in a murine UTI model. While ciprofloxacin promoted clearance of uropathogenic *E. coli* (UPEC), it did not reduce pelvic tactile allodynia, a measure of visceral pain. In contrast, ASB *E. coli* administered intravesically or intravaginally provided comparable reduction of allodynia similar to intravesical lidocaine. Moreover, ASB *E. coli* were similarly effective against UTI allodynia induced by *Proteus mirabilis*, *Enterococcus faecalis* and *Klebsiella pneumoniae*. Therefore, ASB *E. coli* have anti-infective activity comparable to the current standard of care yet also provide superior analgesia suggesting that ASB *E. coli* represent novel LBPs for UTI..

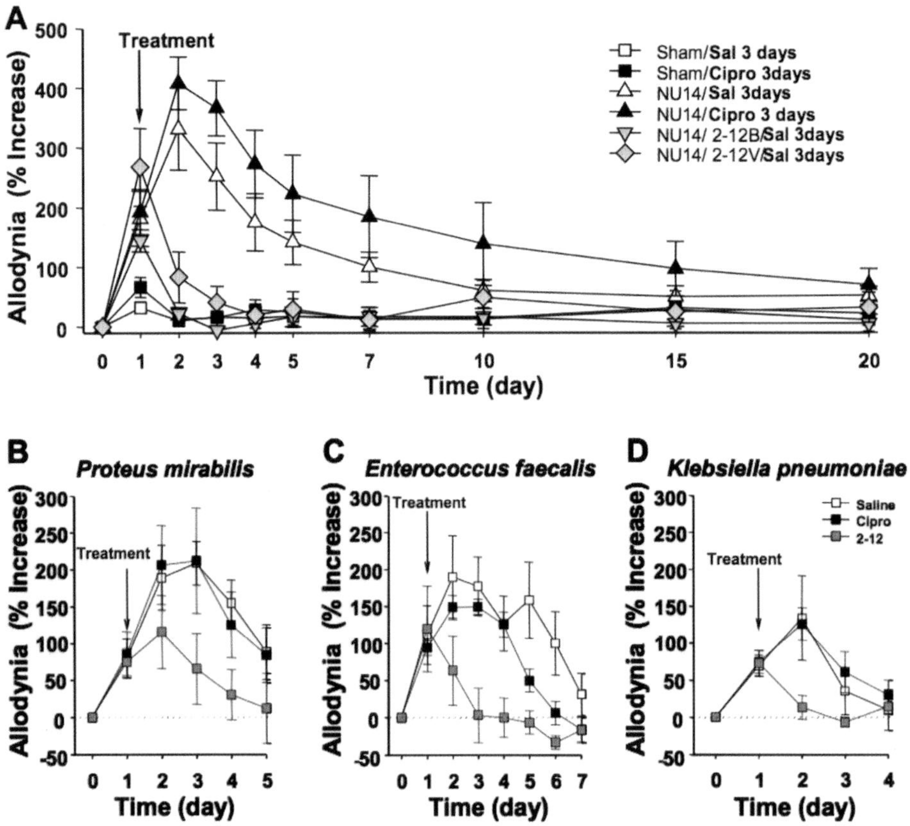

Figure 4. ASB *E. coli* isolate 2–12 rapidly attenuates UTI visceral pain of diverse uropathogens. A) Allodynia was quantified daily in groups of sham- or NU14-infected mice that were then treated at PID1 with saline, a three-day course of ciprofloxacin, or a single dose of intravesical or intravaginal 2–12 as described in Figure 2A (n = 8 in all groups except the 2–12 intravaginal group where n = 6). NU14-infected mice exhibited a significant decrease in pelvic pain 24 hours following treatment with 2–12 via the bladder or vaginal introitus ($P<0.05$). Allodynia was quantified in mice infected via transureathral catheter with *Proteus mirabilis* (PM1), *Enterocccus faecalis* (EF1) and *Klebsiella pneumoniae* (KP1) and then treated with a three-day course of ciprofloxacin initiated at PID1 or a single intravesical dose of 2–12 (n = 5). B) PM1 induced pelvic allodynia that was significantly attenuated on PID3 and PID4 by 2–12 treatment, relative to the ciprofloxacin or saline groups ($P<0.05$). C) EF1 induced allodynia that was significantly attenuated on PID2-PID4 by 2–12 treatment, relative to ciprofloxacin or saline groups ($P<0.05$). Allodynia was also significantly reduced on PID5–6 compared to the saline group ($P<0.05$). D) KP1 induced allodynia that was significantly attenuated on PID2 by 2–12 treatment, relative to ciprofloxacin or saline groups ($P<0.05$).

UTI is associated with a leukocytic influx dominated by neutrophils to drive clearance of UPEC [32,33]. Quantifying urinary myeloperoxidase (MPO) as a marker of bladder neutrophil influx, we previously found that 83972 and UPEC strain NU14 similarly induce MPO and inflammation [7,19]. We also observed that purified LPS preparations from 83972 and NU14 resulted in similar levels of neutrophil recruitment when instilled into the bladder and similarly activated splenic macrophages in culture [19], so it is unlikely that 83972 markedly enhances neutrophil influx. Another potential mechanism is the rapid urothelial apoptotic host defense response that is induced by the interaction of the UPEC type 1 pilus adhesin (FimH) with uroplakins [20,34–36], however 83972 do not express type 1 pili. We speculate that one anti-infective effect of ASB *E. coli* is to function as an adjuvant that enhances immune responses to uropathogens.

Ciprofloxacin and other antimicrobials sterilize the urine of susceptible bacteria, but the relationship between antimicrobial activity and symptomatic relief is increasingly unclear. A recent study revealed that ibuprofen was as effective as ciprofloxacin at ameliorating symptoms of dysuria and frequency during acute, uncomplicated UTI [37]. This is consistent with previous observations that UTI symptoms resolve spontaneously in the majority of patients and do not correlate with urinary bacterial loads [38,39]. We observed that ciprofloxacin did not alter pelvic allodynia in murine UTI (Fig. 4A), reinforcing clinical findings and consistent with our recent report that pelvic allodynia can persist long after bacterial clearance [7]. In contrast, we find ASB *E. coli* significantly reduce UPEC-induced allodynia, suggesting analgesic activity that is not unique to a single ASB strain but rather but varies across a spectrum. We find several aspects of this analgesic effect remarkable. First, ASB *E. coli* can exhibit analgesic activity comparable to intravesical lidocaine (Figs. 1E and F), suggesting clinical utility. Second, the significant reduction in allodynia when 83972 was administered in the vagina or colon indicates that the analgesic activity against UPEC can be mediated via organ crosstalk, similar to lidocaine (Fig. 1E and F; [30]). The physiologic basis for organ crosstalk is visceral convergence of sensory pathways among pelvic organs such as the bladder and bowel [40–42] and this observation of organ crosstalk in ASB *E. coli* analgesia is evidence that ASB *E. coli* may mediate effects independent of bacterial interference. Since prior clinical studies of 83972 and HU2117 demonstrated significant reduction in symptomatic events in patients prone to recurrent UTI [17,18,43], an alternative explanation for those findings is that

83972 analgesic activity masked symptoms that would have been scored as a symptomatic recurrence. Third, 2–12 reduced allodynia induced by infection with non-UPEC uropathogens, demonstrating that ASB *E. coli* exhibit analgesic activity against diverse insults. Since we reported that LPS purified from 83972 reduced allodynia in NU14 infection [19], it is likely that the analgesic activity of other ASB *E. coli* strains is generally mediated by LPS through the cognate receptor TLR4 [7,19].

The anti-infective and analgesic properties of ASB *E. coli* described here suggest several clinical applications, in addition to the use as a prophylactic for catheterized patients as reported previously [16,43]. The anti-infective activity of 83972 was comparable to ciprofloxacin in promoting clearance for acute UTI, suggesting that ASB *E. coli* could be administered as a therapy of uncomplicated UTI. In both acute and recurrent UTI, the analgesic effect would be an advantage of ASB *E. coli* therapy over conventional antimicrobials. Finally, we observe that ASB *E. coli* reduced allodynia associated with diverse acute insults, suggesting general analgesic effects could be exploited to treat non-infectious pain conditions. Patients suffering chronic pelvic pain of interstitial cystitis/bladder pain syndrome (IC) can gain temporary relief from intravesical lidocaine [44]. Since ASB strains exert analgesic activity comparable to lidocaine and mediate these effects via organ crosstalk, ASB *E. coli* therapy could be used for chronic pelvic pain conditions such as IC, vulvodynia, or endometriosis.

The U.S. FDA classifies whole, live microorganisms that exhibit drug activities as LBPs. LBPs are subject to FDA oversight using the same Investigational New Drug regulatory pathway as small molecule drugs [45]. Given that ASB *E. coli* are considered harmless and clinical guidelines are to not treat ASB, therapeutic use of ASB *E. coli* would be safe. We find that ASB *E. coli* is cleared from the urinary tracts of healthy mice within days and consistent with clinical studies revealing the prevalence of ASB among healthy young women is approximately 5% [46]. Thus, the urinary tract appears similarly resistant to stable colonization by ASB *E. coli* in both healthy young women and mice, suggesting that ASB *E. coli* would be safe for clinical use as an LBP. ASB *E. coli* therapy also would not contribute to resistance against conventional antimicrobials. Finally, ASB *E. coli* address unmet needs for effective therapies against recurrent UTI and chronic pelvic pain, representing novel LBP candidates for urologic disease.

Acknowledgments

We thank Dr. Catharina Svanborg for generously providing the asymptomatic bacteriuria strain 83972. We thank Joseph Done for assistance quantifying allodynia and Eduardo and Faye Sarmiento for identifying uropathogens. These studies were as part of the NIH/NIDDK Multi-Disciplinary Approaches to Chronic Pelvic Pain (MAPP) Research Network (www.mappnetwork.org).

Author Contributions

Conceived and designed the experiments: CNR AKT REY AJS DJK. Performed the experiments: CNR AKT REY. Analyzed the data: CNR AKT REY AJS DJK. Contributed reagents/materials/analysis tools: AJS. Wrote the paper: CNR AKT REY AJS DJK.

References

1. Foxman B, Barlow R, D'Arcy H, Gillespie B, Sobel JD (2000) Urinary tract infection: self-reported incidence and associated costs. Ann Epidemiol 10: 509–515.
2. Schappert SM (1999) Ambulatory care visits to physician offices, hospital outpatient departments, and emergency departments: United States, 1997. PG - i–iv. Vital Health Stat 13.
3. Schaeffer AJ, Schaeffer EM (2012) Infections of the urinary tract. In: Wein A, Kavoussi L, Novick A, Partin A, Peters C, editors. Campbell-Walsh Urology. 8th ed. Philadelphia: Elsevier. pp. 223–303.
4. Foxman B (2010) The epidemiology of urinary tract infection. Nat Rev Urol 7: 653–660.
5. Karlowsky JA, Kelly LJ, Thornsberry C, Jones ME, Sahm DF (2002) Trends in antimicrobial resistance among urinary tract infection isolates of Escherichia coli from female outpatients in the United States. Antimicrob Agents Chemother 46: 2540–2545.
6. Hunstad DA, Justice SS (2010) Intracellular lifestyles and immune evasion strategies of uropathogenic Escherichia coli. Annu Rev Microbiol 64: 203–221.
7. Rudick CN, Jiang M, Yaggie RE, Pavlov VI, Done J, et al. (2012) O-antigen modulates infection-induced pain States. PLoS ONE 7: e41273.
8. Stewardson AJ, Huttner B, Harbarth S (2011) At least it won't hurt: the personal risks of antibiotic exposure. Curr Opin Pharmacol 11: 446–452.
9. Naber KG, Wullt B, Wagenlehner FM (2011) Antibiotic treatment of uncomplicated urinary tract infection in premenopausal women. Int J Antimicrob Agents 38 Suppl: 21–35.
10. Wise BL, Peloquin C, Choi H, Lane NE, Zhang Y (2012) Impact of age, sex, obesity, and steroid use on quinolone-associated tendon disorders. Am J Med 125: 1228 e1223–1228 e1228.
11. Looft T, Allen HK (2012) Collateral effects of antibiotics on mammalian gut microbiomes. Gut Microbes 3: 463–467.
12. Gupta K, Stapleton AE, Hooton TM, Roberts PL, Fennell CL, et al. (1998) Inverse association of H2O2-producing lactobacilli and vaginal Escherichia coli colonization in women with recurrent urinary tract infections. J Infect Dis 178: 446–450.
13. Czaja CA, Stapleton AE, Yarova-Yarovaya Y, Stamm WE (2007) Phase I trial of a Lactobacillus crispatus vaginal suppository for prevention of recurrent urinary tract infection in women. Infect Dis Obstet Gynecol 2007: 35387.
14. Stapleton A (2003) Novel approaches to prevention of urinary tract infections. Infect Dis Clin North Am 17: 457–471.
15. Reid G, Bruce AW (2006) Probiotics to prevent urinary tract infections: the rationale and evidence. World J Urol 24: 28–32.
16. Hull R, Rudy D, Donovan W, Svanborg C, Wieser I, et al. (2000) Urinary tract infection prophylaxis using Escherichia coli 83972 in spinal cord injured patients. J Urol 163: 872–877.
17. Sunden F, Hakansson L, Ljunggren E, Wullt B (2010) Escherichia coli 83972 bacteriuria protects against recurrent lower urinary tract infections in patients with incomplete bladder emptying. J Urol 184: 179–185.
18. Darouiche RO, Green BG, Donovan WH, Chen D, Schwartz M, et al. (2011) Multicenter Randomized Controlled Trial of Bacterial Interference for Prevention of Urinary Tract Infection in Patients With Neurogenic Bladder. Urology 78: 341–346.
19. Rudick CN, Billips BK, Pavlov VI, Yaggie RE, Schaeffer AJ, et al. (2010) Host-pathogen interactions mediating pain of urinary tract infection. J Infect Dis 201: 1240–1249.
20. Klumpp DJ, Weiser AC, Sengupta S, Forrestal SG, Batler RA, et al. (2001) Uropathogenic Escherichia coli potentiates type 1 pilus-induced apoptosis by suppressing NF-kappaB. Infect Immun 69: 6689–6695.
21. Lindberg U (1975) Asymptomatic bacteriuria in school girls. V. The clinical course and response to treatment. Acta Paediatr Scand 64: 718–724.
22. Andersson P, Engberg I, Lidin-Janson G, Lincoln K, Hull R, et al. (1991) Persistence of Escherichia coli bacteriuria is not determined by bacterial adherence. Infect Immun 59: 2915–2921.
23. Klemm P, Hancock V, Schembri MA (2007) Mellowing out: adaptation to commensalism by Escherichia coli asymptomatic bacteriuria strain 83972. Infect Immun 75: 3688–3695.
24. Bergsten G, Wullt B, Schembri MA, Leijonhufvud I, Svanborg C (2007) Do type 1 fimbriae promote inflammation in the human urinary tract? Cell Microbiol 9: 1766–1781.
25. Hultgren SJ, Schwan WR, Schaeffer AJ, Duncan JL (1986) Regulation of production of type 1 pili among urinary tract isolates of Escherichia coli. Infect Immun 54: 613–620.
26. Old DC, Duguid JP (1970) Selective outgrowth of fimbriate bacteria in static liquid medium. J Bacteriol 103: 447–456.
27. Billips BK, Schaeffer AJ, Klumpp DJ (2008) Molecular basis of uropathogenic Escherichia coli evasion of the innate immune response in the bladder. Infect Immun 76: 3891–3900.
28. Hopkins WJ, Hall JA, Conway BP, Uehling DT (1995) Induction of urinary tract infection by intraurethral inoculation with Escherichia coli: refining the murine model. J Infect Dis 171: 462–465.
29. Rudick CN, Bryce PJ, Guichelaar LA, Berry RE, Klumpp DJ (2008) Mast cell-derived histamine mediates cystitis pain. PLoS ONE 3: e2096.

30. Rudick CN, Chen MC, Mongiu AK, Klumpp DJ (2007) Organ Crosstalk Modulates Pelvic Pain. Am J Physiol Regul Integr Comp Physiol 293: R1191–1198.
31. Mulvey MA, Schilling JD, Hultgren SJ (2001) Establishment of a persistent Escherichia coli reservoir during the acute phase of a bladder infection. Infect Immun 69: 4572–4579.
32. Hang L, Frendeus B, Godaly G, Svanborg C (2000) Interleukin-8 receptor knockout mice have subepithelial neutrophil entrapment and renal scarring following acute pyelonephritis. J Infect Dis 182: 1738–1748.
33. Mulvey MA, Schilling JD, Martinez JJ, Hultgren SJ (2000) From the cover: bad bugs and beleaguered bladders: interplay between uropathogenic Escherichia coli and innate host defenses. Proc Natl Acad Sci U S A 97: 8829–8835.
34. Klumpp DJ, Rycyk MT, Chen MC, Thumbikat P, Sengupta S, et al. (2006) Uropathogenic Escherichia coli induces extrinsic and intrinsic cascades to initiate urothelial apoptosis. Infect Immun 74: 5106–5113.
35. Mulvey MA, Lopez-Boado YS, Wilson CL, Roth R, Parks WC, et al. (1998) Induction and evasion of host defenses by type 1-piliated uropathogenic Escherichia coli. Science 282: 1494–1497.
36. Thumbikat P, Berry RE, Zhou G, Billips BK, Yaggie RE, et al. (2009) Bacteria-induced uroplakin signaling mediates bladder response to infection. PLoS Pathog 5: e1000415.
37. Bleidorn J, Gagyor I, Kochen MM, Wegscheider K, Hummers-Pradier E (2010) Symptomatic treatment (ibuprofen) or antibiotics (ciprofloxacin) for uncomplicated urinary tract infection?—results of a randomized controlled pilot trial. BMC Med 8: 30.
38. Christiaens TC, De Meyere M, Verschraegen G, Peersman W, Heytens S, et al. (2002) Randomised controlled trial of nitrofurantoin versus placebo in the treatment of uncomplicated urinary tract infection in adult women. Br J Gen Pract 52: 729–734.
39. Ferry SA, Holm SE, Stenlund H, Lundholm R, Monsen TJ (2004) The natural course of uncomplicated lower urinary tract infection in women illustrated by a randomized placebo controlled study. Scand J Infect Dis 36: 296–301.
40. Malykhina AP, Wyndaele JJ, Andersson KE, De Wachter S, Dmochowski RR (2012) Do the urinary bladder and large bowel interact, in sickness or in health? ICI-RS 2011. Neurourol Urodyn 31: 352–358.
41. McMahon SB, Morrison JF (1978) Convergence of visceral and somatic axons on neurones which ascend in the lateral funiculus of the cat [proceedings]. J Physiol 275: 56P.
42. Pezzone MA, Liang R, Fraser MO (2005) A model of neural cross-talk and irritation in the pelvis: implications for the overlap of chronic pelvic pain disorders. Gastroenterology 128: 1953–1964.
43. Darouiche RO, Thornby JI, Cerra-Stewart C, Donovan WH, Hull RA (2005) Bacterial interference for prevention of urinary tract infection: a prospective, randomized, placebo-controlled, double-blind pilot trial. Clin Infect Dis 41: 1531–1534.
44. Parsons CL (2006) Advances in the treatment of interstitial cystitis. Expert Opin Pharmacother 7: 411–419.
45. Fiore C (2010) Regulatory considerations for the safety assessment of live biotherapeutic products in clinical trials. New York Academy of Sciences: U.S. Food and Drug Administration.
46. Hooton TM, Scholes D, Stapleton AE, Roberts PL, Winter C, et al. (2000) A prospective study of asymptomatic bacteriuria in sexually active young women. N Engl J Med 343: 992–997.

A Comparative Study on the Efficacy of Solifenacin Succinate in Patients with Urinary Frequency with or without Urgency

Ji-Yeon Han[1], Kyu-Sung Lee[2], Won Hee Park[3], Choal Hee Park[4], Jeong Gu Lee[5], Jeong Zoo Lee[6], Duk Yoon Kim[7], Yong Gil Na[8], Dong Deuk Kwon[9], Myung-Soo Choo[10]*

1 Department of Urology, Pusan National University Yangsan Hospital, Yangsan, Korea, **2** Department of Urology, Samsung Medical Center, Sungkyunkwan University School of Medicine, Seoul, Korea, **3** Department of Urology, Inha University College of Medicine, Incheon, Korea, **4** Department of Urology, Keimyung University School of Medicine, Daegu, Korea, **5** Department of Urology, Korea University College of Medicine, Seoul, Korea, **6** Department of Urology, Pusan National University Hospital, Busan, Korea, **7** Department of Urology, Catholic University of Daegu School of Medicine, Daegu, Korea, **8** Department of Urology, Chungnam National University School of Medicine, Daejeon, Korea, **9** Department of Urology, Chonnam National University Hwasun Hospital, Chonnam National University Medical School, Gwangju, Korea, **10** Department of Urology, University of Ulsan College of Medicine, Asan Medical Center, Seoul, Korea

Abstract

Objectives: Patients with overactive bladder (OAB) often have trouble perceiving urgency because of difficulties in distinguishing between urgency and desire to void. Empirical antimuscarinic treatment of patients with frequency only may be reasonable if conservative management has failed. We compared the efficacy of solifenacin in patients with frequency with or without urgency.

Materials and Methods: This multicenter, 12-week, open-label, comparative, non-inferiority clinical trial assessed whether the solifenacin efficacy for frequency without urgency is non-inferior to its efficacy for frequency with urgency. All patients had micturition frequency ≥8 voids/day with or without urgency. Primary efficacy variable: daily frequency change at 12 weeks relative to baseline. Secondary efficacy variables: change at 12 weeks relative to baseline in Patients' Perception of Bladder Condition (PPBC), OAB Symptom Score (OABSS), and Benefit, Satisfaction, Willingness to continue (BSW) questionnaire.

Results: Of the 286 enrolled patients, 240 (83.9%) completed the study (without urgency n = 115; with urgency n = 125). Full dataset analysis revealed that the groups without and with urgency exhibited significant reductions in daily micturition frequency of -2.49 ± 0.35 (mean ± standard error) and -2.63 ± 0.37, respectively. The lower limit of the 95% two-sided CI of the comparison of the two group means was −1.14, which is smaller than the −0.8 margin of clinical equivalence. The two groups did not differ in improvement in PPBC, OABSS, or BSW scores. Both tolerated the treatment well.

Conclusions: It was not possible to verify that the solifenacin efficacy for frequency alone was non-inferior to its efficacy for OAB. Nevertheless, solifenacin tended to be effective for frequency regardless of urgency.

Editor: Stephen L. Atkin, Weill Cornell Medical College Qatar, Qatar

Funding: Funding provided by Astellas Pharma, Korea. The funders had no role in study design, data collection and analysis, decision to publish, or preparation of the manuscript.

Competing Interests: This study was funded by Astellas, Korea.

* Email: mschoo@amc.seoul.kr

Introduction

Overactive bladder (OAB) is defined by the International Continence Society (ICS) as urgency [with or without urgency urinary incontinence (UUI)] that is usually associated with frequency and nocturia [1]. This definition suggests that urgency is the key symptom for a diagnosis of OAB, and as such, OAB cannot be diagnosed in the absence of urgency and is thought to be a driver for all other symptoms of OAB including frequency, nocturia, and UUI [2]. Due to its primary role in defining the OAB syndrome, it is important for clinicians to have a reasonable understanding of the definition of urgency.

The ICS defines urgency as "the complaint of a sudden compelling desire to pass urine which is difficult to defer" [1]. This assumes that urgency is an abnormal or pathological bladder sensation that is distinguishable from the normal physiological sensation of urge to void [2,3]. In most studies of OAB, diagnosis was based on physician identification of urgency according to the ICS definition, and urgency was the primary endpoint. However, greater clarity has been needed in the development of instruments for measuring urgency, because it is generally difficult for patient with OAB to perceive urgency and to differentiate urgency from urge to void [4].

In clinical experience, it seems that many patients who present with urinary frequency complain of a desire to void without urgency as defined by ICS, yet it is not suited for the current ICS definition of OAB. Nevertheless, despite the fact that urgency is the key symptom in OAB, frequency is also regarded as one of the most bothersome OAB symptom [5]. Despite this, the pathophysiology of frequency only and treatment guidelines for the management of patients with frequency only have not been established.

We hypothesized that the some of the patients who complained of only frequency without urgency may be actually OAB patient who cannot perceive or express their urgency symptoms, and antimuscarinic drugs may be effective in patients who complained of only urinary frequency without urgency, as they are in patients with urgency. Thus, we compared the efficacy of solifenacin in patients with frequency only and frequency with urgency.

Materials and Methods

The protocol for this trial and supporting CONSORT checklist are available as supporting information; see Checklist S1, Protocol S1 and Protocol S2.

2.1. Study design

This multicenter, 12-week, open-label, comparative, non-inferiority study was based on the hypothesis, "The efficacy of solifenacin for frequency only is non-inferior to the efficacy of solifenacin for frequency with urgency". It was conducted at nine sites between April 2009 and September 2011 in Korea. The study was conducted in accordance with the ethical principles in Korean Good Clinical Practice, the Declaration of Helsinki, and the International Conference of Harmonization Guidelines. This study was approved by the Institutional Review Board of Asan Medical Center (No. 2009-0014). Before enrollment in the study, all patients provided written informed consent.

2.2. Study patients

The study population consisted of men and women aged ≥18 years with symptoms of frequency for more than 3 months. All patients were assessed by a 3-day voiding diary and the urinary sensation scale (USS) [6]. The voiding diary and USS were carefully instructed by a study nurse who had been trained and explained the meaning of urgency and USS to all patients. Recording in voiding diary included day and night frequency, voided volume, and USS for each void. In the USS, the grade of urinary sensation perception was defined by scores from 1 to 5 as follows: 1 = no urgency: no feeling of urgency (can continue activities until it is convenient to use bathroom); 2 = mild urgency: feel urgency (can easily tolerate; can finish usual activity and tasks quickly, and then go straight to the bathroom); 3 = moderate urgency: enough urgency discomfort (need to stop usual activity and tasks, and go straight to the bathroom); 4 = severe urgency: strong urgency discomfort (almost cannot hold urine; need to stop usual activity and tasks immediately, and run to bathroom to avoid a micturition accident); and 5 = urge incontinence: extreme urgency discomfort (cannot hold urine, and has a micturition accident before reaching the bathroom). The mean score of USS recorded on the 3-day voiding diary was considered as the USS for the patient, and urgency was defined as USS ≥3 based on a voiding diary.

The Patients were excluded if they had: significant stress urinary incontinence, an average total daily urine volume >3000 ml, serum liver enzymes or creatinine level >2 times the upper limit of normal, symptomatic urinary tract infection at screening, recurrent urinary tract infections (defined as receiving treatment for symptomatic urinary tract infections >4 times in the last year), interstitial cystitis, urothelial tumor, a post-void residual (PVR) urine volume >100 ml, clinically relevant bladder outlet obstruction, clinically significant pelvic organ prolapse, electrostimulation treatment, undergone bladder training in the preceding 2 weeks, received antimuscarinic medication in the preceding 2 weeks, and/or neurological conditions that can specifically affect bladder function.

2.3. Interventions

We classified the patients with average micturition frequency ≥ 8/24 hours without urgency as Group 1, and patients with average micturition frequency ≥8/24 hours with urgency (USS ≥3/3 days) as Group 2, based on a 3-day voiding diary. Patients received solifenacin 5 mg once daily. At the week 4 visit, the dose could be increased to 10 mg based on discussion between the subject and investigator regarding treatment efficacy and tolerability.

2.4. Efficacy and safety assessments

To assess efficacy, the patients completed a 3-day voiding diary before the clinic visits at baseline and at weeks 4 and 12 (final visit). The primary efficacy variable was change in daily micturition frequency at 12 weeks relative to baseline. The secondary efficacy variables were change from baseline in Patients' Perception of Bladder Condition (PPBC) [7], OAB Symptom Score (OABSS) [8], and Benefit, Satisfaction, and Willingness to continue (BSW) scores, as determined by questionnaires completed at baseline and the end of treatment. Safety was evaluated by recording adverse events and measuring maximal urinary flow rate (MFR) and PVR.

2.5. Statistical analyses

Sample size was calculated by using the Power Analysis and Sample Size (PASS) statistical software package (PASS 11, NCSS, LLC, Kaysville, UT, USA). Sample sizes of 128 evaluable patients per treatment group were deemed to provide approximately 80% power to detect a non-inferiority margin of equivalence of −0.8 (standard deviation: 2.56 [9]) in terms of change in mean micturitions per 24 hours when Group 1 was compared to Group 2. Thus, 256 subjects were required. Based on an estimated 10% dropout rate, it was planned to recruit 286 subjects.

To analyze the efficacy data, the full analysis set (FAS) was used, namely, all patients who took the study medication and completed at least one efficacy evaluation. Per protocol (PP) analysis was performed for evaluation of changes in MFR and PVR relative to baseline. Categorical data were compared with chi-square statistics or Fisher's exact test and presented as frequencies. Continuous variables were analyzed using unpaired Student t- test and presented as mean ± standard error. All statistical tests had a two-sided significance level of 0.05 and were performed by using SPSS statistical software package (SPSS 21.0, SPSS, Chicago, IL).

Results

3.1. Baseline demographic data

A total of 286 patients were enrolled and 240 (83.9%) successfully completed the 12-week treatment period (Group 1:

115; Group 2: 125) (Figure 1). Twenty-six (18.4%) in Group 1 and 20 (13.8%) Group 2 patients dropped out. The two groups were similar in terms of baseline demographic and clinical characteristics (Table 1). Compliance for solifenacin at 12 weeks was 97.5% and there was no significantly difference between the two groups (97.0% vs. 98.0%, $p=0.408$).

3.2. Treatment efficacy

At 12 weeks, Groups 1 and 2 both exhibited statistically significant reductions in average daily micturition frequency relative to baseline (-2.49 ± 0.35 and -2.63 ± 0.37; all $p<0.001$); Table 2). There was no significantly difference between two groups. However, the lower limit of the 95% two-sided CI of the comparison of the two group means was -1.14, which is smaller than the -0.8 margin of clinical equivalence (non-inferior p-value $=0.099$). Therefore, it cannot be said that the efficacy of solifenacin for frequency alone was non-inferior to the efficacy of solifenacin for frequency with urgency.

The two groups did not differ significantly in improvement in OABSS, PPBC, or BSW scores (Table 3).

After 4 weeks of treatment, nine patients (7.8%) in Group 1 and four (3.2%) in Group 2 requested a dose escalation to 10 mg. This difference was not statistically significant. In Group 1, the solifenacin escalators had significantly more micturition episodes at baseline than the non-escalators (12.10 ± 1.07 *vs.* 14.81 ± 1.56, $p=0.019$). The solifenacin escalators and non-escalators in Group 2 did not differ significant in terms of this variable.

3.3. Safety

Adverse events were reported in 25.5% (36/141) in Group 1 and 39.3% (57/145), and the difference was not significant. However, these adverse events were generally mild (Table 4). Dry mouth was the most frequently reported adverse reaction. The two groups did not differ significantly in terms of MFR and PVR changes relative to baseline (-1.4 ± 1.05 *vs.* -0.11 ± 0.92 ml/s and 5.5 ± 2.99 *vs.* 9.3 ± 3.94 ml, respectively).

Discussion

To the best of our knowledge, this is the first trial to evaluate the efficacy of an antimuscarinic agent for frequency without urgency. We demonstrated a reduction of approximately two frequency episodes per day in patients with frequency without urgency at week 12, which was similar to that in patients with frequency with urgency, as well as the mean change in daily micturition of antimuscarinic treatment in meta-analysis [10]. The PPBC and BSW questionnaires revealed that the treatment had positive effects in the patients with frequency without urgency, which indicates that the treatment induced clinical meaningful improvements in micturition frequency in this group.

Urinary urgency is the cornerstone of the definition of OAB that is estimated to affect 10% of the worldwide population [11], however yet we know little about the definite cause, effect on voiding behavior, or proper measurement of urgency. OAB patients might modify voiding behavior to avoid showing urgency

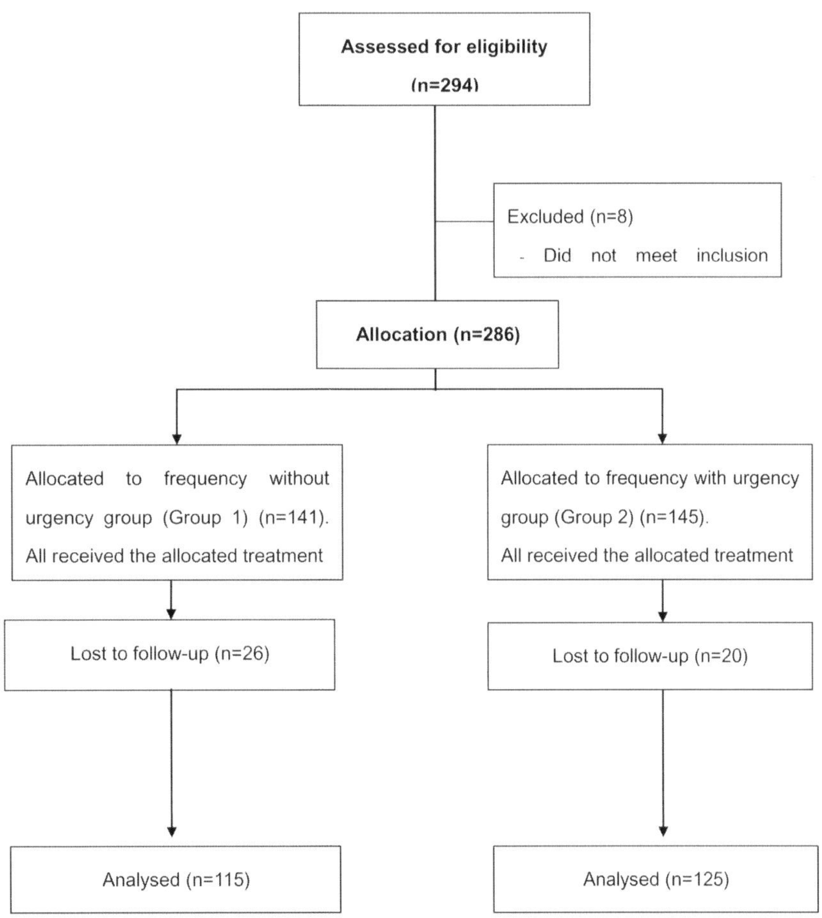

Figure 1. Participant flowchart.

Table 1. Demographics and baseline characteristics.

Variables	Frequency without urgency group (Group 1, n = 115)	Frequency with urgency group (Group 2, n = 125)	*p*-value
Age, years, mean (range)	57.46 (26–86)	56.60 (22–82)	0.60
Sex, n (%)			0.14
Men	26 (22.61)	19 (15.20)	
Women	89 (77.39)	106 (84.80)	
Symptom duration, months, mean (range)	56.46 (3–480)	65.93 (3–720)	0.42
Voiding diary/24 hour			
Frequency, mean (range)	12.32 (8.33–22.67)	13.16 (8–32)	0.09
Nocturia, mean (range)	1.86 (0–10.33)	1.74 (0–6)	0.45
Bladder volume, ml, mean (range)	138.34 (32.22–292.31)	136.78 (42.5–315.56)	0.83
OABSS grade, n (%)			
Mild	80 (69.57)	15 (12.00)	<0.0001
Moderate	32 (27.83)	89 (71.20)	
Severe	3 (2.61)	21 (16.80)	
Uroflowmetry parameters			
Maximal flow rate, ml/s, mean (range)	19.24 (10.4–61.6)	21.53 (10.3–56.5)	0.12
Voided volume, ml, mean (range)	229.75 (122.5–871.5)	215.72 (122.7–831)	0.45
Post-voided residual, ml, mean (range)	25.18 (0–92)	23.35 (0–99)	0.65

or urgency incontinence. Therefore, their episodes of urgency may be underestimated or hidden behind frequency only. This can lead to confusion in diagnosis and treatment decision of OAB.

At present, the pathophysiology of frequency without urgency is poorly understood. The most common cause of frequency only would be that the vast majority of patients do not understand the subtle diagnostic nuances of urinary urgency. Indeed, a study on patient understanding of lower urinary tract symptoms showed that the term "urgency" was correctly defined by only 46% of the subjects [12]. A study examining how patients described their urge or desire to urinate reported diverse descriptions, including frequency, full bladder, relief, necessity, and must go [13]. Although the USS has good content validity, discriminated validity, and test-retest reliability [14], it may not capture the patient's experience of urinary urgency thoroughly as other current urgency scales [15]. It may be that these patients void frequently with no preceding desire to void to avoid more compelling situations; this is known as convenience voiding [16]. Healthy volunteers may empty their bladders early for social reasons, such as before joining a meeting, going out on a long journey, or retiring to bed at night [17]. Specifically, OAB patients go to the toilet more often to avoid urgency or leakage because they know of their sudden urgency or urgency incontinence. In these patients, once this decision to convenience void is made, most voiding may be initiated with mild sensations rather than sensation of immediate needing to void. The third explanation of frequency only is the lack of the progressive increase in bladder awareness [18]. These subjects report frequent voiding, which appears to originate from their cognitive strategies to avoid intense urge sensation and incontinence. Thus, interpreting bladder awareness may be depressed in pathological states. Further study is necessary to confirm this modified view for determining the decision to void.

The clinically significant efficacy of an antimuscarinic agent in our patients with frequency without urgency may be explained by an inhibitory effect of this agent on afferent bladder nerves. Antimuscarinic treatment is believed to repress the detrusor overactivity associated with OAB by blocking the muscarinic receptors in the detrusor muscle. However, several studies [19–21] have shown that antimuscarinic treatment also significantly improves sensory functions, as shown by increased time to first sensation to void and reduced voiding frequency. On the basis of these observations, we proposed that solifenacin treatment may improve the frequency symptoms of subjects without urgency.

Table 2. Non-inferior analysis of solifenacin in patients with urinary frequency with or without urgency.

Variables	Frequency without urgency group (Group 1)	Frequency with urgency group (Group 2)	*p*- value
Baseline	12.32±0.31	13.16±0.38	0.09
Week 12	9.82±0.36	10.52±0.42	0.21
Change from baseline	−2.49±0.35	−2.63±0.37	0.78
95% CI	−3.17, −1.81	−3.37, −1.90	-
95% CI for difference	−3.37, −1.90		

Table 3. Patients' perception of treatment benefit, satisfaction, and willing to have retreatment and Changes in Patients' Perception of Bladder Condition scores.

Variables	Frequency without urgency group (Group 1, n = 115)	Frequency with urgency group (Group 2, n = 125)	*p*-value
Treatment benefit, satisfaction, and willing to have retreatment			
Benefit	69.9%	73.8%	0.55
Satisfaction	66.3%	75.7%	0.15
Retreatment	83.1%	88.8%	0.26
Change in Patients' Perception of Bladder Condition scores			
Deterioration	6.0%	6.5%	0.84
No change	16.9%	17.6%	0.72
1-point improvement	30.1%	24.1%	0.41
≥2-point improvement	47.0%	51.9%	0.51

Overall, the 12-week solifenacin treatment was well tolerated in the patients with frequency with and without urgency.

One limitation of this study was that we did not find that solifenacin had a non-inferior effect on frequency without urgency relative to its effect on frequency with urgency in terms of change in daily micturition frequency (the primary endpoint of this study). However, our study did show that solifenacin treatment significantly decreased the daily micturition frequency in patients with frequency regardless of urgency. Moreover, the difference between the urgency and non-urgency groups in terms of micturition frequency change did not achieve statistical significance. The inability of this study to detect non-inferiority may reflect the wide standard deviation (−2.56) associated with the mean number of micturitions per 24 hour that was reported by the study that was used to establish the margin of clinical equivalence for the present study [9]. The second limitation was that there was no placebo

Table 4. Treatment-emergent adverse events in both groups.

Variables	Frequency without urgency group (Group 1, n = 115)	Frequency with urgency group (Group 2, n = 125)
Subjects with AEs, n (%)	36 (25.5)	57 (39.3)
Dry mouth	13 (36.1)	32 (56.2)
Mild	11	25
Moderate	2	6
Severe	-	1
Constipation	2 (5.6)	5 (8.8)
Mild	1	4
Moderate	1	1
Severe	-	-
Blurred vision	1 (2.8)	4 (7.0)
Mild	1	4
Dyspepsia	6 (16.6)	5 (8.8)
Mild	4	4
Moderate	2	1
Dizziness	1 (2.8)	1 (1.7)
Moderate	1	1
Voiding difficulty	7 (19.4)	8 (14.1)
Mild	6	6
Moderate	1	2
Headache	1 (2.8)	-
Mild	1	
Fatigue	2 (5.6)	1 (1.7)
Mild	2	1
Itching	3 (8.3)	1 (1.7)
Mild	3	1

group. The placebo response for OAB symptoms is a well-known occurrence during drug trials. Although this was not a placebo-controlled study, we tried to eliminate the effects of the placebo response by recording the voiding diary during the screening period. The placebo response during drug trials in OAB can be partly attributable to the bladder training effect of completing a voiding diary [22]. Through the process of recording and reviewing the voiding diary, patients can become more aware of voiding frequency and they may establish more appropriate voiding intervals. At the initial screening visit, the lifestyle modification (avoidance of bladder irritants such as caffeine), bladder training, and voiding diary were explained, and during the 3 days before the next visit, patients recorded episodes in a 3-day voiding diary. Patients were then assigned to one of two groups. And, a total of 256 subjects enrolled could not reach 80% power to detect non-inferiority because of unexpected subject dropout. We assumed that, although we showed that solifenacin tended to be effective for frequency regardless of urgency, we could not have shown non-inferiority because of low power.

Conclusions

It was not possible to verify that the solifenacin efficacy for frequency alone was non-inferior to its efficacy for OAB. Nevertheless, solifenacin tended to be effective for frequency regardless of urgency.

Author Contributions

Conceived and designed the experiments: MSC. Performed the experiments: KSL WHP CHP JGL JZL DYK YGN DDK. Analyzed the data: MSC JYH. Contributed reagents/materials/analysis tools: MSC. Wrote the paper: MSC JYH.

References

1. Abrams P, Cardozo L, Fall M, Griffiths D, Rosier P, et al. (2002) The standardisation of terminology of lower urinary tract function: report from the Standardisation Sub-committee of the International Continence Society. Neurourol Urodyn 21: 167–178.
2. Chapple CR, Artibani W, Cardozo LD, Castro-Diaz D, Craggs M, et al. (2005) The role of urinary urgency and its measurement in the overactive bladder symptom syndrome: current concepts and future prospects. BJU Int 95: 335–340.
3. Brubaker L (2004) Urgency: the cornerstone symptom of overactive bladder. Urology 64: 12–16.
4. Abrams P, Chapple CR, Junemann KP, Sharpe S (2012) Urinary urgency: a review of its assessment as the key symptom of the overactive bladder syndrome. World J Urol 30: 385–392.
5. Elinoff V, Bavendam T, Glasser DB, Carlsson M, Eyland N, et al. (2006) Symptom-specific efficacy of tolterodine extended release in patients with overactive bladder: the IMPACT trial. Int J Clin Pract 60: 745–751.
6. Coyne KS, Margolis MK, Hsieh R, Vats V, Chapple CR (2011) Validation of the urinary sensation scale (USS). Neurourol Urodyn 30: 360–365.
7. Coyne KS, Matza LS, Kopp Z, Abrams P (2006) The validation of the patient perception of bladder condition (PPBC): a single-item global measure for patients with overactive bladder. Eur Urol 49: 1079–1086.
8. Homma Y, Yoshida M, Seki N, Yokoyama O, Kakizaki H, et al. (2006) Symptom assessment tool for overactive bladder syndrome–overactive bladder symptom score. Urology 68: 318–323.
9. Lee KS, Lee HW, Choo MS, Paick JS, Lee JG, et al. (2010) Urinary urgency outcomes after propiverine treatment for an overactive bladder: the 'Propiverine study on overactive bladder including urgency data'. BJU Int 105: 1565–1570.
10. Chapple CR, Khullar V, Gabriel Z, Muston D, Bitoun CE, et al. (2008) The Effects of Antimuscarinic Treatments in Overactive Bladder: An Update of a Systematic Review and Meta-Analysis. Eur Urol 54: 543–562.
11. Irwin DE, Kopp ZS, Agatep B, Milsom I, Abrams P (2011) Worldwide prevalence estimates of lower urinary tract symptoms, overactive bladder, urinary incontinence and bladder outlet obstruction. BJU Int 108: 1132–1138.
12. Digesu GA, Khullar V, Panayi D, Calandrini M, Gannon M, et al. (2008) Should we explain lower urinary tract symptoms to patients? Neurourol and Urodyn 27: 368–371.
13. Coyne KS, Harding G, Jumadilova Z, Weiss JP (2012) Defining urinary urgency: Patient descriptions of "gotta go". Neurourol and Urodyn 31: 455–459.
14. Nixon A, Colman S, Sabounjian L, Sandage B, Schwiderski UE, et al. (2005) A validated patient reported measure of urinary urgency severity in overactive bladder for use in clinical trials. J Urol 174: 604–607.
15. Starkman JS, Dmochowski RR (2008) Urgency assessment in the evaluation of overactive bladder (OAB). Neurourol Urodyn 27: 13–21.
16. Darling R, Neilson D (2005) Convenience voids: an important new factor in urinary frequency volume chart analysis. J Urol 173: 487–489.
17. Honjo H, Kawauchi A, Nakao M, Ukimura O, Kitakoji H, et al. (2010) Impact of convenience void in a bladder diary with urinary perception grade to assess overactive bladder symptoms: A community-based study. Neurourol and Urodyn 29: 1286–1289.
18. Harvey J, Finney S, Stewart L, Gillespie J (2012) The relationship between cognition and sensation in determining when and where to void: the concept of cognitive voiding. BJU Int 110: 1756–1761.
19. Finney SM, Andersson KE, Gillespie JI, Stewart LH (2006) Antimuscarinic drugs in detrusor overactivity and the overactive bladder syndrome: motor or sensory actions? BJU Int 98: 503–507.
20. Panayi DC, Tekkis P, Fernando R, Khullar V (2010) Is the beneficial effect of antimuscarinics related to motor or sensory changes in the bladder? Int Urogynecol J 21: 841–845.
21. Yamaguchi O (2010) Antimuscarinics and overactive bladder: other mechanism of action. Neurourol Urodyn 29: 112–115.
22. Stav K, Dwyer PL, Rosamilia A (2009) Women Overestimate Daytime Urinary Frequency: The Importance of the Bladder Diary. J Urol 181: 2176–2180.

Aetiology of Acute Febrile Episodes in Children Attending Korogwe District Hospital

Coline Mahende[1,2]*, Billy Ngasala[2], John Lusingu[1], Allvan Butichi[1], Paminus Lushino[1], Martha Lemnge[1], Zul Premji[2]

1 Korogwe Research Laboratory, National Institute for Medical Research, Tanga, Tanzania, **2** Department of Medical Entomology and Parasitology, School of Public Health, Muhimbili University of Health and Allied Sciences, Dar es Salaam, Tanzania

Abstract

Introduction: Although the burden of malaria in many parts of Tanzania has declined, the proportion of children with fever has not changed. This situation underscores the need to explore the possible causes of febrile episodes in patients presenting with symptoms at the Korogwe District Hospital (KDH).

Methods: A hospital based cross-sectional study was conducted at KDH, north-eastern Tanzania. Patients aged 2 to 59 months presenting at the outpatient department with an acute medical condition and fever (measured axillary temperature ≥37.5°C) were enrolled. Blood samples were examined for malaria parasites, human immunodeficiency virus (HIV) and bacterial infections. A urine culture was performed in selected cases to test for bacterial infection and a chest radiograph was requested if pneumonia was suspected. Diagnosis was based on both clinical and laboratory investigations.

Results: A total of 867 patients with a median age of 15.1 months (Interquartile range 8.6–29.9) were enrolled from January 2013 to October 2013. Respiratory tract infections were the leading clinical diagnosis with 406/867 (46.8%) of patients diagnosed with upper respiratory tract infection and 130/867 (15.0%) with pneumonia. Gastroenteritis was diagnosed in 184/867 (21.2%) of patients. Malaria infection was confirmed in 72/867 (8.3%) of patients. Bacterial infection in blood and urine accounted for 26/808 (3.2%) infections in the former, and 66/373 (17.7%) infections in the latter. HIV infection was confirmed in 10/824 (1.2%) of patients. Respiratory tract infections and gastroenteritis were frequent in patients under 36 months of age (87.3% and 91.3% respectively). Co-infections were seen in 221/867 (25.5%) of patients. The cause of fever was not identified in 65/867 (7.5%) of these patients.

Conclusions: The different proportions of infections found among febrile children reflect the causes of fever in the study area. These findings indicate the need to optimise patient management by developing malaria and non-malaria febrile illnesses management protocols.

Editor: Ana Paula Arez, Instituto de Higiene e Medicina Tropical, Portugal

Funding: The study was sponsored by Swedish International Development Cooperation Agency (SIDA) through Muhimbili University of Health and Allied Sciences. The funders had no role in study design, data collection and analysis, decision to publish, or preparation of the manuscript.

Competing Interests: The authors have declared that no competing interests exist.

* Email: cbdmahende@yahoo.co.uk

Introduction

More than half of the children presenting at health facilities in Africa are estimated not to have a malaria infection [1,2]. The lack of knowledge on the prevalence of the causative agents of other febrile illnesses, the limited access to affordable diagnostic tests as well as the fear of overlooking a life threatening malaria infection, result in most febrile cases being treated and managed as malaria [3,4].

Fever commonly accompanies a wide range of childhood illnesses and if the patient is not properly managed, this can have potentially serious outcomes including death [5]. In malaria endemic countries, febrile episodes are commonly associated with malaria infection [6,7]. As current epidemiological data indicates a decline in malaria infections in many parts of sub Saharan Africa, including Tanzania, other causative agents of febrile illnesses should be investigated [8,9].

Acute febrile episodes are caused by various pathogenic organisms (such as viruses and bacteria), and infections with these agents result in patients presenting with clinical symptoms which resemble those of a malaria infection [10]. An accurate clinical diagnosis without laboratory confirmation can be difficult to make and misleading [11,12]. Despite efforts by the World Health Organisation (WHO) to improve the diagnosis of malaria through its updated integrated management of childhood illness (IMCI) guidelines, confirmatory diagnosis of malaria is still not adequately carried out. In routine practice, clinicians have continued prescribing antimalarial drugs to malaria negative patients [13,14]. As IMCI approach is apparently not specific on the diagnosis of non-malarial febrile illnesses [15]. This results in the inappropriate use of antimalarial drugs, possible development of antimicrobial drug resistance and also elevates treatment costs due to unnecessary prescriptions. Incorrect prescriptions may leave patients untreated, thereby unnecessarily increasing morbidity and mortality in these resource poor settings [16].

There is limited data on the epidemiological causes of febrile illnesses (other than malaria) among outpatient children, as well as a lack of reliable surveillance data in Tanzania. A recent study conducted in Tanzania found that malarial infections were no longer a major cause of fever among outpatient children [17]. Disease-specific studies among febrile patients have been conducted in few settings across Sub Saharan Africa. These studies focused mainly on malaria, bacteraemia and human immunodeficiency virus (HIV) infection among inpatients [18–20].

Information on the prevalence of local infections, that is based on diagnosis using both clinical presentation and laboratory confirmatory tests is critical for correct management of both malarial and non-malarial febrile illnesses. The main objective of this study was to describe the common causes of fever in children presenting at an outpatient department at the Korogwe District Hospital, north-eastern Tanzania.

Methods

Study area

The study was conducted at Korogwe District Hospital (KDH) in Korogwe District, Tanga Region, north-eastern part of Tanzania. The Korogwe District has a population of approximately 73,275 children under the age of five years according to the Tanzanian population and housing census of 2012 [21]. The District has a population growth rate of 2.7% per annum [21]. The environment is characterised by daily temperatures varying from 18°C to 20°C during the rainy season and 26°C to 30°C during the dry season. The annual rainfall ranges from 700–1000 mm with long rainy seasons extending from March to May. The majority of the inhabitants reside in rural settings, practicing subsistence farming and informal trade. The hospital receives 6000 (2010 estimates) children under the age of five years as outpatients annually. The most common clinical diagnoses among children under the age of five years have been malaria, pneumonia, gastroenteritis, septicaemia, anaemia and diarrhoea (Korogwe District Medical Officer, personal communication).

The prevalence of *Plasmodium falciparum* malaria parasitaemia from the community in lowland villages has decreased from 78% in 2003 to 13% in 2008, whereas in the highland villages, the decrease was from 25% to 3% during the same time period [22]. The prevalence of HIV infection among women attending the antenatal clinic at KDH was 2.5% for 2010 [23]. Pneumococcal and rotavirus vaccines were introduced into Tanzania in January 2013 as part of the Expanded Program on Immunization. Vaccine coverage for other vaccines in the Expanded Program on Immunization (EPI) has been above 80%. These vaccines include; Bacille Calmette–Guérin, pentavalent vaccine (diphtheria–tetanus–pertussis, hepatitis B and haemophilus influenza type B), poliovirus and measles vaccines.

Study population

Sick children aged between 2 and 59 months presenting at KDH outpatient department were assessed for study eligibility from January 2013 to October 2013. Enrolment took place Mondays to Fridays every week. The inclusion criteria were: children aged 2 to 59 months of age presenting at KDH with an acute medical condition and a history of fever in the last 48 hours or measured axillary temperature of ≥37.5°C. The visit should be their first consultation for the present problem. Patients younger than 2 months of age were excluded in the study. Patients were excluded if they had planned admissions (e.g. elective surgery), trauma/injury, if they required an emergency intervention or if they had taken antimalarial drugs and/or antibiotics within the last seven days.

Ethics statement

The study obtained ethical clearance with reference number NIMR/HQ/R.8a/Vol.IX/1373 from the Tanzanian Medical Research Coordinating Committee. A written informed consent form was issued and signed by the parent/legal guardian of every child enrolled in the study.

Study procedure

A detailed medical history and a thorough clinical examination were performed on each patient and this information was recorded on a standardised Case Report Form (CRF). This information included: demographic information, clinical history and physical examination data (including weight, axillary temperature and respiratory rate). A chest radiograph was requested if pneumonia was suspected. A clinical diagnosis was made based on the presenting signs and symptoms according to the IMCI guidelines [24]. This ensured that patients could be appropriately managed according to national standard practice while laboratory tests were being processed. Patients who had positive culture results were contacted and the necessary required treatment provided. The Final diagnosis was based on both the clinical presentation and the laboratory findings for malaria microscopy, bacteriology, radiology and HIV testing.

Laboratory investigations

A maximum of 5 mL venous blood for laboratory investigations was drawn from every patient once inclusion criteria had been met. Each blood draw was conducted aseptically in order to avoid contamination. The venipuncture site was disinfected with 70% isopropyl alcohol and allowed to dry prior to blood drawing.

Diagnosis of Plasmodium species and *Borrelia* parasitic infection

Thick and thin blood smears were prepared (in duplicate) from the blood collected in the ethylene diamine tetra acetic acid (EDTA) tubes. The thin film was fixed with methanol and blood slides were stained with a 5% Giemsa solution for identification and quantitation of asexual *Plasmodium falciparum* and other *Plasmodium* species. The blood slides were read by two expert microscopists and in case of discrepancy, a third reading was performed. Asexual parasites were counted against 200 (500 if parasite count was <10) white blood cells. A blood slide was considered negative for *Plasmodium* species if no parasites were seen in at least 100 oil-immersion high power fields on the thick film. During examination of the slides for *Plasmodium* species, *Borrelia* species were also screened. *Borrelia* species are seen as spirochaetes under microscopy.

Differential complete blood count

Blood collected in anticoagulated EDTA tubes was analysed for differential complete blood count using automated MS4s haematology analyser (Melet Schloesing Diamond Diagnostics, USA).

Aerobic blood culturing

Blood collected in commercially available BD BACTEC PEDS PLUS culture bottles were incubated in an automated blood culture system BACTEC 9050 (Becton Dickinson, Sparks, Maryland, USA). A single blood culture bottle was used per patient. The minimal volume inoculated was 2 mL (3 mL was an ideal volume) and blood culture bottles were incubated for a maximum of five days (unless they flag positive). The BACTEC 9050 detects positive cultures based on CO_2 production. Blood culture bottles which flagged positive were cultured on standard media with the use of routine microbiological techniques. Analytical Profile Index (API) biochemical test kit (BioMérieux, France) and/or serological tests were used to confirm suspected pathogens.

Definition of positive and negative culture

A blood culture was considered positive when: a definite pathogen was isolated (e.g. *Streptococcus pneumoniae*, *Streptococcus agalactiae*, *Streptococcus pyogenes*, *Haemophilus influenzae*, *Salmonella* species), a bacteria that could be either a pathogen or a contaminant was isolated within 48 hours of blood culture incubation (e.g. *Escherichia coli*, *Klebsiella pneumoniae*, *Staphylococcus aureus*, *Enterococcus faecalis* group D). Blood cultures were considered to be negative if there were no bacteria isolated after five days incubation.

Definition of contamination

A blood culture was considered to be contaminated if one or more of the following organisms were identified; coagulase-negative *Staphylococcus* species, *Corynebacterium* species, *alpha- or gamma-hemolytic streptococci*, *Micrococcus* species, *Bacillus* species and *Propionibacterium* species. However, a definitive diagnosis of a contaminant was decided by a clinician based on the clinical presentation of the patient due to the fact that these organisms could be the cause of an opportunistic infection.

Urine culturing

Urine was collected from patients presenting with fever, dysuria and/or no obvious cause of fever on clinical examination. A midstream urine was collected in a sterile container. The perineum was swabbed with chlorhexidine and the sample was collected using a sterile urine collector for the younger patients who were not able to follow instructions. Urinalysis by dipstick (URiScan, YD Diagnostics, Korea) was used for presumptive diagnosis of urinary tract infections for early initiation of therapy while urine cultures were being processed. The urine was cultured by inoculation onto cysteine lactose electrolyte deficient agar, MacConkey agar and sheep blood agar. An API biochemical test kit (BioMérieux, France) was used to confirm suspected pathogens. A definitive diagnosis of urinary tract infection was based on the isolation of a bacteria pathogen from the positive culture containing $>10^5$ colony-forming units (CFU)/ml [25].

Antimicrobial susceptibility testing

The Kirby-Bauer disc diffusion method was used for in-vitro antimicrobial susceptibility testing for all pathogenic bacterial isolates from blood and urine cultures. The testing was performed on the following antimicrobial agents; amoxicillin, chloramphenicol, ceftriaxone, ciprofloxacin, co-trimoxazole, gentamicin and penicillin. Reading and interpretation of zone sizes was performed using criteria stipulated by the Clinical and Laboratory Standards Institute (CLSI).

Human immunodeficiency virus (HIV) testing

HIV antibody testing was performed after patients were informed and counselled as per the National Health Guidelines. Blood drawn from patients was tested for the presence of HIV-1 and HIV-2 antibodies according to the National HIV rapid testing algorithm using the Determine HIV-1/2 Assay Kit (Abbott Laboratories, Abbott Park, IL, USA) [26]. If this was positive, confirmation was carried out using the Uni-Gold HIV (Trinity Biotech, Bray, Co Wicklow, Ireland). For children under the age of 18 months, HIV testing was performed using HIV-1 RNA PCR.

Case definitions

Fever was defined as history of abnormally high body temperature as reported by the parent/guardian and/or measured axillary temperature ≥37.5°C on presentation. Malaria infection was defined as fever with the presence of asexual *Plasmodium falciparum* parasites in a blood smear confirmed by microscopy. Bacteremia was defined as fever with isolation of pathogenic bacteria from blood culture. Anaemia was defined as haemoglobin concentration below 9.3 g/dL. Clinical diagnoses of respiratory infections and gastroenteritis were defined according to the IMCI guidelines [24].

Data management and statistical analysis

Data management involved double entry and validation using Microsoft Access 2007. Data analysis was done by STATA version 11.2 (Stata Corp LP, College Station, Texas, USA). Variables were summarized as frequencies and proportions and medians and inter-quartile ranges, as appropriate. Data was compared using the chi-square (X^2) test when comparing proportions. Odds ratios (OR) and 95% confidence intervals (95% CI) were calculated as appropriate. The value of $p<0.05$ was considered statistically significant.

Results

Demographic characteristics of the study population

A total of 1380 patients attending the outpatient department at KDH from January 2013 to October 2013 were screened. Of these, 867/1380 (62.8%) were febrile children who were eligible for enrolment (Figure 1). The median age was 15.1 months (Interquartile range (IQR): 8.6–29.9) and girls comprised of 459/867 (52.9%) patients as shown on Table 1. Median axillary body temperature was 38.1°C (IQR 37.5–38.7). The common presenting clinical symptoms other than fever were cough 411/867 (47.4%) and diarrhoea 174/867 (20.1%).

Malaria infection

Malaria infection due to *Plasmodium falciparum* was confirmed in 72/867 (8.3%, 95%CI, 6.5–10.1) of the patients identified by thick and thin blood smears. Anaemia was found in 226/841 (26.9%) patients, of whom 36/226 (15.9%) had malaria which increased the risk of anaemia (OR: 3.6 [95%CI: 2.1–6.1] p<0.01). No other *Plasmodia* species or *Borrelia* species were found. Overlap of clinical symptoms was observed among patients with malaria infection; 14/72 (19.4%) and 4/72 (5.6%) patients had clinical symptoms of respiratory tract infections and gastroenteritis respectively.

Bacteremia

Blood cultures were collected and analysed from 808 patients, of which 26/808 (3.2%, 95%CI, 1.9–4.4) were positive for pathogenic bacterial growth. *Salmonella typhi* was the predominant

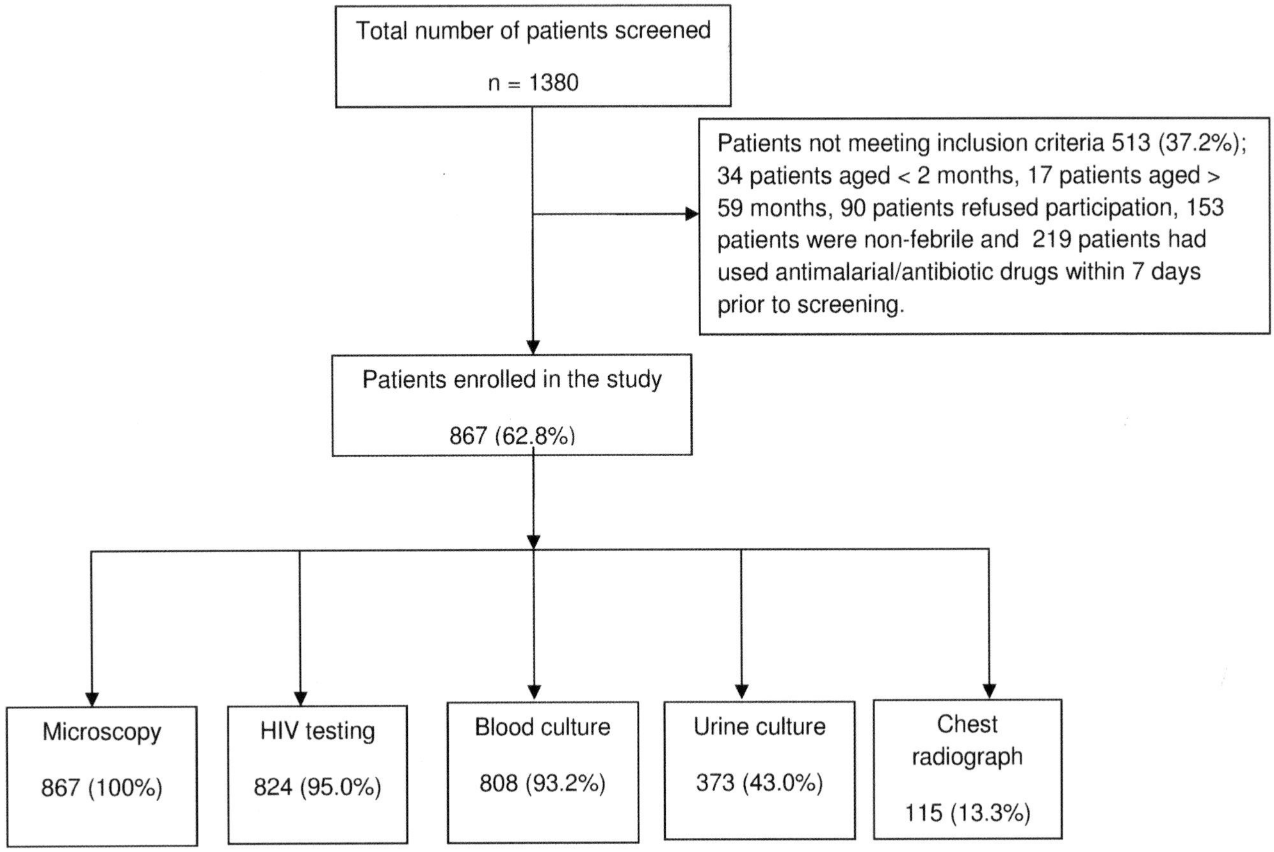

Figure 1. Study flow diagram of patient enrollment at KDH and the investigations performed.

bacteria isolated in 17/26 (65.4%) of cases followed by *Streptococcus pneumoniae* 4/26 (15.4%) as shown in Table 1.

Urinary tract infection

A Urinary tract infection was confirmed in 66/373 (17.7%, 95%CI, 14.0–22.0) of patients and there was no significant association with gender (36 boys, 30 girls, $X^2 = 0.074$, $P = 0.786$). The most commonly isolated bacteria were *Escherichia coli* 37/66 (56.1%) followed by *Klebsiella pneumoniae* 7/66 (10.6%), *Staphylococcus aureus* 6/66 (9.1%) and *Proteus mirabilis* 5/66 (7.6%).

HIV infection

HIV testing was performed in 824/867 (95.0%) patients and among them, 10/824 (1.2%, 95%CI, 0.6–2.2) were confirmed positive for infection with HIV. None of the HIV infected patients had either a malarial or a bacterial infection.

Clinical diagnoses

Respiratory tract infections. Upper respiratory tract infections were the most common clinical diagnoses presenting in 406/867 (46.8%, 95%CI, 43.5–50.2) of patients. Pneumonia was clinically diagnosed in 130/867 (15.0%, 95%CI, 12.7–17.5) of patients. Pneumonia confirmed by chest radiograph was accounted in 54/130 (41.5%) of these cases and five patients had diagnosis of severe pneumonia. *Salmonella typhi* (n = 2) and *Escherichia coli* (n = 1) were isolated from single blood cultures of patients with upper respiratory tract infections. *Streptococcus pneumoniae* (n = 1) and *Staphylococcus aureus* (n = 1) were isolated from single blood cultures of patients with pneumonia diagnosis. One patient was suspected to have pulmonary tuberculosis from clinical symptoms and chest radiograph results.

Gastroenteritis. Gastroenteritis was diagnosed in 184/867 (21.2%, 95%CI, 18.5–24.1) of patients. Dysentery was diagnosed in 6 patients. *Salmonella typhi* (n = 6) and non-typhi salmonella (n = 1) were isolated from the blood cultures of patients with gastroenteritis.

Other infections. Other infections are summarised on Table 1. The cause of fever could not be identified in 65/867 (7.5%, 95%CI, 5.8–9.5) of the patients.

Distribution of diagnoses according to age. The majority of the patients under the age of 36 months presented with respiratory tract infections 468/536 (87.3%). The second most common diagnosis was gastroenteritis 168/184 (91.3%) and thirdly, urinary tract infections 57/66 (86.4%). Malaria infection 8/72 (11.1%) was less common in patients under the age of 12 months (Figure 2).

Diagnosis of hospitalised patients

Following enrolment, 141/867 (16.3%) patients were hospitalised, of whom 2/141 (1.4%) died from severe pneumonia and upper respiratory tract infection. Malaria infection was a leading cause of admission with 53/141 (37.6%) of patients, followed by pneumonia 35/141 (24.8%), gastroenteritis 27/141 (19.1%) and other infections as indicated in Figure 3.

Co- infections

Co-infections were common and were observed in 221/867 (25.5%, 95%CI, 22.6–28.5) of the patients. Urinary tract

Table 1. Demographic characteristics, clinical diagnosis and laboratory findings of patients enrolled at KDH.

Patient characteristics	n, n/N	Proportions (%)
Gender		
Girls	408	47.1
Age		
2–11 months	356	41.1
12–35 months	370	42.7
36–59 months	141	16.3
Fever		
Duration of fever in days, median (IQR)	2 (1–2)	-
Axillary temperature ≥37.5°C	627	72.3
Common symptoms		
Cough	411	47.4
Diarrhoea	174	20.1
Difficulty breathing	97	11.2
Clinical diagnosis		
Respiratory infections		
Upper respiratory tract infection	406/867	46.8
Pneumonia	130/867	15
Pulmonary Tuberculosis	1/867	0.1
Asthma	19/867	2.2
Gastroenteritis	184/867	21.2
Dysentery	6/867	0.7
Otitis media	5/867	0.6
Fungal infections	6/867	0.7
Skin infections/soft tissue infections	33/867	3.8
Other infections	44/867	5.1
Laboratory findings		
Plasmodium falciparum	72/867	8.3
Geometric mean parasitemia (range)	37635 (159–1656400)	-
Human immunodeficiency virus	10/824	1.2
Anaemia	226/841	26.9
Blood culture positive	26/808	3.2
Non-typhi salmonella	2/26	7.7
Salmonella typhi	17/26	65.4
Streptococcus pneumoniae	4/26	15.4
Other[†]	3/26	11.5
Urine culture	66/373	17.7
Escherichia coli	37/66	56.1
Klebsiella pneumoniae	7/66	10.6
Proteus mirabilis	5/66	7.6
Other[‡]	17/66	25.7
Pyrexia of Unknown Origin	65/867	7.5

[†] *Escherichia coli* (1), *Enterobacter cloacae* (1), *Staphylococcus* aureus (1).
[‡] *Acinetobacter baumanii* (1), *Citrobacter koseri* (1), *Pseudomonas aeruginosa* (2), *Staphylococcus aureus* (6) *Staphylococcus saprophyticus* (3), *Streptococcus faecalis* (1), *Streptococcus mitis* (1), *Streptococcus viridans* (2).

infections were present in 33/436 (7.6%) patients with respiratory tract infections and in 19/184 (10.3%) patients with gastroenteritis (Figure 4). Five patients had multiple diagnoses of urinary tract infection, respiratory tract infection and gastroenteritis. Among patients with malaria, 8/72 (11.1%) patients had urinary tract infections. Sixty patients had both respiratory tract infections as well as gastroenteritis.

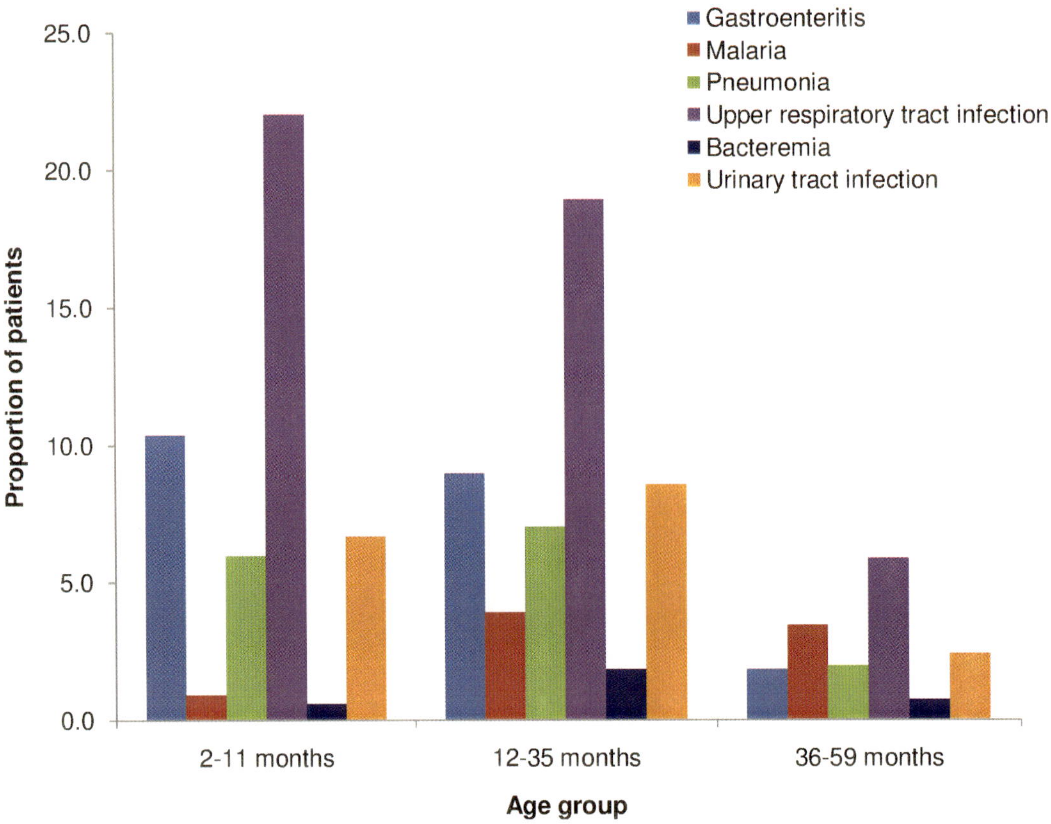

Figure 2. Distribution of common diagnosis according to age group.

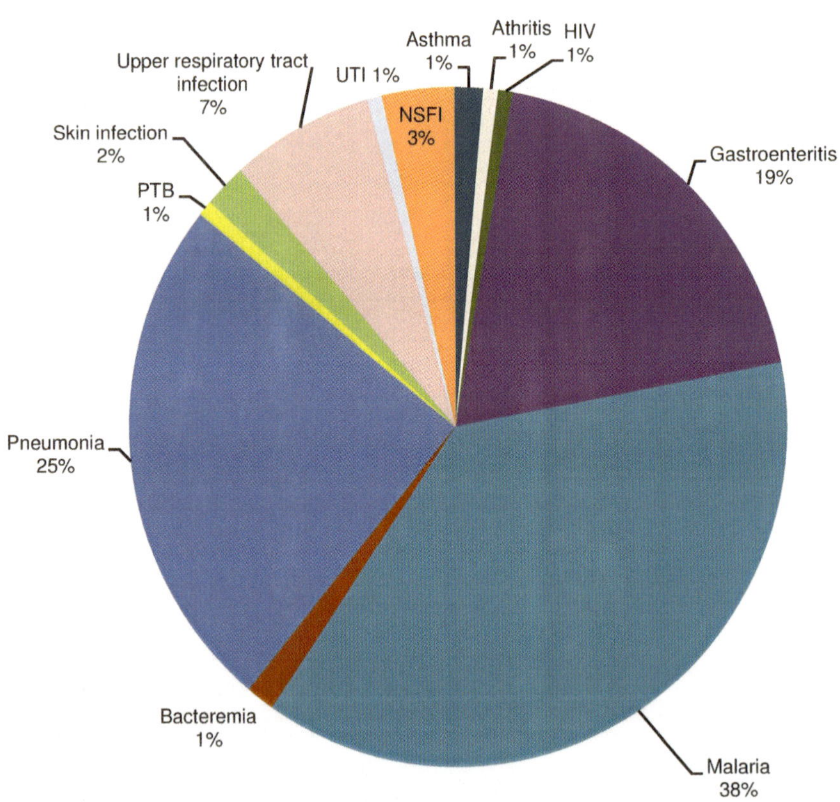

Figure 3. Distribution of illnesses among hospitalised patients at KDH (n = 141).

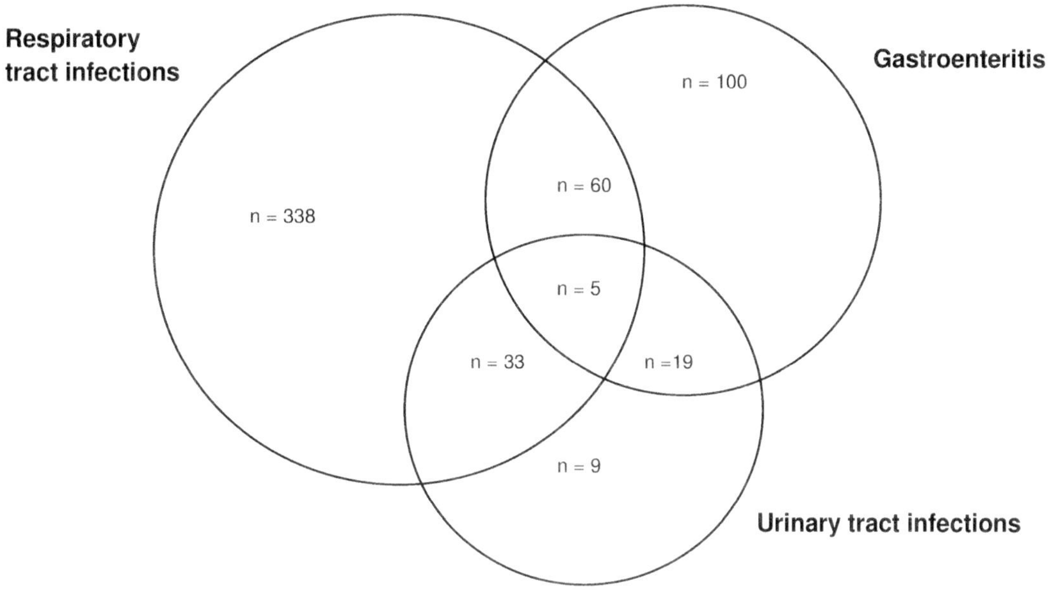

Figure 4. Co-infections of common diagnosis.

Antimicrobial susceptibility pattern

Gram negative bacterial isolates demonstrated good susceptibility to ciprofloxacin (80%–100%), moderate susceptibility to gentamicin (50%–72%) and poor susceptibility to amoxicillin, chloramphenicol and co-trimoxazole (3%–14%). *Escherichia coli* and *Klebsiella pneumoniae* demonstrated poor susceptibility to ceftriaxone (35.1% and 14.3% respectively). *Klebsiella pneumoniae* was the only Gram negative bacteria with good susceptibility to chloramphenicol (71.4%). The Gram positive bacterial isolates were observed to have good susceptibility to ceftriaxone and chloramphenicol (75%–100%) and poor susceptibility to co-trimoxazole and penicillin (0%–50%).

Discussion

This study has been able to contribute information on the prevalence of the possible causes of common febrile episodes among children less than five years of age, attending an outpatient department at KDH in north-eastern Tanzania. Over three quarters of children presenting with fever were under the age of 36 months and the majority had respiratory tract infections and gastroenteritis as the leading clinical diagnosis. Younger children under the age of 36 months tend to be more vulnerable to infections due to their immature immunity, different modes of exposure to pathogenic organisms and possibly due to a low rate of immunisation [27,28].

Plasmodium falciparum malaria, invasive community-acquired bacteria and HIV infections were uncommon among febrile children in the study with a prevalence of 8.3%, 3.2% and 1.2%, respectively. These findings are consistent with other studies on the declining malaria and community-acquired bacterial infections in the region [29,30]. The low malaria prevalence rate might partly be due to current interventions which include use of insecticide treated nets, the wide availability of effective antimalarial drugs, residual spraying and change of malaria vector behaviour [31,32]. This underscores the importance of the rational use of antibiotic and antimalarial drugs in evidence based medicine among less severely ill patients in order to counteract the problem of drug resistance.

This study found an increasing prevalence of *Salmonella typhi* among young children compared with that of non-typhi salmonella. These findings are in keeping with those of Biggs and colleagues, who found similar changing pattern of bacterial infections where *Salmonella typhi* compared with non-typhi salmonella was more common in lower malaria prevalent areas [20]. The observed prevalence of *Salmonella typhi* indicates the presence of typhoid fever among these young rural patients. The following critical measures can be implemented in preventing typhoid fever in this resource poor area through improving the quality of life. This can be done by ensuring good sanitation, safe water supply and public health education on personal as well as food hygiene.

Amoxicillin, chloramphenicol and co-trimoxazole are the most widely available antimicrobial agents in the community. These were shown to demonstrate poor susceptibility to the leading Gram negative bacterial isolates from both blood and urine cultures. Ciprofloxacin was effective but not recommended for use in children under the age of five years [33,34]. The findings support previously published work and emphasize the increasing problem of antimicrobial drug resistance [35,36]. Specific identification of bacteria causing infections is important for understanding and monitoring of antimicrobial drug resistance patterns. This will ensure patients especially children are provided with appropriate and effective treatment.

The prevalence of urinary tract infections in this study was higher among children under 36 months of age and these patients were often co-infected. The lack of access to clean water and good sanitation in this rural community might be the reason for the higher prevalence of infections observed. As in most studies conducted on urinary tract infections, *Escherichia coli* were found to be the predominant isolate. This study did not find any significant difference in gender among children with urinary tract infection. The burden of urinary tract infections in young children living in developing countries remains undefined, despite being the most common bacterial infections in childhood. The diagnosis of urinary tract infection is important in young children since if left untreated can cause nephrourologic abnormalities and impaired renal function in future [37]. With an increase in the prevalence of urinary tract infections among young children, findings from this study recommend routine urine testing of febrile children from rural communities where living conditions are poor [17,36].

Half of the febrile children in the study were clinically diagnosed with respiratory tract infections and nearly a quarter had gastroenteritis making these the leading clinical diagnoses. The observations were more frequent in children under the age of 36 months. The majority of respiratory tract infections and diarrhoea in children are known to be of viral origin [38–40,40–42]. A recent study conducted in Tanzanian children has indicated nearly half of acute respiratory infections were caused by respiratory viruses [17]. Unfortunately, antibiotics are routinely and continuously used to treat these viral infections, contributing to the increase burden of antimicrobial drug resistance. The current study provides preliminary data for future evidence-based research on respiratory and enteric viruses in the community.

Co-infections were observed in a quarter of the patients, mostly among those with urinary tract infections, respiratory tract infections and gastroenteritis. Existence of multiple infections is a challenging issue when developing fever management guidelines, especially in poor rural areas which are usually at higher risks of numerous kinds of infections [43]. This study has underlined the prevalence of co-infections that exist among patients enrolled in the study area.

The causative agents of febrile infections documented in this study can be considered as representative of the causes of fever in this specific area. Despite recommendations by WHO on the parasitological evidence for malaria treatment, management of fever cases in Tanzania is still challenging [44,45]. Furthermore, IMCI guidelines remain unspecific for the management of non-malaria febrile illnesses. Evidence based findings on bacterial infections from the current study can contribute to the revision of clinical algorithms for management of febrile illnesses. There is a need for guidelines that would assist in the management of non-malarial febrile illnesses given the declining malaria trend. Febrile illnesses, especially in children, require proper management so as to avoid unnecessary morbidity and mortalities, antimicrobial abuse and unnecessary expense. Investment in diagnostic facilities, such as adequate microbiology laboratories, qualified and trained laboratory personnel is needed. Furthermore, availability of rapid diagnostic tests for malaria, bacterial and viral infections, is required for rapid and accurate diagnoses of paediatric infections. A possible recommendation is that fever surveillance be conducted along side the existing malaria surveillance systems in future clinical research on vaccines and drugs.

The study had a number of limitations. Firstly, the study was conducted for the period of ten months and therefore could not assess seasonality of febrile episodes. Secondly, the study relied on verbal information provided by parents and guardians on the prior use of antimalarial drugs and antibiotics. This means that some of the children enrolled may well have been on antimicrobial therapy and this will have contributed to the low yield of positive cultures. In addition, the collection of only a single blood culture is known to reduce the possibility of isolating the organisms present in the bloodstream. The volume of blood inoculated into culture bottles was sometimes low due to difficulty in getting venous access especially from young patients and this might have contributed to the low bacterial yield. The study could not provide evidence-based data on respiratory and enteric viruses which are thought to cause majority of respiratory tract infections and diarrhoea in young children. Causative agents of zoonosis among outpatient children from this particular study community were not investigated. Understanding their prevalence would be of advantage despite not being investigated routinely at health facilities in the country.

Acknowledgments

We would like to thank all children and their parents/guardians who participated in the study. We thank Korogwe District Hospital management, NIMR employees; Samwel Gesase, Samuel Sembuche, Monica Billa and Boniface Eustack for their clinical assistance; Neema Malle, Theresia Joseph and Thabita Joseph for blood drawing and sample collection; Geofrey Lyimo, Jerome Msamba, Jackson Kimaro and Grayson Mwakalindile for chest radiographs; Zeno Manjulungu, Peter Gondwe, Gerson Goodluck Maro, Martin George, Joyce Mbwana and Lincoln Malle for laboratory sample analysis; Mohammed Mapondela, Neema Barua and Mary Lukindo for database and data entry; Filbert Francis and Brunno Mmbando for statistical assistance. We thank RTS,S project, PATH-MVI and Afrique-One Project for their support during the study. We thank NIMR Director General for permission to publish this work.

Author Contributions

Conceived and designed the experiments: CM BN JL AB PL ML ZL. Performed the experiments: CM AB PL. Analyzed the data: CM BN JL. Contributed reagents/materials/analysis tools: CM BN JL. Contributed to the writing of the manuscript: CM. Reviewed the manuscript and provided critical inputs: CM BN JL AB PL ML ZL. Read and approved the final manuscript: CM BN JL AB PL ML ZL.

References

1. Gething PW, Kirui VC, Alegana VA, Okiro EA, Noor AM, et al. (2010) Estimating the number of paediatric fevers associated with malaria infection presenting to Africa's public health sector in 2007. PLoS Med 7: e1000301. doi:10.1371/journal.pmed.1000301
2. Osei-Kwakye K, Asante KP, Mahama E, Apanga S, Owusu R, et al. (2013) The benefits or otherwise of managing malaria cases with or without laboratory diagnosis: the experience in a district hospital in Ghana. PLoS One 8: e58107.;PONE-D-12-26544 [pii]. doi:10.1371/journal.pone.0058107
3. Archibald LK, Reller LB (2001) Clinical microbiology in developing countries. Emerg Infect Dis 7: 302–305. doi:10.3201/eid0702.700302
4. Gwer S, Newton CR, Berkley JA (2007) Over-diagnosis and co-morbidity of severe malaria in African children: a guide for clinicians. Am J Trop Med Hyg 77: 6–13. 77/6_Suppl/6 [pii].
5. Petit PL, van Ginneken JK (1995) Analysis of hospital records in four African countries, 1975–1990, with emphasis on infectious diseases. J Trop Med Hyg 98: 217–227.
6. Ye Y, Madise N, Ndugwa R, Ochola S, Snow RW (2009) Fever treatment in the absence of malaria transmission in an urban informal settlement in Nairobi, Kenya. Malar J 8: 160. 1475-2875-8-160 [pii]; doi:10.1186/1475-2875-8-160
7. Hertz JT, Munishi OM, Sharp JP, Reddy EA, Crump JA (2013) Comparing actual and perceived causes of fever among community members in a low malaria transmission setting in northern Tanzania. Trop Med Int Health 18: 1406–1415. doi:10.1111/tmi.12191
8. D'Acremont V, Lengeler C, Genton B (2010) Reduction in the proportion of fevers associated with Plasmodium falciparum parasitaemia in Africa: a systematic review. Malar J 9: 240. 1475-2875-9-240 [pii]; doi:10.1186/1475-2875-9-240
9. Rutta AS, Francis F, Mmbando BP, Ishengoma DS, Sembuche SH, et al. (2012) Using community-owned resource persons to provide early diagnosis and treatment and estimate malaria burden at community level in north-eastern Tanzania. Malar J 11: 152. 1475-2875-11-152 [pii]; doi:10.1186/1475-2875-11-152
10. Were T, Davenport GC, Hittner JB, Ouma C, Vulule JM, et al. (2011) Bacteremia in Kenyan children presenting with malaria. J Clin Microbiol 49: 671–676. JCM.01864-10 [pii]; doi:10.1128/JCM.01864-10
11. Petti CA, Polage CR, Quinn TC, Ronald AR, Sande MA (2006) Laboratory medicine in Africa: a barrier to effective health care. Clin Infect Dis 42: 377–382. CID37615 [pii]; doi:10.1086/499363
12. Urdea M, Penny LA, Olmsted SS, Giovanni MY, Kaspar P, et al. (2006) Requirements for high impact diagnostics in the developing world. Nature 444 Suppl 1: 73–79. nature05448 [pii]; doi:10.1038/nature05448

13. Strom GE, Haanshuus CG, Fataki M, Langeland N, Blomberg B (2013) Challenges in diagnosing paediatric malaria in Dar es Salaam, Tanzania. Malar J 12: 228. 1475-2875-12-228 [pii]; doi:10.1186/1475-2875-12-228
14. Moon AM, Biggs HM, Rubach MP, Crump JA, Maro VP, et al. (2014) Evaluation of In-Hospital Management for Febrile Illness in Northern Tanzania before and after 2010 World Health Organization Guidelines for the Treatment of Malaria. PLoS One 9: e89814. doi:10.1371/journal.pone.0089814; PONE-D-13-35569 [pii].
15. World Health Organisation (WHO) (2010) Guidelines for the treatment of malaria, 2nd edition.
16. Reyburn H, Mbatia R, Drakeley C, Carneiro I, Mwakasungula E, et al. (2004) Overdiagnosis of malaria in patients with severe febrile illness in Tanzania: a prospective study. BMJ 329: 1212. bmj.38251.658229.55 [pii]; doi:10.1136/bmj.38251.658229.55
17. D'Acremont V, Kilowoko M, Kyungu E, Philipina S, Sangu W, et al. (2014) Beyond malaria–causes of fever in outpatient Tanzanian children. N Engl J Med 370: 809–817. doi:10.1056/NEJMoa1214482
18. Nadjm B, Amos B, Mtove G, Ostermann J, Chonya S, et al. (2010) WHO guidelines for antimicrobial treatment in children admitted to hospital in an area of intense Plasmodium falciparum transmission: prospective study. BMJ 340: c1350.
19. Crump JA, Ramadhani HO, Morrissey AB, Msuya LJ, Yang LY, et al. (2011) Invasive bacterial and fungal infections among hospitalized HIV-infected and HIV-uninfected children and infants in northern Tanzania. Trop Med Int Health 16: 830–837. doi:10.1111/j.1365-3156.2011.02774.x
20. Biggs HM, Lester R, Nadjm B, Mtove G, Todd JE, et al. (2014) Invasive salmonella infections in areas of high and low malaria transmission intensity in Tanzania. Clin Infect Dis 58: 638–647. cit798 [pii]; doi:10.1093/cid/cit798
21. National Bureau of Statistics Ministry of Finance Tanzania (2013) 2012 Population and housing census.
22. Mmbando BP, Vestergaard LS, Kitua AY, Lemnge MM, Theander TG, et al. (2010) A progressive declining in the burden of malaria in north-eastern Tanzania. Malar J 9: 216. 1475-2875-9-216 [pii]; doi:10.1186/1475-2875-9-216
23. Schmiegelow C, Minja D, Oesterholt M, Pehrson C, Suhrs HE, et al. (2013) Malaria and fetal growth alterations in the 3(rd) trimester of pregnancy: a longitudinal ultrasound study. PLoS One 8: e53794. doi:10.1371/journal.-pone.0053794; PONE-D-12-29446 [pii].
24. World Health Organisation (WHO) (2005) Intergrated Managemnet of Childhood Illness.
25. Kwon JH, Fausone MK, Du H, Robicsek A, Peterson LR (2012) Impact of laboratory-reported urine culture colony counts on the diagnosis and treatment of urinary tract infection for hospitalized patients. Am J Clin Pathol 137: 778–784. 137/5/778 [pii]; doi:10.1309/AJCP4KVGQZEG1YDM
26. National Aids Control Programme Ministry of Health and Social Welfare Tanzania (2012) Guideline for HIV testing.
27. Liu L, Johnson HL, Cousens S, Perin J, Scott S, et al. (2012) Global, regional, and national causes of child mortality: an updated systematic analysis for 2010 with time trends since 2000. Lancet 379: 2151–2161. S0140-6736(12)60560-1 [pii]; doi:10.1016/S0140-6736(12)60560-1
28. Hamilton JL, John SP (2013) Evaluation of fever in infants and young children. Am Fam Physician 87: 254–260. d10789 [pii].
29. Mmbando BP, Vestergaard LS, Kitua AY, Lemnge MM, Theander TG, et al. (2010) A progressive declining in the burden of malaria in north-eastern Tanzania. Malar J 9: 216. 1475-2875-9-216 [pii]; doi:10.1186/1475-2875-9-216
30. Mtove G, Amos B, Nadjm B, Hendriksen IC, Dondorp AM, et al. (2011) Decreasing incidence of severe malaria and community-acquired bacteraemia among hospitalized children in Muheza, north-eastern Tanzania, 2006–2010. Malar J 10: 320. 1475-2875-10-320 [pii]; doi:10.1186/1475-2875-10-320
31. Murray CJ, Rosenfeld LC, Lim SS, Andrews KG, Foreman KJ, et al. (2012) Global malaria mortality between 1980 and 2010: a systematic analysis. Lancet 379: 413–431. S0140-6736(12)60034-8 [pii]; doi:10.1016/S0140-6736(12)60034-8
32. Aregawi MW, Ali AS, Al-mafazy AW, Molteni F, Katikiti S, et al. (2011) Reductions in malaria and anaemia case and death burden at hospitals following scale-up of malaria control in Zanzibar, 1999–2008. Malar J 10: 46. 1475-2875-10-46 [pii]; doi:10.1186/1475-2875-10-46
33. The United Republic of Tanzania MoHaSW (2007) Standard Treatment Guidelines (STG) and The National Essential Medicines List (NEMLIT) for Mainland Tanzania (Page 6).
34. Choi SH, Kim EY, Kim YJ (2013) Systemic use of fluoroquinolone in children. Korean J Pediatr 56: 196–201. doi:10.3345/kjp.2013.56.5.196
35. Thriemer K, Ley B, Ame S, von SL, Pak GD, et al. (2012) The burden of invasive bacterial infections in Pemba, Zanzibar. PLoS One 7: e30350. doi:10.1371/journal.pone.0030350; PONE-D-11-19140 [pii].
36. Msaki BP, Mshana SE, Hokororo A, Mazigo HD, Morona D (2012) Prevalence and predictors of urinary tract infection and severe malaria among febrile children attending Makongoro health centre in Mwanza city, North-Western Tanzania. Arch Public Health 70: 4. 0778-7367-70-4 [pii]; doi:10.1186/0778-7367-70-4
37. Montini G, Tullus K, Hewitt I (2011) Febrile urinary tract infections in children. N Engl J Med 365: 239–250. doi:10.1056/NEJMra1007755
38. Feikin DR, Njenga MK, Bigogo G, Aura B, Aol G, et al. (2013) Viral and bacterial causes of severe acute respiratory illness among children aged less than 5 years in a high malaria prevalence area of western Kenya, 2007–2010. Pediatr Infect Dis J 32: e14–e19. doi:10.1097/INF.0b013e31826fd39b
39. Niang MN, Diop OM, Sarr FD, Goudiaby D, Malou-Sompy H, et al. (2010) Viral etiology of respiratory infections in children under 5 years old living in tropical rural areas of Senegal: The EVIRA project. J Med Virol 82: 866–872. doi:10.1002/jmv.21665
40. Bonkoungou IJ, Haukka K, Osterblad M, Hakanen AJ, Traore AS, et al. (2013) Bacterial and viral etiology of childhood diarrhea in Ouagadougou, Burkina Faso. BMC Pediatr 13: 36. 1471-2431-13-36 [pii]; doi:10.1186/1471-2431-13-36
41. Sire JM, Garin B, Chartier L, Fall NK, Tall A, et al. (2013) Community-acquired infectious diarrhoea in children under 5 years of age in Dakar, Senegal. Paediatr Int Child Health 33: 139–144. doi:10.1179/2046905512Y.0000000046
42. Moyo SJ, Gro N, Matee MI, Kitundu J, Myrmel H, et al. (2011) Age specific aetiological agents of diarrhoea in hospitalized children aged less than five years in Dar es Salaam, Tanzania. BMC Pediatr 11: 19. 1471-2431-11-19 [pii]; doi:10.1186/1471-2431-11-19
43. Alemu A, Shiferaw Y, Addis Z, Mathewos B, Birhan W (2013) Effect of malaria on HIV/AIDS transmission and progression. Parasit Vectors 6: 18. 1756-3305-6-18 [pii]; doi:10.1186/1756-3305-6-18
44. Mubi M, Kakoko D, Ngasala B, Premji Z, Peterson S, et al. (2013) Malaria diagnosis and treatment practices following introduction of rapid diagnostic tests in Kibaha District, Coast Region, Tanzania. Malar J 12: 293. 1475-2875-12-293 [pii]; doi:10.1186/1475-2875-12-293
45. Baltzell K, Elfving K, Shakely D, Ali AS, Msellem M, et al. (2013) Febrile illness management in children under five years of age: a qualitative pilot study on primary health care workers' practices in Zanzibar. Malar J 12: 37. 1475-2875-12-37 [pii]; doi:10.1186/1475-2875-12-37

Lower Blood Glucose and Variability Are Associated with Earlier Recovery from Renal Injury Caused by Episodic Urinary Tract Infection in Advanced Type 2 Diabetic Chronic Kidney Disease

Ping-Fang Chiu[1,2,3], Chia-Lin Wu[3], Ching-Hui Huang[4], Hung-Hsiang Liou[3], Chirn-Bin Chang[3], Horng-Rong Chang[1,2,5¶], Chia-Chu Chang[2,3,6*¶]

1 Institute of Medicine, Chung Shan Medical University, Taichung, Taiwan, **2** School of Medicine, Chung Shan Medical University, Taichung, Taiwan, **3** Nephrology Division, Department of Internal Medicine, Changhua Christian Hospital, Changhua, Taiwan, **4** Division of Cardiology, Department of Internal Medicine, Changhua Christian Hospital, Changhua, Taiwan, **5** Division of Nephrology, Department of Internal Medicine, Chung Shan Medical University Hospital, Taichung, Taiwan, **6** Ph.D. Program for Aging, College of Medicine, China Medical University, Taichung, Taiwan

Abstract

Purpose: In our previous study, type 2 diabetic chronic kidney disease (CKD) patients with glomerular filtration rates of <30 mL/min upon hospitalization for urinary tract infection (UTI) were at a risk for acute kidney injury. This study aimed to clarify the effect of glucose and its variability on renal outcomes during admission for the treatment of UTI.

Materials and Methods: Based on the date of renal recovery (RIFLE criteria: acute kidney injury occurred within 1–7 days and was sustained over 1 day), we divided these patients into early- (≤9 days, Group A) and late-recovery (>9 days, Group B) groups. The differences in the continuous and categorical variables of the two groups were assessed separately. The mean glucose levels and their variability (using the standard deviation and the coefficient of standard deviation) were compared at the fasting, midday pre-meal, evening pre-meal, and evening post-meal time points during hospitalization. We have organized the manuscript in a manner compliant with the STROBE (Strengthening the Reporting of Observational Studies in Epidemiology) statement.

Results: Acute kidney injury occurred within the two groups ($p = 0.007$ and $p = 0.001$, respectively). The early-morning blood glucose levels (149.7±44.0 mg/dL) and average blood glucose levels (185.6±52.0 mg/dL) were better in Group A ($p = 0.01$, $p = 0.02$). Group A patients also had lower glucose variability than Group B at the different time points ($p < 0.05$). Group A also had earlier renal recovery. More relevant pathogens were identified from blood in Group B ($p = 0.038$).

Conclusions: Early-morning fasting and mean blood glucose levels and their variability can be good indicators of severe infection and predictors of renal outcome in type 2 diabetic patients with CKD and UTI.

Editor: Francesca D'Addio, San Raffaele Hospital, Italy

Funding: The study was supported by a research grant (97CCHIRP-31) from Changhua Christian Hospital. The funders had no role in study design, data collection and analysis, decision to publish, or preparation of the manuscript.

Competing Interests: The authors have declared that no competing interests exist.

* Email: 27509@cch.org.tw

¶ These authors contributed equally to this work.

Introduction

Urinary tract infection (UTI) is a common disease in type 1 and 2 diabetic patients, and diabetic patients are prone to UTI as well [1]. Among diabetic patients, 9–20% of women and 3–11% of men may develop UTI [2], which may result in longer hospitalizations (3- to 5-fold) [3] and higher mortality (7.6% versus 1.6%) [4] in patients with diabetes than in those without diabetes. Additionally, in a previous study, we found that UTI can also lead to acute kidney injury (AKI) in type 2 diabetic chronic kidney disease (CKD) patients who had an estimated glomerular filtration rate (eGFR) of <30 mL/min on admission [5]. Furthermore, AKI episodes can be independent risk factors for renal progression in diabetes CKD patients [6]. The RIFLE criteria for AKI were defined according to the Acute Dialysis Quality Initiative consensus in 2002, and denoted that GFR can abruptly decrease by more than 25% within 1–7 days after admission and may be sustained for longer than 1 day. For almost all type 2 diabetic patients with advanced CKD, renal dysfunction did gradually revert within 6 months after the UTI if they survived and were free from long-term dialysis [5]. The rate of renal recovery was also essential; a shorter recovery period would

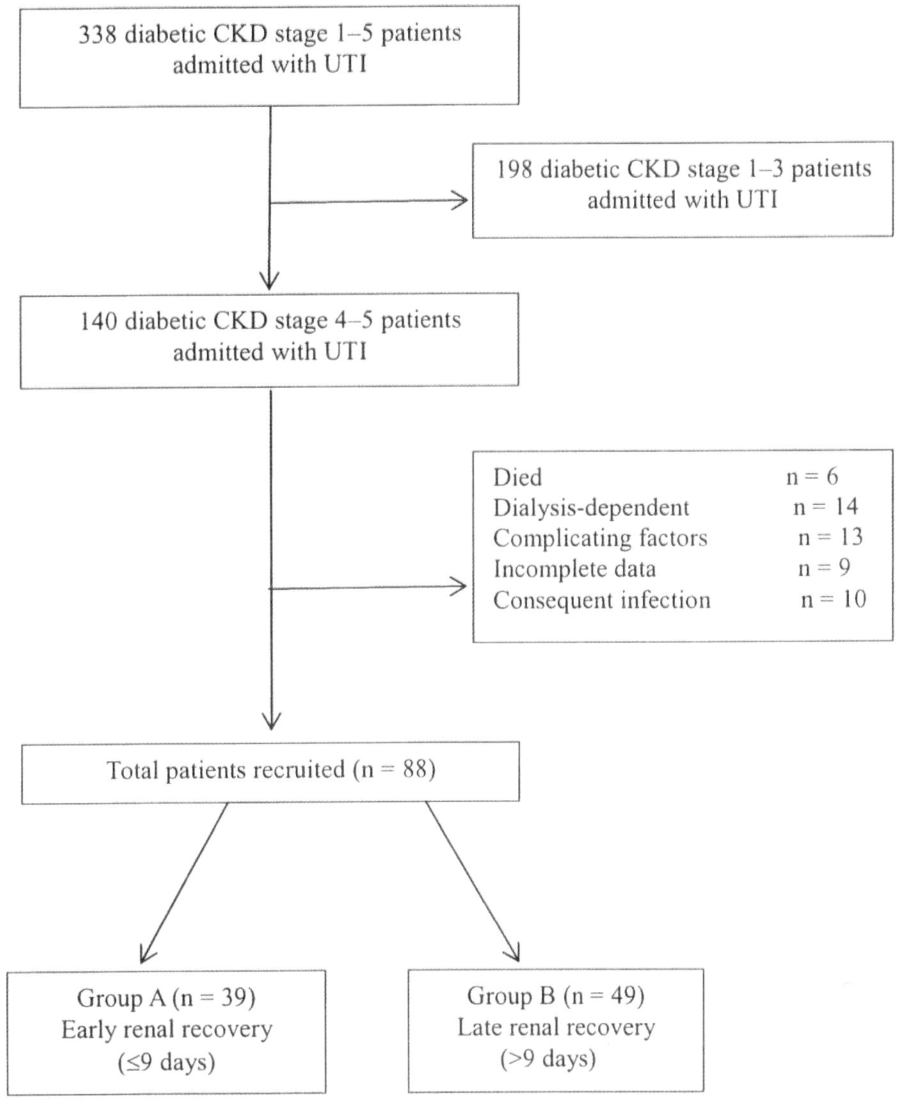

Figure 1. Participant flow diagram depicting the screening/enrollment process.

improve health and reduce the risk of another episode of infection. Possible factors that could affect renal recovery included the baseline GFR, severity or duration of sepsis, and concurrent co-morbidities. Critically ill patients with lower glucose variability have lower short-term or hospital mortality than patients with higher glucose variability [7]. However, the impact of glucose and its fluctuations on renal function during hospitalization from nonfatal infection has not been reported. This study aimed to clarify the association of glucose and its variability during admission and renal outcome in type 2 diabetic patients with CKD and episodic UTI.

Materials and Methods

We enrolled patients that had been managed under CKD care programs, who also had UTI and were admitted to our hospital from 2001 to November 2013. The admission criteria for UTI in our hospital included the presence of a systemic inflammatory response syndrome or a complicated condition involving a major organ. We excluded patients who had untreated obstructive uropathy, those who died, those who were dialysis-dependent after infection, or those who had subsequent hospital-acquired infections. To improve the quality of reporting in observational studies, the manuscript was organized in a manner compliant with the STROBE (Strengthening the Reporting of Observational Studies in Epidemiology) statement [8]. The patient flow chart is shown in Figure 1, which includes the number of patients recruited and excluded from the study. The Modification of the Diet in Renal Disease (MDRD) formula was applied for GFR estimation. The formula used for eGFR was the following:

$$\begin{aligned} \text{GFR (mL/min/1.73 m}^2) &= 186 \times \text{serum creatinine}^{-1.154} \\ &\times \text{age}^{-0.203} \\ &\times 1.212 \text{ (if black)}. \end{aligned}$$

AKI was defined using the RIFLE criteria. When the decrease in eGFR returned to <10% of baseline renal function, the patient was determined to be in renal recovery as defined in previously published manuscripts [9,10]. Based on the date of renal recovery

Table 1. Patient characteristics.

	Group A (n = 39)		Group B (n = 49)		
	Mean	**SD**	**Mean**	**SD**	*p*
Age‡	67.8	8.7	68.4	14.1	0.80
Gender, male†	26.3%		26.5%		0.98
Hypertension†	76.3%		63.3%		0.009*
CVD†	23.7%		24.5%		0.86
Hyperlipidemia†	18.4%		16.3%		0.61
Liver†	15.8%		16.3%		0.89
Stroke†	21.1%		22.5%		0.75
SBP (mmHg)‡	135	26	121	17	0.057
DBP (mmHg)‡	73	17	72	13	0.78
eGFR (ml/mln)‡	16.9	7.9	15.4	7.7	0.47
BUN (mg/dL)‡	61.4	41.7	59.6	33.6	0.84
Cr (mg/dL)‡	4.09	2.9	3.99	2.3	0.86
ALT (U/L)‡	23.3	12.3	34.6	29.6	0.03*
HbA1C (%)‡	7.7	2.0	8.2	2.8	0.30
Cholesterol (mg/dL)‡	150.8	62.1	169.6	60	0.79
Triglyceride (mg/dL)‡	170.3	77.9	209.5	80.1	0.51
HDL (mg/dL)‡	37.7	12.8	39.4	17.7	0.90
LDL (mg/dL)‡	89.8	35.6	102.9	44.8	0.76
Uric acid (mg/dL)‡	6.3	1.6	7.9	2.2	0.08
Albumin (g/dL)‡	2.8	0.7	2.7	0.6	0.37
Na (mEq/dL)‡	132.3	6.8	133.0	7.0	0.61
K (mEq/dL)‡	4.6	1.0	4.2	1.1	0.15
WBC ($\times 10^3$)‡	11.3	5.5	13.5	8.3	0.10
Hemoglobin (g/dL)‡	10.4	2.4	10.2	2.5	0.72
Hematocrit (%)‡	30.5	7.7	30.0	7.4	0.77
UPCR (g/g)‡	1.8	2.0	1.1	1.2	0.31
Hospital days§	6.78	3.68	11.5	10.8	0.019*
(median)	6.0		7.5		

Abbreviations: CVD, cardiovascular disease; ALT, alanine aminotransferase; WBC, white blood cell; UPCR, urine protein–creatinine ratio; SBP, systolic blood pressure; DBP, diastolic blood pressure.
†chi-square test.
‡student's t-test.
§Mann–Whitney U test.
*$p<0.05$.

Table 2. Blood glucose levels and renal outcome.

	Group A		Group B		
Glucose (mg/dL)	**mean**	**SD**	**mean**	**SD**	*p*
Fasting	149.7	44.0	181.2	64.5	0.01*
Midday pre-meal	203.7	60.8	228.5	81.9	0.17
Evening pre-meal	209.9	62.5	234.6	74.4	0.11
Evening post-meal	216.0	54.5	228.2	68.8	0.41
mean	185.6	52.0	216.7	69.5	0.02*

Abbreviation: SD, standard deviation.
*$p<0.05$.

Table 3. Glucose variability: standard deviation (SD) and renal outcome.

	Group A		Group B		
Glucose (mg/dL)	**SD mean**	**SD**	**SD mean**	**SD**	*p*
Fasting	46.6	37.9	64.0	32.6	0.03*
Midday pre-meal	64.6	40.1	72.1	40.2	0.46
Evening pre-meal	66.1	37.4	84.6	40.5	0.04*
Evening post-meal	64.0	37.7	83.0	38.3	0.04*

*$p<0.05$.

(GFR decrease within 1–7 days and that was sustained for longer than 1 day) after admission, we divided these patients into early- (≤9 days, Group A) and late-recovery (>9 days, Group B) groups. The basic characteristics of these patients were collected and analyzed in Table 1. The continuous and categorical variable differences, including blood glucose (Table 2–4) and bacteriology (Table 5), of the two groups were assayed separately by the Student's t-test, the Mann–Whitney U test, and the chi-squared test. The mean glucose level and its variability (calculated by the standard deviation and the coefficient of standard deviation: SD/mean) at four fixed time points (fasting, midday pre-meal, evening pre-meal, evening post-meal) during the hospitalization were compared. The patients' survival rates after episodic UTI were analyzed using the Kaplan–Meier method.

Ethics Statement

The CKD care program including ethics and patients' right was guided by the Clinical Care Program Certification and Joint Commission International. This protocol was also approved by the Institutional Review Board of the Changhua Christian Hospital, Taiwan. All subjects gave written informed consent to participate. If patients could not be contacted in any way, the data were categorized as incomplete.

Results

One hundred and forty diabetic CKD patients with eGFR of <30 mL/min who were admitted to the hospital with UTI during the 13 years were evaluated for the study. Fifty-two patients had been excluded because of various causes as reported in Figure 1. Eighty-eight patients (65 females, 23 males) were included. Thirty-nine patients had recovered renal function early (≤9 days, Group A), and 49 patients recovered function late (>9 days, Group B). The baseline characteristics of the patients are listed in Table 1. The age and incidence of comorbidities, such as cardiovascular disease, stroke, and liver disease, were compared between the two groups. The biochemical and hematological data were balanced in both groups, with the exception of alanine aminotransferase (ALT). The estimated GFR series are illustrated in Figure 2. AKI occurred during admission in the two groups ($p=0.007$ and $p=0.001$, respectively), and almost all diabetic patients gradually recovered within 6 months. In contrast, 34 non-diabetic CKD stage 4–5 patients (n = 544; 0.063%, data not shown) were admitted for urosepsis during this period. No significant AKI was observed ($p=0.39$, data not shown).

Microorganisms detected in blood were more notable in Group B (Table 5; $p=0.038$). Urine pathogen culture rates found between both groups were comparable. E. coli was the most commonly isolated pathogen. Moreover, approximately 32% (12 in Group A; 16 in Group B) of patients had cystitis within 3 months before the urosepsis episodes. Two-week antibiotic regimens were prescribed at least for patients with complicated UTI, including first- and second-generation cephalosporins and third-generation cephalosporin/or quinolone (33, 6 in group A; 38, 11 in Group B, respectively). Aminoglycosides were avoided owing to their nephrotoxicity.

The mean early-morning blood glucose levels (149.7±44.0 mg/dL) and average blood glucose levels (185.6±52.0 mg/dL) were better in Group A ($p=0.01$, $p=0.02$; Table 2). Patients in Group A also had lower glucose variability based on the differences in the standard deviation and the coefficient of variation (SD/mean) than patients in Group B at the different time points. There was more relevance in the fasting and the evening post-meal blood glucose levels (Table 3 and 4; $p<0.05$). The trend of glucose variability was also consistently observed at the midday pre-meal and evening pre-meal time points.

The two groups had equivalent long-term patient survival (data not shown). We also adjusted for possible confounding factors that may have contributed to renal recovery using multivariate cox

Table 4. Glucose variability: coefficient of variation (CV) and renal outcome.

	Group A		Group B		
Glucose (mg/dL)	**CV mean**	**SD**	**CV mean**	**SD**	*p*
Fasting	0.29	0.19	0.36	0.14	0.001*
Midday pre-meal	0.30	0.15	0.32	0.16	0.03*
Evening pre-meal	0.32	0.18	0.36	0.15	0.13
Evening post-meal	0.28	0.13	0.35	0.15	0.02*

*$p<0.05$.

Table 5. Bacteriology.

	Group A	Group B	*p*
Blood culture	7	17	0.038*
GNB	5	15	
GPC	2	2	
Urine culture	34	39	0.18
GNB	21	30	
GPC	5	6	
fungus	5	2	
others	3	1	

Abbreviations: GNB, gram-negative bacillus; GPC, gram-positive cocci.
chi-square test.
*$p<0.05$.

proportional hazard regression, including age, severity of infection, and glucose and blood pressure control (Table 6).

Discussion

Diabetes and its complications are the leading cause of end-stage renal disease worldwide. Diabetes patients are vulnerable to UTI. Further, UTI may cause AKI in diabetic CKD patients with an eGFR of <30 mL/min. Furthermore, repeated episodes of AKI are related to rapid progression of renal-failure. The main finding of this study was that better blood glucose control and lower glucose variability during hospitalization in type 2 diabetic patients with CKD could predict earlier renal recovery from UTI.

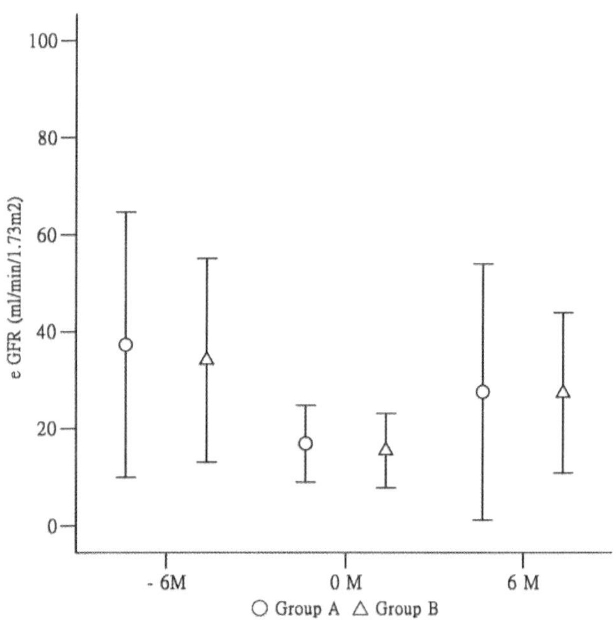

Figure 2. Changes in estimated glomerular filtration rate (eGFR) over time within the early- and late-recovery groups. T (0) represents the time point on admission from urinary tract infection; the "plus" and "minus" symbols represent the time interval after and before admission, respectively. Acute kidney injury occurred in diabetic patients with chronic kidney disease [eGFR at T (0) versus T (−6); $p=0.007$ in Group A; $p=0.001$ in Group B], and eGFR reverted to the trend 6 months later if urinary tract infection was cured.

Because these patients were not critically ill and remained in the ward, glucose measurement at four different time points (fasting, midday pre-meal, evening pre-meal, evening post-meal) was applicable, instead of continued glucose monitoring.

High glycosylated hemoglobin in the diabetic population has been associated with a high incidence of microangiopathy, macroangiopathy, and mortality [11]. Long-term glucose variability has also played a role in the development of microangiopathy and macroangiopathy [12,13]. A study by Monnier et al even suggested that glucose variability may be more deleterious than chronic hyperglycemia in the development of diabetic complications [14]. Acute blood glucose fluctuations during hospitalization for various critical conditions have predicted short-term or in-hospital mortality [15]. The better outcomes were obtained in critical patients with lower glucose variability. This scenario was also found in non-diabetic critically ill patients [16]. Jeon et al demonstrated that pre- and post-operative glucose levels and their variability were associated with the risk of surgical site infection or in-hospital death [17]. Additionally, increased blood glucose variability during hospitalization has been a precursor of sepsis and mortality in burn patients as reported by Alexander et al [18]. Furthermore, a meta-analysis by Haga et al revealed that tight glycemic control might reduce early mortality, the incidence of atrial fibrillation, and the time spent in the intensive care unit after cardiac surgery [19].

In contrast, in data from the reanalysis of the HEART2D study, Siegelaar et al found that a decrease in glucose variability did not reduce cardiovascular events in type 2 diabetic patients after an acute myocardial infarction [20]. The tight blood glucose control in critical patients does not reduce mortality but does increase the risk of hypoglycemia according to meta-analysis studies [21,22]. In the NICE-SUGAR Study, a blood glucose target of 180 mg/dL or less resulted in lower mortality than did a target of 81–108 mg/dL [23]. For non-critically-ill patients treated with insulin, according to the Standards of Medical Care in Diabetes 2013, the pre-meal glucose target should be around 140 mg/dL and post-meal glucose target should be around 180 mg/dL [24]. However, because advanced CKD diabetic patients can be at higher risk of hypoglycemia, sugar control that is less tight seems reasonable. Nevertheless, no current guidelines have been recommended for these patients.

Several possible mechanisms may account for chronic glucose variability. Short-term Type 1 diabetes mellitus (DM) participants with residual β-cell function had lower glucose variability than longer-term Type 1 DM participants (27% versus 42%, respec-

Table 6. Cox proportional hazard regression: hazard ratio of variables and renal injury.

Variable	HR	95% CI	p
Glucose (mean)	1.006	1.002–1.010	0.003*
Age	0.979	0.951–1.008	0.150
Hypertension	0.329	0.174–0.619	0.001*
WBC	0.955	0.889–1.025	0.202
HbA1C	0.957	0.844–1.086	0.498

*$p<0.05$.

tively; $p<0.001$) [25]. An autonomic imbalance from increased hypothalamic-pituitary axis activity and cortisol levels can also lead to worsening glucose variability and neuropathy [26,27]. The study by Monnier et al indicated that acute glucose excursion triggered more oxidative stress than chronic sustained hyperglycemia in type 2 diabetic patients. There is a linear correlation between 24-hour urinary excretion rates of 8-Iso Prostaglandin F2 and glycemic variability [28]. The antidiabetic agents, dipeptidyl peptidase IV inhibitors, were found to reduce glucose fluctuations and plasma nitrotyrosine, IL-6, and IL-18 levels ($p<0.05$) in type 2 diabetic patients after 3 months of treatment [29]. Additionally, acute glucose elevation can be highly predictive of infection in critically injured trauma patients, as reported by Bochicchio et al [30]. In our study, it was evident that increased glucose variability in type 2 diabetic patients with CKD and eGFR of <30 mL/min could have delayed the renal recovery from UTI. Additionally, those who had delayed renal recovery also had longer hospital stays.

Another interesting finding was the remarkable pathogen identification rate from blood in Group B. Both C-reactive protein and procalcitonin concentrations can suggest bacterial infection in emergency patients [31,32]. This may imply that hospitalized patients with higher blood glucose and greater variability were in course of more severe inflammation and oxidative stress. Perhaps, infections with concurrent glucose variability may simultaneously influence renal injury and recovery. Elevated liver enzymes were frequently found in septic conditions. Several hepatic biomarkers, including bilirubin, albumin, alkaline phosphatase, aspartate, ALTs, and lactate dehydrogenase, had been evaluated in association with the mortality rate in the intensive care unit by Marshall et al. However, no ideal biomarker has been identified at this time [33].

Several methods were applied for measuring the glucose variability [34]. However, from previous systematic reviews and our study, the magnitude of glycemic variability was highly correlated with the level of the mean glucose value. The degree of correlation of the different measures of glycemic variability was also high [35].

Some limitations in our current study included the following: (1) relative small sample size; (2) single-center evaluation; (3) retrospective analysis; and (4) the use of monitored glucose at fixed time points, instead of continuous glucose monitoring. Whether aggressive control of blood glucose levels during ward hospitalization could improve the recovery of the renal dysfunction would need to be evaluated in a controlled study in the future. However, at least, the glucose levels are a good indicator of severe infection, organ dysfunction, and renal outcome in type 2 diabetic patients with CKD and UTI.

Conclusions

Early-morning fasting and mean blood glucose levels and glucose variability during hospitalization are good indicators of severe infection, and also predictors of renal outcome in type 2 diabetic patients with CKD and UTI.

Author Contributions

Conceived and designed the experiments: PFC CLW CHH CCC HRC. Performed the experiments: PFC CLW CHH CCC HRC. Analyzed the data: PFC CLW HHL CBC. Contributed reagents/materials/analysis tools: CHH CCC. Wrote the paper: PFC CLW CHH CCC.

References

1. Muller LM, Gorter KJ, Hak E, Goudzwaard WL, Schellevis FG, et al. (2005) Increased Risk of Common Infections in Patients with Type 1 and Type 2 Diabetes Mellitus. Clin Infect Dis 41: 281–288.
2. Balachandar MS, Pavković P, Metelko Ž (2002) Kidney infections in diabetes mellitus. Diabetologia Croatica 31: 85–103.
3. Nicolle LE, Friesen D, Harding GK, Roos LL (1996) Hospitalization for acute pyelonephritis in Manitoba, Canada, during the period from 1989 to 1992; impact of diabetes, pregnancy, and aboriginal origin. Clin Infect Dis 22: 1051–1056.
4. Robbins SL, Tucker AW (1944) The cause of death in diabetes. A report of 307 autopsied cases. N Engl J Med 231: 865–868.
5. Chiu PF, Huang CH, Liou HH, Wu CL, Wang SC, et al. (2013) Long-term renal outcomes of episodic urinary tract infection in diabetic patients. J Diabetes Complications 27: 41–43.
6. Thakar CV, Christianson A, Himmelfarb J, Leonard AC (2011) Acute kidney injury episodes and chronic kidney disease risk in diabetes mellitus. Clin J Am Soc Nephrol 6: 2567–2572.
7. Eslami S, Taherzadeh Z, Schultz MJ, Abu-Hanna A (2011) Glucose variability measures and their effect on mortality: a systematic review. Intensive Care Med 37: 583–593.
8. von Elm E, Altman DG, Egger M, Pocock SJ, Gotzsche PC, et al. (2007) The Strengthening the Reporting of Observational Studies in Epidemiology (STROBE) statement: guidelines for reporting observational studies. BMJ 335: 806–808.
9. Bouman CS, Oudemans-Van Straaten HM, Tijssen JG, Zandstra DF, Kesecioglu J (2002) Effects of early high-volume continuous venovenous hemofiltration on survival and recovery of renal function in intensive care patients with acute renal failure: A prospective, randomized trial. Crit Care Med 30: 2205–2211.
10. Luckraz H, Gravenor MB, George R, Taylor S, Williams A, et al. (2005) Long and short-term outcomes in patients requiring continuous renal replacement therapy post cardiopulmonary bypass. Eur J Cardiothorac Surg 27: 906–909.
11. Zhang Y, Hu G, Yuan Z, Chen L (2012) Glycosylated hemoglobin in relationship to cardiovascular outcomes and death in patients with type 2 diabetes: a systematic review and meta-analysis. PLoS One 7: e42551. doi: 10.1371/journal.pone.0042551.
12. Bragd J, Adamson U, Bäcklund LB, Lins PE, Moberg E, et al. (2008) Can glycaemic variability, as calculated from blood glucose self-monitoring, predict the development of complications in type 1 diabetes over a decade? Diabetes Metab 34: 612–616.
13. Di Flaviani A, Picconi F, Di Stefano P, Giordani I, Malandrucco I, et al. (2011) Impact of glycemic and blood pressure variability on surrogate measures of cardiovascular outcomes in type 2 diabetic patients. Diabetes Care 34: 1605–1609.

14. Monnier L, Colette C, Owens DR 2008) Glycemic variability: the third component of the dysglycemia in diabetes. Is it important? How to measure it? J Diabetes Sci Technol 2: 1094–1100.
15. Eslami S, Taherzadeh Z, Schultz MJ, Abu-Hanna A (2011) Glucose variability measures and their effect on mortality: a systematic review. Intensive Care Med 37: 583–593.
16. Krinsley JS (2008) Glycemic variability: a strong independent predictor of mortality in critically ill patients. Crit Care Med 36: 3008–3013.
17. Jeon CY, Furuya EY, Berman MF, Larson EL (2012) The role of pre-operative and post-operative glucose control in surgical-site infections and mortality. PLoS One 7: e45616. doi: 10.1371/journal.pone.0045616.
18. Pisarchik AN, Pochepen ON, Pisarchyk LA (2012) Increasing blood glucose variability is a precursor of sepsis and mortality in burned patients. PLoS One 7: e46582. doi: 10.1371/journal.pone.0046582
19. Haga KK, McClymont KL, Clarke S, Grounds RS, Ng KY, et al. (2011) The effect of tight glycaemic control, during and after cardiac surgery, on patient mortality and morbidity: A systematic review and meta-analysis. J Cardiothorac Surg 6: 3. Available: http://www.cardiothoracicsurgery.org/content/6/1/3. Accessed 2011 Jan 10.
20. Siegelaar SE, Kerr L, Jacober SJ, Devries JH (2011) A decrease in glucose variability does not reduce cardiovascular event rates in type 2 diabetic patients after acute myocardial infarction. Diabetes Care 34: 855–857.
21. Wiener RS, Wiener DC, Larson RJ (2008) Benefits and risks of tight glucose control in critically ill adults. JAMA 8: 933–944.
22. Griesdale DE, de Souza RJ, van Dam RM, Heyland DK, Cook DJ, et al. (2009) Intensive insulin therapy and mortality among critically ill patients: a meta-analysis including NICE-SUGAR study data. CMAJ 8: 821–827.
23. Finfer S, Chittock DR, Su SY, Blair D, Foster D, et al. (2009) Intensive versus conventional glucose control in critically ill patients. N Engl J Med 360: 1283–1297.
24. American Diabetes Association (2013) Standards of medical care in Diabetes-2013. Diabetes Care 36: S11–S66
25. Sherr J, Tamborlane WV, Xing D, Tsalikian E, Mauras N, et al. (2012) Achievement of target A1C levels with negligible hypoglycemia and low glucose variability in youth with short-term type 1 diabetes and residual β-cell function. Diabetes Care 35: 817–820.
26. Chiodini I, Di Lembo S, Morelli V, Epaminonda P, Coletti F, et al. (2006) Hypothalamic-pituitary-adrenal activity in type 2 diabetes mellitus: role of autonomic imbalance. Metabolism 55: 1135–1140.
27. Tsigos C, Young RJ, White A (1993) Diabetic neuropathy is associated with increased activity of the hypothalamic-pituitary-adrenal axis. J Clin Endocrinol Metab 76: 554–558.
28. Monnier L, Mas E, Ginet C, Michel F, Villon L, et al. (2006) Activation of Oxidative Stress by Acute Glucose Fluctuations Compared With Sustained Chronic Hyperglycemia in Patients With Type 2 Diabetes. JAMA 295:1681–1687
29. Rizzo MR, Barbieri M, Marfella R, Paolisso G (2012) Reduction of oxidative stress and inflammation by blunting daily acute glucose fluctuations in patients with type 2 diabetes: role of dipeptidyl peptidase-IV inhibition. Diabetes Care 35: 2076–2082.
30. Bochicchio GV, Bochicchio KM, Joshi M, Ilahi O, Scalea TM (2010) Acute glucose elevation is highly predictive of infection and outcome in critically injured trauma patients. Ann Surg 252: 597–602.
31. Tudela P, Prat C, Lacoma A, Mòdol Deltell JM, Domínguez J, et al. (2012) Biological markers for predicting bacterial infection, bacteremia, and severity of infection in the emergency department. Emergencias 24: 348–356
32. Riedel S, Melendez JH, An AT, Rosenbaum JE, Zenilman JM (2011) Procalcitonin as a marker for the detection of bacteremia and sepsis in the emergency department. Am J Clin Pathol 135: 182–189
33. Marshall JC, Cook DJ, Christou NV, Bernard GR, Sprung CL, et al. (1995) Multiple organ dysfunction score: a reliable descriptor of a complex clinical outcome. Crit Care Med 23: 1638–1652.
34. Siegelaar SE, Holleman F, Hoekstra JB, DeVries JH (2010) Glucose variability; does it matter? Endocr Rev 31: 171–182.
35. Rodbard D (2012) The challenges of measuring glycemic variability. J Diabetes Sci Technol 6: 712–715.

Extended-Spectrum-Beta-Lactamase Producing Bacteria Related Urinary Tract Infection in Renal Transplant Recipients and Effect on Allograft Function

Poornima Ramadas[1], Prejith P. Rajendran[1], Prathik Krishnan[1], Asha Alex[1], Eric Siskind[2], Aditya Kadiyala[3], Vivek Jayaschandran[1], Amit Basu[1], Madhu Bhaskaran[1]*, Ernesto P. Molmenti[1]

1 Transplant Program, North Shore University Hospital, Manhasset, New York, United States of America, **2** Department of Surgery, North Shore University Hospital, Manhasset, New York, United States of America, **3** Department of Nephrology, North Shore University Hospital, Manhasset, New York, United States of America

Abstract

Background: Urinary tract infection (UTI) is a well-recognized early complication in renal transplant recipients (RTR) and can have significant bearing on their outcome. The recent rise in incidence of extended spectrum beta lactamase (ESBL) producing bacteria causing UTI among RTR poses new and significant challenges in terms of management and outcome. Our aim is to analyze the effect of ESBL producing bacteria causing UTI in these patients and its impact on allograft function.

Methods: We reviewed the medical records of 147 RTR who were followed at a tertiary care hospital affiliated transplant center between January 2007 and May 2013 and noted five RTR who developed episodes of ESBL producing bacteria related UTI during follow up. Multiple patient characteristics including demographics, immunosuppression, recurrences, allograft function and outcome were analyzed.

Results: Five patients (3.4%) out of 147 had ESBL producing bacteria related UTI. We found all patients to be above 60 years of age, with three out of five being females, and all five patients had diabetes mellitus. We identified a total of 37 episodes of UTI among these five patients during this period. Two of these patients had elevated creatinine values during the episodes of UTI and three of them developed bacteremia. Of the five patients, four of them had a favorable outcome except for one patient who developed persistent allograft dysfunction.

Conclusion: RTR are at a higher risk for developing ESBL producing bacteria associated UTI. Early diagnosis along with appropriate and judicious use of antibiotics will ensure long term success in allograft and patient outcome.

Editor: Paola Romagnani, University of Florence, Italy

Funding: These authors have no support or funding to report.

Competing Interests: The authors have declared that no competing interests exist.

* E-mail: mbhaskar@nshs.edu

Introduction

Renal transplants have become the standard of care for end stage renal transplant (ESRD), thereby increasing the number of patients on immunosuppressive regimen who are extremely susceptible to a host of infections in the post-transplant phase [1]. Urinary tract infection (UTI) is a common infection in these patients and their effect on the allograft kidney has been well documented in previous studies [2,3]. Approximately 70% of these UTI's are caused by gram-negative bacteria and can predispose to dehydration, allograft rejection, transplant pyelonephritis and reactivation of Cytomegalovirus (CMV) infection, all subsequently leading to allograft dysfunction and graft failure [4,5].

We would like to address the issue of extended-spectrum-beta-lactamase (ESBL) producing bacteria causing UTI among renal transplant recipients (RTR) [6]. ESBL is essentially an enzyme located on transferrable bacterial plasmid DNA, capable of hydrolyzing penicillins, extended spectrum cephalosporins as well as monobactams [7]. ESBL is commonly expressed by organisms belonging to Enterobacteriaceae, mainly Escherichia coli and Klebsiella species, both of which are frequently associated with UTI in RTR [6,7]. RTR have multiple local and systemic risk factors, which predispose them to UTI [8]. Timely intervention and appropriate management of the condition is essential to avoid exacerbation of the clinical course in these patients.

Subjects and Methods

We reviewed the medical records of 147 renal transplant recipients (RTR) who were followed at a tertiary care hospital affiliated transplant center between January 2007 and May 2013 and noted five RTR who developed episodes of extended-spectrum-beta-lactamase (ESBL) producing bacteria related urinary tract infection (UTI) during follow up. This study was approved by the Institutional review board at North Shore LIJ Hospital, NY. The patient records/information was anonymized and de-identified prior to analysis. The general policy for urinalysis for post-transplant visits at our center is as follows:

Table 1. Patient characteristics, episodes of UTI, treatment and outcome.

	PATIENT 1	PATIENT 2	PATIENT 3	PATIENT 4	PATIENT 5
AGE (Years)	62	74	60	73	69
GENDER	M	F	F	M	F
RACE	Hispanic	Caucasian	Caucasian	South Asian	Persian
CAUSE OF ESRD	DM, HTN	DM, HTN	Autoimmune interstitial nephritis	DM, HTN	DM, HTN
YEAR OF TRANSPLANT	2011	2011	2010	2006	2005
TYPE OF DONOR	Cadaveric	Live	Live	Live	Live
COMORBIDITIES	DM, HTN, Hypothyroidism	DM, HTN, Hypothyroidism, Hepatitis C	DM, HTN, Hypothyroidism, CMV viremia	DM, HTN	DM, HTN
IMMUNOSUPPRESSION PROTOCOL	Tacrolimus, Mycophenolate mofetil, Prednisone	Tacrolimus, Mycophenolate mofetil, Prednisone	Tacrolimus, Mycophenolate mofetil, Prednisone	Tacrolimus, Mycophenolate mofetil, Prednisone	Cyclosporine, Mycophenolate mofetil, Prednisone
BASELINE CREATININE POST TRANSPLANT (mg/dl)	1.62	1.09	0.9	0.8	1.1
TIME OF FIRST EPISODE OF UTI SINCE TRANSPLANT	2 weeks	2 weeks	3 months	30 months	36 months
DETECTION OF ESBL BACTERIA (EPISODE)	First	Third	Fourth	First	Second
NO OF UTI RECURRENCES WITH ESBL BACTERIA	All	4	All	All	5
OBSTRUCTION	Stone in the transplanted ureter on CAT scan and ureteral stent inserted. Removed 4 weeks later.	No	No	No	No
TREATMENT	Imipenem-cilastatin, Ertapenem (2 weeks)	Pireracillin tazobactam, Meropenem (2 weeks)	Ertapenem (2 weeks)	Imipenem-cilastatin, Ertapenem (2 weeks)	Piperacillin tazobactam, Ertapenem (2 weeks)
OUTCOME	Chronic allograft dysfunction	Improved	Improved	Improved	Improved

M-Male, F-Female, ESRD-End stage renal disease, DM-Diabetes mellitus, HTN-Hypertension, CMV-Cytomegalovirus, UTI-Urinary tract infection, ESBL-Extended spectrum beta lactamase.

First 2 weeks - twice a week
2–4 weeks - once a week
4–12 weeks - once in 2 weeks
3 months-1 year - once a month
1–2 year - once in 2 months
2–5 years - once in 3 months
>5 years - once in 6 months

Clean catch mid-stream urine sample is taken. If there is any evidence of UTI such as leukocytosis or positive nitrites/leukocyte esterase, then a reflex culture is sent. All these patients presented with fever and dysuria and were diagnosed with UTI based on urine microscopy and culture results. Antibiotic sensitivity testing of the cultures was used to confirm the presence of ESBL producing bacteria. All patients were on routine immunosuppression protocol consisting of tacrolimus or cyclosporine, mycophenolate mofetil, and prednisone and prophylactic regimen against bacterial infections consisting of cefazolin 1 gm preoperatively and Trimethoprim-Sulfamethoxazole (80/400) one tab daily life long post-transplant. After the treatment of an episode of UTI, urine cultures are done to confirm resolution of the infection. Subsequent episodes were identified when symptoms of UTI occurred with positive urine cultures for the bacteria. These patients are followed lifelong like other RTR, with concern for the recurrence of UTI. This study was approved by the Institutional review board at this health system.

Results

Five patients (3.4%) out of 147 had extended-spectrum-beta-lactamase (ESBL) producing bacteria related urinary tract infection (UTI). All patients were above 60 years of age and included 3 female and 2 male patients. Of the two male patients, one was diagnosed with benign prostatic hyperplasia (BPH). Four of them underwent live donor renal transplantation and one received kidney from a deceased donor. All the patients in our study were diabetic. None of them had a ureteral stent inserted in the immediate post-transplant phase. In our study 3 out of 5 patients had episodes of UTI due to non ESBL producing bacteria prior to contracting the ESBL producing one. We identified a total of 37 episodes of UTI among these five patients between January 2007 and May 2013. One of our patients required a ureteral stent later in the post-transplant phase during the course of treatment of urinary stone in the transplanted ureter. None of them were noted to have an episode of rejection. Interestingly two of these patients had elevated creatinine values during the episodes of UTI. One patient was noted to have progressively elevated creatinine during successive episodes of UTI resulting in persistent allograft

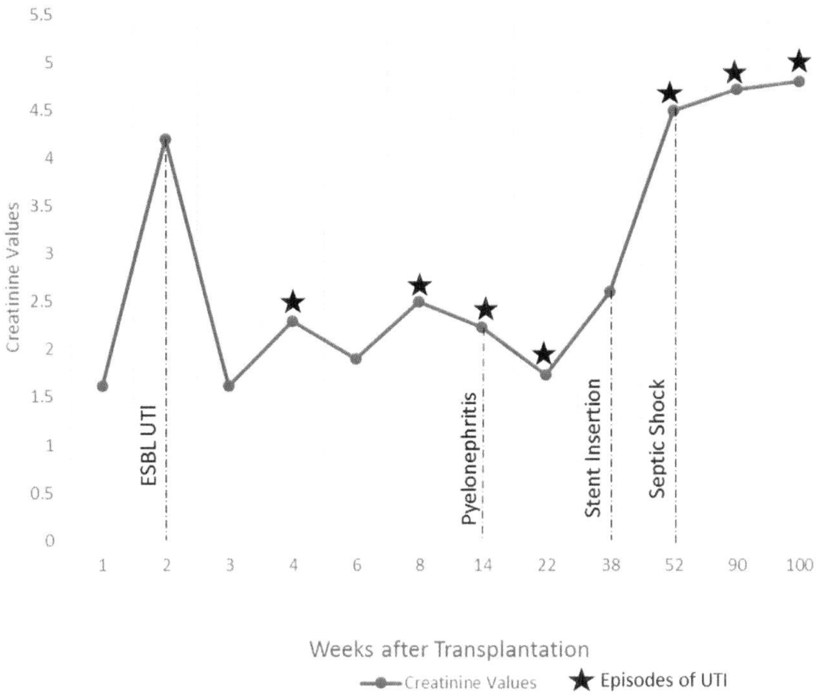

Figure 1. Creatinine Values and Clinical Events of Patient 1.

dysfunction. Of the five patients described in this case study, three developed bacteremia and sepsis. One of them had acute pyelonephritis which progressed into full blown septicemia and shock requiring long term hospitalization and later on developed chronic allograft dysfunction. Carbapenems were the most commonly used treatment in our patients (1 gram ertapenem/meropenem intravenously once daily or 1 gram imipenem intravenously twice daily for 14 days). The potential risk factors we observed in patients other than the genitourinary surgery (kidney transplant) and bladder catheterization were diabetes, prior episodes of non ESBL UTI, ureteral obstruction and ureteral

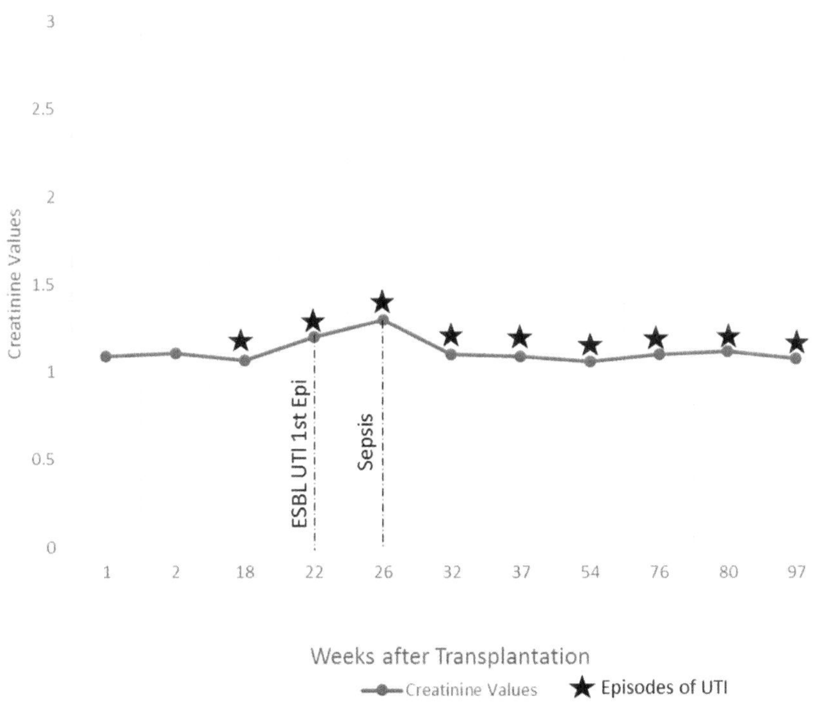

Figure 2. Creatinine Values and Clinical Events of Patient 2.

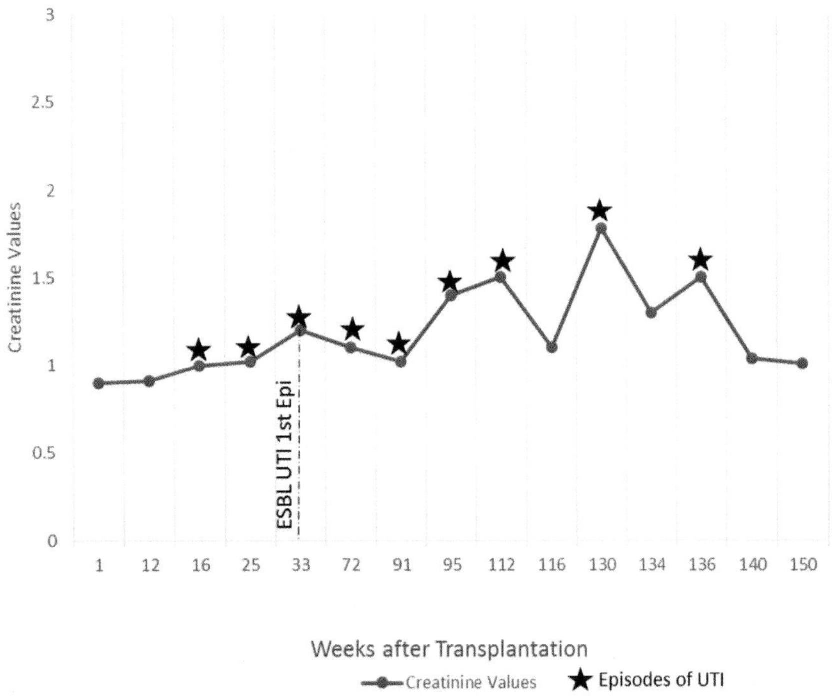

Figure 3. Creatinine Values and Clinical Events of Patient 3.

stent, of which all except the prior episodes of non ESBL UTI is applicable to UTI in general.

Refer to Table 1 for details regarding patient characteristics, episodes of UTI, treatment and outcome.

Refer to Figures 1 to 5 for graphical representation of the creatinine values and the clinical events of the five patients.

Discussion

Urinary tract infection (UTI) is the most common bacterial infection, representing 40 to 50% of all post-transplant infections [9] and is most commonly seen in the first few weeks following transplantation [4]. Gram-negative bacteria are the culprits in 70

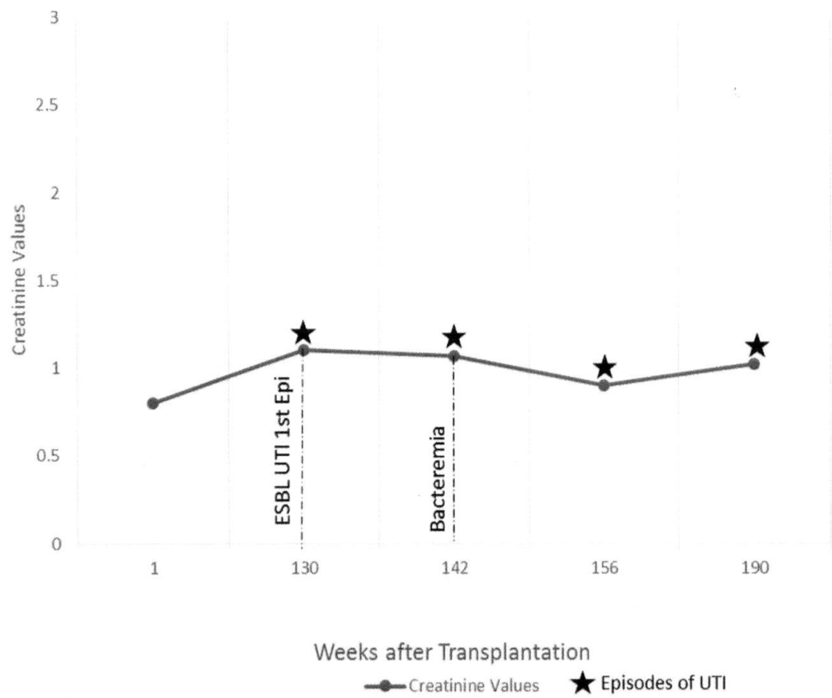

Figure 4. Creatinine Values and Clinical Events of Patient 4.

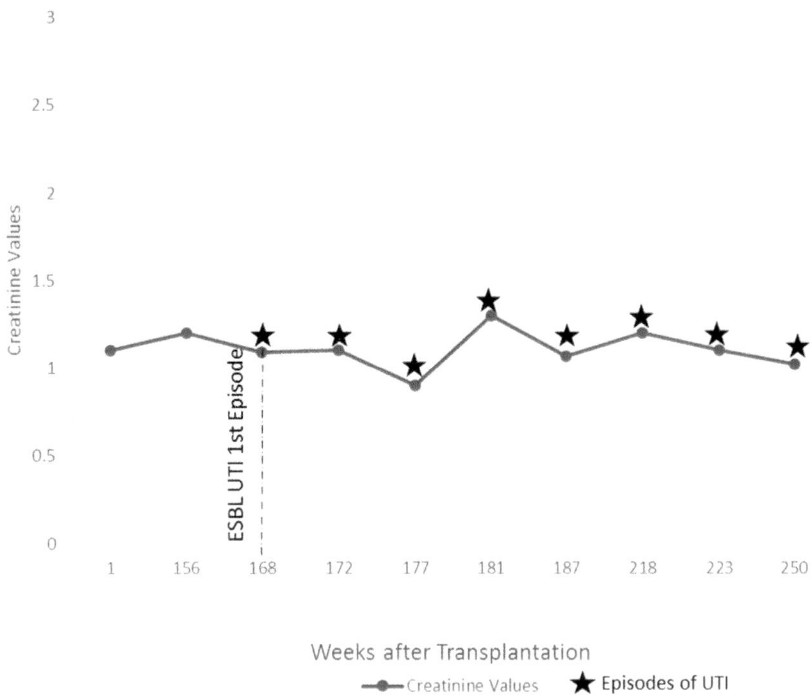

Figure 5. Creatinine Values and Clinical Events of Patient 5.

percent of the cases, with E coli being the most common etiology [10]. Antibiotics such as 3rd generation cephalosporins used preoperatively [11] and Trimethoprim-Sulfamethoxazole used in the post-transplant phase have been found to reduce the incidence of UTI [12]. However antibiotic prophylaxis induces bacterial resistance and has led to the emergence of extended-spectrum-beta-lactamase (ESBL) producing bacteria [13]. ESBL resistance has been increasingly reported around the world in recent years. A study in 2010 has shown a 14 percent increase in ESBL bacteria over the time period of 2007–2010 [14]. The choice of antibiotics we have for this condition is limited [15]. In addition ESBL UTI is associated with significant patient mortality and morbidity, which poses a challenge in proper evaluation and management [16].

As in general community acquired UTI, ESBL producing bacterial UTI is associated with numerous risk factors. In our case analysis we focused on age, gender, living or cadaveric donor kidneys, stent insertion during or post transplantation, antibiotic prophylaxis, immunosuppression, diabetes mellitus, rejection, recurrent episodes of UTI and urinary tract obstruction as possible risk factors in this patient population.

There are contradicting data regarding the correlation of age and UTI. A study done in Spain found that age over 60 years is a significant risk factor for ESBL UTI [17]. UTI in elderly patients also have a high risk for septic shock and death [9]. A study at Mayo Clinic in 2009 found that there was no difference in rates of UTI in women over the age of 65 as compared to younger women [18].

It is a well-known fact that female patients have a higher risk of developing UTI, which is mostly due to difference in anatomy [19]. In spite of protective barriers in men, it has been found that ESBL producing bacteria do in fact penetrate this barrier, thus increasing the incidence in males [20].

Studies which correlate the type of donor to the incidence of UTI are rare. A study in 2005 noted an increased incidence in UTI in patients who had cadaveric donors [21].The type of donor is also a major risk factor for chronic allograft dysfunction [22].

Ureteral stents are usually placed intraoperatively to reduce urologic complications post-transplant, the risk of infection being taken into consideration. Studies show that stenting predisposes to UTI and a high recurrence rate of UTI was seen even after stent removal [23]. Early removal of the stent by the end of 2 weeks post-transplant has reduced incidence of UTI compared to late removal [24].

Antibiotic therapy is a significant risk factor for development of ESBL producing bacteria [25]. A study in 2011 suggested an association between UTI and perioperative cephalosporin prophylaxis in renal transplant patients [26].

Immunosuppression is an important risk factor for ESBL UTI. A study done by in 2010 showed a higher incidence of UTI in patients who had cyclosporine in their immunosuppression protocol [27]. Tacrolimus and prednisone have also been associated with an increased risk of infections of which UTI is the most common [28].

Diabetes mellitus predisposes to UTI in general due to decreased local cytokine secretion in the urinary tract and this relationship has been proven by several studies [22]. The reduced local immunity augments the risk of infection by multidrug resistant microorganisms including ESBL producing organisms.

Recurrent UTI can act as predisposing factor for development of ESBL UTI. A study done in 2011 showed over 75% of patients with ESBL had recurrent UTI in the past [29]. Another study done in 2010 also documented increased incidence of ESBL UTI in patients with recurrent UTI [14]. This association could be due to prior use of multiple antibiotics.

Functional or mechanical disorders of urinary tract are other risk factors associated with an increased risk of developing UTI [30]. It has also been found that all patients with vesicoureteral strictures had recurrent UTI [31].

UTI in RTR can have significant negative effects on the allograft kidney and can even lead to allograft failure [32]. UTI can even trigger the onset of acute allograft rejection [33]. UTI is a risk factor for the onset of chronic rejection and requires early and intense treatment [3]. It can also predispose to acute pyelonephritis [34] of the transplant kidney which may progress to systemic bacteremia and septic shock associated with significant morbidity and mortality in these patients [5]. A study using United States Renal Data System Treatment data showed that RTR had a higher incidence of hospitalization due to septicemia, 30.6% of which were secondary to UTI [2].

ESBL producing bacteria related UTI is extremely difficult to treat given the very few drug options available to treat the condition [35,36]. Two most commonly used antibiotic choices are piperacilin-tazobactam and imipenem [37]. Currently carbapenems are considered as the preferred drug of choice for infections due to ESBL-producing organisms as they are generally resistant to ESBL-mediated hydrolysis [38]. Ertapenem and faropenem are newer carbapenems which are being used more commonly and have excellent activity against ESBL-producing organisms [7]. Fosfomycin, the latest addition has shown to have a high level of broad spectrum antimicrobial activity against ESBL producing enterobacteriacae [39].

Conclusion

Renal transplant recipients are at a higher risk of developing UTI due to ESBL producing bacteria. As many of the inherent risk factors are non-modifiable, this situation poses a special challenge. Potential adverse consequences of ESBL UTI may include sepsis as well as acute and chronic allograft dysfunction. Efficient management of these patients with a high index of suspicion, prompt diagnosis and use of appropriate antibiotics can result in successful allograft and patient outcome. Continued monitoring on a large scale with close attention to the treatment outcome will help understand and manage this evolving disease.

Acknowledgments

We thank all the staff at the Transplant Program, NSUH for their whole hearted support.

Author Contributions

Conceived and designed the experiments: PR PPR PK MB. Performed the experiments: PR PPR PK AA ES AK. Analyzed the data: PR PPR PK AK VJ AB EPM. Contributed reagents/materials/analysis tools: AB MB EPM. Wrote the paper: PR PPR PK MB.

References

1. Kee T, Lu YM, Vathsala A (2004) Spectrum of severe infections in an Asian renal transplant population. Transplant Proc. 36(7):2001–3.
2. Abbott KC, Oliver JD 3rd, Hypolite I, Lepler LL, Kirk AD, et al. (2001) Hospitalizations for bacterial septicemia after renal transplantation in the united states. Am J Nephrol. 21(2):120–7.
3. Müller V, Becker G, Delfs M, Albrecht KH, Philipp T, et al. (1998) Do urinary tract infections trigger chronic kidney transplant rejection in man? J Urol. 159(6):1826–9.
4. Dantas SR, Kuboyama RH, Mazzali M, Moretti ML (2006) Nosocomial infections in renal transplant patients: risk factors and treatment implications associated with urinary tract and surgical site infections. J Hosp Infect. 63(2):117–23.
5. Tolkoff-Rubin NE, Rubin RH (1997) Urinary tract infection in the immunocompromised host. Lessons from kidney transplantation and the AIDS epidemic. Infect Dis Clin North Am. 11(3):707–17.
6. Rodríguez-Baño J, Navarro MD, Romero L, Muniain MA, Perea EJ, et al. (2006) Clinical and molecular epidemiology of extended-spectrum beta-lactamase-producing Escherichia coli as a cause of nosocomial infection or colonization: implications for control. Clin Infect Dis. 42(1):37–45.
7. Rupp ME, Fey PD (2003) Extended spectrum beta-lactamase (ESBL)-producing Enterobacteriaceae: considerations for diagnosis, prevention and drug treatment. Drugs. 63(4):353–65.
8. de Souza RM, Olsburgh J (2008) Urinary tract infection in the renal transplant patient. Nat Clin Pract Nephrol. 4(5):252–64. doi: 10.1038/ncpneph0781
9. Cove-Smith A, Almond MK (2007) Management of urinary tract infections in the elderly. Trends in Urology, Gynaecology & Sexual Health. 12(4): 31–34.
10. Rice JC, Peng T, Kuo YF, Pendyala S, Simmons L, et al. (2006) Renal allograft injury is associated with urinary tract infection caused by Escherichia coli bearing adherence factors. Am J Transplant. 6(10):2375–83.
11. Naber KG, Bergman B, Bishop MC, Bjerklund-Johansen TE, Botto H, et al. (2001) EAU guidelines for the management of urinary and male genital tract infections. Urinary Tract Infection (UTI) Working Group of the Health Care Office (HCO) of the European Association of Urology (EAU). Eur Urol. 40(5):576–88.
12. Fox BC, Sollinger HW, Belzer FO, Maki DG (1990) A prospective, randomized, double-blind study of trimethoprim-sulfamethoxazole for prophylaxis of infection in renal transplantation: clinical efficacy, absorption of trimethoprim-sulfamethoxazole, effects on the microflora, and the cost-benefit of prophylaxis. Am J Med. 89(3):255–74.
13. Säemann M, Hörl WH (2008) Urinary tract infection in renal transplant recipients. Eur J Clin Invest. 38 Suppl 2:58–65. doi: 10.1111/j.1365-2362.2008.02014.x
14. Pinheiro HS, Mituiassu AM, Carminatti M, Braga AM, Bastos MG (2010) Urinary tract infection caused by extended-spectrum beta-lactamase-producing bacteria in kidney transplant patients. Transplant Proc. 42(2):486–7.doi: 10.1016/j.transproceed.2010.02.002
15. Kader AA, Kumar A (2005) Prevalence and antimicrobial susceptibility of extended-spectrum beta-lactamase-producing Escherichia coli and Klebsiella pneumoniae in a general hospital. Ann Saudi Med. 25(3):239–42.
16. Rodríguez-Baño J, Pascual A (2008) Clinical significance of extended-spectrum beta-lactamases. Expert Rev Anti Infect Ther. 6(5):671–83. doi: 10.1586/14787210.6.5.671
17. Calbo E, Romaní V, Xercavins M, Gómez L, Vidal CG, et al. (2006) Risk factors for community-onset urinary tract infections due to Escherichia coli harbouring extended-spectrum beta-lactamases. J Antimicrob Chemother. 57(4):780–3.
18. Grover ML, Bracamonte JD, Kanodia AK, Edwards FD, Weaver AL (2009) Urinary tract infection in women over the age of 65: is age alone a marker of complication? J Am Board Fam Med. 22(3):266–71. doi: 10.3122/jabfm.2009.03.080123
19. Domann E, Hong G, Imirzalioglu C, Turschner S, Kühle J, et al. (2003) Culture-independent identification of pathogenic bacteria and polymicrobial infections in the genitourinary tract of renal transplant recipients. J Clin Microbiol. 41(12):5500–10.
20. Yilmaz E, Akalin H, Ozbey S, Kordan Y, Sinirtaş M, et al. (2008) Risk factors in community-acquired/onset urinary tract infections due to extended-spectrum beta-lactamase-producing Escherichia coli and Klebsiella pneumoniae. J Chemother. 20(5):581–5.
21. Chuang P, Parikh CR, Langone A (2005) Urinary tract infections after renal transplantation: a retrospective review at two US transplant centers. Clin Transplant. 19(2):230–5.
22. Abbott KC, Swanson SJ, Richter ER, Bohen EM, Agodoa LY, et al. (2004) Late urinary tract infection after renal transplantation in the United States. Am J Kidney Dis. 44(2):353–62.
23. Ranganathan M, Akbar M, Ilham MA, Chavez R, Kumar N, et al. (2009) Infective complications associated with ureteral stents in renal transplant recipients. Transplant Proc. 41(1):162–4. doi: 10.1016/j.transproceed.2008.10.022
24. Coskun AK, Harlak A, Ozer T, Eyitilen T, Yigit T, et al. (2011) Is removal of the stent at the end of 2 weeks helpful to reduce infectious or urologic complications after renal transplantation? Transplant Proc. 43(3):813–5. doi: 10.1016/j.transproceed.2010.11.016
25. Colodner R, Rock W, Chazan B, Keller N, Guy N, et al. (2004) Risk factors for the development of extended-spectrum beta-lactamase-producing bacteria in nonhospitalized patients. Eur J Clin Microbiol Infect Dis. 23(3):163–7.
26. Kawecki D, Kwiatkowski A, Sawicka-Grzelak A, Durlik M, Paczek L, et al. (2011) Urinary tract infections in the early posttransplant period after kidney transplantation: etiologic agents and their susceptibility. Transplant Proc. 43(8):2991–3. doi: 10.1016/j.transproceed.2011.09.002
27. Khanna P, Abraham G, Mohamed Ali AA, Miriam PE, Mathew M, et al. (2010) Urinary tract infections in the era of newer immunosuppressant agents: a tertiary care center study. Saudi J Kidney Dis Transpl. 21(5):876–80.
28. Bloom RD, Crutchlow MF (2008) New-onset diabetes mellitus in the kidney recipient: diagnosis and management strategies. Clin J Am Soc Nephrol. 3 Suppl 2:S38–48. doi: 10.2215/CJN.02650707
29. Özçakar ZB, Yalçınkaya F, Kavaz A, Kadıoğlu G, Elhan AH, et al. (2011) Urinary tract infections owing to ESBL-producing bacteria: microorganisms change—clinical pattern does not. Acta Paediatr. 100(8):e61–4. doi: 10.1111/j.1651-2227.2011.02262.x

30. Goya N, Tanabe K, Iguchi Y, Oshima T, Yagisawa T, et al. (1997) Prevalence of urinary tract infection during outpatient follow-up after renal transplantation. Infection. 25(2):101–5.
31. Gołębiewska J, Dębska-Ślizień A, Komarnicka J, Samet A, Rutkowski B (2011) Urinary tract infections in renal transplant recipients. Transplant Proc. 43(8):2985–90. doi: 10.1016/j.transproceed.2011.07.010
32. John U, Everding AS, Kuwertz-Bröking E, Bulla M, Müller-Wiefel DE, et al. (2006) High prevalence of febrile urinary tract infections after paediatric renal transplantation. Nephrol Dial Transplant. 21(11):3269–74.
33. Charfeddine K, Kharrat M, Yaich S, Jarraya F, Mkawar K, et al. (2002) Infection in kidney transplant recipients in Tunisia. Saudi J Kidney Dis Transpl. 13(2):195–8.
34. Valera B, Gentil MA, Cabello V, Fijo J, Cordero E, et al. (2006) Epidemiology of urinary infections in renal transplant recipients. Transplant Proc. 38(8):2414–5.
35. Paterson DL, Ko WC, Von Gottberg A, Casellas JM, Mulazimoglu L, et al. (2001) Outcome of cephalosporin treatment for serious infections due to apparently susceptible organisms producing extended-spectrum beta-lactamases: implications for the clinical microbiology laboratory. J Clin Microbiol. 39(6):2206–12.
36. Jacoby GA (1997) Extended-spectrum beta-lactamases and other enzymes providing resistance to oxyimino-beta-lactams. Infect Dis Clin North Am. 11(4):875–87.
37. Patterson JE, Hardin TC, Kelly CA, Garcia RC, Jorgensen JH (2000) Association of antibiotic utilization measures and control of multiple-drug resistance in Klebsiella pneumoniae. Infect Control Hosp Epidemiol. 21(7):455–8.
38. Livermore DM (1995) beta-Lactamases in laboratory and clinical resistance. Clin Microbiol Rev. 8(4):557–84.
39. Falagas ME, Kastoris AC, Kapaskelis AM, Karageorgopoulos DE (2010) Fosfomycin for the treatment of multidrug-resistant, including extended-spectrum beta-lactamase producing, Enterobacteriaceae infections: a systematic review. Lancet Infect Dis. 10(1):43–50. doi: 10.1016/S1473-3099(09)70325-1.

The Age-Related Risk of Co-Existing Meningitis in Children with Urinary Tract Infection

Marc Tebruegge[1,2,3]*, Anastasia Pantazidou[2], Vanessa Clifford[3,4], Gena Gonis[4], Nicole Ritz[1,2,3], Tom Connell[1,2,3], Nigel Curtis[1,2,3]

1 Department of Paediatrics, The University of Melbourne, Parkville, Victoria, Australia, **2** Infectious Diseases Unit, Department of General Medicine, Royal Children's Hospital Melbourne, Parkville, Victoria, Australia, **3** Murdoch Children's Research Institute, Parkville, Victoria, Australia, **4** Department of Microbiology, Royal Children's Hospital Melbourne, Parkville, Victoria, Australia

Abstract

Objective: The primary aim of this study was to determine age-stratified rates of co-existing bacterial meningitis in children with urinary tract infection (UTI). The secondary aims of this study were to determine the causative pathogens of UTI, and the clinical features and outcome of children with co-existing meningitis.

Methods: Analysis of data collected over a nine-year period at a tertiary pediatric hospital in Australia. Study population: children below 16 years of age with culture-confirmed UTI and a paired CSF sample.

Results: A total of 748 episodes in 735 cases were included in the final analysis. The commonest pathogens causing UTI were *Escherichia coli* (67.4%), *Enterococcus faecalis* (8.4%), *Klebsiella oxytoca* (3.5%) and *Klebsiella pneumoniae* (3.5%). Only two (1.2%; 95% CI: 0.15–4.36%) of 163 neonates (between 0 and 28 days of age) with UTI had co-existing meningitis. Both presented with pyrexia, irritability and lethargy, and recovered uneventfully with antibiotic treatment. There were no cases of co-existing meningitis among 499 infants (between 29 days and 12 months of age) with UTI (95% CI: 0.00–0.74%), or any of the 86 children aged 12 months or over (95% CI: 0.00–4.20%).

Conclusions: These findings indicate that clinicians should have a low threshold to perform a lumbar puncture in neonates with UTI, as the risk of co-existing meningitis is not insignificant in this age group. In contrast, beyond the neonatal period, the risk is small and a more selective approach is warranted.

Editor: Adam J. Ratner, Columbia University, United States of America

Funding: No external funding was received for this study. MT and NR were supported by Fellowship awards from the European Society for Paediatric Infectious Diseases and International Research Scholarships provided by the University of Melbourne. The funders had no role in study design, data collection and analysis, decision to publish, or preparation of the manuscript.

Competing Interests: The authors have declared that no competing interests exist.

* E-mail: marc.tebruegge@rch.org.au

Introduction

Urinary tract infection (UTI) is common in infants and young children. Between 1% and 15% of young children presenting to hospital with pyrexia have an underlying UTI [1,2]. Previous studies show that bacteremia in association with UTI is not uncommon in infants, occurring in 4% to 10% [3–7]. As meningitis is generally the result of dissemination of bacteria via the bloodstream and subsequent penetration of the blood-brain barrier [8,9], it has been suggested that young children with UTI are therefore at higher risk of co-existing meningitis.

A study by Bergstrom *et al.* published in 1972, which is frequently referred to in this context, suggests that co-existing meningitis is very common in infants with UTI [10]. The authors reported that co-existing bacterial meningitis was present in six (19.4%) of the 31 infants with UTI who had a lumbar puncture. Subsequent studies have reported considerably lower estimates for the risk of co-existing meningitis in children presenting with UTI [3–7,11–19]. However, the majority of studies have significant limitations, including small sample size [4,6,13,15–19] and absence of a precise definition for UTI [12,17]. Furthermore, in the majority of previous studies, the study population exclusively comprised infants younger than three months of age, [3–6,12,14–18] and therefore only limited data exist regarding older infants, as well as children outside infancy.

Accurately determining the rate of co-existing meningitis in children with UTI is clinically highly relevant. In the absence of reliable data, it remains uncertain whether young children with UTI should always have a lumbar puncture to rule out co-existing meningitis [20]. The age after which the risk of co-existing meningitis becomes negligible is also unknown. Identification of co-existing meningitis is critically important, as failure to diagnose central nervous system (CNS) infection may result in partial or incomplete treatment, particularly in view of the fact that several national guidelines suggest that uncomplicated UTI in children can be treated with short courses of oral antibiotics, some of which have poor CNS penetration [21,22].

The primary aim of our study was to determine accurate, age-stratified rates of co-existing meningitis in children with culture-proven UTI. Secondarily the study aimed to determine the spectrum of bacteria causing UTI in children, and to describe the clinical features and outcome of children with co-existing meningitis.

Methods

Study design and setting

The study was conducted at the Royal Children's Hospital Melbourne, the largest pediatric referral center in the state of Victoria, Australia (estimated population 1.19 million children between 0 and 18 years of age). We analyzed data collected over a nine-year period (1st Jan 2001 to 1st Jan 2010). The following data were extracted from the hospital microbiology department database: patient age, date and type of sample, and bacterial culture results. In patients who potentially fulfilled the case definition of UTI and co-existing meningitis, additional clinical and laboratory data were extracted from the patient's record by one of the investigators.

Inclusion criteria and definitions

Patients between one day and 16 years of age were eligible for inclusion if they had a positive urine culture and a cerebrospinal fluid (CSF) sample obtained within 48 hours of the urine sample being collected. Cases were identified by matching all children with a positive urine culture result during the study period with CSF culture results.

In this study, 'neonate' was defined as a patient between 0 and 28 days of age; 'infant' was defined as a patient between 29 days and 12 months of age. UTI was defined as: i) a pure growth of a single bacterial pathogen with $\geq 10^2$ colony forming units (CFU)/ml from a urine sample obtained by suprapubic aspirate or catheterization, ii) $\geq 10^3$ CFU/ml from a clean catch urine sample or, iii) $\geq 10^5$ CFU/ml from a bag urine sample. In cases with more than one UTI, these were included in the analysis as separate episodes if they occurred more than 14 days apart. For each episode, only the result of the first positive urine culture was included in the data analysis. In the event that two different bacterial pathogens were isolated from two separate urine samples during one episode, the culture result of the more reliable sample was included in the final analysis (suprapubic aspirate>catheter urine>clean catch urine>bag urine).

CSF pleocytosis was defined as a CSF white blood cell (WBC) count on microscopy of $>19/\mu l$ during the first month of life, and $>9/\mu l$ thereafter, based on recently published data [23]. In blood-stained CSF samples, the WBC count was corrected according to the number of red blood cells using a fixed ratio of 1:500 [24]. Definite meningitis was defined as the growth of a single bacterial pathogen from a CSF sample. Co-existing meningitis was defined as a positive CSF culture with a pure growth of the same bacterial pathogen that was isolated from the patient's urine culture. *Micrococcus* species, *Bacillus* species, coagulase-negative staphylococci and viridans streptococci isolated from CSF were considered to be contaminants [25], unless the same organism was simultaneously isolated from urine.

Exclusion criteria

Episodes with urine cultures that showed mixed growth (ie two or more organisms in one sample) were excluded, as these are likely to represent contaminated samples. Episodes with urine samples growing fungal organisms (ie possible fungal UTI) were also excluded.

Assays for antimicrobial activity

CSF samples were routinely tested for antimicrobial activity to identify samples which may yield false-negative culture results due to the presence of antibiotics administered prior to the CSF being obtained, as previously described with minor modifications [26]. Briefly, the antimicrobial activity assays were done by adding one drop of CSF to Mueller-Hinton agar plates (Oxoid, Adelaide, Australia) enriched with a fully sensitive strain (ATCC 6633) of *Bacillus subtilis* (Chrisope Technologies, Louisiana, USA). Presence of antibiotics leads to inhibition of bacterial growth resulting in a zone of clearing around the inoculated CSF, which is assessed after overnight incubation at 35°C.

Data analysis

Data analysis and the construction of the figures were done using Prism (GraphPad Software Inc., La Jolla, California) and Excel (Microsoft, Redmond, Washington). Nonparametric statistics were used for age-related data, as these data were not normally distributed. The 'exact' method was used to calculate 95% confidence intervals (CI). A two-sided chi-square test was used to compare the rate of co-existing meningitis between different age groups.

Ethical approval

The study was approved by the Human Research Ethics Committee of the Royal Children's Hospital Melbourne (HREC 30062A).

Results

A total of 735 cases who fulfilled the inclusion criteria were identified. Thirteen of these cases had two episodes of UTI during which CSF had been obtained. None of the cases had three or more episodes. Therefore, a total of 748 episodes were included in the final analysis. Table 1 shows the demographic characteristics of the study population. The majority of cases (88.5%) were below the age of 12 months.

In 607 (81.1%) episodes, urine and CSF samples had been obtained on the same day, in 114 (15.2%) episodes within one day, and in 27 (3.6%) episodes within two days. The most common type of urine sample was catheter urine (31.1%), followed by clean catch urine (28.2%), and suprapubic aspirates (20.9%) (Table 2).

The spectrum and frequency of bacterial pathogens isolated from urine cultures are summarized in Table 2. *Escherichia coli* was by far the commonest isolate, accounting for 67.4% of positive urine cultures, followed by *Enterococcus faecalis* (8.4%), *Klebsiella oxytoca* (3.5%) and *Klebsiella pneumoniae* (3.5%).

Cases with UTI and definite co-existing meningitis

There were two cases of UTI with definite co-existing bacterial meningitis. Case 1 was a male neonate who had been diagnosed with bilateral renal dysplasia antenatally. On day 15 of life he presented with pyrexia, poor feeding, irritability and lethargy. The serum C-reactive protein (CRP) concentration was elevated (36 mg/L); the peripheral blood WBC was within normal limits. A catheter urine sample was obtained and a lumbar puncture was done at the same time. A pure growth of *Staphylococcus aureus* was detected in both the urine and the CSF sample. The patient received two weeks of intravenous flucloxacillin and gentamicin. Case 2 was a 19-day-old male neonate who presented with pyrexia, poor feeding, irritability and lethargy. A catheter urine sample was obtained and a lumbar puncture done 12 hours later. The CRP was within normal range (<8 mg/L), but the full blood count revealed neutrophilia (total WBC $12.0 \times 10^9/L$, neutrophils $9.0 \times 10^9/L$). A pure growth of *E. coli* was detected in both the urine and the CSF sample; an assay for *E. coli* K1 antigen in CSF was also positive. The patient received two weeks of ceftriaxone

Table 1. Baseline characteristics and rate of definite co-existing meningitis according to age group.

Age (months)		
median	2.2	
IQR	1.1–4.6	
range	0.1–191.2	
Gender		
male:female	1.8:1	
Age group	**Number of episodes (n = 748)**	**Number of cases with co-existing meningitis (n = 2)**
<1 month	163 (21.8%)	2 (1.2%; 95% CI: 0.15–4.36%)
1–2 months	304 (40.6%)	0 (95% CI: 0.00–1.25%)
3–5 months	129 (17.2%)	0 (95% CI: 0.00–2.82%)
6–11 months	66 (8.8%)	0 (95% CI: 0.00–5.44%)
12–23 months	32 (4.3%)	0 (95% CI: 0.00–10.89%)
24–59 months	21 (2.8%)	0 (95% CI: 0.00–16.11%)
≥5 years	33 (4.4%)	0 (95% CI: 0.00–10.58%)

CI: confidence interval; IQR: interquartile range.

and gentamicin, followed by a further two weeks of ceftriaxone monotherapy. Both patients had an uncomplicated clinical course, and were discharged without evidence of neurological sequelae.

Table 1 shows the rate of definite co-existing meningitis according to age group. The overall rate of definite co-existing meningitis in infants under the age of 12 months was 0.30% (95% CI: 0.04–1.09%); for all ages combined the incidence was 0.27% (95% CI: 0.03–0.96%). There were no cases of definite co-existing meningitis among the 499 infants with UTI that presented outside the neonatal period (95% CI: 0.00–0.74%). Further analysis confirmed that the rate of definite co-existing meningitis was significantly higher in neonates than in infants outside the neonatal period ($p = 0.013$).

Table 2. Urine sampling technique and urine culture isolates.

Type of urine sample (n = 748)	
Suprapubic aspirate	156 (20.9%)
Catheter	233 (31.1%)
Clean catch	211 (28.2%)
Urine bag	7 (0.9%)
Nephrostomy/ureterostomy	6 (0.8%)
Not stated	135 (18.0%)
Pathogen isolated in urine culture (n = 748)	
Escherichia coli	504 (67.4%)
Enterobacter faecalis	63 (8.4%)
Klebsiella oxytoca	26 (3.5%)
Klebsiella pneumoniae	26 (3.5%)
Enterobacter cloacae	19 (2.5%)
Proteus mirabilis	18 (2.4%)
Group B streptococci	17 (2.3%)
Pseudomonas aeruginosa	13 (1.7%)
Staphylococcus aureus	12 (1.6%)
Citrobacter species	9 (1.2%)
Serratia marcescens	5 (0.7%)
Other	36 (4.8%)

Description of additional cases with positive CSF cultures

In an additional four patients, pathogenic bacteria were isolated from the CSF sample, but these did not fulfill the case definition for definite co-existing meningitis.

In two cases, it is likely that the children did not have meningitis. In an 8-day-old, previously healthy term neonate, *Enterococcus faecalis* was isolated from urine obtained by suprapubic aspirate. The CSF sample did not show pleocytosis (CSF analysis: WBC 10/µl (neutrophils 0; lymphocytes 10), RBC 18,750/µl, protein 1.18 g/L, glucose 2.6 mmol/L) and no antimicrobial activity was detected. *Micrococcus* species were grown from CSF within 48 hours. The following day, a scanty growth of *E. faecalis* was detected in CSF enrichment cultures. In a 40-day-old infant with congenital posterior urethral valves, a urine sample obtained by suprapubic aspirate grew *E. coli*; the CSF grew scanty mixed *E. coli* and *E. faecalis* (CSF analysis: WBC 8/µl (neutrophils 6; lymphocytes 2), RBC 6,410/µl, protein 0.42 g/L, glucose 2.5 mmol/L). In both cases CSF findings were not suggestive of meningitis making contamination of the CSF sample likely.

In the other two cases the children had bacterial meningitis, but their urine sample was likely contaminated. In a two-month-old infant with Down's syndrome and complex cardiac malformation, a catheter urine sample grew *E. coli*, while group B streptococci were isolated from blood cultures and the CSF. In a 16-month-old child with a ventriculo-peritoneal shunt, *E. coli* was isolated from a urine sample (sampling method not stated on the request form), while CSF cultures grew *S. aureus*.

Antimicrobial activity assay results

Antimicrobial activity assays were done on the CSF samples from 730 (97.6%) episodes (Figure 1). In 658 (90.1%) of these CSF

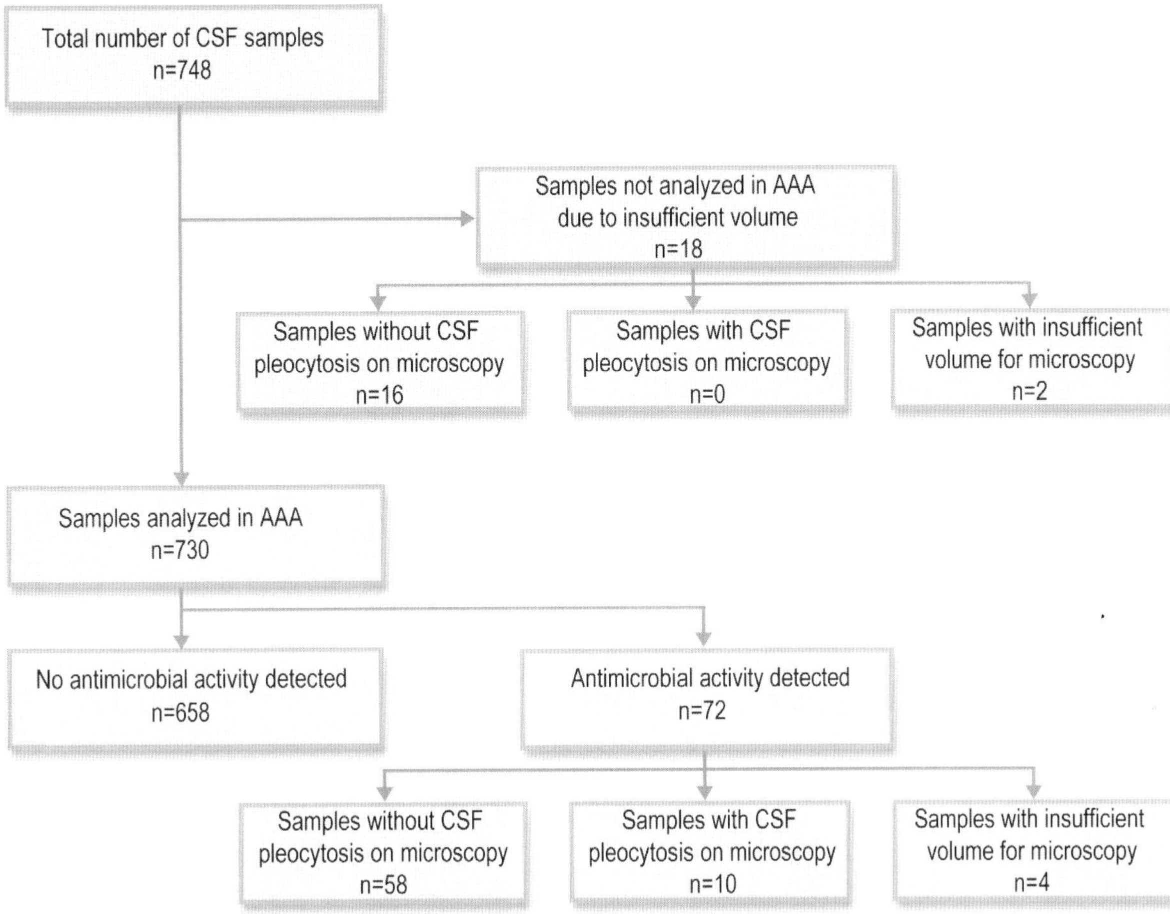

Figure 1. Summary of antimicrobial activity assays done on cerebrospinal fluid samples. Summary of the results of the antimicrobial activity assays (AAA) in relation to cerebrospinal fluid (CSF) microscopy results.

samples, no antimicrobial activity was detected. In the 72 remaining CSF samples, antimicrobial activity was detected. Four of these samples were clotted and could not be analyzed by microscopy. Of the remaining 68 samples, only 10 had a corrected WBC count consistent with pleocytosis (Table 3). One of these patients was case 2 described above. In five patients, an alternative diagnosis explaining the CSF pleocytosis was identified, comprising meningococcal sepsis/meningitis, ventriculo-peritoneal shunt infection, CNS lymphoma, miliary tuberculosis and cytomegalovirus infection. In none of the remaining four patients were microscopy and biochemical findings characteristic of bacterial meningitis.

Discussion

To our knowledge this study is the first to provide age-stratified data on co-existing meningitis in children of all ages with UTI. Our study is considerably larger than any previous study in this area with the exception of the recent study by Schnadover *et al.* that exclusively investigated patients between 29 and 60 days of age [3].

The aforementioned study by Bergstrom *et al.* is frequently quoted as evidence that young children with UTI are at significant risk of co-existing meningitis [10]. However, the limitations of this study have previously been highlighted, and it is likely that it considerably overestimates the risk of co-existing meningitis [6,14]. Firstly, all urine samples in this study were obtained using urine bags, which are far more prone to contamination than samples obtained by sterile techniques (ie suprapubic aspiration or catheterization) [27]. This may have led to a considerable number of false-positive urine culture results. Consequently, a significant proportion of patients with meningitis could falsely have been classified as having co-existing UTI. Secondly, only 31 (38.8%) of the 80 neonates with UTI in this study had a lumbar puncture. As it is likely that lumbar punctures were predominantly performed on the 'sicker'-appearing neonates, this could have introduced a significant selection bias and skewed the reported rate of co-existing meningitis even further.

Since the publication by Bergstrom *et al.*, several other studies have investigated co-existing meningitis in children with UTI [3,7,11–19]. However, the majority are limited by the size of the study population, which in most instances comprised fewer than 200 patients with UTI who had a lumbar puncture [4,14,17,19], or even less than 100 patients [6,13,15,16,18]. This is a significant limitation, in the light of more recent data suggesting that co-existing meningitis is uncommon in patients with UTI.

The majority of previous studies have exclusively focused on infants under three months of age [3–6,10,12,14–18], and the available data in older children are limited. In previous reports, the rates of co-existing meningitis in children with UTI varied between 0% [6,12–15,17,19] and 2% [18]. However, a further limitation of previous studies is that only few have reported

Table 3. Cerebrospinal fluid findings and diagnoses in patients with CSF antimicrobial activity detected and CSF pleocytosis.

Case	Age (months)	WBC * (/μl)	Neutrophils (/μl)	Lymphocytes (/μl)	RBC (/μl)	Protein (g/L)	Glucose (mmol/L)	Diagnosis
A	9.5	7690	7290	400	60	1.49	2.8	Meningococcal sepsis (blood culture: *N. meningitidis*; CSF microscopy: Gram-negative diplococci)
B	0.7	1820	1590	230	700	1.62	4.2	Co-existing *E. coli* UTI and meningitis ('Case 2' described in results section)
C	2.4	1674	1557	117	36	1.00	2.6	VP shunt infection (CSF microscopy: Gram-positive cocci; urine culture: *K. pneumoniae*)
D	184.3	620	0	620	30	2.87	<1.2	CNS lymphoma
E	2.7	447	183	264	1760	0.14	2.7	
F	27.2	144	83	61	24	n.d.	n.d.	Miliary tuberculosis
G	63.5	92	15	77	68	1.66	3.2	
H	4.1	19	2	17	4250	0.42	3.1	
I	10.6	16	0	16	0	1.04	3.0	Cytomegalovirus Infection
J	1.1	12	2	10	16	0.88	2.8	

CNS: central nervous system; CSF: cerebrospinal fluid; n.d.: not done; RBC: red blood cell count; VP: ventriculo-peritoneal; WBC *: white blood cell count (uncorrected).

confidence intervals [4,6], which are critically important for the interpretation of incidence data related to uncommon events. Our data show that the risk of co-existing meningitis in infants with UTI below the age of one month is not insignificant, with the true risk being between 0.15% and 4.36%. In contrast, in infants outside the neonatal age this risk is relatively small (between 0.00% and 0.74%).

Ginsburg and McCracken, who reported a study in 100 infants with UTI, found that the proportion of positive blood cultures correlated inversely with age [13]. Positive blood cultures were observed in 31.4% of cases aged below 1 month, in 18.4% of cases aged 1 to 3 months, and in only 5.6% of cases aged 3 to 12 months. In view of the fact that co-existing bacterial meningitis in patients with UTI is generally the result of bacterial dissemination via the blood stream, this observation further supports the notion that the risk of co-existing meningitis declines significantly with increasing age.

While it could be argued that universal lumbar puncture would be the safest strategy in infants with UTI, this procedure is uncomfortable and can be associated with rare, but potentially serious complications, such as brainstem herniation, introduction of infectious organisms into the CSF and epidermoid tumors [28–30]. Based on our data, in conjunction with the results from other studies, we do not believe that universal lumbar puncture in children with UTI outside the neonatal age is necessary. This does not imply that lumbar puncture is not warranted in patients outside the neonatal period who have symptoms or signs indicating possible meningitis.

In our study, both patients with co-existing meningitis were neonates who presented with features suggestive of meningitis, including pyrexia, poor feeding, irritability and lethargy. However, clinical features are insufficiently sensitive to reliably rule out meningitis in neonates and typical meningeal signs are often absent in this age group [9,31].

It is important to highlight that our study only includes data from patients who had paired urine and CSF results. Patients with UTI who did not have a lumbar puncture were not included, as the presence or absence of meningitis cannot be established. Consequently, our data are more likely to overestimate rather than underestimate the risk of co-existing meningitis, as clinicians are likely to have done a lumbar puncture preferentially on 'sicker'-appearing children.

The spectrum and frequency of bacterial pathogens causing UTI in our study is consistent with previous pediatric studies, with *E. coli* accounting for more than two thirds of infections [3–6,13,14,16,18,32,33]. Similar to other reports *Enterococcus*, *Klebsiella* and *Enterobacter* species were also commonly implicated [3,5–7,14,16,18].

Strengths and limitations

The strengths of our study include the large sample size, the age-stratification of data and the quality of the urine samples included. More than half of the urine samples were obtained by suprapubic aspirate or catheterization, which are less prone to contamination than other sampling methods [27]. Only a small proportion were documented to be bag urine samples. In addition, we excluded all urine samples with mixed growth to prevent the inclusion of patients with false-positive urine culture results.

Limitations of our study include its retrospective nature. We cannot exclude with absolute certainty the possibility that some patients had received antibiotics prior to the CSF sample being obtained, thereby potentially rendering their CSF culture false-negative, as we did not have data regarding the timing of the lumbar puncture and the initiation of antibiotic treatment. However, in the large majority (81.1%) of episodes CSF cultures were obtained on the same day as the urine sample. Also, antimicrobial activity was detected in the CSF in only 9.9% of the episodes. The vast majority of these patients had a normal CSF WBC count, while only ten had CSF pleocytosis. In only four of these could no alternative diagnosis be established; in none of these patients were microscopy and biochemical findings characteristic of bacterial meningitis. By assessing these aspects in detail we have limited the number of potentially false-negative CSF culture results, which adds to the robustness of our data. Notably, only one previous study, which included only 106 patients, has attempted to identify patients who had received antibiotics prior to lumbar puncture [19].

Conclusions

Identification of co-existing meningitis in children presenting with UTI is critically important, as failure to detect CNS infection can result in partial treatment of meningitis with potentially severe long-term consequences [8,9,31]. Our findings suggest that the risk of co-existing meningitis in infants with UTI under the age of one month is not insignificant. In contrast, outside the neonatal period this risk is small, indicating that a selective, rather than universal, approach to lumbar puncture is warranted.

Author Contributions

Conceived and designed the experiments: MT NC. Analyzed the data: MT AP VC GG NR TC NC. Wrote the paper: MT AP VC GG NR TC NC. Data collection: MT AP VC GG.

References

1. Lin DS, Huang SH, Lin CC, Tung YC, Huang TT, et al. (2000) Urinary tract infection in febrile infants younger than eight weeks of Age. Pediatrics 105(2): E20.
2. Hoberman A, Wald ER (1997) Urinary tract infections in young febrile children. Pediatr Infect Dis J 16(1): 11–17.
3. Schnadower D, Kuppermann N, Macias CG, Freedman SB, Baskin MN, et al. (2010) Febrile infants with urinary tract infections at very low risk for adverse events and bacteremia. Pediatrics 126(6): 1074–1083.
4. Dayan PS, Hanson E, Bennett JE, Langsam D, Miller SZ (2004) Clinical course of urinary tract infections in infants younger than 60 days of age. Pediatr Emerg Care 20(2): 85–88.
5. Bonsu BK, Harper MB (2007) Leukocyte counts in urine reflect the risk of concomitant sepsis in bacteriuric infants: a retrospective cohort study. BMC Pediatr 7: 24.
6. Vuillermin PJ, Starr M (2007) Investigation of the rate of meningitis in association with urinary tract infection in infants 90 days of age or younger. Emerg Med Australas 19(5): 464–469.
7. Bachur R, Caputo GL (1995) Bacteremia and meningitis among infants with urinary tract infections. Pediatr Emerg Care 11(5): 280–284.
8. de Louvois J (1994) Acute bacterial meningitis in the newborn. J Antimicrob Chemother 34 Suppl A: 61–73.
9. Kim KS (2010) Acute bacterial meningitis in infants and children. Lancet Infect Dis 10(1): 32–42.
10. Bergstrom T, Larson H, Lincoln K, Winberg J (1972) Studies of urinary tract infections in infancy and childhood. XII. Eighty consecutive patients with neonatal infection. J Pediatr 80(5): 858–866.
11. Adler-Shohet FC, Cheung MM, Hill M, Lieberman JM (2003) Aseptic meningitis in infants younger than six months of age hospitalized with urinary tract infections. Pediatr Infect Dis J 22(12): 1039–1042.
12. Finkelstein Y, Mosseri R, Garty BZ (2001) Concomitant aseptic meningitis and bacterial urinary tract infection in young febrile infants. Pediatr Infect Dis J 20(6): 630–2.
13. Ginsburg CM, McCracken GH, Jr. (1982) Urinary tract infections in young infants. Pediatrics 69(4): 409–412.
14. Goldman RD, Matlow A, Linett L, Scolnik D (2003) What is the risk of bacterial meningitis in infants who present to the emergency department with fever and pyuria? CJEM 5(6): 394–399.
15. Magin EC, Garcia-Garcia JJ, Sert SZ, Giralt AG, Cubells CL (2007) Efficacy of short-term intravenous antibiotic in neonates with urinary tract infection. Pediatr Emerg Care 23(2): 83–86.
16. Shah SS, Zorc JJ, Levine DA, Platt SL, Kuppermann N (2008) Sterile cerebrospinal fluid pleocytosis in young infants with urinary tract infections. J Pediatr 153(2): 290–292.
17. Syrogiannopoulos GA, Grivea IN, Anastassiou ED, Triga MG, Dimitracopoulos GOg (2001) Sterile cerebrospinal fluid pleocytosis in young infants with urinary tract infection. Pediatr Infect Dis J 20(10): 927–930.
18. Wang SF, Huang FY, Chiu NC, Tsai TC, Ho UY, et al. (1994) Urinary tract infection in infants less than 2 months of age. Zhonghua Min Guo Xiao Er Ke Yi Xue Hui Za Zhi 35(4): 294–300.
19. Yam AO, Andresen D, Kesson AM, Isaacs D (2009) Incidence of sterile cerebrospinal fluid pleocytosis in infants with urinary tract infection. J Paediatr Child Health 45(6): 364–367.
20. Tebruegge M, Pantazidou A, Curtis N (2011) How common is co-existing meningitis in infants with urinary tract infection? Arch Dis Child 96(6): 602–606.
21. National Institute for Health and Clinical Excellence UK (2007) Clinical guideline: Urinary tract infection in children - diagnosis, treatment and long-term management (CG54). Available: http://www.nice.org.uk/nicemedia/pdf/CG54fullguideline.pdf. Accessed 2011 Sep 30.
22. American Academy of Pediatrics, Committee on Quality Improvement & Subcommittee on Urinary Tract Infection (1999) Practice parameter: the diagnosis, treatment, and evaluation of the initial urinary tract infection in febrile infants and young children. Pediatrics 103(4 Pt 1): 843–852.
23. Kestenbaum LA, Ebberson J, Zorc JJ, Hodinka RL, Shah SS (2010) Defining cerebrospinal fluid white blood cell count reference values in neonates and young infants. Pediatrics 125(2): 257–264.
24. Connell T, Curtis N (2005) How to interpret a CSF- the art and the science. Adv Exp Med Biol 568: 199–216.
25. Greisen K, Loeffelholz M, Purohit A, Leong D (1994) PCR primers and probes for the 16S rRNA gene of most species of pathogenic bacteria, including bacteria found in cerebrospinal fluid. J Clin Microbiol 32(2): 335–351.
26. Erickson RC, Hildebrand AR, Hoffman PF, Gibson CB (1989) A sensitive bioassay for teicoplanin in serum in the presence or absence of other antibiotics. Diagn Microbiol Infect Dis 12(3): 235–241.
27. Infectious Diseases and Immunization Committee, Canadian Paediatric Society (2004) Bag urine specimens still not appropriate in diagnosing urinary tract infections in infants. Paediatr Child Health 9(6): 377–378.
28. Batnitzky S, Keucher TR, Mealey J, Jr., Campbell RL (1977) Iatrogenic intraspinal epidermoid tumors. JAMA 237(2): 148–150.
29. Teele DW, Dashefsky B, Rakusan T, Klein JO (1981) Meningitis after lumbar puncture in children with bacteremia. N Engl J Med 305(18): 1079–1081.
30. Joffe AR (2007) Lumbar puncture and brain herniation in acute bacterial meningitis: a review. J Intensive Care Med 22(4): 194–207.
31. Heath PT, Nik Yusoff NK, Baker CJ (2003) Neonatal meningitis. Arch Dis Child Fetal Neonatal Ed 88(3): F173–178.
32. Honkinen O, Jahnukainen T, Mertsola J, Eskola J, Ruuskanen O (2000) Bacteremic urinary tract infection in children. Pediatr Infect Dis J 19(7): 630–634.
33. Hsiao AL, Chen L, Baker MD (2006) Incidence and predictors of serious bacterial infections among 57- to 180-day-old infants. Pediatrics 117(5): 1695–1701.

The Ability of Virulence Factor Expression by *Pseudomonas aeruginosa* to Predict Clinical Disease in Hospitalized Patients

Michel Ledizet[1], Thomas S. Murray[2¤a], Sailaja Puttagunta[3¤b], Martin D. Slade[4], Vincent J. Quagliarello[3], Barbara I. Kazmierczak[3,5]*

1 L2 Diagnostics, New Haven, Connecticut, United States of America, **2** Department of Pediatrics (Infectious Diseases), Yale University School of Medicine, New Haven, Connecticut, United States of America, **3** Department of Medicine, Sections of Infectious Diseases, Yale University School of Medicine, New Haven, Connecticut, United States of America, **4** Department of Occupational & Environmental Medicine, Yale University School of Medicine, New Haven, Connecticut, United States of America, **5** Department of Microbial Pathogenesis, Yale University School of Medicine, New Haven, Connecticut, United States of America

Abstract

Background: *Pseudomonas aeruginosa* is an opportunistic pathogen that frequently causes hospital acquired colonization and infection. Accurate identification of host and bacterial factors associated with infection could aid treatment decisions for patients with *P. aeruginosa* cultured from clinical sites.

Methods: We identified a prospective cohort of 248 hospitalized patients with positive *P. aeruginosa* cultures. Clinical data were analyzed to determine whether an individual met predefined criteria for infection versus colonization. *P. aeruginosa* isolates were tested for the expression of multiple phenotypes previously associated with virulence in animal models and humans. Logistic regression models were constructed to determine the degree of association between host and bacterial factors with *P. aeruginosa* infection of the bloodstream, lung, soft tissue and urinary tract.

Results: One host factor (i.e. diabetes mellitus), and one bacterial factor, a Type 3 secretion system positive phenotype, were significantly associated with *P. aeruginosa* infection in our cohort. Subgroup analysis of patients with *P. aeruginosa* isolated from the urinary tract revealed that the presence of a urinary tract catheter or stent was an additional factor for *P. aeruginosa* infection.

Conclusions: Among hospitalized patients with culture-documented *P. aeruginosa,* infection is more likely to be present in those with diabetes mellitus and those harboring a Type 3 secretion positive bacterial strain.

Editor: Gunnar F Kaufmann, The Scripps Research Institute and Sorrento Therapeutics, Inc., United States of America

Funding: This work was supported by National Institutes of Health (NIH) grants T32 AI007517 (to SP), T32 AI07210 (to TSM), R42 AI058659 (to BIK) and the Patrick and Catherine Weldon Donaghue Medical Research Foundation (to BIK). The funders had no role in study design, data collection and analysis, decision to publish, or preparation of the manuscript.

* E-mail: barbara.kazmierczak@yale.edu

¤a Current address: Department of Basic Medical Sciences, Frank H. Netter MD School of Medicine, Quinnipiac University, Hamden, Connecticut, United States of America
¤b Current address: Durata Therapeutics, Branford, Connecticut, United States of America

Introduction

Hospital acquired infections (HAI) are estimated to complicate 5–10% of hospitalizations in the United States annually, leading to increased health care costs and prolonged hospitalizations [1]. *Pseudomonas aeruginosa* is a frequent cause of HAI, isolated in 16% of urinary tract infections and 18% of pneumonias, particularly ventilator-associated pneumonia [2,3]. A combination of several factors–intrinsic antibiotic and microbicide resistance, prevalence and persistence in the hospital environment, and a propensity to form biofilms on medical devices–lead to relatively high colonization rates by this organism. Prospective studies have shown that a subgroup of colonized patients develop clinically significant disease, such as ventilator-associated pneumonia. However, many patients do not progress to invasive disease, suggesting that differences in bacterial virulence and/or host susceptibility influence clinical course [4–7].

Many *P. aeruginosa* virulence factors have been identified over the past decades. The most robust virulence factor in animal models and human studies is the Type 3 secretion system (T3SS), a specialized protein secretion apparatus that allows Gram-negative bacteria such as *P. aeruginosa* to translocate a specific subset of bacterial effector proteins into the host cell cytosol [8]. Only four *P. aeruginosa* effectors have been identified to date: Exotoxin Y (ExoY), an adenylate cyclase; ExoT and Exo S, related proteins that exhibit both GTPase activating activity and ADP-ribosyl transferase activity; and ExoU, a phospholipase A_2 [9–15]. Carefully controlled studies examining virulence of isogenic T3SS mutants in murine models of acute pneumonia have demonstrated that two secreted effectors, ExoU and ExoS, are independently associated with increased virulence in this model. Other virulence factors identified in animal models include those promoting bacterial motility and adhesion (i.e., flagella and Type IV pili) [16–21], degradative enzymes [22–25], and genomic pathogenicity islands [26–31].

Bacterial expression of the T3SS is co-regulated with expression of many bacterial traits associated with acute infection (flagella, type IV pili, secreted proteases) or chronic colonization (biofilm formation). As inverse regulation of acute vs. chronic virulence factors is a feature of many of these regulatory networks, some authors have postulated that bacteria may switch their behavior to favor acute infection or chronic colonization [32]. The natural history of *P. aeruginosa* in Cystic Fibrosis patients is thought to illustrate such a switch, as younger CF patients are usually acutely infected by T3SS-positive strains, but progress to long-term colonization by T3SS-negative strains that usually display mucoid or hyper-biofilm phenotypes [33,34]. No study has asked, however, whether bacterial expression of particular virulence factors is associated with infection vs colonization in non-CF patients. Identifying such associations might have significant utility for clinical decision-making for hospitalized patients with positive *P. aeruginosa* cultures. Discriminating between patients at high vs. low risk of acute infection could improve delivery of effective anti-pseudomonal therapy to infected patients, but decrease inappropriate antibiotic use in colonized patients.

In this study, we prospectively enrolled 248 unique hospitalized patients with *P. aeruginosa* cultured from blood, airway secretions, urine, or deep wound specimens, excluding individuals with Cystic Fibrosis. Subjects were followed clinically for five days after their positive culture to determine whether they met pre-determined clinical criteria for infection vs. colonization with *P. aeruginosa*. Selected bacterial phenotypes associated in the literature with virulence or colonization were assayed for each bacterial isolate. We employed the statistical tool of factor analysis to determine whether any of the measured bacterial variables grouped together in orthogonal "factors" [35]. The primary endpoint of our study was to determine which, if any, readily measured bacterial traits were associated with *P. aeruginosa* infection versus colonization of the respiratory or urinary tract.

Methods

Cohort Assembly

This study was approved by the Institutional Review Board of Yale University School of Medicine (HIC #0411027243). All pediatric and adult patients hospitalized at Yale New Haven Hospital (New Haven, CT) with a positive culture for *P. aeruginosa* from the respiratory tract, urinary tract, blood, or deep tissue were eligible for study enrollment if they, or designated proxies, provided written consent. Clinical isolates were identified as *P. aeruginosa* if they grew as non-lactose fermenting colonies on MacConkey agar, were oxidase positive, could utilize acetamide as a sole carbon source, and gave a characteristic zone of inhibition to colistin on Kirby-Bauer plates. The presence of characteristic "grape-like" odor, pigment production and ability to grow at 42°C were also noted. Isolates from enrolled patients were subcultured from either primary specimen plates (i.e. blood or MacConkey agar) or from Kirby-Bauer plates generated by the Clinical Microbiology laboratory to Luria Broth (LB) agar, then coded and banked as 15% glycerol stocks at −80°C. Patient demographics, risk factors for infection, co-morbid medical conditions, prior and concurrent antibiotic exposure, history of prior *P. aeruginosa* cultures, clinical and laboratory features were collected at baseline and for 5 days after the initial culture date. Patients were excluded from the study if they had Cystic Fibrosis (n = 5), had *P. aeruginosa* isolates that would not grow in the defined media required for the Type 3 phenotypic assay (n = 2), or had isolates cultured from a non-eligible site (i.e. a biliary catheter drainage bag) (n = 1).

Clinical Outcomes

Anonymously coded data collection forms were reviewed independently by two Infectious Diseases physicians to determine whether patients met criteria for infection of the respiratory tract (pneumonia), urinary tract (cystitis or pyelonephritis) or soft tissue/bone (abscess or osteomyelitis), based on definitions established by the National Nosocomial Infection Surveillance (NNIS) system (Table 1) [36]; reviewing physicians were blinded to virulence testing results. Patients who met clinical criteria were categorized as infected; those who did not were categorized as colonized. Bloodstream isolates were considered indicative of infection. If the patient met the criteria for infection, but other potential pathogens were co-cultured with *P. aeruginosa*, the patient was categorized as "infection, possibly due to *Pseudomonas*". Potential pathogens were considered to be: (1) any other organism isolated from blood or an intraoperative tissue culture, (2) any organism present in $>10^5$ cfu/ml in urine, or (3) *Staphylococcus aureus*, *Streptococcus pneumoniae*, *Hemophilus influenzae*, *Moraxella catarhalis*, any Gram-negative rod not normally isolated from the oropharynx, *Mycobacterium tuberculosis*, and dimorphic fungi or molds in respiratory tract specimens. The report of "normal respiratory flora" without the specific identification of one of these microorganisms, or the isolation of *Candida albicans* in sputum, was not interpreted as indicating the presence of another potential pathogen. When the two reviewers disagreed, a third independent review was performed to determine clinical assignment of infection versus colonization.

Testing of Type III Protein Secretion by ELISA

Components of the T3SS were detected quantitatively by an ELISA assay as described previously [37]. Monoclonal antibodies against ExoS (SD1, SE1) were used to detect ExoS simultaneously with the other antigens.

Isolation of Monoclonal Antibodies Against ExoS

Monoclonal antibodies against ExoS were isolated using techniques described in detail previously [37]. Briefly, ExoS was partially purified from culture supernatants of PA103 Δ*exoU* Δ*exoT attB::exoS*. Splenocytes were isolated from immunized mice and fused to myeloma cells. Antibody-producing cell lines were identified by performing ELISAs on hybridoma culture supernatants. Two monoclonal antibodies, SD1 and SE1, were selected for the immunoassay described here. The specificity of the antibodies was ascertained by demonstrating that they reacted in ELISAs against culture supernatants of PA103 Δ*exoU* Δ*exoT attB::exoS* and PAO1, but not PA103 Δ*exoU* Δ*exoT*, PA14 or PA103. In immunoblots, both antibodies recognized a single protein with a molecular weight of 48,000, consistent with the known structure of ExoS. Isotyping of the purified immunoglobulins was performed with a kit (Pierce) according to the manufacturer's instructions. Both SD1 and SE1 are IgG1 and contain a kappa light chain. Competition experiments showed that SD1 and SE1 recognize different epitopes on the ExoS molecule.

Table 1. Clinical criteria for infection based on site of culture.

Respiratory tract: Infection (pneumonia)	*P. aeruginosa* cultured from respiratory specimen containing fewer than 25 epithelial cells/HPF.
	New and persistent infiltrates are noted on chest x-ray or computed tomography (CT).
	Two of the following three criteria are met: (1) fever >38.3°C; (2) WBC>12,000 or bands/metamyelocytes ≥6% or 1500/µl; (3) altered mental status (patient >70 y).
	Symptoms referable to the respiratory tract, evidenced by at least one of the following: (1) new purulent sputum OR increased sputum, secretions or suctioning; (2) new/worsening cough OR dyspnea OR tachypnea; (3) worsening gas exchange (increased requirement for supplemental oxygen, increased ventilator support, $PaO_2/FiO_2 \leq 240$).
Urinary tract: Infection (cystitis or pyelonephritis & urosepsis)	Greater than 10^5 cfu *P. aeruginosa*/ml urine
	Pyuria (>10 WBC/HPF)
Soft tissue/bone: Infection (abscess or osteomyelitis)	*P. aeruginosa* cultured from deep wound or intraoperative tissue specimen
	Clinical evidence of infection (purulent drainage, pain/erythema/dehiscence) or histopathological confirmation of infection

Motility Assays

Swimming, twitching and swarming motility were measured as previously described [38]. Each isolate was independently assayed twice.

Static Biofilm Formation

Static biofilm formation on polystyrene was measured in triplicate using the method of O'Toole [39].

Secreted Protease Activity

Protease production was measured by a casein proteolysis microplate assay as previously described [38]. The LasB elastase, alkaline protease, and protease IV are all capable of degrading casein [40].

Pathogenicity Island Loci

Genomic DNA was amplified by PCR using primers specific for PAPI-I pathogenicity island loci RL033 (RL033F: 5′ AAAGTTTAGCGCCGACTTCA; RL033R: 5′ GAAGTGAGTTGGGCACCATT) or RL112 (RL112F: 5′ GACTGGAATAGACGCCCAAG; RL112R: 5′AAACCTTCGACGGTGATCTG). This pathogenicity island was interrogated based on its association with virulence in several distinct animal models of virulence; the queried loci encode two experimentally identified "pathogenicity genes" [26,31].

Statistical Analysis

Values obtained for all measured bacterial virulence phenotypes were subjected to an exploratory factor analysis [35]. The principal factor method was used to extract factors, followed by promax (oblique) rotation. A "scree" test was used to determine the number of meaningful factors retained for rotation. An item was considered to load on a given factor if the factor loading was 0.50 or greater for that factor and was less than 0.50 for all other factors.

Unadjusted and adjusted logistic regression models were conducted. Parsimonious models were obtained through the use of a forward selection strategy with a significance-to-enter defined as 0.06. The outcome was defined as infection or sepsis caused by *P. aeruginosa* vs. colonization. Patients in whom infection was present but could not be attributed to *P. aeruginosa* (i.e. another potential pathogen was co-cultured) were coded as unknown and excluded from our analysis. All statistical analyses were performed using SAS 9.1.

Results

Patient Characteristics

A total of 248 patients with *P. aeruginosa* cultured from blood, urine, respiratory secretions or tissue provided written informed consent and were enrolled in this study at Yale New Haven Hospital (YNHH) from July 2005 through March 2007. Eight patients were found to be ineligible based on defined exclusion criteria. One eligible *P. aeruginosa* isolate was discarded by the Clinical Microbiology laboratory. Two additional individuals were enrolled twice, during independent hospitalizations under different medical record numbers; the second enrollment event was not analyzed in this study, resulting in a total of 237 unique participants.

Patient age ranged between <1 to 96 years at the time of enrollment (mean, 58.6 years). One hundred sixty (68%) patients were admitted to YNHH from home, while 48 (20%) were admitted from rehabilitation or extended care facilities. Twenty-six (11%) patients were transferred from other hospitals, while three patients remained at YNHH since their birth. The median elapsed time between hospital admission and the positive *P. aeruginosa* culture that triggered enrollment was 4 days (range, 0 to 1749); for 79 patients (33%), a prior positive culture for *P. aeruginosa* was documented during either the index or a previous hospitalization.

Host factors historically associated with increased risk of *P. aeruginosa* infection were assessed in our cohort [41]. Sixty-five (27%) patients carried a diagnosis of Type I or Type II diabetes mellitus. Fifty-five (23%) patients were deemed immunocompromised as a result of chronic steroid use (≥10 mg prednisone per day for 30 days or longer), post-transplant immunosuppression, marrow suppressive chemotherapy or HIV/AIDS. Seventy-two patients (30%) carried a diagnosis of asthma, chronic obstructive pulmonary disease or emphysema, or had radiologic evidence of bronchiectasis; these individuals were considered to have "chronic lung disease" in our analysis. The majority of patients (183/237; 77%) had at least one medical device that might be expected to predispose to infection of the respiratory tract (i.e., endotracheal tube or tracheostomy), urinary tract (i.e., bladder catheter or nephrostomy tube) or blood (i.e., central intravascular catheter). In 144 patients (61%) such a device was present at the anatomical site from which *P. aeruginosa* was cultured, and was considered a "relevant foreign device" in our analysis.

Clinical Characteristics of Patients

Seventy-one patients (30%) met the criteria for infection of bloodstream, respiratory tract, urinary tract or soft tissue/bone, and had no other potential pathogens cultured from these sites except for *P. aeruginosa*. An additional 52 patients (22%) met criteria for infection, but at least one other potential pathogen was cultured from the site of infection in addition to *P. aeruginosa*. One hundred fourteen patients (48%) did not meet the criteria for infection despite a positive culture for *P. aeruginosa* and were classified as "colonized". This group included 65 individuals with pure *P. aeruginosa* cultures (urine or wound) or normal respiratory flora plus *P. aeruginosa*, and 49 patients whose cultures yielded a potential pathogen in addition to *P. aeruginosa*. Table 2 shows the distribution of patient age, gender, ethnicity and selected comorbidities among the groups.

Bacterial Isolates

We collected sputum isolates from 136 patients, urine isolates from 65 patients, and deep wound/tissue isolates from 22 patients. Ten patients had blood isolates; in addition, one patient had positive cultures from both sputum and blood, two from both urine and blood, and one from wound and blood. Table 3 shows the distribution of clinical outcomes by site of culture. Each bacterial isolate was assayed for each virulence phenotype as described in Methods. For the first 75 individuals enrolled in the study, we collected 10 independent *P. aeruginosa* colonies from the primary culture plates and assayed each individually. Although heterogeneity of T3SS phenotype expression has been reported among isolates cultured from patients with CF [34], we found that only 4 (5.3%) of our tested samples harbored mixtures of T3SS-positive and -negative strains. Given this low rate of T3SS phenotype heterogeneity, only one isolate per unique anatomic site was collected and phenotyped in subsequently enrolled patients.

A number of the bacterial variables that we measured in our study are likely to be biologically interrelated. We applied the statistical tool of factor analysis to identify which variables were most highly interdependent, and found that most of the bacterial phenotypes loaded into three mathematically defined factors [35]. Factor 1 ("Type 3 secretion") reflected secretion of the two T3SS structural proteins, PopD and PcrV, and of the T3SS substrates ExoT, ExoS and ExoU. Factor 2 ("Flagellar motility & proteases") consisted of two flagellar based forms of motility (swimming and swarming) and protease production. Factor 3 ("Fimbriae") consisted of twitching motility and the presence of two loci, RL033 and RL112, within the PAPI-1 pathogenicity island. Equations for factors 1, 2 and 3 are listed in Figure S1. Biofilm formation did not load strongly onto any of the three factors and was thus evaluated as an independent variable in our models.

Bacterial and Host Variables Associated with Increased Risk of Infection

We tested the measured bacterial phenotypes, as well as host variables potentially associated with altered risk of infection, in both an unadjusted (bivariate) logistic regression model and a parsimonious model resulting from multivariate logistic regression models using a forward selection strategy. All tested model variables are listed in Table 4. Patients with infections that could not be definitely attributed to *P. aeruginosa* because another potential pathogen was co-cultured were considered to have an "unknown" clinical categorization, and their records were excluded from analysis, lowering the sample size from 237 to 185. Results of the parsimonious (forward selection) model are presented in Table 4. Only two variables, diabetes mellitus and "Type 3 secretion" (Factor 1) showed a significant association with infection vs. colonization ($p \leq 0.05$). We also ran our models on the subsets of patients with positive cultures from the respiratory tract ($n = 105$) or urine ($n = 59$). In patients with positive respiratory specimens, no host or bacterial variable was significantly associated with patient outcome (infection vs. colonization) in the multivariate analysis, and no variables entered the parsimonious model. In patients with positive urine cultures, two independent parsimonious models could be constructed. Both contained diabetes mellitus and the presence of a urinary catheter or stent as host variables significantly associated with increased risk of infection, plus a bacterial variable which was either "Flagellar motility & proteases" (odds ratio 2.3; $p = 0.02$) or "Type 3 secretion" (odds ratio 1.9; $p = 0.05$).

Discussion

In this study, we hypothesized that distinct virulence traits of the opportunistic pathogen *P. aeruginosa* would be associated with increased risk of infection vs. colonization in hospitalized patients with positive *P. aeruginosa* cultures. The presence of *P. aeruginosa* in conjunction with evidence of host tissue impairment and a local or systemic immune response was indicative of infection (Table 1), while the presence of bacteria with no or minimal tissue damage or inflammation was taken to represent colonization. We assayed a set of bacterial phenotypes, primarily chosen on the basis of their prior association with virulence in animal models of acute infection

Table 2. Patient characteristics as a function of colonization vs. infection status.

	Colonization (n = 114)	*P. aeruginosa* Infection/ Sepsis (n = 71)	Infection, possibly due to *P. aeruginosa* (n = 52)	*p* value (chi square)
Gender	51 (45%) female	24 (34%) female	24 (46%) female	0.26
Mean age, yrs (95% CI)	58.0 (53.3–62.7)	61.4 (56.4–66.4)	58.3 (51.4–65.2)	–
Ethnicity (Hispanic)	21 Hispanic (18%)	5 Hispanic (7.0%)	5 Hispanic (9.6%)	0.06
Diabetes	26 (23%)	27 (38%)	12 (23%)	0.06
Immunocompromised	31 (27%)	17 (24%)	17 (33%)	0.56
Relevant foreign device	67 (59%)	46 (65%)	31 (60%)	0.70

Table 3. Sources of bacterial isolates as a function of clinical categorization.

Site	Colonization (n = 114)	*P. aeruginosa* Infection/Sepsis (n = 71)	Infection, possibly due to *P. aeruginosa* (n = 52)
Respiratory	80	25*	32
Urine	30	29*	8
Soft tissue/bone	4	9*	10
Blood		12	2

*Patients with *P. aeruginosa* isolated concurrently from blood and another site (n = 4) are analyzed with both blood and non-blood sites.

or their co-regulation with such virulence traits. Bacterial phenotypes predominantly associated with persistence in chronic infection models (e.g. production of quorum sensing molecules or pyocyanin) were not considered. Factor analysis of the measured bacterial variables revealed interrelationships between several of these phenotypes. Some groupings were expected, such as that of the five measured T3SS proteins that loaded onto Factor 1. Others were not anticipated, such as the association of twitching motility with the PAPI-1 loci RL033 and RL112 within Factor 3, but are biologically plausible given the recent finding that the PAPI-1 pathogenicity island is transferred by conjugation via a Type IV pilus encoded therein [42]. The association of two flagellar-based forms of motility with protease secretion in Factor 2 may reflect the co-regulation of both flagellar genes and the Type II secretion system by the cyclic AMP dependent transcriptional activator Vfr [43].

Most published studies report bacterial virulence phenotypes as a binary variable (i.e., present/absent). Our study differed in providing quantitative measures for most variables, and this information was retained in the statistically defined factors used in our analysis. Although studies commonly stratify risk factors when considering association with risk of disease (e.g., CD4 count and risk of opportunistic infection, LDL cholesterol and risk of coronary artery disease), this approach is not widespread in studies of microbial pathogenesis, where two-way comparisons are often made between bacteria that do or do not express a putative virulence trait.

Production and secretion of T3SS components and effectors as measured by Factor 1 was the only bacterial variable that was associated with increased risk of infection in our total cohort (odds ratio 1.4), albeit with a p value = 0.5. The host risk factor diabetes mellitus was also associated with an increased risk of infection (odd ratio 2.1; $p<0.05$) in this parsimonious model. The association of T3SS with clinical infection was weaker than we expected based on data from animal models of acute pulmonary infection. Indeed, in the subset of patients with respiratory tract *P. aeruginosa* isolates, no association between pneumonia and T3SS was observed. Reanalysis of the data applying a less stringent definition of infection, which allowed patients with tracheobronchitis to be classified as infected, did not result in the association of T3SS or any other bacterial variable with increased risk of infection in the multivariate or parsimonious models (data not shown). In the subset of patients with urinary tract infections, two independent parsimonious models could be constructed. The host factors of diabetes mellitus and the presence of a urinary tract catheter or stent were associated with increased risk of infection in both models, along with either bacterial T3SS protein secretion (Factor 1) or the expression of flagellar based motility and protease

Table 4. Parsimonious multivariate analysis of factors associated with risk of *P. aeruginosa* infection.

Parameter	Level	Parsimonious (forward selection), All culture sites				Parsimonious (forward selection), Urinary tract cultures			
		p-value	Odds Ratio			*p*-value	Odds Ratio		
			estimate	L95%	U95%		estimate	L95%	U95%
Gender	female v male	–	–	–	–	–	–	–	–
Ethnicity	hispanic v non-hispanic	–	–	–	–	–	–	–	–
Race	nonwhite v white	–	–	–	–	–	–	–	–
Relevant foreign device	yes v no	–	–	–	–	0.03	6.3	1.2	34
Any chronic lung disease	yes v no	–	–	–	–	–	–	–	–
Immunocompromised	yes v no	–	–	–	–	–	–	–	–
Solid tumor	yes v no	–	–	–	–	–	–	–	–
Diabetes mellitus	yes v no	0.03	2.1	1.1	4.3	0.006	12	2.1	70
Age	per year	–	–	–	–	–	–	–	–
Biofilm	per unit	–	–	–	–	–	–	–	–
Factor 1	per unit	0.05	1.4	1.0	1.8	0.05	1.9	0.99	3.8
Factor 2	per unit	–	–	–	–	–	–	–	–
Factor 3	per unit	–	–	–	–	–	–	–	–

secretion (Factor 2). A greater propensity for protease secretion by human urinary tract isolates, as opposed to isolates from other body sites, has been reported in several studies (recently reviewed in [44]), suggesting that this group of virulence factors may play a specific role in causing disease at this anatomic site. It is not known whether decreased protease secretion by quorum-sensing mutants underlies the observed attenuation of quorum-sensing deficient *P. aeruginosa* strains in murine models of acute ascending pyelonephritis [45].

Several series have examined whether T3SS production by *P. aeruginosa* is associated with poor outcomes for human pulmonary infection. Roy-Burman et al. reported an association between increased mortality and bacterial secretion of one or more T3SS proteins in a study of 108 patients with lower respiratory tract or blood isolates of *P. aeruginosa* [11]. The interpretation of this study is confounded by the inclusion of patients with Cystic Fibrosis, whose chronic pulmonary colonization by T3SS-negative strains rarely results in severe, systemic disease. Hauser and colleagues studied a more homogeneous retrospective cohort of 35 patients with an established diagnosis of *P. aeruginosa* ventilator-associated pneumonia, and reported that infection with a T3SS-positive isolate was significantly associated with severe disease, defined as death or relapse despite appropriate therapy [10]. These findings were corroborated by a recent study demonstrating increased risk of persistence and relapse associated with T3SS-positive *P. aeruginosa* strains in patients with ventilator-associated pneumonia [9]. These latter two studies supported an association between T3SS and more severe disease in patients with ventilator-associated pneumonia, but their design did not allow them to assess the influence of this bacterial variable on the risk of infection vs. colonization in the respiratory tract (as was considered in the current study). These studies also did not consider a role for other potential virulence factors in human respiratory infection.

Limitations and Strengths of the Current Study

Our study has limitations. First, all assays required culture and isolation of *P. aeruginosa* from primary clinical specimens, and all bacterial virulence phenotypes were measured in vitro. Although bacterial phenotypes of banked isolates were stable and reproducible upon repeat assay, we only determined whether an isolate could express a particular virulence factor under defined in vitro conditions. Thus our assays measured the potential for an isolate to express a virulence factor in the human host, but did not determine whether those virulence factors were actually expressed in the host. This limitation also applies to other studies that measure virulence factor expression of clinical isolates. Second, the definitions for infection that we applied were based on NNIS system criteria and are congruent with clinical practice. However, our definition of respiratory tract infection was rigorous in requiring radiographic findings consistent with pneumonia, and was not met by patients with tracheobronchitis; in contrast, our definition of urinary tract infection was satisfied by evidence of a local inflammatory response even in patients with a urinary catheter. Nonetheless, our findings did not change when we broadened our criteria for respiratory tract infection to include tracheobronchitis. Third, patients were followed clinically for only 5 days after the *P. aeruginosa* culture that triggered enrollment was obtained. Any individual who met criteria for infection after this time would nonetheless be considered "colonized" in our analysis.

P. aeruginosa causes nosocomial infections at sites beyond the respiratory tract. A strength of our study cohort is inclusion of patients with positive cultures from lung, urine and deep wound or tissue, making it more representative of patients with positive cultures for *P. aeruginosa* seen in tertiary care hospitals. Despite the heterogeneity of this patient population, we observed an increased risk of *P. aeruginosa* infection associated with T3SS-positive isolates. This association persisted in the subgroup of patients with a urinary tract source of *P. aeruginosa*, arguing that T3SS-associated virulence is not specific to the respiratory tract.

Concluding Observations

The T3SS of *P. aeruginosa* is a dominant virulence factor in acute infections of model organisms that range from insects [46] to mice [8]. In our study, the T3SS was associated with increased risk of infection, but the magnitude of the effect was smaller than might be predicted from studies with inbred mice. Our result illustrates that in human patients, host-related variability has an equal or greater influence on the outcome of host-pathogen encounters than production of virulence factors by bacterial isolates.

Although the culture of certain organisms from clinical specimens, e.g. *M. tuberculosis*, is diagnostic of infection, the prognostic implications of culturing organisms such as *P. aeruginosa* are less clear. The identification of microbial virulence factors that influence the development of infection in humans may aid clinician decision-making in such a setting, and prompted us to undertake this study. Consideration of patient comorbidities that increase the risk and severity of infection, such as diabetes mellitus, is an integral part of treatment algorithms used by clinicians. Our findings suggest that an intrinsic bacterial factor, namely production of T3SS proteins, is also associated with an increased risk of *P. aeruginosa* infection in a heterogeneous cohort of hospitalized patients. By considering the T3SS phenotype of a clinical *P. aeruginosa* isolate, clinicians may be able to direct appropriate antimicrobial therapy to patients at higher risk of infection while still limiting the indiscriminate use of antimicrobials associated with increased antibiotic resistance [47]. Our findings also support further investigation into therapeutic strategies that target the T3SS and its effectors [48–52].

Acknowledgments

We would like to thank all of the patients who participated in this study. We gratefully acknowledge Roberta Willenkin for assistance with patient consent and enrollment, Maria Lebron and Xiao Bai for technical assistance with bacterial phenotyping assays, and the staff of the Clinical Microbiology Laboratory of Yale-New Haven Hospital.

Author Contributions

Conceived and designed the experiments: ML BIK. Performed the experiments: ML TSM SP BIK. Analyzed the data: ML TSM MDS VJQ BIK. Contributed reagents/materials/analysis tools: MDS. Wrote the paper: ML BIK.

References

1. Wenzel RP, Edmond MB (2001) The impact of hospital-acquired bloodstream infections. Emerging Infect Dis 7: 174–177.
2. Gaynes R, Edwards JR, National Nosocomial Infections Surveillance System (2005) Overview of nosocomial infections caused by gram-negative bacilli. Clin Infect Dis 41: 848–854.

3. Chastre J, Fagon JY (2002) Ventilator-associated pneumonia. Am J Respir Crit Care Med 165: 867–903.
4. Lambert PA (2002) Mechanisms of antibiotic resistance of *Pseudomonas aeruginosa*. J Royal Soc Med 95: 22–26.
5. Cortes P, Mariscal D, Valles J, Rello J, Coll P (2001) Presence of polyclonal *Pseudomonas aeruginosa* in an intensive care unit: a 27-month prospective study on molecular epidemiology. Infect Control Hosp Epidemiol 22: 720–723.
6. Parsek MR, Singh PK (2003) Bacterial biofilms: an emerging link to disease pathogenesis. Ann Rev Microbiol 57: 677–701.
7. Talon D, Mulin B, Rouget C, Bailly P, Thouverez M, et al. (1998) Risks and routes for ventilator-associated pneumonia with *Pseudomonas aeruginosa*. Am J Respir Crit Care Med 157: 978–984.
8. Hauser AR (2009) The type III secretion system of *Pseudomonas aeruginosa*: infection by injection. Nat Rev Microbiol 7: 654–665.
9. El Solh AA, Akinnusi ME, Wiener-Kronish JP, Lynch SV, Pineda LA, et al. (2008) Persistent infection with *Pseudomonas aeruginosa* in ventilator-associated pneumonia. Am J Respir Crit Care Med 178: 513–519.
10. Hauser A, Cobb E, Bodi M, Mariscal D, Valles J, et al. (2002) Type III protein secretion is associated with poor clinical outcomes in patients with ventilator-associated pneumonia caused by *Pseudomonas aeruginosa*. Crit Care Med 30: 521–528.
11. Roy-Burman A, Savel RH, Racine S, Swanson BL, Revadigar NS, et al. (2001) Type III protein secretion is associated with death in lower respiratory and systemic *Pseudomonas aeruginosa* infections. J Infect Dis 183: 1767–1774.
12. Vance RE, Rietsch A, Mekalanos JJ (2005) Role of the Type III secreted exoenzymes S, T and Y in systemic spread of *Pseudomonas aeruginosa* PA01 in vivo. Infect Immun 73: 1705–1713.
13. Lee VT, Smith RS, Tummler B, Lory S (2005) Activities of *Pseudomonas aeruginosa* effectors secreted by the Type III secretion system in vitro and during infection. Infect Immun 73: 1695–1705.
14. Shaver CM, Hauser AR (2004) Relative contributions of *Pseudomonas aeruginosa* ExoU, ExoS and ExoT to virulence in the lung. Infect Immun 72: 6969–6977.
15. El-Solh AA, Hattemer A, Hauser AR, Alhajhusain A, Vora H (2012) Clinical outcomes of type III *Pseudomonas aeruginosa* bacteremia. Crit Care Med 40: 1157–1163.
16. Nguyen D, Emond MJ, Mayer-Hamblett N, Saiman L, Marshall BC, et al. (2007) Clinical response to azithromycin in cystic fibrosis correlates with in vitro effects on *Pseudomonas aeruginosa* phenotypes. Pediatric Pulmonology 42: 533–541.
17. Mahenthiralingam E, Campbell ME, Speert DP (1994) Nonmotility and phagocytic resistance of *Pseudomonas aeruginosa* isolates from chronically colonized patients with cystic fibrosis. Infect Immun 62: 596–605.
18. Arora SK, Neely AN, Blair B, Lory S, Ramphal R (2005) Role of motility and flagellin glycosylation in the pathogenesis of *Pseudomonas aeruginosa* burn wound infections. Infect Immun 73: 4395–4398.
19. Balloy V, Verma A, Kuravi SK, Si-Tahar M, Chignard M, et al. (2007) The role of flagellin versus motility in acute lung disease caused by *Pseudomonas aeruginosa*. J Infect Dis 196: 289–296.
20. Feldman M, Bryan R, Rajan S, Scheffler L, Brunnert S, et al. (1998) Role of flagella in pathogenesis of *Pseudomonas aeruginosa* pulmonary infection. Infect Immun 66: 43–51.
21. Tang H, Kays M, Prince A (1995) Role of *Pseudomonas aeruginosa* pili in acute pulmonary infection. Infect Immun 63: 1278–1285.
22. Hamood AN, Griswold JA, Duhan CM (1996) Production of extracellular virulence factors by *Pseudomonas aeruginosa* isolates obtained from tracheal, urinary tract, and wound infections. J Surg Res 61: 425–432.
23. Mun JJ, Tam C, Kowbel D, Hawgood S, Barnett MJ, et al. (2009) Clearance of *Pseudomonas aeruginosa* from a healthy ocular surface involves surfactant protein D and is compromised by bacterial elastase in a murine null-infection model. Infect Immun 77: 2392–2398.
24. Preston M, Seed P, Toder D, Iglewski B, Ohman D, et al. (1997) Contribution of Proteases and LasR to the Virulence of *Pseudomonas aeruginosa* during Corneal Infections. Infection and Immunity 65: 3086–3090.
25. Woods DE, Schaffer MS, Rabin HR, Campbell GD, Sokol PA (1986) Phenotypic comparison of *Pseudomonas aeruginosa* strains isolated from a variety of clinical sites. J Clin Microbiol 24: 260–264.
26. He J, Baldini RL, Deziel E, Saucier M, Zhang Q, et al. (2004) The broad host range pathogen *Pseudomonas aeruginosa* strain PA14 carries two pathogenicity islands harboring plant and animal virulence genes. Proc Natl Acad Sci U S A 101: 2530–2535.
27. Battle SE, Meyer F, Rello J, Kung VL, Hauser AR (2008) Hybrid pathogenicity island PAGI-5 contributes to the highly virulent phenotype of a *Pseudomonas aeruginosa* isolate in mammals. J Bacteriol 190: 7130–7140.
28. Kulasekara BR, Kulasekara HD, Wolfgang MC, Stevens L, Frank DW, et al. (2006) Acquisition and Evolution of the exoU Locus in Pseudomonas aeruginosa. J Bacteriol 188: 4037–4050.
29. Lee DG, Urbach JM, Wu G, Liberati NT, Feinbaum RL, et al. (2006) Genomic analysis reveals that *Pseudomonas aeruginosa* virulence is combinatorial. Genome Biol 7: R90.91–R90.14.
30. Wiehlmann L, Wagner G, Cramer N, Siebert B, Gudowius P, et al. (2007) Population structure of *Pseudomonas aeruginosa*. Proceedings of the National Academy of Sciences 104: 8101–8106.
31. Harrison EM, Carter ME, Luck S, Ou HY, Deng Z, et al. (2010) Pathogenicity islands PAPI-1 and PAPI-2 contribute individually and synergistically to the virulence of *Pseudomonas aeruginosa* strain PA14. Infect Immun 78: 1437–1446.
32. Mikkelsen H, Sivaneson M, Filloux A (2011) Key two-component regulatory systems that control biofilm formation in *Pseudomonas aeruginosa*. Environ Microbiol 13: 1666–1681.
33. Hu H, Harmer C, Anuj S, Wainwright CE, Manos J, et al. (2012) Type 3 secretion system effector genotype and secretion phenotype of longitudinally collected *Pseudomonas aeruginosa* isolates from young children diagnosed with cystic fibrosis following newborn screening. Clin Microbiol Infect: no-no.
34. Jain M, Ramirez D, Seshadri R, Cullina JF, Powers CA, et al. (2004) Type III secretion phenotypes of *Pseudomonas aeruginosa* strains change during infection of individuals with Cystic Fibrosis. J Clin Microbiol 42: 5229–5237.
35. Hatcher L (1994) A Step-by-Step Approach Using the SAS System for Factor Analysis and Structural Equation Modeling. Cary, NC: SAS Institute, Inc.
36. Garner JS, Jarvis WR, Emori TG, Horan TC, Hughes JM (1988) CDC definitions for nosocomial infections, 1988. Am J Infect Control 16: 128–140.
37. Li L, Ledizet M, Kar K, Koski RA, Kazmierczak BI (2005) An indirect enzyme-linked immunosorbent assay for rapid and quantitative detection of type III virulence phenotypes of *Pseudomonas aeruginosa* isolates. Ann Clin Microbiol Antimicrobiol 4: 22–35.
38. Murray TS, Ledizet M, Kazmierczak BI (2010) Swarming motility, secretion of type 3 effectors and biofilm formation phenotypes exhibited within a large cohort of *Pseudomonas aeruginosa* clinical isolates. J Med Microbiol 59: 511–520.
39. Merritt JH, Kadouri DE, OToole GA (2005) Growing and analyzing static biofilms. In: Coico R, Kowalik T, Quarles J, Stevenson B, Taylor RK, editors. Current Protocols in Microbiology: John Wiley & Sons, Inc. 1B.1.1–1B.1.17.
40. Caballero AR, Moreau JM, Engel LS, Marquart ME, Hill JM, et al. (2001) *Pseudomonas aeruginosa* protease IV enzyme assays and comparison to the Pseudomonas proteases. Anal Biochem 290: 330–337.
41. Pier GB, Ramphal R (2010) *Pseudomonas aeruginosa*. In: Mandell GL, Bennett JE, Dolin R, editors. Mandell, Douglas, and Bennett's principles and practice of infectious diseases. 7th ed. Philadelphia, PA: Churchill Livingstone Elsevier. 2835–2860.
42. Carter MQ, Chen J, Lory S (2010) The *Pseudomonas aeruginosa* pathogenicity island PAPI-1 is transferred via a novel type IV pilus. J Bacteriol 192: 3249–3258.
43. Wolfgang MC, Lee VT, Gilmore ME, Lory S (2003) Coordinate regulation of bacterial genes by a novel adenylate cyclase signaling pathway. Devlop Cell 4: 253–263.
44. Mittal R, Aggarwal S, Sharma S, Chhibber S, Harjai K (2009) Urinary tract infections caused by *Pseudomonas aeruginosa*: a minireview. J Infect Public Health 2: 101–111.
45. Kumar R, Chhibber S, Harjai K (2009) Quorum sensing is necessary for the virulence of *Pseudomonas aeruginosa* during urinary tract infection. Kidney Int 76: 286–292.
46. Miyata S, Casey M, Frank DW, Ausubel FM, Drenkard E (2003) Use of the *Galleria mellonella* Caterpillar as a Model Host To Study the Role of the Type III Secretion System in *Pseudomonas aeruginosa* Pathogenesis. Infect Immun 71: 2404–2413.
47. National Nosocomial Infection Surveillance System (2004) National Nosocomial Infection Surveillance (NNIS) System report, data summary from January 1992 through June 2004, issued October 2004. Am J Infect Control 32: 470–485.
48. Arnoldo A, Curak J, Kittanakom S, Chevelev I, Lee VT, et al. (2008) Identification of small molecule inhibitors of *Pseudomonas aeruginosa* exoenzyme S using a yeast phenotypic screen. PLoS Genet 4: e1000005.
49. Lee VT, Pukatzki S, Sato H, Kikawada E, Kazimirova AA, et al. (2007) Pseudolipasin A is a specific inhibitor for phospholipase A2 activity of *Pseudomonas aeruginosa* cytotoxin ExoU. Infect Immun 75: 1089–1098.
50. Sawa T, Yahr TL, Ohara M, Kurahashi K, Gropper MA, et al. (1999) Active and passive immunization with the *Pseudomonas* V antigen protects against type III intoxication and lung injury. Nat Med 5: 392–398.
51. Holder IA, Neely AN, Frank DW (2001) PcrV immunization enhances survival of burned *Pseudomonas aeruginosa*-infected mice. Infect Immun 69: 5908–5910.
52. Francois B, Luyt CE, Dugard A, Wolff M, Diehl JL, et al. (2012) Safety and pharmacokinetics of an anti-PcrV PEGylated monoclonal antibody fragment in mechanically ventilated patients colonized with *Pseudomonas aeruginosa*: A randomized,double-blind, placebo-controlled trial*. Crit Care Med 40: 2320–2326.

26

Prostatic Stones: Evidence of a Specific Chemistry Related to Infection and Presence of Bacterial Imprints

Arnaud Dessombz[1]*, Paul Méria[2], Dominique Bazin[1,2,3], Michel Daudon[4]

1 Laboratoire de Physique des Solides, Université Paris Sud, Centre National de la Recherche Scientifique, Orsay, France, **2** Service d'Urologie, Hôpital Saint-Louis, Assistance Publique-Hôpitaux de Paris, Paris, France, **3** Laboratoire de la Chimie de la Matière Condensée de Paris, Université Pierre et Marie Curie, Collège de France, Centre National de la Recherche Scientifique, Paris, France, **4** Service d'Explorations Fonctionnelles, Hôpital Tenon, Assistance Publique-Hôpitaux de Paris, Paris, France

Abstract

Prostatic stones are a common condition in older men in industrialized countries. However, aging appears not to be the unique pathogenesis of these calcifications. Our morpho-constitutional investigation of 23 stone samples suggested that infection has a significant role in the lithogenic process of prostate calcifications, even without detection of infection by clinical investigation. Most stones (83%) showed bacterial imprints and/or chemical composition, suggestive of a long-term infection process. Chronic infection may induce persistent inflammation of the tissue and secondarily, a cancerization process within a few years. Thus, the discovery of prostate calcifications by computerized tomodensitometry, for example, might warrant further investigation and management to search for chronic infection of the prostate gland.

Editor: Niels Olsen Saraiva Câmara, Universidade de Sao Paulo, Brazil

Funding: This work was supported by the physic and chemistry institutes of CNRS (Centre National de la Recherche Scientifique) and by an Agence Nationale de la Recheche contract (grant number: ANR-09-BLAN-0120-02). The funders had no role in study design, data collection and analysis, decision to publish, or preparation of the manuscript. All the supporters have no commercial interests.

Competing Interests: The authors have declared that no competing interests exist.

* E-mail: arnaud.dessombz@u-psud.fr

Introduction

Prostate cancer is the second most frequent cause of mortality due to cancer in males in the United States [1]. Transuretral resection, radical prostatectomy, radiation therapy and hormone therapy are the usual prostate cancer treatments [2]. Prostate removal leads to the observation of prostatic calculi. Because almost 99% of surgically removed prostates contain stones, these stones are generally considered clinically insignificant [3]. Therefore, only a few papers have investigated these calcifications.

We noted the large chemical diversity of these prostatic stones. Carbonated calcium phosphate apatite (carbapatite; CA) seems to be the major component, but several investigations show the presence of other mineral phases such as calcium oxalate monohydrate and dihydrate [4], brushite [5], and whitlockite [6]. More recently, several other mineral phases previously not reported in prostatic calculi were octacalcium phosphate pentahydrate and amorphous carbonated calcium phosphate [7]. Such chemical diversity indicates significant variations in the local biochemistry, which may be linked to different conditions.

A previous investigation involving stone culture revealed that infected calculi in the prostate were implicated in relapsing urinary tract infection [6]. This work aimed to assess a possible relationship between infection and prostatic calculi, taking into account the chemical and structural characteristics of such calculi. We combined chemical analysis with Fourier transform infra-red (FTIR) spectroscopy and structural investigation at the mesoscopic scale by scanning electron microscopy (SEM). FTIR spectroscopy has helped us to examine the presence of chemical phases involved in infection of other organs [8,9]. Moreover, SEM observations allowed for assessing the presence of bacterial imprints on prostatic calculi [10]. FTIR spectroscopy and SEM have been used in several studies of pathological calcifications [11,12,13,14,15].

Materials and Methods

Samples

We investigated 23 prostatic stones obtained from the Saint-Louis and Tenon hospitals in Paris. The calcifications were collected from the prostate after radical prostatectomy or transuretral resection. The mean age of the patients was 71 years (range 35 to 87 years). All participants gave their verbal consent for use of the material. Samples were examined without knowledge of the name of the patient or other identifying data. Ethical approval for the study was obtained from the ethics committee of Tenon Hospital.

FTIR Spectroscopy

The FTIR spectroscopy was performed at Tenon Hospital. Each sample was analysed in absorbance mode on a Bruker Vector 22 spectrometer by accumulation of 32 spectra between 4000 and 400 cm^{-1}, with resolution 4 cm^{-1} and time acquisition 1 sec/spectrum. The analysis was as previously described [16]. For each sample, the inner and surface compositions were established. The compounds were identified by comparing them to reference spectra [17].

SEM

Each prostatic stone was observed by Field-effect SEM (Zeiss SUPRA55-VP with an Everhart-Thornley secondary electron detector). To maintain sample integrity, each measurement was

Table 1. Major phases in inner and peripheral layers (minor phases in italics) in 23 samples of prostate stones, along with presence of urinary infection and bacterial imprints.

N°	Age	Core	Periphery	Urinary infection	Bacterial imprints
1	81	WK>ACCP>*CA>PROT*	CA>OCP>*ACCP>PROT*	ND	Yes
2	68	CA>ACCP>>*MAP, COM, PROT*	CA>=ACCP>>*PROT*	ND	Yes
3	78	CA>>COD>*PROT>COM*	CA>>*COD, PROT*	Yes	No
4	78	CA>>COD>*COM>>MAP,PROT*	CA>=PROT>>*COD*	No	Yes
5	79	CA>WK>*PROT*	CA>=*WK>PROT*	ND	Yes
6	81	CA>COD>>*COM, PROT*	CA>>PROT>*COM, COD*	No	No
7	53	CA>COD>>*PROT, COM*	CA>>*COD, PROT, COM*	Yes	No
8	63	CA>>PROT>*COM*	CA>PROT>>*COM*	Yes	Yes
9	69	WK>CA>>*ACCP>PROT>COM, COD*	WK>CA>>*ACCP*	Yes	Yes
10	71	CA>WK>=PROT>*COM*	PROT>CA>*ACCP>=WK*	Yes	Yes
11	42	CA>>Br>*WK>COD>PROT, COM*	CA>>*WK>PROT*	No	Yes
12	58	CA>>PROT	CA>PROT	ND	No
13	70	ACCP>CA>*PROT>COM*	ACCP>>CA>*PROT*	No	Yes
14	58	WK>CA>>*ACCP>PROT*	WK>>CA>*PROT*	ND	Yes
15	76	CA>>WK>*OCP>PROT, ACCP*	PROT>CA>*OCP>WK, ACCP*	No	Yes
16	59	ACCP>CA>>*PROT, MAP*	PROT>>ACCP>CA	ND	Yes
17	75	WK>PROT>*ACCP>CA>COD*	WK>ACCP>*PROT>CA*	Yes	Yes
18	35	WK>> CA>*ACCP>COM, PROT*	CA>WK>>*ACCP, PROT*	No	No
19	77	WK>ACCP>>*CA>PROT*	CA>>PROT>*ACCP, WK*	ND	Yes
20	68	CA>Br>COD>*PROT>COM*	CA>Br>>*PROT*	No	Yes
21	72	WK>>CA>*PROT*	CA>WK>>*PROT, ACCP*	ND	Yes
22	74	ACCP>CA>>*WK, PROT*	PROT>ACCP>>*CA*	No	Yes
23	67	WK>CA>*ACCP>>COD, PROT*	WK>>CA>*PROT*	No	Yes

Br = brushite, ACCP = amorphous carbonated calcium phosphate, CA = carbapatite (carbonated calcium phosphate), COD = calcium oxalate dihydrate, COM = calcium oxalate monohydrate, OCP = octacalcium phosphate pentahydrate, Prot = proteins, WK = whitlockite. ND: not determined.

taken at low voltage (≤ 2 keV). Stones were imaged at similar magnification for comparison.

Results

Table 1 summarizes the age of patients, the chemical components of the 23 samples in the core and peripheral layers (main phases [>5%], minor phase [<5%]), the clinical data regarding urinary tract and prostate infection, and the presence of bacterial imprints seen by SEM. Several chemical phases (9 phases) were identified by FTIR spectroscopy. All stones mainly consisted of calcium phosphate, with CA the most common. Interestingly, the frequency of 2 phases, namely whitlockite and amorphous carbonated calcium phosphate (ACCP), as the main components was higher but not significantly in the core than in peripheral layers (48% vs 21%, $p = 0.07$). SEM revealed bacterial imprints in 18 stones (78%, $p = 0.001$), but clinical signs of urinary tract infection were reported for only 6 patients.

Table 2 shows the proportion and frequencies of the main chemical phases in the 23 stones. Whitlockite was detected in the

Table 2. Nature and frequency of main chemical phases in 23 prostatic stones.

Chemical phase	Core phase (%)	Main core phase (%)	Peripheral phase (%)	Main peripheral phase (%)
Carbapatite	21 (91%)	12 (52%)	17 (68%)	14 (62%)
Whitlockite	11 (48%)	8 (35%)	7 (30%)	4 (17%)
Amorphous carbonated calcium phosphate	6 (26%)	3 (13%)	5 (22%)	1 (4%)
Octacalcium phosphate pentahydrate	1 (4%)	0	2 (9%)	0
Brushite	2 (9%)	0	1 (4%)	0
Proteins	4 (17%)	0	8 (35%)	4 (17%)

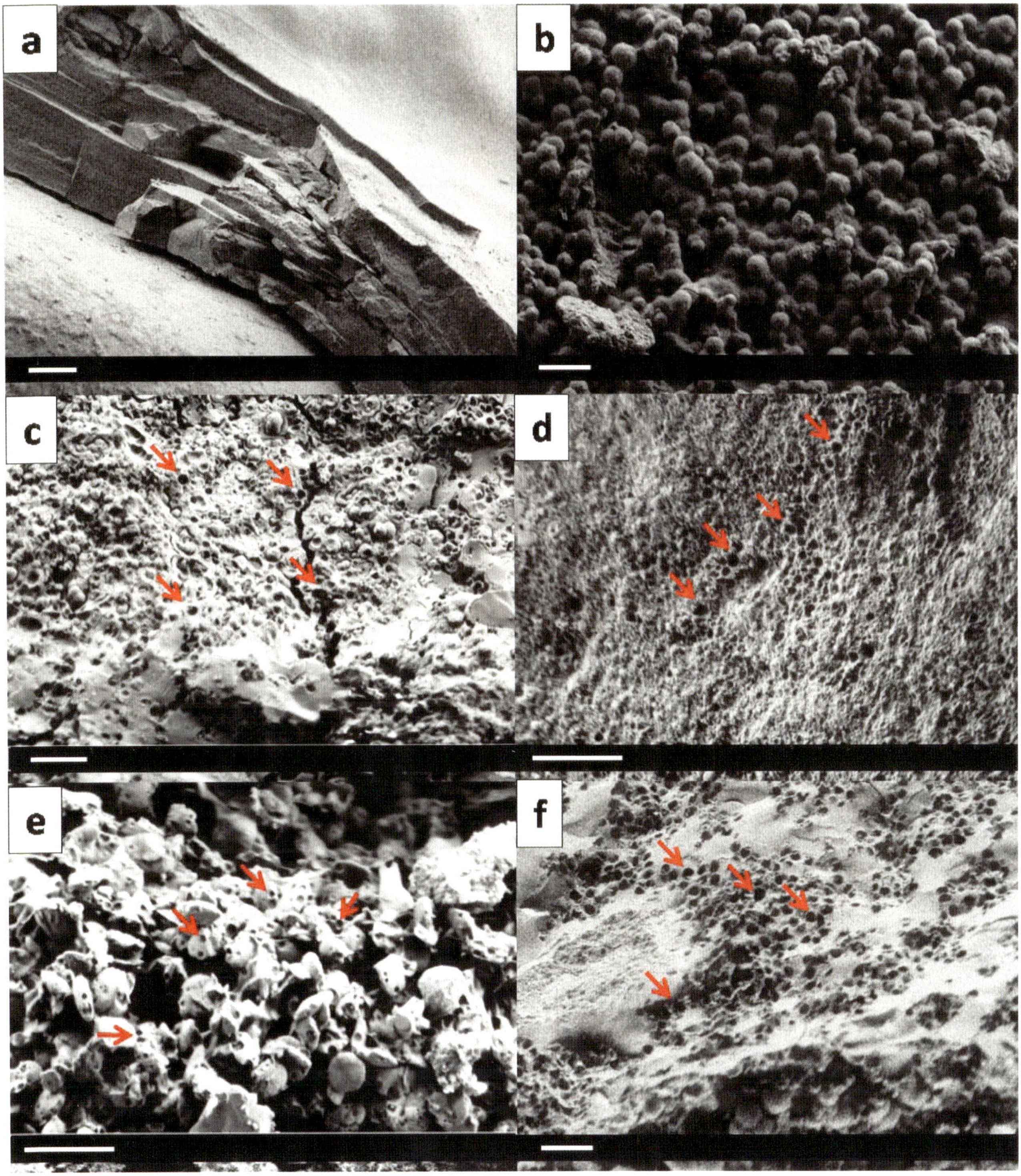

Figure 1. Fixed-effects SEM of prostatic stones. Red arrows show bacterial imprints. a) prostatic carbapatite-amorphous carbonated calcium phosphate (CA-ACCP) stone without any visible imprint; b) spherical prostatic CA stones without any visible imprint; c) prostatic CA-ACCP stone; d) prostatic ACCP stone, e) prostatic CA stone; f) prostatic CA-whitlockite stone. Bar, 4 μm.

core of 11 stones (48%) and as the main component in 8 (35%) but was the main component of the stone surface in only 4 stones (17%). ACCP was identified in the core of 6 stones (26%) and was the main phase in 3 (13%). ACCP was the main component of the stone surface in only 1 stone (4%).

Representative SEM images of normal stones and those with bacterial imprints (size about 500 nm) on the surface and in the core of stones are in Figure 1.

Discussion

Our SEM study revealed a high occurrence of bacterial imprints (78%) in 23 prostatic stones, which reveals a past or present infection of the prostate tissue; however, urinary tract infection was detected in only 6 (26%) cases. The large difference between number of reported infections and markers of infection within stones implies that aging may not be the only cause of prostatic calcifications. Infection and a lithogenic process induced by infection may play a role in most of the 99% of surgically removed prostate-containing stones.

The bacterial imprints had a specific spherical shape, which suggests infection by cocci germs. More precisely, the grape-like clustering, shape and size are common with staphylococci infection [18]. In 2 cases of proven infection, the species was *Staphylococcus aureus*. Nevertheless, these imprints were not seen on all stone surfaces. Similarly to kidney stones, the bacteria can imprint on a particle surface such as CA or ACCP but not other crystal types such as whitlockite, octacalcium phosphate or brushite. Indeed, the size of CA and ACCP crystals is smaller than that of other phases, such as struvite [19]. As well, SEM examination was restricted to some parts of small and partial samples collected during prostate removal. However, all stones contained at least 15% CA or ACCP, so a careful observation by SEM allows for detection of bacterial imprints on the surface of these minerals.

We discuss only the major phases. As previously reported, the main compounds of prostatic stones are calcium phosphate [20]. The most common and abundant phase is CA, well known as a common form of ectopic calcification in the kidney [21], vascular system [22,23] or breast [24]. Particular crystalline phases, namely whitlockite and ACCP, a marker of infection stones in the urinary tract, were identified in the core of 17 (74%) prostatic stones. Whitlockite is an infrequent component of kidney stones and has been associated with chronic urinary tract infection in most calculi from women [8]. This phase has been also found in infections such as tuberculosis [9]. These different markers (imprints, specific phases, etc.) led to the conclusion that 83% of calculi (19 stones, $p<0.0001$) could be linked to an infection process.

The deleterious consequences of chronic infection and inflammation have been well described in the cellular model [25] and chemical model [26]. A number of papers have highlighted the relation between infection-related inflammation and cancer in various organs such as stomach, liver, lung, colon or bladder [27,28]. The same reasoning may be applied to prostatic stones. Moreover, recent studies suggest epidemiological and pathologic links between benign prostate hypertrophy and prostate cancer [29]. Chronic infection, as well as the resulting stones, may induce persistent inflammation and could contribute to prostatic hypertrophy. In fact, the inflammatory process, associated with tumor phenomena, seems to influence the formation and evolution of these concretions [30]. We previously reported a high content of proteins in prostate stones [7]. Lactoferrin was found among proteins identified in both corpora amylacea and stones. This protein is considered a marker of inflammation and infiltration by neutrophil polynuclear factors and is implicated in the cancerization process [30].

The clinical interest of this paper is to draw attention to the high occurrence of asymptomatic infection of the prostate.

History of urinary tract infection and risk of renal cell carcinoma have been found to be related. As reported by Parker et al. [31], analysis of epidemiological data suggests a positive association of history of urinary tract infection and renal cell carcinoma development. Similar results were reported by MacLaughin et al. [32] and by Meares for prostate tissue [6]. Clearly more research is needed to establish a relationship because intratissular infection necessitates antibiotic treatment during several weeks. Our data suggest that the presence of stones or calcifications within the prostate could indicate chronic, often asymptomatic infection, the consequence of which remains to be assessed for medical management.

Conclusions

Prostatic stones are often considered to have no clinical significance, but the use of SEM showed for the first time the high frequency of bacterial imprints in these stones. Moreover, our data underline the specific chemistry of calcium phosphate phases, particularly the preponderance of whitlockite and ACCP in these calcifications. These results demonstrate the high occurence of bacterial infections in the prostate, often without any clinical symptoms.

Inflammation induced by an infection may lead to cancerization of the tissue. Early detection of prostatic calcifications or stones could suggest a search for asymptomatic chronic infection. If an infection is detected, medical management and antibiotic treatment could avoid chronic inflammation of the tissue and further deleterious consequences. Thus, we suggest that discovery of prostate calcifications by imaging such as computerized tomodensitometry might warrant further investigations and management to search for chronic infection of the prostate gland.

Author Contributions

Conceived and designed the experiments: AD PM DB MD. Performed the experiments: AD PM DB MD. Analyzed the data: AD PM DB MD. Contributed reagents/materials/analysis tools: AD PM DB MD.

References

1. Jemal A, Siegel R, Xu J, Ward E (2010) Cancer statistics, 2010. CA Cancer J. Clin. 60: 277–300.
2. Oh S, Shin S, Janknecht R (2012) ETV1, 4 and 5: An oncogenic subfamily of ETS transcription factors. Biochimica et Biophysica Acta 1826: 1–12.
3. Søndergaard G, Vetner M, Christensen PO (1987) Prostatic calculi. Acta Pathol Microbiol Immunol Scand A 95: 141–145.
4. Hsu THS, Lin SY, Lin CC, Cheng WT (2011) Preliminary feasibility study of FTIR microscopic mapping system for the rapid detection of the composited components of prostatic calculi. Urol. Res. 39: 165–170.
5. Kato H, Ogawa A (1987) Large brushite stone in a dilated prostatic urethra. The Journal of Urology 138: 154–155.
6. Meares EM (1974) Infection Stones of Prostate Gland. Urology 4: 560–567.
7. Dessombz A, Méria P, Bazin D, Foy E, Rouzière S, et al. (2011) Revisiting the chemical diversity in prostatic calculi: An SEM and FT-IR investigation. Progrès en Urologie 21: 940–945.
8. Maurice-Estepa L, Levilain P, Lacour B, Daudon M (1999) Crystalline phase differentiation in urinary calcium phosphate and magnesium phosphate calculi. Scan J. Urol Nephrol 33: 299–305.
9. Lagier R, Baud CA (2003) Magnesium whitlockite, a calcium phosphate crystal of special interest in pathology. Pathology, Research and Practice 199: 329–335.
10. Carpentier X, Daudon D, Traxer O, Jungers P, Mazouyes A, et al. (2009) Relationships Between Carbonation Rate of Carbapatite and Morphologic Characteristics of Calcium Phosphate Stones and Etiology. Urology 73: 968–975.
11. Daudon M, Junger P, Bazin D (2008) Peculiar Morphology of Stones in Primary Hyperoxaluria. New England Journal of Medecine, 359: 100–102.
12. Li C, Ebenstein D, Xu C, Chapman C, Saloner D, et al. (2003) Biochemical characterization of atherosclerotic plaque constituents using FTIR spectroscopy and histology. Biomed. Mater. Res. 64: 197–206.
13. Mendelsohn R, Hassankhani A, DiCarlo E, Boskey A (1989) FT-IR microscopy of endochondral ossification at 20 mu spatial resolution. Calcif Tissue Int. 44: 20–24.
14. Bazin D, Daudon M (2012) Pathological calcifications and selected examples at the medicine solid-state physics interface. J. Phys. D: Appl. Phys. 45: 383001–383010.

15. Bazin D, Daudon M, Combes Ch, Rey Ch (2012) Characterization and some physicochemical aspects of pathological microcalcifications. Chem Rev. DOI: 10.1021/cr200068d.
16. Estepa L, Daudon M (1997) Contribution of Fourier transform infrared spectroscopy to the identification of urinary stones and kidney crystal deposits. Biospectroscopy 3: 347–369.
17. Quy-Dao N, Daudon M (1997) Infrared and Raman Spectra of Calculi. Elsevier.
18. Freeman-Cook L, Freeman-Cook K (2005) Staphylococcus Aureus Infections, Chelsea House Publications.
19. Bazin D, André G, Weil R, Matzen G, Emmanuel V et al. (2012) Absence of bacterial imprints on struvite-containing kidney stones: a structural investigation at the mesoscopic and atomic scale. Urology 79: 786–790.
20. Sutor DJ, Wooley SE (1974) The Crystalline composition of prostatic calculi. British Journal of Urology 46: 533–535.
21. Dessombz A, Bazin D, Dumas P, Sandt C, Sule-Suso J, et al. (2011) Shedding Light on the Chemical Diversity of Ectopic Calcifications in Kidney Tissues: Diagnostic and Research Aspects. PLoS ONE 6.
22. Dorfmüller P, Bazin D, Aubert S, Weil R, Brisset F, et al. (2010) Crystalline ultrastructures, inflammatory elements and neoangiogenesis are present in inconspicuous aortic valve tissue. Cardiology Research and practice, 685926.
23. Reid JD, Andersen ME (1993) Medial calcification (whitlockite) in the aorta. Atherosclerosis. 101: 213–224.
24. Kopans D, Gavenonis S, Halpern E, Moore R (2011) Calcifications in the breast and digital breast tomosynthesis. Breast J. 17: 638–644.
25. Karin M, Lawrence T, Nizet V (2006) Innate Immunity Gone Awry: Linking Microbial Infections to Chronic Inflammation and Cancer. Cell 124: 823–835.
26. Hussain P, Harris C (2007) Inflammation and cancer: An ancient link with novel potentials. Int. J. Cancer 121: 2373–2380.
27. Engels EA (2008)Inflammation in the development of lung cancer: epidemiological evidence. Experet Rev Anticancer Ther. 8: 605–615.
28. Grivennikov SI, Greten FR, Karin M (2010) Immunity, inflammation, and cancer. Cell 140: 883–899.
29. Alcaraz A, Hammerer P, Tubaro A, Schröder FH, Castro R (2009) Is there evidence of a relationship between benign prostate hyperplasia and prostate cancer? Findings of a literature review. Eur Urol 55: 864–875.
30. Sfanos KS, Wilson BA, De Marzo AM, Isaacs WB (2009) Acute inflammatory proteins constitute the organic matrix of prostatic corpora amylacea and calculi in men with prostate cancer. PNAS 106: 3443–3448.
31. Parker AS, Cerhan JR, Lynch CF, Bradley BC, Cantor KP (2004) History of urinary tract infection and risk of renal cell carcinoma. Am J Epidemiol 159: 42–48.
32. McLaughlin JK, Mandel JS, Blot WJ, Schuman LM, Mehl ES, et al. (1984) A population-based case control study of renal cell carcinoma. J. Natl Cancer Inst. 72: 275–284.

Permissions

All chapters in this book were first published in PLOS ONE, by The Public Library of Science; hereby published with permission under the Creative Commons Attribution License or equivalent. Every chapter published in this book has been scrutinized by our experts. Their significance has been extensively debated. The topics covered herein carry significant findings which will fuel the growth of the discipline. They may even be implemented as practical applications or may be referred to as a beginning point for another development.

The contributors of this book come from diverse backgrounds, making this book a truly international effort. This book will bring forth new frontiers with its revolutionizing research information and detailed analysis of the nascent developments around the world.

We would like to thank all the contributing authors for lending their expertise to make the book truly unique. They have played a crucial role in the development of this book. Without their invaluable contributions this book wouldn't have been possible. They have made vital efforts to compile up to date information on the varied aspects of this subject to make this book a valuable addition to the collection of many professionals and students.

This book was conceptualized with the vision of imparting up-to-date information and advanced data in this field. To ensure the same, a matchless editorial board was set up. Every individual on the board went through rigorous rounds of assessment to prove their worth. After which they invested a large part of their time researching and compiling the most relevant data for our readers.

The editorial board has been involved in producing this book since its inception. They have spent rigorous hours researching and exploring the diverse topics which have resulted in the successful publishing of this book. They have passed on their knowledge of decades through this book. To expedite this challenging task, the publisher supported the team at every step. A small team of assistant editors was also appointed to further simplify the editing procedure and attain best results for the readers.

Apart from the editorial board, the designing team has also invested a significant amount of their time in understanding the subject and creating the most relevant covers. They scrutinized every image to scout for the most suitable representation of the subject and create an appropriate cover for the book.

The publishing team has been an ardent support to the editorial, designing and production team. Their endless efforts to recruit the best for this project, has resulted in the accomplishment of this book. They are a veteran in the field of academics and their pool of knowledge is as vast as their experience in printing. Their expertise and guidance has proved useful at every step. Their uncompromising quality standards have made this book an exceptional effort. Their encouragement from time to time has been an inspiration for everyone.

The publisher and the editorial board hope that this book will prove to be a valuable piece of knowledge for researchers, students, practitioners and scholars across the globe.

List of Contributors

Andreas Oberbach, Nadine Schlichting and Matthias Blüher
Department of Medicine, University of Leipzig, Leipzig, Germany

Peter Kovacs
Faculty of Medicine, Interdisciplinary Centre for Clinical Research, University of Leipzig, Leipzig, Germany

Holger Till
Department of Pediatric Surgery, University of Leipzig, Leipzig, Germany

Jens-Uwe Stolzenburg and Jochen Neuhaus
Department of Urology, University of Leipzig, Leipzig, Germany

Catherine Huoi, Philippe Vanhems, Marie-Christine Nicolle and Thomas Bénet
Infection Control and Epidemiology Unit, Edouard Herriot Hospital, Hospices Civils de Lyon, Lyon, France

Philippe Vanhems and Thomas Bénet
Epidemiology and Public Health Group, Centre National de la Recherche Scientifique, Unité Mixte de Recherche 5558, University of Lyon 1, Lyon, France

Mauricette Michallet
Haematology Department, Edouard Herriot Hospital, Hospices Civils de Lyon, Lyon, France

John David Spencer and Brian Becknell
Pediatric Nephrology Fellowship Program, Nationwide Children's Hospital, Columbus, Ohio, United States of America

John David Spencer, David S. Hains, Brian Becknell and Andrew L. Schwaderer
Division of Nephrology, Department of Pediatrics, Nationwide Children's Hospital, Columbus, Ohio, United States of America

David S. Hains, Julianne DiRosario, Huanyu Wang and Andrew L. Schwaderer
Center for Clinical and Translational Research, The Research Institute at Nationwide Children's Hospital, Columbus, Ohio, United States of America

Edith Porter
Department of Biological Sciences, California State University Los Angeles, Los Angeles, California, United States of America

Charles L. Bevins
Department of Microbiology and Immunology, School of Medicine, University of California Davis, Davis, California, United States of America

Bibi C. G. C. Slingerland, Mehri Tavakol, Susan V. Snijders, Alex van Belkum, Margreet C. Vos, Henri A. Verbrugh and Willem J. B. van Wamel
Department of Medical Microbiology and Infectious Diseases, Erasmus MC, Rotterdam, The Netherlands

Alex J. McCarthy and Jodi A. Lindsay
Division of Clinical Sciences, Centre for Infection, St George's University of London, London, United Kingdom

Jaap A. Wagenaar
Department of Infectious Diseases and Immunology, Faculty of Veterinary Medicine, Utrecht University, Utrecht, The Netherlands
Central Veterinary Institute of Wageningen UR, Lelystad, The Netherlands

Aditya Kadiyala
Department of Nephrology, North Shore University Hospital, Manhasset, New York, United States of America

Chia-Chu Chang
Ph.D. Program for Aging, College of Medicine, China Medical University, Taichung, Taiwan

Poornima Ramadas, Prejith P. Rajendran, Prathik Krishnan, Asha Alex, Vivek Jayaschandran, Amit Basu, Madhu Bhaskaran and Ernesto P. Molmenti
Transplant Program, North Shore University Hospital, Manhasset, New York, United States of America

Eric Siskind
Department of Surgery, North Shore University Hospital, Manhasset, New York, United States of America

Xiaolin Yin, Ying Liu Zhiyan Yao, Cuiqing Ma, Lijuan Yang and Lin Wei
Department of Immunology, Hebei Medical University, Shijiazhuan, China

Tianwen Hou and Jing Chen
Department of Laboratory Medicine, Bethune International Peace Hospital, Shijiazhuan, China

Chi-Hui Cheng
Division of Pediatric Nephrology, Department of Pediatrics, Chang Gung Children's Hospital, Chang Gung Memorial Hospital, Taoyuan, Taiwan

Chi-Hui Cheng and Tzou-Yien Lin
College of Medicine, Chang Gung University, Taoyuan, Taiwan

Yun-Shien Lee
Genomic Medicine Research Core Laboratory (GMRCL), Chang Gung Memorial Hospital, Taoyuan, Taiwan
Department of Biotechnology, Ming-Chuan University, Taoyuan, Taiwan

Chee-Jen Chang
Statistical Center for Clinical Research, Chang Gung Memorial Hospital, Taoyuan, Taiwan

Tzou-Yien Lin
Division of Pediatric Infectious Diseases, Department of Pediatrics, Chang Gung Children's Hospital, Chang Gung Memorial Hospital, Taoyuan, Taiwan

Michel Ledizet
L2 Diagnostics, New Haven, Connecticut, United States of America

Thomas S. Murray
Department of Pediatrics (Infectious Diseases), Yale University School of Medicine, New Haven, Connecticut, United States of America

Sailaja Puttagunta, Vincent J. Quagliarello and Barbara I. Kazmierczak
Department of Medicine, Sections of Infectious Diseases, Yale University School of Medicine, New Haven, Connecticut, United States of America

Martin D. Slade
Department of Occupational and Environmental Medicine, Yale University School of Medicine, New Haven, Connecticut, United States of America

Barbara I. Kazmierczak
Department of Microbial Pathogenesis, Yale University School of Medicine, New Haven, Connecticut, United States of America

Casper D. J. den Heijer, John Penders, Cathrien A. Bruggeman and Ellen E. Stobberingh
Department of Medical Microbiology, Maastricht University Medical Centre/Care and Public Health Research Institute, Maastricht, The Netherlands

GéA. Donker
NIVEL, The Netherlands Institute for Health Services Research, Utrecht, The Netherlands

Sophie Vimont and Guillaume Arlet
AP-HP, Hôpitaux Universitaires Est Parisien - site Tenon, Service de Bactériologie, Paris, France

Sophie Vimont, Anders Boyd and Guillaume Arlet
Université Paris 6 - Pierre et Marie Curie, Paris, France

Anders Boyd
INSERM U707, Paris, France

Alexandre Bleibtreu, Marcelle Bens, Louis Garry, Olivier Clermont, Erick Denamur and Alain Vandewalle
Université Paris Diderot, Sorbonne Paris Cité, Paris, France

Alexandre Bleibtreu, Louis Garry, Olivier Clermont and Erick Denamur
INSERM U722, Paris, France

Marcelle Bens and Alain Vandewalle
INSERM U773, Paris, France

Jean-Michel Goujon
Unité de Pathologie Ultrastructurale et Expérimentale, Centre Hospitalier et Universitaire de Poitiers; Université de Poitiers, Poitiers, France

Marcel E. Curlin and Lawrence Corey
Fred Hutchinson Cancer Research Center, Seattle, Washington, United States of America

Marcel E. Curlin, Meei-Li Huang, Connie L. Celum, Stacy Selke, Jared M. Baeten and Lawrence Corey
Department of Medicine, University of Washington, Seattle, Washington, United States of America

Lawrence Corey
Department of Laboratory Medicine, University of Washington, Seattle, Washington, United States of America

Connie L. Celum
Department of Epidemiology, University of Washington, Seattle, Washington, United States of America

Connie L. Celum and Jared M. Baeten
Department of Global Health, University of Washington, Seattle, Washington, United States of America

Jorge Sanchez
Asociación Civil Impacta Salud y Educación, Lima, Peru

Richard A. Zuckerman
Division of Infectious Diseases, Dartmouth-Hitchcock Medical Center, Lebanon, New Hampshire, United States of America

Xiaoyan Lu and Dean D. Erdman
Centers for Disease Control and Prevention, Atlanta, Georgia, United States of America

Daniel M. Saman, Brian Johnson and M. Nawal Lutfiyya
Essentia Institute of Rural Health, Duluth, Minnesota, United States of America

Daniel M. Saman and Kevin T. Kavanagh
Health Watch USA, Somerset, Kentucky, United States of America

Felix Fluri
Department of Neurology, University Hospital Basel, Basel, Switzerland

Felix Fluri and Mira Katan
Department of Neurology, University Hospital Zürich, Zürich, Switzerland

Nils G. Morgenthaler
Institut für Experimentelle Endokrinologie, Charité, Berlin, Germany

Beat Mueller
Medical University Clinic, Cantonal Hospital Aarau, Aarau, Switzerland

Mirjam Christ-Crain
Department of Endocrinology, University Hospital Basel, Basel, Switzerland

Mira Katan
Columbia University, Department of Neurology, Division of Stroke, New York, New York, United States of America

Savita Jadhav and Nageshwari Gandham
Department of Microbiology, Dr. D. Y. Patil Medical College and Hospital, Pimpri, Pune, India

Arif Hussain, Savita Devi, Ashutosh Kumar, Sana Parveen and Niyaz Ahmed
Pathogen Biology Laboratory, Department of Biotechnology, School of Life Sciences, University of Hyderabad, Hyderabad, India

Lothar H. Wieler and Christa Ewers
Veterinary Faculty, Institute for Microbiology and Epizootics, Freie Universitaet Berlin, Berlin, Germany

Niyaz Ahmed
Institute of Biological Sciences, University of Malaya, Kuala Lumpur, Malaysia
Institute of Life Sciences, University of Hyderabad Campus, Hyderabad, India

Michiel B. Haeseker, Nicole H. T. M. Dukers-Muijrers, Christian J. P. A. Hoebe, Cathrien A. Bruggeman and Annelies Verbon
Department of Medical Microbiology, Maastricht University Medical Centre, Maastricht, The Netherlands

Nicole H. T. M. Dukers-Muijrers and Christian J. P. A. Hoebe
Department of Sexual Health, Infectious Diseases, and Environmental Health, Public Health Service South Limburg, Geleen, The Netherlands

Jochen W. L. Cals
Department of General Practice, Maastricht University, Maastricht, The Netherlands

Michiel B. Haeseker, Nicole H. T. M. Dukers-Muijrers, Christian J. P. A. Hoebe Cathrien A. Bruggeman and Jochen W. L. Cals
School for Public Health and Primary Care (CAPHRI), Maastricht, The Netherlands

Annelies Verbon
Department of Internal Medicine Section, Infectious Disease, Erasmus Medical Centre, Rotterdam, The Netherlands

Jenny Grönberg Hernández, Catharina Svanborg and Björn Wullt
Department of Microbiology, Immunology and Glycobiology, Institute of Laboratory Medicine, Lund University, Lund, Sweden

Fredrik Sundén
Department of Urology, Skåne University Hospital, Malmö, Sweden

John Connolly
Singapore Immunology Network (SIgN), Biomedical Sciences Institutes, Agency for Science, Technology, and Research (A*STAR), Singapore, Singapore

Xiaohua Qin, Fupin Hu, Shi Wu, Xinyu Ye, Demei Zhu, Ying Zhang and Minggui Wang
Huashan Hospital and Key Laboratory of Medical Molecular Virology of the Ministries of Education and Health, Shanghai Medical College, Fudan University, Shanghai, China

Ying Zhang
Department of Molecular Microbiology and Immunology, Bloomberg School of Public Health, Johns Hopkins University, Baltimore, Maryland, United States of America

Taslima T. Lina, Bijay K. Khajanchi, Ishrat J. Azmi, Mohammad Aminul Islam, Belal Mahmood, Mahmuda Akter, Atanu Banik, Rumana Alim, Alejandro Cravioto and Kaisar A. Talukder
Centre for Food and Water Borne Diseases, International Centre for Diarrhoeal Disease Research, Bangladesh, Dhaka, Bangladesh

Armando Navarro and Gabriel Perez
Department of Public Health, Faculty of Medicine, Universidad Nacional Autonoma de Mexico, Mexico City, Mexico

Sohinee Sarkar, Makrina Totsika, Minh-Duy Phan and Mark A. Schembri
Australian Infectious Disease Research Centre, School of Chemistry and Molecular Biosciences, The University of Queensland, Brisbane, Queensland, Australia

Glen C. Ulett
School of Medical Sciences, Griffith Health Institute, Griffith University, Gold Coast, Queensland, Australia

Shuo-Meng Wang, Ya-Yin Chen and Yeong-Shiau Pu
Department of Urology, National Taiwan University Hospital, Taipei, Taiwan

Ming-Nan Lai and Ya-Yin Chen
Department of Statistics, Feng Chia University, Taichung, Taiwan

Alan Wei
School of Medicine, Stony Brook University, Stony Brook, New York, United States of America

Shuo-Meng Wang and Pau-Chung Chen
Institute of Occupational Medicine and Industrial Hygiene, College of Public Health, National Taiwan University, Taipei, Taiwan

Shuo-Meng Wang and Pau-Chung Chen
Institute of Occupational Medicine and Industrial Hygiene, College of Public Health, National Taiwan University, Taipei, Taiwan

Jung-Der Wang
Department of Public Health, National Cheng Kung University Medical College, Tainan City, Taiwan
Departments of Internal Medicine and Occupational and Environmental Medicine, National Cheng Kung University Hospital, Tainan City, Taiwan

Dominique Wobser, Liaqat Ali, Elisabeth Grohmann, Johannes Huebner and Türkan Sakinc
Division of Infectious Diseases, Department of Internal Medicine II, University Hospital Freiburg, Freiburg, Germany

Liaqat Ali and Elisabeth Grohmann
Faculty of Biology, Albert Ludwigs University of Freiburg, Freiburg, Germany

Johannes Huebner
Division of Pediatric Infectious Diseases, Dr. Von Hauner Children's Hospital, Ludwig Maximilian University Munich, Munich, Germany

Antje Berger, Katrin Dohnt, Judith Becker and Christoph Wittmann
Institute of Biochemical Engineering, Technische Universität Braunschweig, Braunschweig, Germany

Petra Tielen and Dieter Jahn
Institute of Microbiology, Technische Universität Braunschweig, Braunschweig, Germany

Judith Becker and Christoph Wittmann
Institute of Systems Biotechnology, Saarland University, Saarbrücken, Germany

Charles N. Rudick, Aisha K. Taylor, Ryan E. Yaggie, Anthony J. Schaeffer and David J. Klumpp
Department of Urology, Feinberg School of Medicine, Northwestern University, Chicago, Illinois, United States of America

David J. Klumpp
Microbiology-Immunology, Feinberg School of Medicine, Northwestern University, Chicago, Illinois, United States of America

Yoichi Matsui, Sohei Satoi, Masaki Kaibori, Hideyoshi Toyokawa, Hiroaki Yanagimoto, Kosuke Matsui, Morihiko Ishizaki and A-Hon Kwon
Department of Surgery, Kansai Medical University, Hirakata, Osaka, Japan

Luke T. Lavallée, Christopher Morash, Ilias Cagiannos and Rodney H. Breau
Division of Urology, Department of Surgery, The Ottawa Hospital, University of Ottawa, Ottawa, Ontario, Canada

Luke T. Lavallée, David Schramm, Kelsey Witiuk, Ranjeeta Mallick, Dean Fergusson and Rodney H. Breau
Clinical Epidemiology Program, Ottawa Hospital Research Institute, Ottawa, Ontario, Canada

David Schramm
Department of Otolaryngology, The Ottawa Hospital, University of Ottawa, Ottawa, Ontario, Canada

Rie Adser Virkus, Ellen Løkkegaard and Thomas Bergholt
Department of Obstetrics and Gynecology, Hillerød Hospital, University of Copenhagen, Hillerød, Denmark

Øjvind Lidegaard and Anne Kristine Nielsen
Gynecological Clinic, Rigshospitalet, University of Copenhagen, Copenhagen, Denmark

Jens Langhoff-Roos
Obstetrical Clinic, Rigshospitalet, University of Copenhagen, Copenhagen, Denmark

Kenneth J. Rothman
Research Triangle Institute, Research Triangle Park, North Carolina, United States of America

Colin Sumpter and Belen Torondel
Department of Disease Control, London School of Hygiene and Tropical Medicine, London, United Kingdom

Ji-Yeon Han
Department of Urology, Pusan National University Yangsan Hospital, Yangsan, Korea

Kyu-Sung Lee
Department of Urology, Samsung Medical Center, Sungkyunkwan University School of Medicine, Seoul, Korea

Won Hee Park
Department of Urology, Inha University College of Medicine, Incheon, Korea

Choal Hee Park
Department of Urology, Keimyung University School of Medicine, Daegu, Korea

Jeong Gu Lee
Department of Urology, Korea University College of Medicine, Seoul, Korea

Jeong Zoo Lee
Department of Urology, Pusan National University Hospital, Busan, Korea

Duk Yoon Kim
Department of Urology, Catholic University of Daegu School of Medicine, Daegu, Korea

Yong Gil Na
Department of Urology, Chungnam National University School of Medicine, Daejeon, Korea

Dong Deuk Kwon
Department of Urology, Chonnam National University Hwasun Hospital, Chonnam National University Medical School, Gwangju, Korea

Myung-Soo Choo
Department of Urology, University of Ulsan College of Medicine, Asan Medical Center, Seoul, Korea

Coline Mahende, John Lusingu, Allvan Butichi, Paminus Lushino and Martha Lemnge
Korogwe Research Laboratory, National Institute for Medical Research, Tanga, Tanzania

Coline Mahende, Billy Ngasala and Zul Premji
Department of Medical Entomology and Parasitology, School of Public Health, Muhimbili University of Health and Allied Sciences, Dar es Salaam, Tanzania

Antoinette A. T. P. Brink, Christian J. H. von Wintersdorff, Christina F. M. van der Donk, Anne M. M. W. Peeters, Patrick S. Beisser, Ellen E. Stobberingh and Petra F. G. Wolffs
Department of Medical Microbiology, Maastricht University Medical Center, Maastricht, The Netherlands

Ellen E. Stobberingh and Petra F. G. Wolffs
School for Public Health and Primary Care, University of Maastricht, Maastricht, The Netherlands

Ping-Fang Chiu and Horng-Rong Chang
Institute of Medicine, Chung Shan Medical University, Taichung, Taiwan

Ping-Fang Chiu, Horng-Rong Chang and Chia-Chu Chang
School of Medicine, Chung Shan Medical University, Taichung, Taiwan

Ping-Fang Chiu, Chia-Lin Wu, Hung-Hsiang Liou, Chirn-Bin Chang and Chia-Chu Chang
Nephrology Division, Department of Internal Medicine, Changhua Christian Hospital, Changhua, Taiwan

Ching-Hui Huang
Division of Cardiology, Department of Internal Medicine, Changhua Christian Hospital, Changhua, Taiwan

Horng-Rong Chang
Division of Nephrology, Department of Internal Medicine, Chung Shan Medical University Hospital, Taichung, Taiwan

Paul Méria and Dominique Bazin
Service d'Urologie, Hôpital Saint-Louis, Assistance Publique-Hôpitaux de Paris, Paris, France

Dominique Bazin
Laboratoire de la Chimie de la Matière Condensée de Paris, Université Pierre et Marie Curie, Collége de France, Centre National de la Recherche Scientifique, Paris, France

Michel Daudon
Service d'Explorations Fonctionnelles, Hôpital Tenon, Assistance Publique-Hôpitaux de Paris, Paris, France

Arnaud Dessombz and Dominique Bazin
Laboratoire de Physique des Solides, Université Paris Sud, Centre National de la Recherche Scientifique, Orsay, France

Index